QUALITY MANAGEMENT IN NURSING AND HEALTH CARE

June A. Schmele, R.N., Ph.D.
Associate Professor
College of Nursing
Adjunct Associate Professor
Department of Health Administration and Policy
College of Public Health
University of Oklahoma
Oklahoma City, Oklahoma

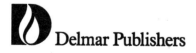 Delmar Publishers

I(T)P™

Albany • Bonn • Boston • Cincinnati • Detroit • London
Madrid • Melbourne • Mexico City • New York • Pacific Grove
Paris • San Francisco • Singapore • Tokyo • Toronto • Washington

NOTICE TO THE READER

Delmar Staff
Publisher: Diane L. McOscar
Senior Acquisitions Editor: Bill Burgower
Assistant Editor: Debra M. Flis
Project Editor: Colleen A. Corrice
Production Coordinator: James Zayicek
Art and Design Coordinator: Timothy J. Conners
Editorial Assistant: Chrisoula Baikos

COPYRIGHT © 1996
By Delmar Publishers
a division of International Thomson Publishing Inc.

The ITP logo is a trademark under license.

Printed in the United States of America

For more information, contact:

Delmar Publishers
3 Columbia Circle, Box 15015
Albany, New York 12212-5015

International Thomson Publishing Europe
Berkshire House 168-173
High Holborn
London, WC1V 7AA
England

Thomas Nelson Australia
102 Dodds Street
South Melbourne, 3205
Victoria, Australia

Nelson Canada
1120 Birchmont Road
Scarborough, Ontario
Canada, M1K 5G4

International Thomson Editores
Campos Eliseos 385, Piso 7
Col Polanco
11560 Mexico D F Mexico

International Thomson Publishing GmbH
Konigswinterer Strasse 418
53227 Bonn
Germany

International Thomson Publishing Asia
221 Henderson Road
#05-10 Henderson Building
Singapore 0315

International Thomson Publishing—Japan
Hirakawacho Kyowa Building, 3F
2-2-1 Hirakawacho
Chiyoda-ku, Tokyo 102
Japan

1 2 3 4 5 6 7 8 9 10 XXX 01 00 99 98 97 96 95

Library of Congress Cataloging-in-Publication Data
Quality management in nursing and health care / [edited by] June A.
  Schmele.
      p. cm.
    Includes bibliographical references and index.
    ISBN 0-8273-6056-8
    1. Medical care — Quality control. 2. Health services.
  administration. I. Schmele, June A., 1935–
    [DNLM: 1. Quality Assurance, Health Care. 2. Delivery of Health
  Care — organization & administration. W 84.1 Q155 1995]
  RA399.A3Q346 1996
  362.1'068'5 — dc20
  DNLM/DLC
  for Library of Congress   94–39828
                                                                        CIP

DEDICATION

This book is dedicated to the special persons who have been my mentors over the years.

To those who are here to share the completion of this endeavor —

> Eva Erickson
>
> Mona Fields
>
> Alice Minthorn-Hall and
>
> Sister Rita Taggart

And to the memory of those who share it from a better place —

> Fred Bozett
>
> Ivan Hanson and
>
> Lorraine Singer

Delmar Publishers' Online Services

To access Delmar on the World Wide Web, point your browser to:

http://www.delmar.com/delmar.html

To access through Gopher: gopher://gopher.delmar.com

(Delmar Online is part of "thomson.com", an Internet site with information on more than 30 publishers of the International Thomson Publishing organization.)

For information on our products and services:

email: info@delmar.com

or call 800-347-7707

CONTRIBUTORS

A. F. Al-Assaf, M.D., M.P.H., C.Q.A.
Assistant Professor
Department of Health Administration and Policy
University of Oklahoma Health Sciences Center
Oklahoma City, Oklahoma
Resident Advisor and Project Director, Quality Assurance Project
Center for Human Services
US AID — Ministry of Health
Hashemite Kingdom of Jordan
Amman, Jordan

Moira Attree, M.Sc., B.Nurs, R.G.N., R.N.T., R.H.V., R.D.N.
Lecturer in Nursing
Department of Nursing
University of Manchester
United Kingdom

Judith Beck, B.S.N., R.N.
Nursing Information Systems Coordinator
University of Minnesota Hospital and Clinic
Minneapolis, Minnesota

G. Ross Baker, Ph.D.
Department of Health Administration
Faculty of Medicine
University of Toronto
Toronto, Ontario, Canada

Michael R. Bleich, M.P.H., R.N., C.N.A.A.
Vice President for Patient Care Services
Bryan Memorial Hospital
Lincoln, Nebraska

Edward N. Brandt, Jr., M.D., Ph.D.
Professor
Department of Health Administration and Policy and Department of Internal Medicine
Co-Director, Center for Health Policy Research and Development
University of Oklahoma Health Sciences Center
Oklahoma City, Oklahoma

Jane M. Bryant, M.H.S.A., F.A.S.H.R.M.
Director of Risk Management
Greenville Hospital System
Greenville, South Carolina

Margaret J. Bull, Ph.D., R.N.
Associate Professor
University of Minnesota, School of Nursing
Minneapolis, Minnesota

Carol Chenoweth, M.D.
Medical Director, Infection Control Services
University of Michigan Medical Center
Ann Arbor, Michigan

Pat Christensen, Ph.D., R.N.
Professor
University of South Carolina-Spartanburg
Spartanburg, South Carolina

Laura L. Cross, J.D., R.N.
Director, Law Firm of Miller, Dollarhide, Dawson & Shaw
Oklahoma City, Oklahoma

Johanna C. M. H. Diepeveen-Speekenbrink, M.Phil., B.S.N., R.N.
Former Project Director for Nursing Science
University of Utrecht
The Netherlands

Avedis Donabedian, M.D., M.P.H.
Nathan Sinai Distinguished Professor of Public Health
University of Michigan
Ann Arbor, Michigan

Betty R. Ferrell, Ph.D., F.A.A.N.
Associate Research Scientist
City of Hope Medical Center
Duarte, California

Mona R. Fields, R.N., Ed.D.
Texas Department of Health
Health Licensure and Certification Division
Arlington, Texas

Candace Friedman, M.P.H., CIC
Manager, Infection Control Services
University of Michigan Medical Center
Ann Arbor, Michigan

Sherril B. Gelmon, Dr.P.H.
Associate Professor of Public Health
Department of Public Administration and Department of Public Health Education
School of Urban and Public Affairs
Portland State University
Portland, Oregon

Hannie Giebing, R.N., B.N., M.N.
Assistant Director and Coordinator
Nursing Programme, CBO
National Association for Quality Assurance in Hospitals
Utrecht, The Netherlands

Robbie Helmich Henson, R.N., M.S.N.
Doctoral Candidate, University of Colorado
Assistant Professor of Nursing
Oklahoma Baptist University
Shawnee, Oklahoma

Joe B. Hurst, Ph.D., Ed.D.
Professor of Education
University of Toledo
Toledo, Ohio

Katherine R. Jones, Ph.D., R.N., F.A.A.N.
Associate Professor
Division of Nursing and Health Care Systems Administration
School of Nursing
University of Michigan
Ann Arbor, Michigan

Mary Keenan, Ed.D., M.S.N., B.S.N.
Associate Professor
School of Nursing
Medical College of Ohio
Toledo, Ohio

K. R. Knapp, M.H.A., C.N.H.A.
Vice President, Life Span Forum, Inc.
Louisville, Kentucky

Mary Jo Kreitzer, Ph.D., R.N.
Associate Director
University of Minnesota Hospital and Clinic
Minneapolis, Minnesota

Connie Leek, R.N., M.S.N.
Clinical Instructor
City of Hope Medical Center
Duarte, California

Amy S. Lesniewski, R.N., M.S.
Head Nurse
Department of Veteran's Affairs Medical Center
Oklahoma City, Oklahoma

Michael Lummis, M.P.A.
Director of Loss Control
Quality Assurance Consultant
Health Midwest
Kansas City, Missouri

Margo MacRobert, M.S., R.N., C.N.A.A.
Director of Nursing
Children's Hospital of Oklahoma
Oklahoma City, Oklahoma

Frances K. Masters, R.N., M.S.
Head Nurse
Department of Veteran's Affairs Medical Center
Oklahoma City, Oklahoma

Claire G. Meisenheimer, Ph.D., R.N., C.N.A.A.
Professor, College of Nursing
University of Wisconsin, Oshkosh
Oshkosh, Wisconsin

John Minnick, B.A.
Vice President of Finance
Medical College of Ohio
Toledo, Ohio

James W. Mold, M.D., CAQ(G)
Director of Research Division
Department of Family Medicine
College of Medicine
University of Oklahoma
Oklahoma City, Oklahoma

Sheila Taylor Myers, R.N., Ph.D.
College of Nursing Associate Professor
University of Oklahoma
Research Consultant
Baptist Medical Center of Oklahoma and Children's Hospital of Oklahoma
Oklahoma City, Oklahoma

Carole H. Patterson, M.N., R.N.
Associate Director, Product Development
Department of Standards
Joint Commission on Accreditation of Healthcare Organizations
Oakbrook Terrace, Illinois

Wanda L. Robinson, R.N., M.S.
Research Assistant
College of Nursing
University of Oklahoma
Oklahoma City, Oklahoma

Phillip Schaedler, B.S., M.A., J.D., F.A.S.H.R.M.
Director of Risk Management
Presbyterian Healthcare Systems Corporation
Charlotte, North Carolina

June A. Schmele, R.N., Ph.D.
Associate Professor
College of Nursing
Adjunct Associate Professor
Department of Health Administration and Policy
College of Public Health
University of Oklahoma
Oklahoma City, Oklahoma

P. Susan Wagner, R.N., M.Sc. (Nursing)
Associate Professor
College of Nursing
University of Saskatchewan
Saskatoon, Saskatchewan, Canada

CONTENTS

FOREWORD

Quality Management may appear to many as a vast, forbidding domain, scarcely explored. In a field where the old has been so assertively challenged by the new, and the new is, itself, constantly being revised, it is no wonder that we often are perplexed, unsure of our bearings. If so, we can find in this volume a map of "quality-land": of its general configuration, of its more detailed features, and of the roads we can take to reach our hoped-for destinations.

It is, of course, a conceptual mapping that we have in mind: an intellectual construct, to which many expert minds have brought their separate, distinctive, but carefully orchestrated, contributions. As a consequence, we are given for each major feature in our metaphorical landscape, a variety of views — coherent rather than contending — allowing us to see more clearly what the landscape is. Nowhere is the method more apparent, or more instructive, than in the presentation of Total Quality Management, a feature so large, so many sided, that it must be seen from many angles to be truly comprehended.

A signal virtue of this book is that it begins with fundamentals, telling us what quality in health care is, and what our responsibilities for it are. We are offered a historical view of how these responsibilities have been defined and discharged, in this country as well as abroad. We are shown the ethical, social, political, and organizational contexts for Quality Management, be they international, national, or institutional. And we are told what contextual changes need to be made if Quality Management is to be introduced and is to flourish.

We see Quality Management not only as a set of techniques but, more fundamentally, as a moral commitment, a culture, a style of management, a means for professional self-realization, and, not least, an expression of consumer sovereignty. But the techniques, themselves, are also exhaustively described, with special attention given to group processes and teamwork, to measurement, and to the acquisition, management, and interpretation of data, so that these later might yield the useful "information" they would otherwise conceal.

As these subjects unfold, always with applications to nursing particularly in mind, we can see how what has been so long established can be welcomed within the new, and how several seemingly disparate enterprises, including cost control and risk management, are, in fact, interrelated. Thus, we end on a note of harmony rather than dissension, facing realistic prospects for a happy collaboration in the pursuit of the general good.

With this felicitous thought, this book is introduced to its many potential readers, to be read either whole or a chapter at a time as the occasion demands — but always with pleasure and profit. As it goes forth, in recognition of the ecumenical nature of the book, we two, a nurse and a physician, join our voices in wishing it Godspeed.

Avedis Donabedian

Dorothy Donabedian   Nathan Sinai Distinguished Professor
Professor Emeritus of Nursing   Emeritus of Public Health
The University of Michigan   The University of Michigan

PREFACE

This book was written in response to the need for an upper-level textbook for Quality-Management courses in nursing and other health-care disciplines. This need first became apparent several years ago when the author taught a graduate-level course in Quality Management, then called Quality Assurance. The students' requests for a course text inspired and stimulated the writing of this book, which is designed around the organizing framework of the course. Thus, one of the unique features of this book is the strong theoretical and historical grounding. It is acknowledged that several other largely practice-oriented Quality-Management books are available. Any one of these books would make an excellent companion source to this text.

The text, which includes an international component, is written from a multi-disciplinary and interdisciplinary perspective. It is suitable for graduate and upper-level nursing students, as well as for students from other health-care disciplines. The rationale for a multidisciplinary approach stems from the philosophy that the current practice of Quality Management and the subsequent improvements in quality of health care are results of the efforts of several disciplines working together, rather than any one discipline working in an isolated or discipline-specific fashion. In addition to the student audience, the book, as a whole or in part, will have value for Quality-Management professionals in practice and for others who view Quality Management as an inherent part of their administrative or management role.

An important feature of the book is the specialized knowledge and varied backgrounds represented by the various contributors. These writers possess unique and distinct expertise in the areas of their respective contributions.

The book is organized in such a way that it can be used in its entirety for a course text or in part as a reference. Each chapter, or each part, is designed to stand alone. It is recognized that with this type of design there is a fine line between redundancy and emphasis. The reader is encouraged to consider the common themes that occur throughout the book as those that deserve emphasis.

In addition to a comprehensive reference list for each chapter, a list of Additional Reading is provided. Chapter contributors consider these resources to be among the most important and/or classic readings addressing the subject of the chapter. This wide array of resources will provide suitable material for student assignments or offer further material for practitioners who wish to pursue a specific topic of interest.

Despite the "semantic jungle" that exists in the field of Quality Management, every effort was made to standardize the use of key terms. In certain instances, however, terms are used differently — for example, in specific geographic locations, within specialty fields, or earlier in time. In these instances, it seemed appropriate to preserve the usage of that country, specialty, or time. It bears emphasis that in the discussion of historical events, terminology pertinent to earlier times is used. Hopefully this will serve to emphasize the evolutionary nature of Quality Management.

A glossary of select key terms relevant to the study of Quality Management is provided. The glossary is presented as the author's representation of the most common

Quality-Management terminology. Just as it is desirable for the staff within an organization to use common terminology to ensure their pursuit of a common goal, readers of this book will benefit from a common understanding of terms. This does not imply that other semantic usage is incorrect; but simply that persons within a specific system, such as an organization or a class, will benefit from common usage of terms.

Part I contains several strong, theoretically focused chapters that provide the conceptual framework for the study of Quality Management. It is fitting that the subject of the first chapter is the consumer. This chapter presents a historical and conceptual view of the concept of consumerism as well as a brief overview of related concepts, which are treated in greater depth throughout the book. This gestalt view envisions the consumer as the raison d'être for the current practice of Quality Management. Chapter 2 deals with the overarching concept of accountability within the health-care system. The four subsequent chapters are theoretically based expositions of various aspects of the concept of quality itself. Part I concludes with consideration of the closely related concepts of program evaluation and interdisciplinarity.

Few would question the current global nature of society and the impact that this has on the operation of all systems, especially the health-care system. During this time of unprecedented change in society and the health-care system, it is vital to understand the broad context within which the quest for quality takes place. Whether the attributes of health-care quality are considered from the perspective of structure, process, or outcome, it is evident that the assessment and improvement process takes place within the broader national and international context. It is important to consider the health-care system as a part of these greater supra systems.

Part II addresses the national context and the historical development of the Quality-Management field. Chapter 9 addresses the changing perspectives and emphasis in the field of health-care quality in the United States. Chapter 10 is a provocative analysis of the evolution of quality improvement from an epidemiological viewpoint. This part concludes with a chapter that examines the current state of the health-care environment and of health-care reform in the United States, including the inherent implications for quality.

An overview of the different types of health-care systems found throughout the world is presented in the first chapter of Part III. Quality implications of each of these systems are described. This description sets the stage for a more specific international perspective that is the subject of the three subsequent chapters on select health-care systems in Western Europe, the Netherlands, and Canada, and their quest for quality.

The organizational context for the implementation of quality is the subject of Part IV. Key contextual considerations are the regulatory and organizational environments, leadership, and the implementation of quality-improvement systems. Chapter 17 is devoted exclusively to describing the current focus of one of the major accrediting agencies in the United States, the Joint Commission on Accreditation of Healthcare Organizations. Although the majority of contextual organizational considerations make reference to the acute-care setting, the applications are considered to be generic in nature and applicable to diverse settings.

The practice of quality is the subject of Part V, which highlights a variety of select models, methods, and approaches for implementing some of the previously described concepts. A comprehensive chapter on data sources, gathering, and management is followed by a chapter focusing on computerization of data for quality-improvement purposes.

Part VI focuses on quality-related processes. Chapter 26 discusses the relationship and linking of research and Quality Management. Subsequent chapters include descriptions of other health-care programs that also deal with approaches to quality improvement. Although the implicit goal of each program is to improve quality, the explicit purpose is usually evident in the title of the program. For example, Risk Management, Infection Control, and Utilization Management are considered the most common quality-related programs. Since the advent of the Total-Quality-Management movement, there has been growing impetus to integrate programs having the common direct or indirect objective of quality improvement.

Part VII includes select topics that can be considered current trends, issues, and opportunities in the rapidly evolving field of Quality Management. This final part presents important, though sometimes controversial, viewpoints, which can serve as material for further discussion. Finally, Chapter 33 focuses on the identification and forecasting of major trends impacting the management of quality in health care. The intent of this last chapter is to encourage the reader to consider the future in a broad and global context. It bears emphasis that the rapidly changing global environment strongly influences the evolving field of Quality Management.

ACKNOWLEDGMENTS

Gratitude is extended to the many students who have taken my course in Quality Management in the past several years. The challenge they have presented and the inspiration they have offered has bolstered my motivation to continue the quest for quality.

With profound gratitude and respect, I acknowledge the expertise, support, and cooperation of all the chapter contributors, who made certain that the whole became greater than the sum of the parts. I recognize that these contributions were above and beyond the contributors' usual and regular professional commitments, so again I thank each of them for their respective contributions to the book and for the privilege of collaborating with them.

I gratefully acknowledge the administration at the University of Oklahoma; Dean Patricia Forni, who furthered this process by granting me a sabbatical leave and by providing other resources; Mary Jane Ward, who offered advice, guidance, and encouragement; and Bonnie Morris-Bright, who has done so much to expedite this process. I express appreciation to faculty colleagues at the College of Nursing, whose regular assignments were extended to absorb my teaching load. I am grateful to other faculty and staff who offered their willing support during this long process.

I wish to express special gratitude to Carol Stephens, who carefully and patiently provided secretarial services for this endeavor, and Deloris Holston, who has always been responsive to the need for additional secretarial support. I gratefully acknowledge Robbie Henson, who assisted me in so many ways including the preparation of the first draft of the manuscript. Special acknowledgement also goes to my Research Assistants, Wanda Robinson and Karen Vessier, who provided thoughtful and able assistance during the final completion of the project.

My gratitude is expressed to Debra Flis, Delmar Assistant Editor, who always provided timely advice and guidance; to Series Editor, Lillian Simms, for the confidence that she expressed in me when she invited me to write this book; and to Bill Burgower, Delmar Senior Acquisitions Editor, who was willing to accept Lillian's recommendation. Special acknowledgment is due to Colleen A. Corrice and Judith B. Thorpe, Project Managers at Flanagan's Publishing Services who offered able assistance and encouragement during the final phases of the project. I offer much appreciation to Danya Plotsky for her very competent copy editing. Although we have not met, nor personally spoken, I have experienced through her able editing, a highly effective form of communication.

A special note of gratitude is extended to those persons who provided thoughtful review and critique of the manuscript. In addition to the three major reviewers, I would especially like to acknowledge the graduate nursing student consumers Pat Barton, Glenda Bell, Tina Collins, Carol Ewing, Donna Haywood, and Marie Mason, who carefully reviewed the manuscript and learned to frequently and endearingly refer to it as "The Book."

I am appreciative of the support of my friends and family, who were understanding of the long-lasting demands of the moment. I extend special gratitude to
my friends, Margarita Blanco and Mary Allen, who were the most likely to have
experienced these long-lasting demands. Especially, I gratefully acknowledge the
sustained interest and encouragement of my brother Bill, who always seemed to
understand the intricacies and challenges of each phase of this project. A special
message of gratitude is extended to the late Ivan Hanson, who provided continuous
inspiration and oversight to this endeavor. And, lastly, my gratitude is conveyed to
the many persons — although unnamed — who by thought, word, or deed, encouraged the completion of this book.

PART I

CONCEPTS IN QUALITY MANAGEMENT

Robbie Helmich Henson
Wanda L. Robinson
June A. Schmele

CHAPTER *1*

Consumerism and Quality Management

INTRODUCTION

In most situations today, consumers are wary buyers. They thump and smell gro-ceries, try on and model clothes, study and compare benefits. Many modern con-sumers are equally diligent when purchasing health care. This, however, was not always the case. It was not until the past decade that an alert was sounded: *Caveat emptor — Let the buyer beware.* Spiraling health care costs combined with diminishing insurance support captured the attention of the consumer public. This public inter-est fostered a steady change of focus in the marketplace to include more consumer input in both decision making and evaluation of the quality of goods and services delivered. Today this trend is noticeable nationally as well as internationally. This chapter addresses the concept of **consumerism** — its history and its relationship to the health-care industry, particularly with regard to the issue of **quality**. Although the **Total Quality Management (TQM)** movement emphasizes both **external** and **internal consumers,** this chapter focuses on the external consumer (i.e., the client or patient) and the provider-consumer relationship.

HISTORY

The development of consumerism in health care is reflected in the societal move-ment toward consumerism over a relatively long historical period. A brief historical synopsis of major happenings in the consumer movement follows.

Early History (Before 1850)

Interest in protecting consumer safety and rights can be traced to the Middle Ages. In 1202 one of the first laws to protect consumers was enacted in England as a result of public outcry. Bakers were routinely cheating customers by using inferior flour and short-weighing bread (Maxwell, 1984). The concept of consumer sovereignty came about much later, driven by the idea that the customer could determine the success or failure of any product or service by choosing whether or not to buy that product or service. This meant that the continuing success of the seller depended on a reputation of quality. The focus for the seller during this period became pleasing the consumer.

Industrial Revolution (1850–1900)

With the industrial revolution came the advent of rapid and anonymous production. Mass production quickly filled the need for goods. This resulted in a postindustrial-revolution view that quality was unnecessary because "everything manufactured was sold" (Widtfelt & Widtfelt, 1992, p. 312). Widespread fraud and monopoly in industry soon greatly undermined consumer power.

Consumer Protection (1870–1910)

It was not until the 1870s that Congress passed the nation's first consumer protection laws, and the consumer movement began again to gain momentum (Maxwell, 1984). These laws, which included postal fraud laws and physician licensing laws, were intended to ensure quality products and consumer access to products. Other efforts to protect consumers included passage of the Pure Food and Drug Law in 1906 and establishment of the Food and Drug Administration in 1931.

Quality Control (1950s)

Consumerism and the demand for quality emerged powerfully in the industrial market of the 1950s and 1960s. During this period, there was an attempt to rebuild the Japanese and international post-war manufacturing industry. American quality expert Deming (1986) and his associates went to Japan to assist in this reconstruction. The successful programs they implemented in Japan included principles such as "applying the ideas of process control, worker involvement in the search for root causes of quality problems, and a systems approach to preventing quality problems" (Widtfelt & Widtfelt, 1992, p. 312). Although the work of Deming and his associates was slow to be recognized in the United States, the following concepts of TQM evolved from their work:

- conformance to customer requirements and specifications
- fitness for use
- buyer satisfaction
- value at an affordable price

In the decades that followed, the success of Deming's work gave consumerism and **Quality Management (QM)** firm roots in the industrial marketplace.

Consumer Rights (1960s)

With the ideas of quality and consumerism gaining strength in the 1960s, President John F. Kennedy offered the Declaration of Rights for all Americans. This document has become known as the Consumer Bill of Rights. In summary, it states that the consumer has:

- the right to safety
- the right to be informed
- the right to choose
- the right to be heard (Consumers' Union, 1989)

Also established at the federal level during the 1960s were the Committee on Consumer Interests, Consumer Advisory Committee, and legislation such as truth in lending, fair packaging, child safety, and hazardous household products (Fine, 1988).

Consumer Advocacy (1970s–1980s)

Strengthening of consumer rights continued in the 1970s through the efforts of consumer advocate groups such as the one headed by Ralph Nader. This period of time saw several advances:

- publication of the Patient's Bill of Rights
- publication of the Rights of Hospital Patients
- consumer participation in the planning and policy making of health maintenance organizations
- the mandate for human subject review committees for all federally funded research
- the mandate for informed consent to ensure that patients received adequate information to make health-care decisions (Fine, 1988)

In the 1980s, consumer participation in QM was exemplified best by consumer advocacy groups and by the significant increase in the dissemination of health care information to consumers and public policy officials.

Global Marketplace (1990s)

Changing global economics of the late 1980s and early 1990s gave the health-care industry a *marketplace orientation* (Fine, 1988). Decreased length of hospital stays, spiraling health-care costs with tighter reimbursement, more uninsured clients, extended lifespans, and changing disease patterns forced health-care administrators to make strategic cuts in cost, and to look to industry for guidance in surviving a competitive, consumer-oriented market. The federal consumer protection/information age of the 1960s and 1970s, and the industrial quality improvement age of the 1980s were pivotal forces in the development of consumerism among health-care clients in the 1990s.

CONCEPTUAL BASE

In 1990 the World Health Organization stated that patient participation in health care is "viewed as not only desirable but as a social, economic, and technical necessity" (Waterworth & Luker, 1990, p. 974). Using consumer participation in health care as a necessary QM tool requires an in-depth look at closely related concepts.

Consumerism

Lancaster and Lancaster (1992) define consumerism as "an organized movement of citizens and government to improve the rights and power of buyers in relation to sellers" (p. 30). The concept of consumerism is exceedingly broad, without a strong specific theoretical or research base. Even the dictionary definitions depict the evolving nature of the consumerism concept. In 1974, Webster's Dictionary defined consumerism as "the promotion of the consumer's interests" (Wolf, p. 244), while today the dictionary definition is "the practice and policies of protecting the consumer by publicizing defective and unsafe products, misleading business practices, etc." (Neufeldt & Guralnik, 1994, p. 299). A discussion of a few significant conceptual underpinnings is necessary to clarify the understanding of the consumer role in health care and quality management.

Paternalism

The issue of consumerism in the health-care industry relates closely to the concept of *paternalism*. Webster (1973) defines paternalism as a system under which an authority undertakes to supply needs or regulate conduct of those under its control in matters affecting them as individuals as well as in their relations to authority and to each other. Bartholome (1992) describes such paternalism in the health-care industry in the following excerpt:

> It was assumed that part of the calling of the health care provider was to take on the burden of responsibility so as to protect the patient . . . It was assumed that the only road to healing required that patients place themselves in the hands of benevolent providers who both know and would do what was best . . . Patients have come to realize that playing along with this parentalism charade required that they remain in the dark, cut off from knowledge of what was really going on in their bodies and lives. (pp. 7–10)

Bartholome suggests that a new model of health care is emerging — one of shared decision making between the consumer of health care and the provider. According to Lehr and Strosberg (1991), the health-care consumer of the 1990s no longer sees himself as a passive patient with limited involvement, but as a therapeutic partner with the health-care provider.

Self-Care

Barofsky (1978) suggests that patient self-care is best understood as a continuum. At one extreme is *compliance*, and at the other extreme is *therapeutic alliance*. Compliance is linked with coercion; the provider takes on a parental role, putting the consumer in the child-like role of having behaviors dictated and being expected to comply with the instructions given. Midway between compliance and therapeutic alliance is *adherence*. Adherence is linked to conformity. The client voluntarily adheres because he realizes the health-care plan is in his best interest, yet there is little intrinsic motivation. Opposite compliance is therapeutic alliance in which the health-care plan is constructed and carried out by the provider-consumer team.

Mutuality

In an analysis of the concept *mutuality*, Henson (1993) also places client-provider health-care participation on a potentially dynamic continuum (see Figure 1-1). At one extreme is *absolute autonomy* in which the client is the only significant referent for the health-care experience. At the other extreme is paternalism in which the provider is the only significant referent for the health-care experience. Mutuality can be seen as a balance between the two: knowledge and expertise of both client and provider are used as resources to achieve health goals.

Autonomy ←—→ Reciprocity ←—→ Mutuality ←—→ Participation ←—→ Paternalism

Figure 1-1 *Model of Client-Provider Mutuality. (Courtesy of Robbie Henson.)*

This emerging paradigm of provider-consumer mutuality brings to light an interesting incongruence. In industry, the consumer and manufacturer together define quality, and the needs and preferences of the consumer are taken seriously. In health care, the provider often defines quality, and consumers are frequently treated in an impersonal manner and given little consideration for anything beyond their immediate needs and preferences (Lehr & Strosberg, 1991).

In spite of a growing consumerism mindset, health-care quality models are obviously not yet consumer driven; they are still clearly provider driven, often in a paternalistic manner. An operational definition of health-care consumerism is needed. It must be based on the new paradigm and the related concepts. Home health-care consumerism is defined as the entering of the consumer/customer (previously called patient) into mutual involvement with the health-care provider related to her/his health needs, goals, and desires.

CONCEPTUAL MODELS OF HEALTH-CARE DELIVERY

The evolution of the concept of health-care consumerism is reflected in the various health-care delivery models. The section that follows discusses selected models that represent various degrees on the consumerism continuum.

Assisted Self-Care Model

Florence Nightingale (1859) was perhaps one of the earliest theorists to write about consumer involvement in health care. With great passion she emphasized active involvement of the sick in their own healing processes.

> It is desirable that the windows in a sick room should be such as that the patient shall, if he can move about, be able to open and shut them easily himself . . . the sick man often says, "This room where I spend 22 hours out of the 24 is fresher than the other where I only spend 2. Because here I can manage the windows myself" . . . Cravings are usually called the "fancies" of the

patients . . . But much more often, their so-called "fancies" are
the most valuable indications of what is necessary for their
recovery. And it would be well if nurses would watch these
so-called "fancies" closely. (pp. 9, 33)

Participative and Guidance-Cooperation Model

As early as 1956, Szasz and Hollender introduced a participative health-care delivery model. In their model, power and authority are shared, being distributed
between patient and provider according to the patient's condition. A second model
discussed in their writings is the guidance-cooperation model. This model best
describes the current health-care delivery system in the United States. In this model,
the physician has responsibility for informed, altruistic guidance, and the patient
has responsibility for unquestioning cooperation. Kasch (1986) suggests that in an
era of increased cost, decreased length of stay, and increased acuity at the time of
discharge, there is necessarily more participation and responsibility for health-care
planning left to the consumer and family. In the guidance-cooperation model,
there is often little previous practice or preparation on the part of the consumer
and family to offset this increased responsibility.

Goal-Oriented Model

In their work, Mold, Blake, and Becker (1991) offered a goal-oriented model of
health-care delivery in which health is defined by the consumer. The plans and
goals to achieve health are mutually constructed based on the combined knowledge
of the consumer and the provider, and the consumer's strengths, resources, interests, needs, and values. Success for both provider and consumer is measured by the
extent to which the consumer's health-related goals are achieved.

Systems-Theory Model

Robinson (1993) describes a systems-theory perspective of consumer-driven health-
care delivery. In her description, the health-care system is seen as a huge, open system
with *input* coming from consumers, who bring their health-care needs into the
system. The boundaries are the laws, while licensing boards and agencies regulate the
health-care industry. *Throughput* is the actual health care that is delivered. The *output*
is both the level of health and wellness that consumers have obtained by proceeding
through the system and consumer satisfaction with the goods and services received.

RELATED RESEARCH

Research dealing with consumerism increases understanding of clients' perceptions
of what is important and substantiates or nullifies proposed hypotheses. The importance of provider perceptions may be only speculative until research is done. The
section that follows summarizes selected research on patient satisfaction as well as
some key findings of outcomes research as it relates to health-care delivery models.

Patient-Satisfaction Research

The study of consumer satisfaction has given providers useful insight into the perceptions and expectations of consumers. Services can then be tailored to match these

perceptions and expectations. Research related to the measurement of consumer satisfaction with health-care services takes various approaches. Some studies and surveys measure satisfaction as a global assessment of all aspects of the patient's hospital experience (Abramowitz, Cote, & Berry, 1987; Cleary & LeRoy, 1989). Others focus specifically on the care patients receive while hospitalized (Hinshaw & Atwood, 1982; LaMonica, Oberst, Madea, & Wolf, 1986). In an extensive review of the literature, McDaniel and Nash (1990) found twenty-one instruments that measure patient satisfaction with health care received. Most of these instruments were designed to be hospital-based and focused on the type of technical and interpersonal care delivered by the institution in which the tool was developed. Few of the studies reported psychometric properties of the instrument, such as reliability and validity. The findings of the studies generally reported high levels of satisfaction with most important aspects of care. When noting the results of these studies, however, it is important to consider the inherent element of responder bias generally present in this type of research.

Outcomes Research

Other research relates to the outcomes of provider-consumer participatory-care delivery models, particularly in the nursing field. Some of the findings include:

- greater satisfaction with health services.
- increased feelings of control and power over one's body and health.
- better compliance with prescribed treatment plan.
- increased rate of recovery.
- increased patient participation after repeated interactions with a service that promotes participation.
- increased effectiveness of provider-patient relationship.
- a reduction in provider power.
- an awkwardness in the provider-consumer relationship.
- decreased stress of provider work.
- decreased risk of lawsuits.
- increased provider creativity.
- increased development of alternative skills in the provider.
- not all patients prefer to participate in their own care. (England & Evans, 1992; Hanucharurnkui & Vinya-nguag, 1991; Krouse & Roberts, 1989; Waterworth & Luker, 1990)

There is a need to replicate studies and develop new research in the area of consumerism in health care. The discovery and exploration of related variables is vital to the growth of the consumer movement in health care.

RELATIONSHIP OF CONSUMERISM TO QUALITY MANAGEMENT

In the current health-care environment few would question that elements of consumerism are vital aspects of health-care quality. Well-recognized authorities point out that the values, expectations, and satisfaction levels of clients are essential components of a comprehensive quality-of-care view.

Definition of Quality

According to Donabedian (1980), "Quality is a property of, and a judgement upon, some definable unit of care that is divisible into at least two parts: technical and interpersonal" (p. 5). There are three approaches to evaluating quality:

- **Structure** — the physical and organizational tools and resources
- **Process** — the activities that occur between the client and provider
- **Outcome** — the changes in the status of the client attributable to antecedent health care

Donabedian also stresses that the client is an expert and the ultimate authority on the quality of care received, based on the values and expectations the client espouses. This is especially true of the interpersonal and communication components of health-care delivery. These components are crucial in augmenting technical care and in demonstrating the caring aspect of services that consumers expect in health-care delivery. Therefore, the consumer's assessment of quality, often measured as patient satisfaction, becomes an important measure of quality.

Consumer Satisfaction

In order to improve competitive edge in the marketplace, it is vital that health-care providers understand the perceptions and expectations of consumers. Obtaining information regarding consumer satisfaction with products or services is one method that manufacturers and service providers frequently use to **evaluate** the quality of a product or service. The feedback they receive from the consumer is used to improve the existing product or service in hopes of increasing customer satisfaction and demand for the product or service, thus increasing revenues (Press, Ganey, & Malone, 1991).

According to Vuori (1991), the satisfaction factor is described most accurately in two facets — the quality of action and, more importantly, the quality of perception of services. Perceptions, Vuori believes, are often even more powerful at guiding clients' behaviors than are the facts in the situation. Quality of care, therefore, cannot be accounted for or measured accurately or fully by anyone but the consumer.

Many studies have been undertaken to determine what satisfies health-care consumers. One such study by Robinson (1994) used "A Client Satisfaction Survey in Home Health Care" (Reeder & Chen, 1990) to determine the level of satisfaction with home health care among older consumers. This client satisfaction survey instrument is one of the few data collection tools available that has documented, acceptable psychometric properties. The satisfaction of elders with nurses who they perceived to be "kind" or "friendly" demonstrates the significant influence of perception and expectation on client satisfaction with health care delivery.

Although patient satisfaction is a central element in QM, there is much more to consider when attempting to understand consumerism as it relates to quality. Information satisfaction serves not only the needs of the recipient of care, but the marketing needs of the institution. To truly address consumerism in health care, it is necessary that quality and mutual participation be addressed at many levels, from individual administrators to individual caregivers, from the one-to-one service unit to the organizational and governmental unit.

Provider Accountability

Provider **accountability** to consumers is the responsibility of all organizations. Each institution and each member of the institution is accountable for consumer involvement and the quality of the programs, services, and facilities provided by the institution and each member of the institution. (See Chapter 2 for a detailed discussion of accountability.) The health-care field today is saturated with highly technical, specifically trained professionals who relate one-to-one with consumers of their products. It is no longer adequate or accurate to attribute solely to an institution or to a physician or to a nurse the responsibility for ongoing, mutually defined processes which are occurring between many varied professionals and the consumer.

Interdisciplinarity

Because of the multiplicity of health-care specialists and the complexity of health-care problems, the model of necessity in a consumer-driven organization is **multi-disciplinary** or **interdisciplinary** in nature. Although each specialist is responsible for and can provide the client with well-defined input regarding the client's health, an interdisciplinary, mutual approach has the best chance for success in a consumer-focused market. In this emerging model, responsibility for decision making and the quality of outcomes is shared between the various providers, the client, and the caregivers. Likewise, the accountability for decision making and the quality of outcomes is shared and synergistic. (See Chapter 8 for a detailed discussion of interdisciplinarity.)

CONSUMER-RELATED TRENDS AND ISSUES

Major societal changes and the health-care reform movement have had a strong impact on the evolution of consumerism in health care. Trends and subsequent issues relating to the growing consumer movement will continue to impact both client and provider behaviors.

Provider Perspective

Over the last century health-care providers often assumed on omniscient, altruistic pater/mater role in their relationships with clients. This offered the providers not only great prestige, but also great power and great economic reward, often at the expense of consumers. The more complex and technical that illness care became, the more willing consumers of that care were to relinquish involvement in their care and, instead, put their trust in the superior abilities of providers. The shift to a mutually participative relationship between the provider and consumer is no small task. The health-care reform movement of the 1990s strongly emphasized the value of the consumer's participation in health-care decisions at various levels. Precisely how this will be brought about remains an issue for the future.

CONSUMER ABILITY TO PARTICIPATE

Ellwood (1988) believes that what providers (particularly physicians)

> find most troubling about restructuring [of the health-care system]
> is not so much sharing decision making and power with patients
> and others; it is the nagging, not entirely arrogant or paternalistic,
> belief that nonphysicians simply do not have the information
> necessary to make rational decisions about medical care. (p. 1550)

Whereas Ellwood questions the consumer's ability to participate, Walker (1991) suggests that not only can consumers participate, but that provider reimbursement should be based on the consumers' evaluation of and satisfaction with their plans of care.

PROVIDER ACCEPTANCE OF CONSUMER ROLE

Bartholome (1992) approached the importance of consumer involvement from a different perspective.

> Professionals have realized that shouldering the burden of decision
> making meant exposing themselves to a kind of strict liability for
> the outcome of treatment which is impossible to endure . . . The
> era of provider knows best has come to an end . . . Both providers
> and patients are increasingly willing to accept the contention that
> providers cannot know what is the best or right treatment without
> the active participation of the patient. (pp. 7–10)

Taking on the new professional role of which Bartholome speaks might prove to be difficult initially. England and Evans (1992) found that reduction of a provider's power led to an initial awkwardness in the provider-client relationship; but, ultimately, providers enjoyed decreased work stress, decreased litigation stress, and an increase in creativity as alternative plans of care became necessary.

CONSUMER WILLINGNESS TO PARTICIPATE

A common response of providers to the challenge of active consumer participation is the suggestion that most patients either do not care to or are unable to participate. As examples these providers cite the comatose client, the critically ill client, or the elder client (who is more comfortable with the paternalistic-care delivery model). In a study by Waterworth and Luker (1990) it was documented that clients were reluctant to collaborate with providers. This finding showed that clients may well agree to participate because they feel it is expected, rather than because they want to be involved.

PROVIDER-CLIENT MUTUALITY

Henson (1993) discussed the elements of true provider-consumer mutuality in an analysis of the concept. Defining attributes of mutuality were identified as:

1. A feeling of intimacy, connection, understanding of the other;

2. A process characterized by an exchange of thoughts, actions, or feelings between two or more people related to a common goal or shared purpose. The exchange is not necessarily equivalent, but is described by both give-and-take behaviors from the involved parties which together facilitate movement toward the shared purpose;

3. The process and the purpose are characterized by a sense of sharing in common, a sense of joint-ness, and by a sense of satisfaction by both/all persons;

4. Mutuality precedes attainment of a goal or purpose that is completely satisfactory to a group of two or more. (p. 11)

By this definition, true mutuality between consumer and provider takes place when an exchange occurs that is appropriate to the circumstances (e.g., increased provider input for the dependent client or for the client who is unable to transition to the participative model) and that relates to a common goal (i.e., health).

EXPANDED VIEW OF CONSUMER

Gustafson (1992) further refines the concept of mutuality when he calls for the expansion of the definition of *consumer* to include family members as well as the patient. It is well recognized that the family/caregiver is oftentimes the consumer who is most able to participate in the planning and caregiving process.

Consumer-Social Perspective

The consumerism movement is greatly influenced by the governmental and policy-making processes of major social institutions. The economic and social power that emanates from large organizations does not necessarily treat consumer interests with the same regard as would the individual consumer (Rosen, Metsch, & Levey, 1977).

WHO IS THE CONSUMER?

Exploring who the consumer actually is reveals that the consumer is not just the individual who is receiving a specific product or service. This fact is particularly true in the health care arena.

Hamilton (1982) remarks,

> In most other situations we call ourselves consumers only when we
> purchase or use specific goods or services. Health care however, is
> not a private affair between provider and patient. In the broadest
> sense we are all consumers, even when we are not patients. (pp. 6–7)

The term *consumer* can be used accurately to describe society because of the insepa-rable nature of the relationship between the individual consumer and factors such as taxes, legislation, monies spent on education of medical professionals, research, insurance, third-party payers, and cost shifting from those who cannot pay to those who are able to pay a large portion. Hence, consumers can be individuals, institu-tions, government, or industry, and the health-care consumer movement can be readily identified as a social issue.

SOCIAL FACTORS

Numerous social trends affect the health-care consumer's perspective. For instance, the demographics of the United States are changing to an increasingly older popu-lation whose health-care issues include disease prevention and accessibility to com-munity-based programs. Further, this particular age group may not be as prepared to participate in health-care matters as are their children and grandchildren. The environmentally concerned baby boomers who grew up in the 1960s and 1970s are more interested in health promotion. They value volunteer activities that reflect their social concerns. They demonstrate a vast potential to influence public opinion and policy, as well as to influence their own individual health care.

Likewise, consumerism trends are appearing elsewhere in society. Changes in the workplace continually reshape the consumer's perspective and expectation of service. For example, industry affects the consumer's perspective through evolving management adaptations, such as flattened administrative hierarchies with responsibility and authority shifted from a centralized power base down to employees (Lefebvre, 1992). Such changes create new expectations in consumers for participative management of health-care systems.

CONSUMER-INITIATED LEGISLATION

In recent years consumers' ideas and activities have been articulated much more by means of legislation and government agencies than by private groups. Consumer advocates do a substantial portion of their work through lobbying efforts with congressional and state legislators. According to Yoho (1988), these lobbyists have been conspicuously successful in getting legislation passed. Among the most socially beneficial outcomes of consumer advocate activities are the laws that have been passed to protect consumers from lack of information, access, and utilization.

INFORMATION ACCESS

Consumers often are not as well-informed about health-care services as they are about many other goods and services. In the 1990s, however, there has been a great upsurge in consumer interest in learning about health-care services (Pear, 1993). Informed consumers are more likely to question providers about the necessity of services offered and about existing alternatives (Inlander & Morales, 1991; Tanne, 1991). Individual and organizational consumers are also becoming more cost conscious, seeking assurance of quality care at the lowest cost (Enthoven & Kronick, 1989; Schiller, 1993; Spencer, 1993).

Consumers must have access to information about health-care costs and concerns in order to meet these objectives. In the past, as is symptomatic of a powerful and paternalistic system, this information has been largely inaccessible to consumers. The current environment of health-care reform and the accompanying media blitz, however, are gradually chiseling away at this bulwark of paternalism.

REGULATORY PROTECTION

In spite of active consumer-interest groups, the consumer's position in the modern economy may be more precarious today than it was 100 years ago. More goods and services, which are more complex in design and operation, are now available. And although more powerful means such as television exist to contact consumers, the contact between the provider/producer of goods and services and consumer is significantly less direct (Yoho, 1988). This anonymity or lack of direct contact creates a major new expense for consumers. Resources must be diverted from the production of goods and services to the provision of regulatory activities for consumer protection. This is clearly evident in the health-care industry which boasts a plethora of regulating bodies and agencies. These regulators establish standards and **monitor** health-care providers' compliance with those standards as some indication of minimal quality. (See Chapter 16 for a detailed discussion of the regulation of the health-care system.)

CONSUMERISM IN THE HEALTH-CARE REFORM AGENDA

The national health-care agenda is also increasingly influenced by concerns for consumer support and input. For example, the basic components of the American Nurses Association's (ANA) *core of care* included recommendations advocating a restructured health-care system that "enhances consumer access to services by delivering primary health care in community-based settings" and "fosters consumer responsibility for personal health, self care and informed decision making in selecting health care services" (ANA, 1991, p. 2). Further, *Healthy People 2000: National Health Promotion and Disease Prevention Objectives* (American Public Health Association, 1990) set the goal to achieve access to preventive services for all Americans. Implicit in such a goal is a transformation in the education of health-care providers from a disease orientation to a health-promotion orientation.

In *Practitioner for 2005* (1991), the Pew Health Professions Commission suggested specific strategies necessary for schools to transform the education of health professionals to a practice that includes the consumer role as a vital element. They have also advocated for public participation in redefining health care and the role of professional providers. Other consumer-related topics addressed by this commission include:

- the demand for responsive providers
- guidance for the use of health resources
- support for health promotion
- increased consumer involvement (p. 8)

Improved education of consumers and a reorientation from a role as passive patient to active participant in health care is warranted because it is expected that consumers will bear a greater share of health-care responsibility and cost in the future. Consumer advocates propose the inclusion of the consumer as a primary player in determining the national health-care policies and the agenda for reform.

INFORMATION ACCESS AND CLIENT/PROVIDER MUTUALITY

This proposition reiterates one of the central social issues embodied in the concept of consumerism in health care: control and access to services and information. For society to become informed as a consumer is a formidable task because information about health care has largely been controlled by health-care professionals, who have been perceived as unwilling to share that information with the general public (Backus & Inlander, 1986).

To compensate for this perceived lack of power in the health-care arena, consumer-focused organizations have actively sought to provide information to empower consumers. This empowerment has begun even with children by attempts to awaken in them a sense of self-care health responsibility and knowledge (Igoe, 1991; Pittman, 1992). Consumer empowerment has produced a deluge of consumer-health-focused literature. Professional and non-professional authors have produced books and magazines to address growing consumer interests and demands. For example, Backus and Inlander (1986), as directors of the Peoples' Medical Society, have published consumer literature endorsing mandated disclosure of information by health-care providers, such as:

- the disclosure of price before services are rendered
- the success rates of various procedures
- information regarding educational background of the provider and any license suspension
- publication of infection rates
- publication of institution policies
- publication of the financial interests of institutional providers (Backus & Inlander, 1986)

Such literature demonstrates a decided societal shift in expectations regarding the relationship between health-care consumers and health-care providers. Igoe (1991) suggests that this societal shift may lead to greater involvement and ultimately improve health care and the quality of life for future generations.

Organizational Response

One of the major tenets of the TQM movement is the recognition of the consumer as a vital force in determining what constitutes quality of care. (See Chapter 5 for a detailed discussion of TQM). Although the TQM movement generally emphasizes both internal and external customers, health-care organizations are increasingly recognizing that the external consumer (i.e., the patient or client) is their raison d'entre. Consequently, the expectations and perceptions of consumers are increasingly influencing definitions of health-care quality. According to Gaucher and Coffey (1993), "Valid customer requirements include any needs, wants, and expectations of customers for which an agreement has been reached between the supplier and the customers" (p. 33). Considering the growing TQM movement, the increase in health-care competition, and the rapidly emerging plans for health-care reform, the consumer's voice will likely grow even stronger in the quest for **Continuous Quality Improvement (CQI)**.

CONCLUSION

In the past, health care has not been seen as a part of the market economy. Today, however, clients are willing to be involved consumers of health care, demanding high quality and positive outcomes for their dollars. Because it is the task of service providers to respond to public demand, health-care professionals must be accountable for the quality of the outcome of their work and to involve clients, the consumers of their goods, as participants in the process of evolving life health patterns that work.

As the health-care industry evolves in the light of expensive high technology and in an era of global economic restraint, consumer involvement in health care can only become more critical. As individual disease patterns change from acute curable illness to chronic lifestyle illness, it is imperative that the health-care delivery systems change to effectively address those patterns. Lifestyle illness can be successfully treated only through the evolution of new patterns of health behaviors in individuals. Lifestyle health behavior changes require personal involvement and commitment. Because the occurrence of tighter reimbursement schedules, decreased length of stay, increased acuity at the time of discharge, and increased responsibility of family caregivers are parts of the current situation, client and caregiver active involvement is inevitable.

With the multiplicity of health-care options available today, each having significantly different outcomes, providers can no longer be expected to know the best choice for clients. The personal and financial ramifications of such an omniscient provider role are staggering. To achieve positive outcomes and high-quality health care, decision making now requires mutuality and responsibility from the consumer and caregiver, accountability for quality of outcomes from individual providers, and mutuality from both. The health-care needs of the world today can no longer be addressed by well-intentioned, altruistic, paternalistic providers. Providers must begin to conceptualize the consumer as a serious partner in the planning and implementation of quality health-care services.

REFERENCES

Abramowitz, S., Cote, A. A., & Berry, E. (1987). Analyzing patient satisfaction: A multianalytic approach. *Quality Review Bulletin, 13*(4), 122–130.

American Nurses Association. (1991). *Nursing's agenda for health care reform* (PR-3220m). Kansas City, MO: Author.

American Public Health Association, Professional Affairs Division. (1990). *Healthy people 2000: National health promotion and disease prevention objectives.* Washington, DC: Author.

Backus, L. V., & Inlander, C. B. (1986). Consumer rights in health care. *Nursing Economics, 4*(6), 314–317, 324.

Barofsky, I. (1978). Compliance, adherence, and the therapeutic alliance: Steps in the development of self-care. *Social Science Medicine, 12,* 369–376.

Bartholome, W. G. (1992). A revolution in understanding: How ethics has transformed health care decision making. *Quality Review Bulletin, 18*(1), 6–11.

Cleary, P. D., & LeRoy, C. (1989). Patient assessments of hospital care. *Quality Review Bulletin, 15*(6), 172–179.

Consumers' Union. (1989). The new medicine show: Consumers' Union's practical guide to some everyday health problems and health products. Mount Vernon, NY: Author.

Deming, W. E. (1986). *Out of the crisis.* Cambridge, MA: Massachusetts Institute of Technology.

Donabedian, A. (1980). *The definition of quality and approaches to its assessment.* Ann Arbor, MI: Health Administration Press.

Ellwood, P. M. (1988). Outcomes management: A technology of patient experience. *New England Journal of Medicine, 318,* 1549–1556.

England, S. L., & Evans, J. (1992). Patients' choices and perceptions after an invitation to participate in treatment decisions. *Social Science Medicine, 34*(11), 1217–1225.

Enthoven, A., & Kronick, R. (1989). A consumer-choice health plan for the 1990s: Universal health insurance in a system designed to promote quality and economy. *New England Journal of Medicine, 320,* 94–102.

Fine, R. B. (1988). Consumerism and information: Power and confusion. *Nursing Administration Quarterly, 12*(3), 66–73.

Gaucher, E. J., & Coffey, R. J. (1993). *Total quality in healthcare.* San Francisco: Jossey-Bass.

Gustafson, D. H. (1991). Expanding on the role of patient as consumer. *Quality Review Bulletin, 17*(10), 324–325.

Hamilton, P. A. (1982). *Health care consumerism.* St. Louis, MO: C. V. Mosby.

Hanucharurnkui, S., & Vinya-nguag, P. (1991). Effects of promoting patients' participation in self-care on postoperative recovery and satisfaction with care. *Nursing Science Quarterly, 4*(1), 14–20.

Henson, R. J. (1993). *Mutuality: An analysis of the concept.* Unpublished manuscript, University of Colorado Health Sciences Center, Denver, CO.

Hinshaw, A. S., & Atwood, J. R. (1982). A patient satisfaction instrument: Precision by replication. *Nursing Research, 31*(3), 170–175.

Igoe, J. (1991). Research agenda: Empowerment of children and youth for consumer self-care. *American Journal of Health Promotion, 6*(1), 55–65.

Inlander, C. B., & Morales, K. (1991). *Getting the most for your medical dollar.* Allentown, PA: People's Medical Society Press.

Kash, C. R. (1986). Establishing a collaborative nurse-patient relationship: A distinct focus of nursing action in primary care. *Image, 18*(2), 44–47.

Krouse, H. J., & Roberts, S. J. (1989). Nurse-patient interactive styles: Power, control, and satisfaction. *Western Journal of Nursing Research, 11*(6), 717–725.

LaMonica, E. L., Oberst, M. T., Madea, A. R., & Wolf, R. M. (1986). Development of a patient satisfaction scale. *Research in Nursing and Health, 9*(1), 43–50.

Lancaster, J., & Lancaster, W. (1992). Current status of the health care system. In M. Stanhope, & J. Lancaster, *Community health nursing: Process and practice for promoting health* (3rd ed., pp. 21–33). St. Louis, MO: C. V. Mosby.

Lefebvre, R. C. (1992). Consumer trends in the 1990's: Implications for health promotion. *American Journal of Health Promotion, 6*, 165–168.

Lehr, H., & Strosberg, M. (1991). Quality improvement in health care: Is the patient still left out? *Quality Review Bulletin, 17*(10), 326–329.

Maxwell, J. A. (Ed.). (1984). *Reader's digest consumer advisor: An action guide to your rights.* Pleasantville, NY: The Reader's Digest Association.

McDaniel, C., & Nash, J. G. (1990). Compendium of instruments measuring patient satisfaction with nursing care. *Quality Review Bulletin, 6*(5), 182–188.

Mold, J. W., Blake, G. H., & Becker, L. A. (1991). Goal-oriented medical care. *Family Medicine, 23*(1), 46–51.

Neufeldt, V., & Guralnik, D. B. (Eds.). (1994). *Webster's new world dictionary* (3rd College ed.). New York: Prentice-Hall.

Nightingale, F. (1859). *Notes on nursing: What it is and what it is not.* London: Edward Stern & Company.

Pear, R. (1993, March 5). White House shuns bigger AMA voice in health changes; talks to be kept secret; consumer groups complain as well of having no role in medical-care overhaul. *New York Times,* p. A1.

Pew Health Professions Commission. (1991). *Practitioners for 2005: An agenda for action for U.S. health professional schools: A report of the Pew Health Professions Commission.* Durham, NC: Duke University Medical Center.

Pittman, K. P. (1992). Awakening child consumerism in health care. *Pediatric Nursing, 18*(2), 132–136.

Press, I., Ganey, R., & Malone, M. (1991). Satisfied patients can spell financial well-being. *Healthcare Financial Management, 45*(2), 34–36, 38, 40–42.

Reeder, P. J., & Chen, S. C. (1990). A client satisfaction survey in home health care. *Journal of Nursing Quality Assurance, 5*(1), 16–24.

Robinson, W. (1993). *Consumerism: The power of information and access.* Unpublished manuscript, University of Oklahoma Health Sciences Center, Oklahoma City, OK.

Robinson, W. (1994). *Satisfaction with home health care among elderly clients.* Unpublished thesis, University of Oklahoma Health Sciences Center, Oklahoma City, OK.

Rosen, H., Metsch, J., & Levey, S. (Eds.). (1977). *The consumer and the health care system: Social and managerial perspectives.* New York: Spectrum.

Schiller, Z. (1993, May 3). A consumer's guide for health-care shoppers: Cleveland's novel study grades local institutions' performance. *Business Week,* pp. 52–54.

Spencer, P. L. (1993, March). Calling all consumers: The hidden costs. *Consumer Research,* p. 38.

Szasz, T., & Hollender, M. (1956). A contribution to the philosophy of medicine: The basic models of the doctor-patient relationship. *Archives of Internal Medicine, 97,* 585–592.

Tanne, J. H. (1991). How to be a savvy medical consumer. *New York, 24*(46), 58–64.

Vuori, H. (1991). Patient satisfaction — Does it really matter? *Quality Assurance in Health Care, 3*(3), 183–189.

Walker, G. C. (1991). Accountability for quality improvement: Patients' rights to assess the plan of care. *Journal of Professional Nursing, 7*(5), 269.

Waterworth, S., & Luker, K. A. (1990). Reluctant collaborators: Do patients want to be involved in decisions concerning care? *Journal of Advanced Nursing, 15*(8), 971–976.

Webster. (1973). *New collegiate dictionary.* Springfield, MA: G. C. Merriam.

Webster. (1989). *New encyclopedic dictionary.* Springfield, MA: G. C. Merriam.

Widtfelt, A. K., & Widtfelt, J. R. (1992). Total quality management in American industry. *American Association of Occupational Health Nursing Journal, 40*(7), 311–318.

Wolf, H. B. (Ed.). (1974). *Webster's new collegiate dictionary.* Springfield, MA: G. & C. Merriam.

Yoho, D. L. (1988). *Study guide for use with economics of social issues* (8th ed, chaps. 8, 10). Plano, TX: Business Publications.

ADDITIONAL READING

Hacquebond, H. (1994). Health care from the perspective of a patient: Theories for improvement. *Quality Management in Health Care, 2*(2), 68–75.

Inlander, C. B. (1993). *This won't hurt (and other lies my doctor told me).* Allentown, PA: Peoples' Medical Society.

King, B. (1994). Techniques for understanding the customer. *Quality Management in Health Care, 2*(2), 61–67.

Mold, J. W., Blake, G. H., & Becker, L. A. (1991). Goal-oriented medical care. *Family Medicine, 23*(1), 46–51.

United States Office of Consumer Affairs. (1990). *Consumers' resource handbook.* Pueblo, CO: Author.

Pat Christensen

CHAPTER *2*

Accountability in the Delivery of Health Services

INTRODUCTION

Accountability means answering for one's actions and the consequences of those actions. Accountability is a "management philosophy that individuals are held liable, or accountable, for how well they use their authority and live up to their responsibility of performing predetermined activities" (Certo, 1989, p. 635). The **Quality Management (QM)** movement has influenced the demand for accountability in health-care practice. The concept of accountability is vital to the paradigm that subscribes to quality as a driving value for the health-care organization.

Accountability is one of the hallmarks of the professions and is especially critical in the delivery of health services. Accountability is increasingly a feature of many disciplines. Because of increasing regulations, the practice professions, notably in the delivery of health care, were early participants in the assignment of accountability to practitioners. The quality movement, liability law suits, escalating costs, and other trends of the 1980s and 1990s brought increased attention to accountability (and liability) in education, business, law, and other professions. Increasingly, nonprofessionals also are being held accountable for their work. Products and services are expected to have a certain level of **quality** and performance. If a product breaks down or does not meet expectations, there is an implied responsibility that the product be replaced or repaired. Likewise, the delivery of services is expected to meet a minimal quality **standard**. According to Certo (1989), the concept of accountability implies that if predetermined activities are not performed, some type of penalty or punishment is justifiably forthcoming. The purpose of this chapter is to explore the concept of accountability and, specifically, the application of accountability to the quality of health care.

HISTORICAL PERSPECTIVES

Historically, accountability for services rendered by health professionals has been linked primarily to personal integrity and professional autonomy. According to

Jones (1989), "Society expected health-care professionals to fulfill their obligation to the public for competent practice through self-regulation. Nurses, traditionally have been granted less autonomy and have been accountable to physicians and to employing agencies" (p. 339).

Traditionally the health services system of the United States has been a personal health system. Prior to 1875 and before private insurance and government funding, the only funding sources were charity and minimal local and state expenditures. Federal government expenditures were for the military, American Indians, and the establishment and maintenance of the public health services (Anderson, 1984).

By the mid nineteenth century physicians and pharmacists were the major dispensers of professionally recognized health services. They were, as they remain today, private entrepreneurs. Persons were cared for at home by family and, if needed (or could be afforded), by private nurses. Religious orders and philanthropic organizations provided care for the poor. Thus, private practice and fee-for-service became firmly embedded in American health tradition (Anderson, 1984).

Blue Cross/Blue Shield

When incomes fell drastically during the Great Depression in the 1930s, hospital admission rates and payments from private patients followed suit (Anderson, 1984). This era saw the start of hospital-sponsored prepayment plans, which eventually became known as Blue Cross. Hospital stays had become costly, and it was believed that the insurance principle could be applied. Later in the 1930s, this same principle was applied to physician's fees (Blue Shield).

During the 1940s private insurance companies, which had insured personal property and life until this time, saw from the Blue Cross/Blue Shield experience that hospital and surgical costs were insurable and could be predicted. The private insurance schemes exploded as labor unions and employers began offering group plans (Anderson, 1984). While the advent of insurance coverage for health care brought about increased accessibility to health care, accountability remained in the realm of professional autonomy in an unregulated health-care industry.

Medicare/Medicaid

In a political climate of social welfare (The Great Society), the Medicare/Medicaid Amendment to the Social Security Act was passed by the United States Congress in 1965. This established a retrospective payment system for health care for the poor and elderly that was to be underwritten by the federal government. These programs ushered in a new era of technology, expanded services, and increased public expectations regarding the right to health care. Enormous sums of money were expended by the unregulated health-care industry after 1965.

During a conservative swing in political thought in the United States, and in an effort to curb soaring health-care costs, the federal government changed to a Prospective Payment System (PPS) for Medicare/Medicaid in 1983. The new system was designed to create an incentive for hospitals and other providers to provide high quality, cost-effective health care (Ginzberg, 1986). The demands for quality *and* cost-effectiveness placed more intense scrutiny on the accountability of providers.

The rising costs of health care and the lack of accountability brought about demands for reform. According to Bice (1988), the reforms which followed the unregulated system established new mechanisms of public accountability. The massive government programs circumvented the traditional delivery of health care and introduced mandatory regulatory accountability. The eras of personal and professional accountability were now eclipsed by statutory and formal accountability schemes.

THEORETICAL ORIENTATION

Various authors have theorized a relationship among authority, responsibility, and accountability. Erickson, a pioneer in the study of accountability in the management of health services, states,

> The existence of any organization, whatever its purposes, goals,
> intended service or products, involves orchestrating many acts by
> many people in relationships that are effective and efficient. *Effective*
> means attaining of a pre-set goal and efficient means doing it with
> the least amount of expenditures (money, time, energy, and other
> resources) and untoward consequences. (Erickson, 1993, p. 1;
> emphasis in original)

For an organization to be effective and efficient, many acts necessitating the use of authority, responsibility, and accountability are needed. Stated simply, these words mean:

   a. authority is the right to do certain acts
   b. responsibility is the internal acceptance of assigned activities
   c. accountability means answering for the performance of these
      assigned acts and their results and consequences.

Accountability is theorized by this author to be at the apex of a triangle of authority, responsibility, and accountability (see Figure 2-1). There is a dynamic interaction

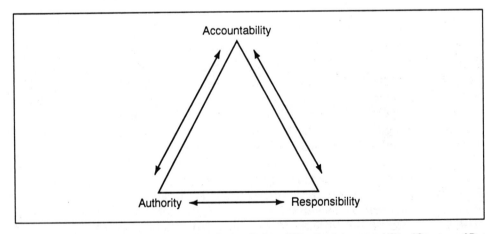

Figure 2-1 *The Dynamic Interaction of Authority, Responsibility, and Accountability. (Courtesy of Pat Christensen.)*

among the concepts of authority, responsibility, and accountability expressed in the professional delivery of health services. Additionally, delegation of authority and tasks is a dimension of accountability. Accountability carries responsibility for one's own actions and for those actions that are delegated. In order to explain the interaction of the central concepts of authority, responsibility, and accountability, these concepts will be briefly explored.

Authority

There are numerous definitions of authority. Fayol, one of the pioneers of administrative theory, defined authority as the right to give orders and the power to exact obedience (Fayol, 1949). Tappen (1989) defined authority as a type of power that originates in the official position a person holds in an organization. In a pure sense it is the right to perform or command. "It allows its holders to act in certain designated ways and to directly influence the actions of others through orders" (Certo, 1989, p. 229).

Barnard (1987) was a major theorist in management. His book *The Function of the Executive* was seminal work in the theory of authority. Barnard states that authority involves two aspects — a subjective and an objective. The subjective aspect is personal and involves the acceptance of a communication as authoritative. According to Barnard, a person will accept an order only if the communication is understood, consistent with the purpose of the organization, compatible with personal interests, and the receiver is mentally and physically able to comply with the order.

Barnard (1987) states, "The objective characteristic of a communication of authority is that aspect which induces acceptance" (p. 93). The principles involve the following:

a. the character of authority in organizational communications lies in the potentiality of assent of those to whom they are sent.

b. the system of communication is a primary continuing problem of a formal organization.

c. there are controlling factors in the character of the communication system as a system of objective authority.

According to Barnard (1987), in practice, "the source of authority is determined not by decree from the formal organization but by whether or not authority is accepted by those existing under it" (p. 230). In other words, authority exists only if it is accepted.

According to Weber (1989), another pioneer in organizational theory, there are three bases of authority. These are:

a. traditional authority, such as a monarchy

b. personal charisma

c. rational legal authority

Like Barnard, Weber theorized that subordinates do not always accept authority, especially if they do not believe a person is qualified for the position of authority (Marriner-Tomey, 1992). Thus, it can be seen that authority implies a reciprocal relationship between those in authority and those who are subordinated to that authority. A person in a position of authority cannot direct the work of others if subordinates do not accept that authority.

DELEGATION

Health-care providers, especially those in supervisory positions, cannot do all the actual work themselves. It becomes necessary and desirable for them to delegate some of the activities. Delegation, a component or subset of authority, involves the assigning of work activities and related authority to specific individuals in an organization (Certo, 1989). According to Newman and Warren (1977), there are three steps in the delegation process. These steps include:

a. the assigning of specific duties

b. granting appropriate authority

c. creating the obligation for the subordinate to perform the duties assigned

By granting authority and creating the obligation for the subordinate to perform the duties, there is a concomitant accountability established. It is vital that the delegation of responsibilities be accompanied by the acceptance of responsibility by the delegatee.

Tappen (1989) stated that there are two criteria of paramount importance in the delegation of responsibilities: "the individual must have the ability to carry out the task, and the assignment must be fair not only for the individual but also for the team as a whole" (p. 385). Individuals should never be assigned tasks that they cannot perform, regardless of professional level.

According to Fayol (1949), one can delegate but not abdicate. Likewise, according to Marriner-Tomey, responsibility and accountability cannot be transferred. While the subordinate carries both conferred authority and individual accountability, the supervising professional is not less accountable for the delivery of health services because some of the activities have been delegated. The delegation of functions with accompanying responsibility and accountability can be difficult for a manager because that manager remains responsible for the actions of the subordinates (Marriner-Tomey, 1992).

Responsibility

There are several dimensions to the concept of responsibility. These include responsibilities, responsibility, and being responsible. The first dimension, according to Erickson (1993), is the act(s) to be done effectively and efficiently. A crucial concern is the delineation of what constitutes the act — what are its parameters, limitations, and boundaries under ordinary and emergency circumstances? Responsibilities are generally considered to be the activities of an assigned role. Job descriptions are examples of the application of this concept. In addition, "policy statements, tradition — what has always been done or never been done, cultural barriers, and resource limitations may be factors that limit the nature of acts to be performed" (Erickson, 1993, p. 1).

The second dimension is responsibility, which is the "obligation to perform assigned activities" (Certo, 1989, p. 223). Responsibility carries a commitment to complete a task to the best of one's ability. While there can be shared responsibilities, the sense of the obligation is essentially a personal and internally controlled function.

According to Certo (1989), "Since responsibility is an obligation that a person accepts, there is no way it can be delegated or passed on to a subordinate" (p. 223).

The final dimension, being responsible, means performing the activities that are assigned. The degree of responsibleness can be determined by the behavior of the person performing the activities, that is, by attitudes and personal values reflected in the **outcomes** and relationships with co-workers.

Accountability

Accountability involves answering for one's actions and the consequences of those actions. Answering for one's actions can take many forms. For example, "in a simple non-complicated act, it may be a yes or no answer to 'did you do what you were assigned to do within limitations of resources available?' and a determination of whether the act was efficient and effective" (Erickson, 1993, p. 2). According to Erickson, accountability becomes much more complex "within a complicated, complex organization structure where no act is isolated, unhampered, free from many kinds of restrictions" (p. 2).

Accountability for delivering quality care is much more complicated because the measurement of quality is not easy to establish. Agreement to what is meant by quality and the standards and **criteria** needed to measure it is very difficult to attain. According to Erickson (1993), quantitative measures may well fall short of measuring quality. Subsequent chapters will address the concept of quality and its assessment. The concept of accountability is both philosophic and pragmatic. It involves a mind set of ethics and decision making and the acting out of those decisions and ethics. According to Tappen and George (1989), the person who is accountable will be able to tell the difference between right and wrong and think and act from a rational perspective.

Accountability has both internal and external locus-of-control aspects. Some persons exhibit accountable behavior with little need for outside regulators; others conform as required by external controls on their work.

Interaction of Concepts

Authority, responsibility, and accountability exist in a dynamic relationship with each other as shown earlier in Figure 2-1. Having authority assumes a measure of responsibility for oneself and others. In turn, responsibility assumes that one will be held accountable for that responsibility. Grohar-Murray and Dicroce (1992) offer a cogent discourse on the interactions of accountability, authority, and responsibility.

> Responsibility is dependent on three coexisting concepts: Authority, Delegation, and Accountability. For example, if a manager is given responsibility for a task, the manager will delegate the responsibility and necessary authority to whomever the task has been delegated. In turn, the employee is accountable to the delegator for completing the task satisfactorily. Accountability is the process of furnishing a justifying explanation for behavior of self or for others. (p. 139)

Overall responsibility continues to reside with the delegator, however. There is an implied trust that the person in charge will support the decisions of the delegated subordinate as long as the subordinate stays within the bounds of the delegated authority.

Central to the interactions of the concepts is the idea that authority must reflect responsibility. Whether delegated or not, there is inherent in authority the idea of responsibility for work done. With responsibility there is accountability or *owning* the results or outcomes of the work done.

APPLICATION OF ACCOUNTABILITY TO HEALTH-CARE SERVICES

The delivery of health-care services carries a heavy burden of responsibility — legal, ethical, and moral. The trust that people put in health professionals, often at times of heightened vulnerability, places those health professionals in uniquely powerful and important positions. The responsibility of health professionals extends beyond the individual client to the wider society. Inherent in the definition of professional is a responsibility to the public. The manner in which health professionals conduct their practices, and the outcomes of their care, are measures of their accountability.

Accountability of health professionals has dimensions of both external and internal controls. Externally imposed accountability has increasingly become a feature of health-care delivery. Issues of public safety, cost control, and the often nebulous concept of quality care are addressed in the forced accountability by the various regulators.

The Role of Regulators

As previously mentioned, health care was largely unregulated until escalating costs demanded an accounting of where funds were being spent; thus government became the major regulator and payer of health care, and the consumer movement demanded that health care be regulated and reformed (Bice, 1988). Historically, the professions of nursing, medicine, and allied health have self regulated practice (in a limited way) through licensing laws.

Beyond the basic legality of licensing laws have been the efforts to establish standards of quality care by the various professional organizations. Professional organizations such as the American Nurses Association (ANA), the American Medical Association (AMA), and other allied-health organizations have developed and published standards of care that offer guides to safe, effective, and optimal practice in the health professions.

Other avenues of regulation of the practice of health professionals are the accreditors of the workplaces of health-care workers. Hospitals are the major employers of nurses and allied-health professionals. There are a plethora of regulators of hospitals, both voluntary and mandatory. In addition, clinics, home-health agencies, and public-health facilities have numerous regulators.

Major regulators in the government sector with broad oversight authority include Medicare, Medicaid, state health departments, the Occupational Safety and Health Administration (OSHA), and others. Increasingly, insurance companies, especially the giant Blue Cross and Blue Shield Companies, are forcing accountability, particularly in the area of health-care financing. Other health-delivery systems which are forcing increased accountability include Health Maintenance Organizations (HMOs) and various employer-sponsored health providers. (See Chapter 16 for a detailed discussion of regulation in health care.)

Increasingly, third-party payers of health care, notably private and public insurance companies, are demanding an accounting of the care that is delivered to their enrollees. Doctors, nurses, social workers, and allied-health professionals are under great pressure to conform to and document the level of care that insurance reviewers determine is adequate and cost effective. Various employer and community-sponsored providers such as HMOs and employee health agencies also have review mechanisms that endeavor to control costs and minimize duplications of coverage. All of these various approaches add layers of accountability to professional health care.

Accountable Practice of Health-Care Professionals

Health-care professionals are entrusted with the health and well-being of those clients under their care. Beyond the external regulatory influences outlined previously, there is an inherent and internally controlled sense of professional responsibility to be accountable for the decisions and conduct of their practices. Most health professionals have a great deal of autonomy in their decision making and practices. Within the framework of accepted practice, state practice laws, and professional standards, professionals often make independent judgments that directly impact the health of their clients. The accountability associated with this autonomy deals with both individual judgments and actions, and those judgments and actions that are delegated.

The professional health-care provider, by definition, must have the ability and willingness to take "responsibility for one's behavior while engaged in the practice of one's profession" (Tappen & George, 1989, p. 475). Consider the nurse who works on a burn unit in a hospital. This nurse has a plan of care that is both standardized and individualized for each patient. In addition, there are medical orders that must be followed. The nursing professional must coordinate and evaluate each aspect of the patient's care in a safe, effective manner with attention paid to the quality of that care. The following case study may serve to illustrate the various dimensions of the nurse's care and accountability.

CASE STUDY: *Clinical Judgment and the Burn Patient*

Ms. G., a fifty-seven-year-old woman, was burned over 25 percent of her body while cooking at a gas stove. She had extensive burns to all her right arm, shoulder, and right upper chest. She was admitted to the burn unit from the emergency department in extreme pain and in a very anxious state. Ms. G. was sedated and medicated for pain and given antibiotics to prevent infection. She had intravenous fluid infusing for nutrition and fluid replacement therapy with an order to progressively advance to a liquid, then to soft, and, finally, to a regular diet as indicated by nursing assessment. Within one week, after the initial period of shock and pain, Ms. G. was considered to be out of immediate danger of death and was advanced to a regular diet by the primary nurse. Because of the burns to her hand and arm, she required assistance with eating.

The primary nurse had delegated the assistance with feeding to a nursing assistant (patient-care technician). The nursing assistant had completed a certified nursing assistant course but had no formal education beyond high school. The nurse's instructions to the assistant were, "Help Ms. G. feed herself." The nursing assistant was also assigned to aspects of care for five other patients and felt very rushed and pushed to complete her care by the end of the day shift. She had concerns that she would not be able to complete all the tasks assigned, but she did not communicate this to the nurse in charge, nor did she document this concern.

Sometime between breakfast at 7:00 A.M. and lunch at 11:30 A.M., Ms. G. had a marked change in her level of consciousness. She slurred her words while talking, lost her train of thought, and had trouble recognizing her daughter when she visited. The nursing assistant noticed these changes, but did not report them right away to the nurse in charge. At lunch, even though the patient was experiencing difficulty in swallowing, the nursing assistant encouraged, cajoled, and pushed food into Ms. G.'s mouth. The nursing assistant later stated that she felt pressured to feed Ms. G. quickly so she could complete her other duties. At approximately 12:00 noon, the patient began wheezing and coughing and lapsed into unconsciousness. The nurse in charge was quickly summoned by the patient's daughter. After an immediate assessment, the nurse ascertained that Ms. G. had vomited and then aspirated her food. The nurse began suctioning the patient's throat and simultaneously called a Code Blue (a call for an emergency resuscitation). Extensive efforts to resuscitate the patient were unsuccessful and she was placed on life-support equipment at 2:00 P.M. After one week of persistent coma and flat brain waves, Ms. G. was taken off life support and pronounced dead.

Immediately, there were demands for an investigation of Ms. G.'s death by all levels of the hospital hierarchy, by the patient's doctor, and the patient's family. "How could this have happened? Ms. G. was getting better," and, "Why was she fed when she was having trouble swallowing?" were among the questions asked.

These events raised questions of accountability of the doctor, the nurse, and the nursing assistant. For the doctor, the medical order to advance the patient to a regular diet was scrutinized. The review of this physician's documentation indicated that the order was within accepted safe practice and that the nurse could be expected to use autonomous clinical judgment in the matter of the patient's ability to handle a regular diet.

Likewise, the actions of the nursing assistant received intense attention. Did the nursing assistant have the knowledge to know that a change in the patient's level of consciousness was an indication that solid food posed a danger of aspiration? Additionally, the nursing assistant's failure to report the change in consciousness to the nurse came under criticism. A review of these actions by a hospital risk-management committee found that the nursing assistant was culpable for failing to report the patient's change in condition, but probably did not have the level of knowledge to predict that the patient could aspirate. The review committee found, however, that the nursing assistant should not have aggressively fed Ms. G.

The actions of the nurse, primarily in the delegation process, were the focus of most of the controversy that swirled around this case. The review committee found that the order to "help Ms. G. feed herself" was too vague and imprecise. While the nurse could not have predicted that the patient would experience a decrease in consciousness, the nursing assistant should have been cautioned that Ms. G. had only been on a regular diet a short time and should be watched closely. Also, the committee found that the process of advancing nutritional methods from intravenous feeding to a regular diet was not sufficiently based on complete assessment data nor properly documented.

The family subsequently sued the hospital and the nurse in charge. A jury found the hospital and the nurse liable for Ms. G.'s death and awarded the family a large sum of money.

Analysis

This case was in many ways unpredictable in that no one could have known that Ms. G.'s condition would suddenly worsen after she appeared to be recovering from her injury. However, the process of advancing nutritional methods and the delegation of feeding points up several areas of accountability.

DELEGATION
In this case, the decision to delegate the feeding of Ms. G. was appropriate; however, the process was flawed. Assistance with feeding is within the accepted practice bounds of nursing assistants. As mentioned earlier, however, three steps are necessary for proper delegation. These steps as applied to this case study are:

1. assigning specific duties to subordinates in operational terms so that the subordinate has a clear understanding of what these duties entail.

2. granting appropriate authority to the subordinate.

3. creating the obligation for the subordinate to perform the duties assigned; the subordinate must accept that responsibility. (Newman & Warren, 1977)

This case shows violations of steps 1 and 3. The assignment of feeding was too vague and did not include the cautionary advice that Ms. G. was only recently advanced to a regular diet and what action should be taken if the patient had difficulty in swallowing. Additionally, it is not clear that the nursing assistant fully accepted the responsibility. She felt overburdened with the work assigned that day, but did not communicate that to the nurse in charge. Thus, while she technically accepted the process of feeding, she did it in an unsafe and rushed manner. This failure to communicate is often a feature of poor delegation, and it occurs frequently, especially in times of staff shortages and overwork.

AUTHORITY, RESPONSIBILITY, AND ACCOUNTABILITY IN PRACTICE

This case illustrates the relationship between authority, responsibility, and accountability in the clinical practice of one nurse. The nurse used authority to advance the patient to a regular diet. Concomitant with this authority was the responsibility, through careful assessment, to ensure that Ms. G. could safely ingest a regular diet. Additionally, this authority and responsibility were not abdicated when the task of feeding was delegated. The responsibility and accountability to feed the patient safely was shared through delegation, but did not suspend the accountability (and liability) of the nurse. While the nursing assistant in this case certainly shared some of the blame, the nurse was held more accountable and liable, by virtue of her professional status and because of the flawed delegation process and the lack of proper justification for advancing the patient to a regular diet.

This case clearly shows the interactivity of authority, responsibility, and accountability. The legal implications are evident, as well. These concepts are linked in a dynamic relationship expressed in the delivery of professional health-care practice.

Continuing Education

Health professionals have a further responsibility to keep their practices current and up-to-date. The science of health care is undergoing rapid changes with new discoveries occurring constantly. According to Cammuso (1993), "Competence in . . . practice and accountability demand a commitment to continued learning" (p. 3). Pursuing post-graduate education, reading current journals, and attending continuing-educational offerings and short-term programs are expected behaviors of all health-care professionals. Lifelong learning is a requirement for maintaining competence in practice (Flynn-McCann & Heffron-Burroughs, 1988). In the current environment, however, the issue often becomes one of allocation of scarce resources for both the institution and the individual. Hence, the question of "accountability" often arises.

TRENDS IN PRACTICE: ISSUES IN ACCOUNTABILITY

Health care is in the process of unprecedented change. Consequently, health-care professionals increasingly find themselves in an environment of rapid change, with high consumer expectations of quality care, and administrative pressures for cost containment (Christensen & Bender, 1994).

Many Americans have come to view health care as a right and not as a privilege of only those who can afford it. Health-care institutions are under pressure to provide quality care to everyone who seeks it, all in a climate of cost restraint. These pressures directly impact health-care professionals and the delivery of care to patients. By establishing the basic tenet that accessibility to health care is a right of all citizens, the United States government has assumed a measure of authority and responsibility to make services available to all. Health-care reforms, initiated in 1993 and 1994, have attempted to bring accountability to bear on health-care organizations and providers to deliver care to all in a cost-effective manner. The various proposed plans call for reducing the amount of time and money spent on paperwork and eliminating duplication of services. A central concept of many health-care reform proposals is coverage for every citizen through some type of health insurance. The impact of these proposals on accountability in the delivery of health services is unknown at this time.

The **Total Quality Management (TQM)** model has become a major paradigm in the management of organizations. Recently, health-care administrators have transferred QM principles to the delivery of health care. These administrators have adopted TQM (or some variation of it) to the missions, philosophies, and objectives of their respective organizations. The quality movement, health-care reform, cost constraints, and consumer expectations have culminated in a demand for increased accountability of health professionals (Christensen & Bender, 1994).

Additional trends that are theorized to impact on accountability include the movement of health care from hospital-based, acute care to community-based acute and chronic care. Health professionals increasingly will work both independently and **interdisciplinarily** in non-traditional settings. The independent, autonomous decision making of professionals will bring about increased authority, responsibility, and accountability.

In place now, and on the horizon, are models which are emerging as frameworks for quality patient-centered health care in the changing health-care environment. Among the emerging models are managed care, case management, patient-focused care, paired practice, cross-training, and collaborative practice (Christensen & Bender, 1994). A mix of employees working across disciplines to deliver quality care is also an emerging trend in health care (Parsons, Scaltrito, & Vondle, 1990).

Since the advent of case management and managed care, the focus on outcomes has increased the authority, responsibility and accountability of health-care professionals. Case managers have responsibility and accountability for care through a system of critical paths derived from standards of care. The collaborative-practice and paired-practice models, as well as the cross-training, requires that health professionals be less specialized and more flexible in taking on new roles. More health-care organizations are introducing and utilizing multi-skilled health practitioners (MHPs) and cross training across disciplines. "Flexibility, efficiency, and cost containment are the major reasons for utilizing such personnel" (Vaughn, Fottler, Bamberg, & Blayney, 1991, p. 397). The trend toward MHPs will require additional education, training, and a new approach to decision making. The utilization of unlicensed assistive personnel will bring about increasing challenges of supervision. These changes in the traditional roles of health professionals may extend authority, responsibility, and accountability well beyond present parameters.

CONCLUSION

The quality movement, lawsuits, ever increasing costs, and the consumer movement have brought scrutiny and focused attention on accountability (and liability) in the delivery of health care. Accountability is linked in a dynamic interaction with responsibility and authority. Health-care providers must be willing to take responsibility for their behavior while engaged in the practice of their professions. Accountability is a hallmark of the professions and is especially critical in the delivery of health services.

New health-care services and delivery systems are rapidly evolving. The outcome of this evolution is yet to be determined, but it appears that the current health-care system will undergo profound changes, forecasted to eventually address universal insurance coverage, a movement toward quality care, collaborative practice, managed care, and community-based, autonomous practice of health professionals. Changes in the traditional roles of health professionals may very well extend authority, responsibility, and autonomy beyond present parameters. The QM movement has been influential in increasing the demand for accountability in the delivery of health care. The concept of accountability is vital to the paradigm that subscribes to quality as a driving value for the delivery of health care.

REFERENCES

Anderson, O. (1984). Health services in the United States: A growth enterprise for a hundred years. In T.J. Litman & L.S. Robins (Eds.), *Health politics and policy*. New York: John Wiley & Sons.

Barnard, C. (1987). The theory of authority. In L.E. Boone & D.D. Bowen (Eds.), *The great writings in management and organizational behavior* (pp. 73–88). New York: Random House.

Bice, T. W. (1988). Health services planning and regulation. In S. J. Williams & P. R. Torrens (Eds.), *Introduction to health services* (3rd ed., pp. 373–405). New York: John Wiley & Sons.

Boone, L. E., & Bowen, D. D. (1987). *The great writings in management and organizational behavior* (2nd ed.). New York: Random House.

Cammuso, B. S. (1993, Spring). Caring and accountability. *Access: Your Nursing Future, 4*(2), 2–3.

Certo, S. (1989). *Principles of modern management: Functions and systems* (4th ed.). Boston: Allyn and Bacon.

Christensen, P., & Bender, L. (1994). Models of delivery: Nursing care in a changing environment: Present problems and future directions. *Orthopaedic Nursing, 13*(2), 64–70.

Erickson, E. (1993). Authority, responsibility, and accountability. Unpublished essay, University of Iowa, Iowa City, IA.

Fayol, H. (1949). *General and industrial management.* London: Sir Isaac Pitman and Sons.

Flynn-McCann, J., & Heffron-Burroughs, P. (1988). *Nursing from concept to practice.* Norwalk, CT: Appleton-Century-Crofts.

Ginzberg, E. (1986). The destabilization of health care. *New England Journal of Medicine, 315*(12), 757–760.

Grohar-Murray, M. E., & Dicroce, H. R. (1992). *Leadership and management in nursing.* Norwalk, CT: Appleton & Lange.

Jones, K. R. (1989). Quality assurance. In B. Henry, C. Arndt., M. DiVincenti, & A. Marriner-Tomey (Eds.), *Dimensions of nursing administration: Theory, research, education, practice* (pp. 339–352). Boston: Blackwell Scientific Publications.

LoGerfo, J. P., & Brook, R. H. (1988). The quality of health care. In S. J. Williams & P. R. Torrens (Eds., 1988), *Introduction to health services* (3rd ed., pp. 406–437). New York: John Wiley & Sons.

Marriner-Tomey, A. (1992). *Guide to nursing management* (4th ed.). St. Louis: Mosby Year Book.

Newman, W., & Warren, E. (1977). The practices of management: Concepts, behavior, and practice. In S. Certo, *Principles of modern management: Functions and systems* (4th ed.). Boston: Allyn and Bacon.

Parsons, M., Scaltrito, S., & Vondle, D. (1990). A program to manage nurse staffing costs. *Nursing Management, 21*(10), 42–44.

Tappen, R. M. (1989). *Nursing leadership and management: Concepts and practice* (2nd ed.). Philadelphia, PA: F. A. Davis.

Tappen, R. M., & George, P. (1989). Accountability and quality assurance. In R. M. Tappen (Ed.), *Nursing leadership and management: Concepts and practice* (2nd ed., pp. 474–488). Philadelphia, PA: F. A. Davis.

Vaughn, D., Fottler, M., Bamberg, R., & Blayney, K. D. (1991). Utilization and management of multiskilled health practitioners in U.S. hospitals. *Hospital & Health Services Administration, 36*(3), 397–417.

Weber, M. (1989). Legitimate authority and bureaucracy. In L. E. Boone & D. D. Bowen (Eds.), *The great writings in management and organizational behavior* (pp. 5–21). New York: Random House.

ADDITIONAL READING

Batey, M., & Lewis, F. (1982). Clarifying autonomy and accountability in nursing service: Part I. *Journal of Nursing Administration, 12*(9), 13–18.

Bergman, R. (1981). Accountability — Definitions and dimensions. *International Nursing Review, 28*(2), 53–59.

Evans, A. (1993). Accountability: A core concept for primary nursing. *Journal of Clinical Nursing, 2*(4), 231–234.

Fiesta, J. (1990). Whistleblowers: Heroes or stool pigeons? *Nursing Management, 21*(6) 16–17.

Fox, D. M., & Leichter, H. M. (1991). Rationing care in Oregon: The new accountability. *Health Affairs, 10*(2), 7–27.

Glazer, S. K., & Gaintner, J. R. (1994). Hospital administrators: The challenge of living in a glass house. *Journal on Quality Improvement, 20*(70), 388–393.

Goodman, J. O. (1993). Key to reforming health care lies in keeping everyone in the system fully accountable. *Modern Healthcare, 23*(49), 34.

Hurst, J., Keenan, M., & Minnick, J. (1992). Healthcare polarities: Quality and cost. *Nursing Management, 23*(9) 40–43.

Jencks, S. F. (1994). The government's role in hospital accountability for quality of care. *Journal on Quality Improvement, 20*(7), 364–369.

Lewis, F., & Batey, M. (1982). Clarifying autonomy and accountability in nursing service: Part II. *Journal of Nursing Administration, 12*(10), 10–15.

Markson, L. E., & Nash, D. B. (1994). Overview: Public accountability of hospitals regarding quality. *Journal on Quality Improvement, 20*(7), 359–363.

Porter-O'Grady, T. (1991). Changing realities for nursing: New models, new roles for nursing care delivery. *Nursing Administration Quarterly, 16*(1) 1–6.

Styles, M. (1985). Accountable to whom? *International Nursing Review, 32*(3), 73–75.

CHAPTER *3*

An Analysis of the Concept *Quality* as It Relates to Contemporary Nursing Care

Abstract This analysis explores the applications and interpretations of the extensively used, but seldom defined, concept of "quality" as it relates to contemporary nursing care. This study employed an inductive approach to describe and explain the use and meaning of the concept; data generated from the literature were also analyzed to identify the predominant attributes or characteristics of the concept quality associated with health care. The analysis yielded data from which modes of conceiving, describing, and explaining the concept *quality nursing care* could be induced and grounded theory could be generated. Quality emerged as a complex, multi-dimensional concept requiring further analysis and clarification. Unaware of, or undeterred by, the conceptual confusion, quality care continues to be assured, controlled, evaluated, and managed in the health service today.

INTRODUCTION

The evaluation of effects or **outcomes** is an essential activity in any organization; however, an unequivocal perception of what is to be assessed is vital before valid and reliable measurement can be achieved. Nursing, according to Taylor and Haussmann (1988), has been "struggling to define quality since the early '60s"; Smith (1987) also acknowledges the "difficulty in operationalizing such complex variables as quality of nursing care." **Quality**, concludes Donabedian (1980), is so "diverse in nature that neither a unifying construct, nor a single empirical measure could be developed." Buchan, Grey, and Hill (1990) submit that there is no single criterion that defines the quality of a health service, in that quality is "essentially a function of many variables."

Note: This chapter is reprinted with permission from the *International Journal of Nursing Studies, 30*(4), 355–369, 1993, Oxford, England: Elsevier Science Ltd.

A preliminary review of the literature relating to *quality of care* revealed the lack of an explicit definition of the concept associated with an implicit assumption that a collective interpretation exists. Confusion and misunderstanding are possible when a concept such as quality, which is abstract, yet familiar, is used without a valid collective definition. Evidently the diversity of dimensions and perspectives of quality complicate efforts to clarify its meaning, and the dearth of conceptual or operational definitions may be a reflection of the difficulties inherent in attempting such a task. Unaware of, or undeterred by, the conceptual confusion, quality of care continues to be assured, controlled, evaluated, and managed in the health service today.

The overall intention of this study was to provide data that could be used to develop nursing theory and inform nursing research in the domain of quality care. The specific aims of this analysis were: firstly, to clarify the applications and interpretations of the concept quality as it relates to contemporary nursing care; secondly, to identify surrogate terms and concepts related to quality currently used in nursing; and thirdly, to identify and classify the **criteria** used to define quality nursing care.

Conscious of the reported difficulties in defining quality, the current analysis was undertaken with the expectation that some of the study aims might not be accomplished entirely; however it was anticipated that valuable insights into the meaning and use of the concept of *quality*, and its related terms, would emerge. The identification and classification of criteria used to describe *quality care* may in itself contribute to the construction of valid and reliable measures.

THE PURPOSE OF CONCEPT ANALYSIS

Walker and Avant (1983) state that concept analysis can "help to clarify overused, vague concepts . . . so that everyone who subsequently uses the term will be speaking of the same thing" (p. 27). They also explain that concept analysis can assist the researcher and theorist to construct "hypotheses which accurately reflect the relationship between the concepts" by the production of "a precise operational definition which by its very nature has construct validity, that is, it will accurately reflect its theoretical base" (p. 28). A concept can only operate as a valid and reliable basis for analysis and measurement when it has been operationally defined and verified. Before a concept can be operationalized it requires conceptual definition; currently no unequivocal definition of the concept of *quality* is evident. Theoretical development is at a preliminary stage where concept clarification and theory generation is required.

Methods used by philosophers of science have been utilized productively by various nursing theorists, for example Walker and Avant (1983) and Chinn and Jacobs (1987). These methods have provided valuable insights into equivocal nursing concepts such as *caring, health,* and *reassurance.* Norris (1982) states that "recent challenges to logical positivism" are emerging; Rodgers (1989) observes that positivist scientific methods have currently fallen into disrepute, and have been displaced by the doctrine of "realism." This latter approach to theoretical clarification explores how a term is utilized, and emphasizes the significance of analyzing concepts as and when they are used by a particular group.

Rodgers (1989) asserts that the nature and meaning of concepts can be altered or lost if they are isolated or removed from their contexts, even for the purpose of analysis. She proposes an "evolutionary view" to analysis which facilitates a broader examination of the circumstances and situation of the concept under investigation. The attributes of a concept are not isolated but appear as a cluster, and are evaluated with reference to their resemblance to the defined concept as it is currently being used in a particular context, time, or place.

DATA ANALYSIS FRAMEWORK

The equivocal nature of the concept *quality* necessitates an analytical framework that would generate both meaningful and context-specific representations of the various applications and interpretations. No single epistemic method appeared to provide a comprehensive framework; therefore, an eclectic model was constructed to provide a more complete evaluation of the concept.

The model adopted an inductive approach that would permit the meaning, uses, and correlates of the concept to be explored. Smith (1987) depicts a methodology that is "more flexible and allows the data to speak for themselves," providing a detailed picture of the variables. This type of approach was integrated into Rodgers' (1989) modifications of the Walker and Avant (1983) framework. The phases of the analytical framework were developed concurrently, but for the purpose of clarity will be presented in the following sequence:

1. identification of the concept to be analyzed
2. identification and selection of an appropriate sample for data collection
3. identification of themes of application and interpretation of the concept
4. identification of surrogate terms and related concepts
5. identification of the attributes or characteristics
6. identification of the antecedents and consequences of the concept

ANALYSIS OF THE CONCEPT *QUALITY*

Identification of the Concept to Be Analyzed

This exploratory review focuses upon the use of the term *quality* as it relates to excellence, value, and worth, as well as describing distinction and superiority. The concept is analyzed as it is commonly used in the particular field of health and nursing. The analysis will not include the use of *quality* in other applications, for example to describe personal qualities.

Identification and Selection of the Sample for Data Collection

The literature survey was conducted via computerized data bases, bibliographies, abstracts, and cumulative indexes. International sources were accessed but data were limited to articles written in the English language. The inquiry covered a span of 30 years, this broad time frame being selected to enable evolution of the concept to be detected, and also to include some of the classic works of the early pioneers upon which the majority of the current quality measurement tools are based.

Data were collected from literature derived from a variety of related disciplines: health care, medicine, and nursing, as well as including material from business and management. Rodgers (1989) recommends sampling from a diverse range of literature to allow for the examination of variations and similarities of use between disciplines. A diversity of data was considered especially important given that use of the concept of *quality*, particularly related to quality control and measurement, appeared to have gained momentum in the business and manufacturing domain.

Empirical studies and operational definitions of the concept *quality* were rare in the literature. Investigators generally focused on the relationships between variables, quality was typically the dependent variable, and construct validity was seldom established. A substantial amount of the literature identified in the search was anecdotal, comprising descriptive accounts, commentaries, or was speculative in nature.

Themes of Application and Interpretation of Quality

APPLICATIONS

The eighth edition of *The Concise Oxford Dictionary* (1990) defines quality in seven senses: (1) degree of excellence; (2a) general excellence (*their work has quality*); (2b) of high quality (*a quality product*); (3) distinctive attribute; a characteristic trait; (4) relative nature or kind of something; (5) timbre of voice or sound; (6) high social standing; (7) "logic — the property of a proposition being affirmative or negative."

The *Collins Dictionary of the English Language* (1984) gives four definitions: (1) a distinguishing characteristic or property or attribute; (2) basic characteristic or nature of something; (3) a degree or standard of excellence [= being exceptionally good], especially a high standard; (4) being associated with high status or distinction. The second edition (1990) develops theme (3), a degree or standard of excellence, but substitutes "a high standard" for "being exceptionally good."

The absence of an articulated opposite or antithetical term to quality is interesting, and may reflect the conceptual confusion surrounding both the general and specific application of the term. Crosby (1979) uses the phrase "un-quality," while Deming (1982) introduces the expression "dis-quality" to represent the antonym to quality. Inferior, inadequate, and poor may seem to be the typical antithetical terms in general use; these antonyms are also used implicitly throughout the health-care and nursing literature.

In everyday language the term *quality* is widely used, especially in business and marketing, with reference to a huge range of goods and services, from telephones to toffees. The conventional uses of the term quality are, as a degree of excellence; skill; or personal quality/trait. Crow (1981) observes that "these meanings are not unitary, at one level quality is used as a value judgment, whereas at another level it is describing discrete characteristics" (p. 493). Examples of each use and level of the term were discovered in the literature when *quality of care* was being discussed. Clarification of which meaning or level of quality was being used, in the same way as explicit definition of the concept, was the exception rather than the rule in the literature.

INTERPRETATIONS

From the literature it emerged that quality is used in the following ways:

Excellence — The "traditional approach" to quality, described by Pfeffer and Coote (1990), is the one most people are familiar with, and relates to the interpretation of quality (usually of products) as superior or special and conveys a notion of prestige and desirability. Taylor and Haussmann (1988) observe that "society attaches importance to the word quality. It is equated with excellence and the belief that the best service or object is being received." The "traditional" view of quality, i.e., "that providers must do everything possible for the patient," was also described by Mitchell (1988).

Lang (1980) describes quality in nursing as "the process for the attainment of the highest degree of excellence in the delivery of patient or client care." The equating of quality with excellence in the delivery of health care is represented implicitly in the works of Phaneuf (1976), Wandelt and Stewart (1975), and Schmadl (1979). McFarlane (1989) compares quality measurement to hotel rating systems, the score or rating representing the prospective standard of excellence.

Patients in Taylor, Hudson, and Keeling's (1991) study equated the nurse's commitment to excellence with quality nursing care using statements such as "doing what's best," "the best care a nurse can give," and "excellence in all areas." The staff nurses in Jackson-Frankl's (1990) study duplicated this notion, describing quality nursing as "the best you can do." The head nurses in the same study, however, "were adamant that quality was *not* perfection" but realistic standards.

Ideal — Van Maanen (1984) states that the most satisfying definition of quality is "the margin between desirability and reality." Bennett (1984) represents the management model of quality as "ideal" or "perfection"; while in health care Berwick's (1989) "Theory of Continuous Improvement" describes quality as the ideal. The nurse executives in Jackson-Frankl's (1990) study also considered quality as "an ideal" or "something that you have a wish list for."

Fitness for purpose and conformance to standards — Crosby (1979) defined quality as a "conformance to requirements," which are specified in **standards**; failures were detected by inspection and improved by deterrence. Quality control using these techniques was prevalent in the manufacturing industries throughout the last three decades; Berwick (1989) calls this the "Theory of Bad Apples" and points out the negative and punitive perspective of quality this approach engenders. Pfeffer and Coote (1990) describe a "scientific" or expert approach to quality based on the idea of fitness for purpose and conformance to standards. Work study methods from the scientific management era and experts were utilized in the early quality **monitoring** tools to establish what nurses did and to what level. The notion that quality is correlated to standards is not new in health care or nursing. As early as 1966 Donabedian had drawn a model for evaluating care quality using standards to express the required level of performance. Confusion and contradictions in the use and meaning of terms was apparent in the medical and nursing literature over the years, both in America and Britain. A discussion of these terms follows in the *Related Concepts* section.

Meeting the customer's requirements — Zierden (1989) contributes one of the rare explicit definitions of quality as "meeting the **customers'** requirements for a product or service." Crosby's (1979) definition of quality as "conformance to requirements" provided the organizational goal, i.e., "to meet the requirements on time, the first time, with no errors or defects." These aims represent the fundamental principle of the **Total Quality Management (TQM)** philosophy espoused by quality theorists Crosby (1979), Juran, Gryna, and Bingham (1979), and Deming (1982). This more positive approach to quality, which Berwick (1989) calls "The Theory of Continuous Improvement," focuses on organization-wide efforts to reduce defects, and to continually improve processes. A managerial or "excellence" approach, described by Pfeffer and Coote (1990), views quality as equated with customers' requirements; this theme is reflected by Coyne (1990) in his "objective definition" of quality as "consistently meeting customers' expectations."

Satisfying need — The British Standards Institute defines quality as "the totality of features of a product or service that bear on its ability to satisfy a given need." The question of who defines need and who constitutes "the customer" did not seem to be addressed and remained obscure. Pfeffer and Coote (1990) describe "the consumerist approach," which follows on from the "excellence" philosophy; however, the focus shifts to the customer's desire to be satisfied. The citizen/consumers' right to quality has been promoted in the Citizens' Charter (1991) in which commercial and public services are being encouraged to publish performance standards to enable the customer to evaluate the quality of the service.

Customer value — Drucker, quoted by Statland (1989), states that "a product or service is quality not because it is hard to make or extremely technical or complicated, but only if it is of use to the customer and gives the customer value." The notion of quality as customer value has become associated with a "marketplace economic philosophy"; that is, if the consumer does not perceive a product or service is [good] value, they take their custom elsewhere. The theme of customer value was implicit in the majority of the current management literature and is becoming more common in the public and health services. The question of who constitutes the "customer," i.e., internal or external users/clients, remains indefinite.

SUMMARY OF THEMES OF APPLICATION AND INTERPRETATION

No unequivocal application or interpretation of the term *quality* emerged from the literature, though common themes of use and meaning were identified. The predominant view of quality from the literature of the 1960s and 1970s was of conformance to standards, while the 1980s was the era of quality assurance. The health and nursing literature appeared to be following a decade behind the pattern of evolution in the general and management paradigm.

The perspective most frequently adopted in the literature was that of the professional/expert, with the producer/provider view following second. In the 1970s and 1980s the purchaser/payer view was becoming predominant in the American health and nursing literature. This trend is becoming apparent in British health policies as the cost of health care soars.

The contemporary management approach to quality emphasizes consumer satisfaction and satisfying customer expectations (Crosby, 1984). The customer/consumer perspective is currently emerging in the health and nursing domains; who "the customer" is remains unspecified.

In Britain the current view of quality in nursing appears to be in transition between standards and **quality assurance (QA)**, with some evidence of a move toward the consumerist view.

Surrogate Terms and Concepts Related to Quality

Conceptual confusion and lack of clarity relate equally to the surrogate terms and related concepts as they do to the term *quality* itself. Uses and interpretations alter over time, and between authors, contexts, and perspectives. A selection of the most common are included here.

SURROGATE TERMS

Roget's Thesaurus (1975) gave the following as synonyms for quality: (1) character (aspects, nature); (2) superiority (greatness, excellence); (3) sort (kind, type); (4) goodness; and (5) nobility (virtue, distinction). The 1988 edition included most of the earlier synonyms, e.g., characteristic nature and type; additional synonyms were power (attribute, capacity) and tendency (characteristic). Further synonyms found elsewhere in the data included distinction, perfection, value, and worth.

RELATED CONCEPTS

Criteria (*criterion*, singular) are defined as predetermined elements against which aspects of service are compared (Donabedian, 1980; Lang, 1980).

Criteria are usually classified as either:

> **Structure** — human and material resources; organizational framework or system.

> **Process** — the actual practice or delivery of care, i.e., action and interaction.

> **Outcome** — effect or end result of the other two criteria on the patient.

> **Indicators** — an objective, measurable dimension that provides information on an important aspect of the quality of care.

> **Norms** — current level of performance corresponding with a criterion.

> **Standards** — precise statements which specify the desired and/or achievable level of performance against which actual performance is compared. (Bloch, 1977)

Bloch (1977), Lang (1980), and Donabedian (1980) sought to clarify the confusion over the use of predominant terms used in America. Donabedian (1980) uses standards to describe an "adequate, acceptable or optimum level of quality"; Lang (1980), however, disagrees, maintaining that a "standard" should be "an agreed on level of excellence," rather than a minimum level of acceptability. The American Nurses Association has adopted Lang's (1980) definition as the basis of its National Quality Assurance strategy.

Wright (1984) clarifies the use of the terms in Britain stating that standards are optimum levels of care against which actual performance is compared, while criteria are variables selected as indicators of care quality. The work of Kitson (1986) led to the development of The Dynamic Standard Setting System of quality monitoring, which utilized standards as the means of specifying care quality. Kitson (1986) maintains that standards describe what care quality *should* be, and recommends that professionals agree on an acceptable level.

Crow (1981) observes that "standards of care" was used synonymously with quality of care and effectiveness of care.

Effectiveness — "doing the right things," Drucker (1974), related to the achievement of intended results, outcome.

Efficiency — "doing things right," Drucker (1974), with processes and often linked with cost, hence:

Economy — careful use of resources, frugality . . . cheapest; this application was standard in management perspectives on quality.

RELATED TERMINOLOGY

Assurance — programs that confirm/ensure the customer of a certain degree of excellence through the evaluation of degree of conformance to pre-established quality standards (Schmadl, 1979)

Circles — group techniques, aiming to identify and solve quality problems

Control — techniques to detect and correct errors, regulate quality of output, usually by statistical sampling techniques

Improvement — increasing the current level of quality

Management — exercise control by implementation of a quality policy, including strategic planning, resource allocation, and monitoring

Monitoring (Audit) — the inspection/observational phase of the assurance/management process

Identification of the Attributes or Characteristics of Quality

Attributes are the observable and quantifiable aspects or features that must be present for a valid description of the concept; an alternative name for attributes or characteristics is criteria. Buchan, Grey, and Hill (1990) submit that there is no single criterion that defines the quality of a health service because quality is "essentially a function of many variables." Donabedian's (1966) structure, process, and outcome criteria have been utilized in this analysis to provide a unifying framework for the identification and classification of the attributes/characteristics of quality nursing care.

STRUCTURAL ATTRIBUTES/CRITERIA

Hagen (1976) identifies the characteristics of the setting or the conditions under which nursing care is delivered as a structural domain of the quality of nursing care. Horn and Swain (1976) identify four main attributes of quality: comprehensiveness; **accountability**; continuity and coordination, which Van Maanen (1984) maintains can be subsumed under structural criteria.

Tools used to measure quality contributed an abundant source of diverse attributes to define nursing care quality. The Rush Medicus Methodology (Jelinek, Haussman, Hegyvary, & Newman, 1974) uses patient- and unit-specific criteria. Structural attributes include hospital/agency characteristics, nursing unit organization, staff attitudes, perceptions, and education levels.

The patients interviewed by Taylor et al. (1991) identified three types of quality care attribute "to do with the nature of nursing practice, the nurse, and the practice setting." Practice setting attributes describe structural characteristics, for example: effective organization and management that incorporated the notion "adequate staffing" with proficient, knowledgeable, and technically competent nurses; as well as the same nurse to care for them for most of their stay; and patient environment, e.g., cleanliness, bed space, and room.

The notion that nursing resources are crucial to the quality of patient care seems commonplace and unexceptionally observed (Giovannetti, 1984). The nurses in Jackson-Frankl's (1990) study identified time to spend with patients talking, teaching, and planning as an essential resource that improved quality of care. Scarcity of this resource, and, as Kitson (1986) discovered, the lack of awareness of its therapeutic function affected the quality of the interpersonal process of nursing. Kitson also includes physical facilities and organizational variables in her structural attributes of quality.

Maxwell (1984) proposes six dimensions of quality health care that can be classified as structural attributes: access to services; relevance to need; effectiveness; equity; social acceptability; and efficiency and economy. Quality, according to Bennett (1984), can be defined from a management perspective by twelve attributes: competitiveness and credibility; a culture of humanism, compassion, good manners, and concern; innovativeness; effective communication, coordination, and control; excellence in management; productive resources; cost effectiveness; operational integrity; meaningful information; attention to the physical context of work; people involvement and participation; and positive attitudes and satisfaction of people at work. These characteristics could be applied equally to nursing and fit into the structure and process elements of the categorizing schema.

These structural attributes have been categorized and are presented as an inventory in Table 3-1.

PROCESS ATTRIBUTES/CRITERIA

Early quality measuring tools, e.g., Qualpacs (Wandelt & Ager, 1974) and Rush Medicus (Jelinek et al., 1974), used criteria founded on the nursing process. The Quality Patient Care Scale (Qualpacs) utilizes standards in six areas for measuring quality of care processes: individual and group psychological care, physical care, general, communication, and professional responsibility (Wandelt & Ager, 1974). These tools also used criteria that embodied judgments of quality or worth of performance; Slater (1975) based one of the first process quality monitoring tools on the competence of the nurse. Felton (1976) declared that "the quality of care can be no better than the competencies of the person giving direct care to that person." Hagen (1976) includes professional practices and processes of nursing as one of her three domains of the quality of nursing care.

Table 3-1 • **ANTECEDENTS OR STRUCTURAL CRITERIA OF QUALITY NURSING CARE**

Criteria Type	Examples
Organizational variables	
Hospital	Ethos; goal/mission/philosophy
	Size: bed numbers, bed occupancy, throughput, activity level
	Competitiveness and credibility
	Resources/funding; cost effectiveness
	Excellence in management; structure and organization; power; authority; coordination: type of accountability (hierarchical versus professional); leadership, supervision; shift length
	Effective communication; social relationships and support structures
	Staff morale, satisfaction, turnover, absenteeism
Nursing unit/practice setting	Concept of care/philosophy of nursing
	Manpower: numbers, grades, competence, level of education and professional development
	Accountability, leadership, and supervision
	Nurse assignment patterns
	Patient care episodes: length of stay
	Patient numbers, acuity/dependency
	Resources: human (i.e., time to care, teach), material (i.e., equipment, physical facilities)
Patient environment	Physical: buildings (type, maintenance, and repair); hygiene, cleanliness; equipment, facilities, services
	Social: atmosphere/climate/milieu
Service attributes	Accessibility, equity
	Relevance to need
	Social acceptability
	Comprehensiveness, continuity, coordination
	Effectiveness, efficiency, and economy

The recording of care was seen by Wandelt and Ager (1974), Jelinek et al. (1974), and Donabedian (1986) as a legitimate dimension for measuring the quality of practice, as well as the medium for evaluating most other dimensions. Phaneuf (1976) asserted that a positive correlation could be demonstrated between the quality of recording in the nursing notes and the actual care given. Whether this is due to the stringent American legal requirements for record keeping or is a function of quality nursing is open to question.

Donabedian (1980) notes that what is judged to be quality is often not the precise care itself, but the person rendering the care. Research by Kitson (1986) extended the personal attribute theme, describing quality nursing care as "more than just tasks," a reflection of the nurses' "therapeutic contribution in each interaction" rather than "merely carrying out activities." Kitson affirmed that the interpersonal skills of the nurse contributed significantly to care quality and characterized these attributes in her description of "Therapeutic Nursing Functions," concluding from her research that "the quality of care was related more to the orientation and perception of the ward sister than to any number of extraneous variables."

Kitson also characterized nursing interventions, i.e., what the nurse actually does to and with the patient, as process criteria of quality nursing. Parish (1986) describes quality nursing care as individualizing the patient's care, and illustrates process criteria of quality care as: taking time to listen to the patient; offering comfort; providing emotional support to patients and family; and involving family members. Valentine (1989) proposes that quality measurement methods that focus on the process of nursing, i.e., "what happens between nurses and patients," are "better predictors" of quality nursing care. Interpersonal aspects of quality care were also reflected in the nurses' views revealed in Jackson-Frankl's (1990) study; quality care was described as a value personified through the attitude and approach of the nurse. These nurses' views correspond with Kitson's (1986) notion that the approach of the nurse is an important attribute of quality nursing care.

A significant proportion (96 percent) of the 144 patients interviewed by Taylor et al. (1991) identified interpersonal aspects of nursing practice as attributes that contributed significantly to the quality of nursing care. These aspects included the personal qualities of the nurse, e.g., caring, compassion, and kindness, as well as the facilitation of positive and therapeutic nurse–patient relationships. Patients in this study also expressed their belief that having "the same nurse to care for them for most of their stay" was an important characteristic of quality care.

Methods used to organize nursing practice were commonly associated with care quality in the literature. Results from research by Shukla (1981) indicated that "people related variables," such as competency, have a greater impact on quality care than primary nursing. Numerous articles discussed the postulated influence of primary nursing on the quality of care; these are summarized elsewhere (Lang & Clinton, 1984; Pearson, 1987). An interesting factor emerged from this data: neither "primary" nor "quality" nursing were consistently conceptually or operationally defined in the literature.

The preceding process attributes are also categorized and presented as an inventory in Table 3-2.

OUTCOME ATTRIBUTES/CRITERIA

Florence Nightingale reviewed nursing outcomes in terms of patient wellness as well as mortality. Lohr (1988) lists "the 5 Ds" as classic outcomes: death, disease, disability, discomfort, and dissatisfaction. She adds that "the importance of outcomes in the quality of care paradigm is unquestioned, because the purpose of health care is patient benefit and well-being." Zimmer (1974) defines outcomes as an alteration in the health/wellness status of the consumer, and described care quality in terms

Table 3-2 • **PROCESS CRITERIA OF QUALITY NURSING CARE**

Criteria Type	Examples
Care functions/processes	Assessment Planning Intervention: physical and psycho-social care, patient education/teaching Recording Evaluation
Interpersonal processes	Effective communication Manner and behavior of care providers Therapeutic interaction Involvement of patient and family Provision of a supportive environment
Method of organizing work	Accountable Effective coordination Individualized, personalized care; patient centered/primary versus task/routine; involvement, partnership, and participation in decision making and care with patient and family
Nurse's professional perspective	Approach to, and philosophy of, nursing Attitudes, beliefs, and values Therapeutic nursing functions: inclination and time to care, listen, talk, and teach
Nurse's professional practices	Knowledgeable, proficient, and technically competent Sound clinical knowledge, skills, and judgment
Nurse's personal characteristics	Qualities: caring; compassion; concern; empathic; integrity; humanism; kindness; respect of individual's rights, dignity, individuality

of the degree of excellence in patient health outcomes. Outcomes were said to represent the end result of care activities and "should always be related to pre-established objectives."

Donabedian (1966) portrayed quality medical care as "a balance of benefits over harms"; he suggested that the outcomes of care will be the answer to the question "what good, if any, are we doing?" Rutstein et al. (1976) described quality medical care as "the effect of care on the health of the individual. . . . Quality is concerned with outcome." The current trend in medical audit is to focus on outcome, however neither the goals nor the outcomes of medical care are made explicit.

The notion that outcomes of care contribute to nursing care quality is identified by Hagen (1976); Lindeman (1976); Mayers, Norby, and Watson (1977); and Van Maanen (1984). The "effects on the consumer" of nursing are seen by Hagen (1976) as a domain of the quality of nursing care. Lindeman (1976) defines quality of care as the "effectiveness of nursing care in terms of maintaining or improving health status," while Mayers (1977) states that "the production of good patient outcomes" is a measure of nursing quality care. Kitson (1986) recognizes change in patient health state, functioning, or knowledge as outcomes, and believes that patient satisfaction is the ultimate outcome.

The consensus of opinion was that outcome criteria are significant for a full assessment of quality, although where outcomes were acknowledged as being correlates of quality of care the criteria were rarely made explicit. The work of Marek (1989) was the exception: she analyzed the nursing literature and classified outcome criteria as physiological, psychological, functional, behavioral, knowledge, symptom control, home maintenance, well-being, goal attainment, patient satisfaction, safety, nursing diagnosis resolution, frequency of service, cost, and rehospitalization.

In America the current trend appears to be toward patient outcome measures; in Britain the outcomes movement is in its infancy. The various issues involved in measuring outcomes are beyond the scope of this chapter but are discussed by Bond and Thomas (1991).

The outcome attributes identified in the preceding literature analysis are categorized and listed in Table 3-3.

Table 3-3 • CONSEQUENCES OR OUTCOME CRITERIA OF QUALITY NURSING CARE

Criteria Type	Examples
Health/wellness level	Death, disease, disability, discomfort, and dissatisfaction
	Improvement/maintenance of health; morbidity; mortality; peaceful death; problem resolution, goal attainment; rehabilitation; survival rates; symptom control; control of illness
Functional ability	Physiological, psychological, social functioning; self-care ability; patient health knowledge; motivation; skill; low stress levels
Patient satisfaction	Access, availability complaints, compliments, coordination, communication, timing
Resource utilization/cost effectiveness/efficiency	Benefit versus harm; cost of correction, repetition, or compensation; compliance; patient return rate; effect for individual patients; quality of life
Undesirable events	Accidents and incidents: falls
	Complications: contractures, nosocomial infections, pressure sores, iatrogenic diseases
	Readmission, return to theater, patient self-harm, suicides, post-mortems, untimely deaths
Undesirable processes	Medication and recording errors, uncoordinated services; unmanaged pain

The Antecedents and Consequences of Quality

The identification and classification of antecedents and consequences is an important and significant activity in the process of concept analysis because they provide fundamental data that can be used to develop nursing theory and inform nursing research.

As a result of this analysis it is postulated that the antecedents (phenomena that precede quality) are synonymous with, and equivalent to, the attributes of quality previously identified in this analysis as "structural criteria." These structural attributes or criteria have been categorized and are presented as an inventory in Table 3-1.

Similarly the consequences of quality are postulated as corresponding to the "outcome criteria" identified earlier in this analysis. The outcome attributes identified in the literature analysis were categorized and presented in Table 3-3.

In this analysis Donabedian's (1966) structure, process, and outcome criteria were adopted as a unifying framework for the identification and classification of the attributes/characteristics of quality nursing care; for consistency and ease of reference the remaining "process criteria" identified in this study have also been categorized and are presented in summary form in Table 3-2.

CONCLUSION

The intention of this analysis was to clarify the uses and meaning of the concept *quality* as it relates to contemporary nursing. Applications and interpretations varied significantly according to the perspective of the observer, and corresponded with the context, time, and place. Various subtle, yet important, distinctions between interpretations implicit in the literature were exposed and analyzed.

The questions "what attributes/criteria of quality care should be measured?" and "whose perspective should be adopted?" were not explored in the literature reviewed. These issues require urgent attention if the various perspectives of quality, i.e., patient; professional; provider/producer; purchaser/payer and public/society, are to be represented in the evaluation of "quality care."

During the process of analysis it became apparent that to propose a single definition would be a contradiction of the ethnographic principles underpinning the study. Although no operational definition was proposed, the complexities of the concept *quality* have been demonstrated, thus raising awareness of the diversity of perspectives on quality. The concept *quality of care* is not used consistently; it is enigmatic and multidimensional, requiring examination in context, and as it correlates with other concepts. The conceptual confusion and lack of clarity that surrounds quality affects the related concepts; these were identified and described to distinguish them from the concept of *quality*.

The final aim of this analysis was to lay conceptual foundations for the development of nursing theory and research. Hypotheses were not proposed in this analysis, however the potential exists to explore the postulated relationships between concepts. This analysis yielded data from which modes of conceiving, describing, and explaining the concept *quality nursing care* could be induced, and grounded theory could be generated. The attributes or characteristics of the concept *quality nursing care* were identified and classified providing a basis for the development of both theory and research. It is proposed that evaluation and verification of the attributes of quality through theory development and research will improve conceptual clarity and aid operational definition, thus contributing to the construction of valid and reliable measures of quality nursing care.

REFERENCES

Bennett, A. (1984). Quality of care: Bridging the gap between promise and performance. *Trustee, 37*(10), 29–32.

Berwick, D. (1989). Continuous improvement as an ideal in health care. *New England Journal of Medicine, 320*(1), 53–56.

Bloch, D. (1977). Criteria, standards and norms: Crucial terms in quality. *Journal of Nursing Administration, 7*(7), 20–30.

Bond, S., & Thomas, L. (1991). Issues in measuring outcomes of nursing. *Journal of Advanced Nursing, 16,* 1492–1502.

Buchan, H., Grey, M., & Hill, A. (1990). Score on quality. *Health Services Journal, 8*(3), 362–363.

Chinn, P., & Jacobs, A. (1987). *Theory and nursing: A systematic approach* (2nd ed.). St. Louis, MO: C. V. Mosby.

Coyne, W. (1990). Nurses are the key to quality. *Registered Nurse, 53*(2), 69–74.

Crosby, P. (1979). *Quality is free: The art of making quality certain.* New York: New American Library.

Crosby, P. (1984). *Quality without tears.* New York: New American Library.

Crow, R. (1981). Research and the standards of nursing care: What is the relationship. *Journal of Advanced Nursing, 6,* 491–496.

Deming, W. E. (1982). *Quality, productivity and competitive position.* Cambridge, MA: Massachusetts Institute of Technology.

Donabedian, A. (1966). Some issues in evaluating the quality of nursing care. *American Journal of Public Health, 59,* 1833.

Donabedian, A. (1980). Criteria, norms and standards of quality: What do they mean. *American Journal of Public Health, 71*(4), 409–412.

Donabedian, A. (1986). Criteria and standards for quality assessment and monitoring. *Quality Review Bulletin, 12*(3), 99–108.

Drucker, P. (1974). *Management.* New York: Harper and Row.

Felton, G., Frevert, E., Galligan, K., Neill, M., & Williams, L. (1976). Implementation of a quality assurance program. *Journal of Nursing Administration, 6*(1), 20–24.

Giovannetti, P. (1984). Staffing methods — Implications for quality. In L. Willis & M. Linwood (Eds.), *Measuring the quality of care.* Edinburgh, Scotland: Churchill Livingstone.

Hagen, E. (1976). Appraising the quality of nursing care. *Nursing Research Conference, 8,* 1–8.

Horn, B., & Swain, M. (1976). An approach to development of criterion measures for quality health care. In American Nurses Association, *Issues in evaluation research* (pp. 74–82). Kansas City, MO: Author.

HMSO. (1991). *The Citizen's Charter.* London: Cabinet Office.

Jackson-Frankl, M. A. (1990). The language and meaning of quality. *Nursing Administration Quarterly, 14*(3), 52–65.

Jelinek, R., Haussmann, R., Hegyvary, S., & Newman, J. (1974). *A methodology for monitoring the quality of care.* Bethesda, MD: United States Department of Health, Education and Welfare.

Juran, J. M., Gryna, F. M., & Bingham, R. S. (1979). *Quality control handbook.* New York: McGraw-Hill.

Kitson, A. (1986). Indicators of quality in nursing care — An alternative approach. *Journal of Advanced Nursing, 11,* 133–144.

Lang, N. (1980). *Quality assurance in nursing: A selected bibliography* (DHEW Pub HRA 80–30). Bethesda, MD: United States Department of Health, Education and Welfare.

Lang, N., & Clinton, J. (1984). Assessment of quality of nursing care. *Annual Review of Nursing Research, 2,* 135–163.

Lindeman, C. (1976). Measuring the quality of nursing care. *Journal of Nursing Administration, 6*(5), 16–19.

Lohr, K. (1988). Outcome measurements: Concepts and questions. *Inquiry, 25,* 37–50.

Marek, K. (1989). The measurement of patient outcomes. *Journal of Nursing Quality Assurance, 4*(3), 1–9.

Maxwell, R. J. (1984). Quality assessment in health. *British Medical Journal, 288,* 1470–1472.

Mayers, M., Norby, R., & Watson, A. (1977). *Quality assurance for patient care.* New York: Appleton-Century-Crofts.

McFarlane, J. (1989). *Forming links between quality and research.* Paper presented at Nursing Research and Quality Conference. Newcastle Health Authority.

Mitchell, M. K. (1988). *The community health accreditation programme. Caring, 7*(10), 20–24.

Norris, C. (Ed.). (1982). *Concept clarification in nursing.* Rockville, MD: Aspen.

Parish, S. (1986). Quality vs. quantity: Which type of nursing do you practice? *Journal of Practical Nursing, 36*(2), 30–31.

Pearson, A. (Ed.). (1987). *Nursing quality measurement: Quality assurance methods for peer review.* Chichester: John Wiley & Sons.

Pfeffer, N., & Coote, A. (1990). *Is quality good for you?* Social Policy Paper No. 5, IPPR, London.

Phaneuf, M. (1976). *The nursing audit — Self regulation in practice* (2nd ed.). New York: Appleton-Century-Crofts.

Rodgers, B. (1989). Concepts, analysis and the development of nursing knowledge: The evolutionary cycle. *Journal of Advanced Nursing, 14,* 330–335.

Rutstein et al. (1976). Measuring the quality of medical care. *New England Journal of Medicine, 29*(11), 582–588.

Schmadl, J. (1979). Quality assurance: Examination of the concept. *Nursing Outlook, 27*(7), 462–465.

Shukla, R. (1981). Structure vs. people in primary nursing: An inquiry. *Nursing Research, 30,* 236–241.

Slater. (1975). Cited in Wandelt and Stewart (1975).

Smith, P. (1987). The relationship between quality of nursing care and the ward as a learning environment: Developing a methodology. *Journal of Advanced Nursing, 12*(4), 413–430.

Statland, B. (1989). Quality management: Watchword for the '90s. *Medical Lab Observer, 21*(7), 33–40.

Taylor, A., & Haussmann, G. (1988). Meaning and measurement of quality nursing care. *Applied Nursing Research, 1*(2), 84–88.

Taylor, A., Hudson, K., & Keeling, A. (1991). Quality nursing care: The consumers' perspective revisited. *Journal of Nursing Quality Assurance, 5*(2), 23–31.

Valentine, K. (1989). Caring is more than kindness: Modelling its complexities. *Journal of Nursing Administration, 19*(11), 28–35.

Van Maanen, H. (1984). Evaluation of nursing care: Quality of nursing evaluated. In L. Willis & M. Linwood (Eds.), *Measuring the quality of care.* Edinburgh, Scotland: Churchill Livingstone.

Walker, L., & Avant, K. (1983). *Strategies for theory construction in nursing.* Norwalk, CT: Appleton-Century-Crofts.

Wandelt, M., & Ager, J. (1974). *Quality patient care scale.* New York: Appleton-Century-Crofts.

Wandelt, M., & Stewart, D. S. (1975). *The Slater nursing competencies rating scale.* New York: Appleton-Century-Crofts.

Willis, L., & Linwood, M. (Eds.). (1984). *Measuring the quality of care.* Edinburgh, Scotland: Churchill Livingstone.

World Health Organization. (1983). *The principles of quality assurance* (Euro Reports and Studies, 94, WHO). Copenhagen.

Wright, D. (1984). An introduction to the evaluation of nursing care: A review of the literature. *Journal of Advanced Nursing, 9*, 457–467.

Zierden. (1989). Cited by B. Statland. Quality management: Watchword for the '90s. *Medical Lab Observer, 21*(7), 33–41.

Zimmer, M. (1974). Symposium on quality assurance. *Nursing Clinics of North America, 9*(2), 303–379.

ADDITIONAL READING

Bowen, O. R. (1987). Shattuck lecture: What is quality? *The New England Journal of Medicine, 316*(25), 1578–1580.

Donabedian, A. (1980). *The definition of quality and approaches to its assessment: Explanations in quality assessment and monitoring* (Vol. I). Ann Arbor, MI: Health Administration Press.

Frost, M. H. (1992). Quality: A concept of importance to nursing. *Journal of Nursing Care Quality, 7*(1), 64–69.

Katz, J., & Green, E. (1992). In pursuit of a definition of quality. In J. Katz & E. Green, *Managing quality* (pp. 3–12). St. Louis, MO: C. V. Mosby.

Reerink, E. (1990). Defining quality of care: Mission impossible. *Quality Assurance in Health Care, 2*(3/4), 197–202.

Steffen, G. E. (1988). Quality medical care: A definition. *Journal of the American Medical Association, 260*(1), 56–61.

Avedis Donabedian

CHAPTER **4**

The Quality of Care:
How Can It Be Assessed?

Before assessment can begin we must decide how quality is to be defined and that depends on whether one assesses only the performance of practitioners or also the contributions of patients and of the health care system; on how broadly health and responsibility for health are defined; on whether the maximally effective or optimally effective care is sought; and on whether individual or social preferences define the optimum. We also need detailed information about the causal linkages among the structural attributes of the settings in which care occurs, the processes of care, and the outcomes of care. Specifying the components or outcomes of care to be sampled, formulating the appropriate criteria and standards, and obtaining the necessary information are the steps that follow. Though we know much about assessing quality, much remains to be known. (American Medical Association, 1988)

INTRODUCTION

There was a time, not too long ago, when this question could not have been asked. The quality of care was considered to be something of a mystery: real, capable of being perceived and appreciated, but not subject to measurement. The very attempt to define and measure **quality** seemed, then, to denature and belittle it. Now, we may have moved too far in the opposite direction. Those who have not experienced the intricacies of clinical practice demand measures that are easy, precise, and complete — as if a sack of potatoes was being weighed. True, some elements in the quality of care are easy to define and measure, but there are also profundities that still elude us. We must not allow anyone to belittle or ignore them; they are the secret and glory of

Note: This chapter is reprinted with permission from the *Journal of the American Medical Association,* 260(12), 1743–1748, Sept. 23/30, copyright 1988, American Medical Association.

our art. Therefore, we should avoid claiming for our capacity to assess quality either too little or too much. I shall try to steer this middle course.

SPECIFYING WHAT QUALITY IS

Level and Scope of Concern

Before we attempt to assess the quality of care, either in general terms or in any particular site or situation, it is necessary to come to an agreement on what the elements that constitute it are. To proceed to measurement without a firm foundation of prior agreement on what quality consists in is to court disaster (Donabedian, 1980).

As we seek to define quality, we soon become aware of the fact that several formulations are both possible and legitimate, depending on where we are located in the system of care and on what the nature and extent of our responsibilities are. These several formulations can be envisaged as a progression, for example, as steps in a ladder or as successive circles surrounding the bull's-eye of a target. Our power, our responsibility, and our vulnerability all flow from the fact that we are the foundation for that ladder, the focal point for that family of concentric circles. We must begin, therefore, with the performance of physicians and other health-care practitioners.

As shown in Figure 4-1, there are two elements in the performance of practi-

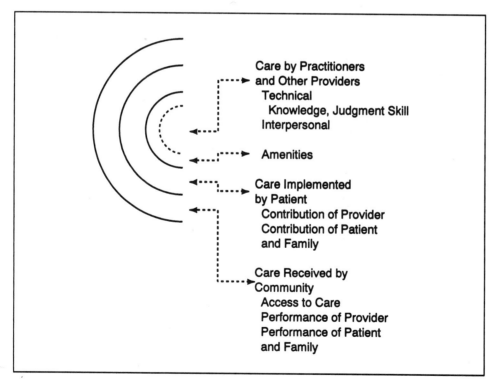

Figure 4-1 *Levels at which Quality May Be Assessed*

tioners: one technical and the other interpersonal. Technical performance depends on the knowledge and judgment used in arriving at the appropriate strategies of care and on skill in implementing those strategies. The goodness of technical performance is judged in comparison with the best in practice. The best in practice, in its turn, has earned that distinction because, on the average, it is known or believed to produce the greatest improvement in health. This means that the goodness of technical care is proportional to its expected ability to achieve those improvements in health status that the current science and technology of health care have made possible. If the realized fraction of what is achievable is called *effectiveness*, the quality of technical care becomes proportionate to its effectiveness (see Figure 4-2).

Here, two points deserve emphasis. First, judgments on technical quality are contingent on the best in current knowledge and technology; they cannot go beyond that limit. Second, the judgment is based on future expectations, not on events already transpired. Even if the actual consequences of care in any given instance prove to be disastrous, quality must be judged as good if care, at the time it was given, conformed to the practice that could have been expected to achieve the best results.

The management of the interpersonal relationship is the second component in the practitioner's performance. It is a vitally important element. Through the interpersonal exchange, the patient communicates information necessary for arriving at a diagnosis, as well as preferences necessary for selecting the most appropriate methods of care. Through this exchange, the physician provides information about the nature of the illness and its management and motivates the patient into collaboration in care. Clearly, the interpersonal process is the vehicle by which technical

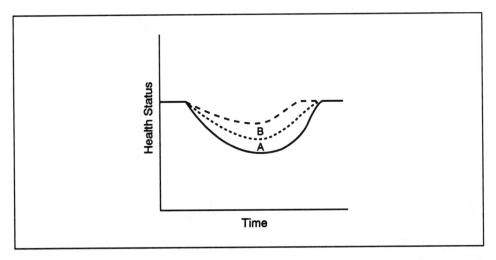

Figure 4-2 *Graphical Presentation of Effectiveness (in a Self-Limiting Disease). Solid line indicates course of illness without care; dotted line, course of illness with care to be assessed; and dashed line, course of illness with "best" care. Effectiveness equals A/(A+B).*

care is implemented and on which its success depends. Therefore, the management of the interpersonal process is to a large degree tailored to the achievement of success in technical care.

But the conduct of the interpersonal process must also meet individual and social expectations and **standards**, whether these aid or hamper technical performance. Privacy, confidentiality, informed choice, concern, empathy, honesty, tact, sensitivity — all these and more are virtues that the interpersonal relationship is expected to have.

If the management of the interpersonal process is so important, why is it so often ignored in assessments of the quality of care? There are many reasons. Information about the interpersonal process is not easily available. For example, in the medical record, special effort is needed to obtain it. Second, the **criteria** and standards that permit precise measurement of the attributes of the interpersonal process are not well developed or have not been sufficiently called upon to undertake the task. Partly, it may be because the management of the interpersonal process must adapt to so many variations in the preferences and expectations of individual patients that general guidelines do not serve us sufficiently well.

Much of what we call the *art of medicine* consists in almost intuitive adaptations to individual requirements in technical care as well as in the management of the interpersonal process. Another element in the art of medicine is the way, still poorly understood, in which practitioners process information to arrive at a correct diagnosis and an appropriate strategy of care (Eraker & Politser, 1982). As our understanding of each of these areas of performance improves, we can expect the realm of our science to expand and that of our art to shrink. Yet I hope that some of the mystery in practice will always remain, since it affirms and celebrates the uniqueness of each individual.

The science and art of health care, as they apply to both technical care and the management of the interpersonal process, are at the heart of the metaphorical family of concentric circles depicted in Figure 4-1. Immediately surrounding the center we can place the amenities of care, these being the desirable attributes of the settings within which care is provided. They include convenience, comfort, quiet, privacy, and so on. In private practice, these are the responsibility of the practitioner to provide. In institutional practice, the responsibility for providing them devolves on the owners and managers of the institution.

By moving to the next circle away from the center of our metaphorical target, we include in assessments of quality the contributions to care of the patients themselves as well as of members of their families. By doing so we cross an important boundary. So far, our concern was primarily with the performance of the providers of care. Now, we are concerned with judging the care as it actually was. The responsibility, now, is shared by provider and consumer. As already described, the management of the interpersonal process by the practitioner influences the implementation of care by and for the patient. Yet, the patient and family must, themselves, also carry some of the responsibility for the success or failure of care. Accordingly, the practitioner may be judged blameless in some situations in which the care, as implemented by the patient, is found to be inferior.

We have one more circle to visit, another watershed to cross. Now, we are concerned with care received by the community as a whole. We must now judge the social distribution of levels of quality in the community (Donabedian, 1972). This depends, in turn, on who has greater or lesser access to care and who, after gaining access, receives greater or lesser qualities of care. Obviously, the performance of individual practitioners and health-care institutions has much to do with this. But, the quality of care in a community is also influenced by many factors over which the providers have no control, although these are factors they should try to understand and be concerned about.

I have tried, so far, to show that the definition of quality acquires added elements as we move outward from the performance of the practitioners, to the care received by patients, and to the care received by communities. The definition of quality also becomes narrower or more expansive, depending on how narrowly or broadly we define the concept of health and our responsibility for it. It makes a difference in the assessment of our performance whether we see ourselves as responsible for bringing about improvements only in specific aspects of physical or physiological function or whether we include psychological and social function as well.

Valuation of the Consequences of Care

Still another modification in the assessment of performance depends on who is to value the improvements in health that care is expected to produce. If it is our purpose to serve the best interest of our patients, we need to inform them of the alternatives available to them, so they can make the choice most appropriate to their preferences and circumstances. The introduction of patient preferences, though necessary to the assessment of quality, is another source of difficulty in implementing assessment. It means that no preconceived notion of what the objectives and accomplishments of care should be will precisely fit any given patient. All we can hope for is a reasonable approximation, one that must then be subject to individual adjustment (McNeil, Pauker, Sox, & Tversky, 1982; McNeil, Weichselbaum & Pauker, 1978, 1981).

Monetary Cost as a Consideration

Finally, we come to the perplexing question of whether the monetary cost of care should enter the definition of quality and its assessment (Donabedian, 1980; Donabedian, Wheeler, & Wyszewianski, 1982). In theory, it is possible to separate quality from inefficiency. Technical quality is judged by the degree to which achievable improvements in health can be expected to be attained. Inefficiency is judged by the degree to which expected improvements in health are achieved in an unnecessarily costly manner. In practice, lower quality and inefficiency coexist because wasteful care is either directly harmful to health or is harmful by displacing more useful care.

Cost and quality are also confounded because, as shown in Figure 4-3, it is believed that as one adds to care, the corresponding improvements in health become progressively smaller while costs continue to rise unabated. If this is true, there will be a point beyond which additions to care will bring about improvements that are too small to be worth the added cost. Now, we have a choice. We can ignore cost and say that the highest quality is represented by care that can be expected to achieve the greatest improvement in health; this is a *maximalist* specification of quality. Alternatively, if we believe that cost is important, we would say that care must stop short of including elements that are disproportionately costly compared with the improvements in health that they produce. This is an *optimalist* specification of quality. A graphical representation of these alternatives is shown in Figure 4-3.

Health-care practitioners tend to prefer a maximalist standard because they only have to decide whether each added element of care is likely to be useful. By contrast, the practice of optimal care requires added knowledge of costs, and also some method of weighing each added bit of expected usefulness against its corresponding cost (Torrance, 1986). Yet, the practice of optimal care is traditional, legitimate, even necessary, as long as costs and benefits are weighed jointly by the practitioner and the fully informed patient. A difficult, perhaps insoluble, problem arises when a third party (for example, a private insurer or a governmental agency) specifies what the optimum that defines quality is (Donabedian, 1983).

Preliminaries to Quality Assessment

Before we set out to assess quality, we will have to choose whether we will adopt a maximal or optimal specification of quality and, if the latter, whether we shall

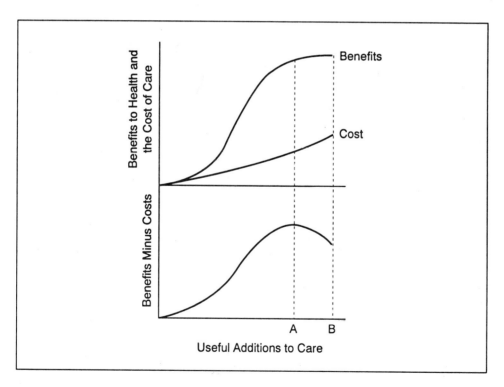

Figure 4-3 *Hypothetical Relations between Health Benefits and Cost of Care as Useful Additions Are Made to Care. A indicates optimally effective care; and B, maximally effective care.*

accept what is the optimum for each patient or what has been defined as socially optimal. Similarly, we should have decided (1) how health and our responsibility for it is to be defined, (2) whether the assessment is to be of the performance of practitioners only or also include that of patients and the health-care system, and (3) whether the amenities and the management of the interpersonal process are to be included in addition to technical care. In a more practical vein, we need to answer certain questions: Who is being assessed? What are the activities being assessed? How are these activities supposed to be conducted? What are they meant to accomplish? When we agree on the answers to these questions we are ready to look for the measures that will give us the necessary information about quality.

Approaches to Assessment

The information from which inferences can be drawn about the quality of care can be classified under three categories: **structure**, **process**, and **outcome** (Donabedian, 1966, 1980).

> *Structure* — Structure denotes the attributes of the settings in which care occurs. This includes the attributes of material resources (such as facilities, equipment, and money), of human resources (such as the number and qualifications of personnel), and of organizational structure (such as medical staff organization, methods of peer review, and methods of reimbursement).
>
> *Process* — Process denotes what is actually done in giving and receiving care. It includes the patient's activities in seeking care and carrying it out as well as the practitioner's activities in making a diagnosis and recommending or implementing treatment.
>
> *Outcome* — Outcome denotes the effects of care on the health status of patients and populations. Improvements in the patient's knowledge and salutary changes in the patient's behavior are included under a broad definition of health status, and so is the degree of the patient's satisfaction with care.

This three-part approach to quality assessment is possible only because good structure increases the likelihood of good process, and good process increases the likelihood of a good outcome. It is necessary, therefore, to have established such a relationship before any particular component of structure, process, or outcome can be used to assess quality. The activity of quality assessment is not itself designed to establish the presence of these relationships. There must be preexisting knowledge of the linkage between structure and process, and between process and outcome, before quality assessment can be undertaken.

Knowledge about the relationship between structure and process (or between structure and outcome) proceeds from the organizational sciences. These sciences are still relatively young, so our knowledge of the effects of structure is rather scanty (Donabedian, 1985; Palmer & Reilly, 1979). Furthermore, what we do know suggests that the relationship between structure characteristics and the process of care is rather weak. From these characteristics, we can only infer that conditions are either inimical or conducive to good care. We cannot assert that care, in fact, has been good or bad. Structural characteristics should be a major preoccupation in system design; they are a rather blunt instrument in quality assessment.

As I have already mentioned, knowledge about the relationship between attributes of the interpersonal process and the outcome of care should derive from the behavioral sciences. But so far, these sciences have contributed relatively little to quality assessment. I cannot say whether this is because of a deficiency in these sciences or a narrowness in those who assess quality.

Knowledge about the relationship between technical care and outcome derives, of course, from the health-care sciences. Some of that knowledge, as we know, is pretty detailed and firm, deriving from well-conducted trials or extensive, controlled observations. Some of it is of dubious validity and open to question. Our assessments of the quality of the technical process of care vary accordingly in their certainty and persuasiveness. If we are confident that a certain strategy of care produces the best outcomes in a given category of patients, we can be equally confident that its practice represents the highest quality of care, barring concern for cost. If we are uncertain of the relationship, then our assessment of quality is correspondingly uncertain. It cannot be emphasized too strongly that our ability to assess the quality of technical care is bounded by the strengths and weaknesses of our clinical science.

There are those who believe that direct assessment of the outcome of care can free us from the limitations imposed by the imperfections of the clinical sciences. I do not believe so. Because a multitude of factors influence outcome, it is not possible to know for certain, even after extensive adjustments for differences in case mix are made, the extent to which an observed outcome is attributable to an antecedent process of care. Confirmation is needed by a direct assessment of the process itself, which brings us to the position we started from.

The assessment of outcomes, under rigorously controlled circumstances, is, of course, the method by which the goodness of alternative strategies of care is established. But, quality assessment is neither clinical research nor technology assessment. It is almost never carried out under the rigorous controls that research requires. It is, primarily, an administrative device used to **monitor** performance to determine whether it continues to remain within acceptable bounds. Quality assessment can, however, make a contribution to research if, in the course of assessment, associations are noted between process and outcome that seem inexplicable by current knowledge. Such discrepancies would call for elucidation through research.

If I am correct in my analysis, we cannot claim either for the measurement of process or the measurement of outcomes an inherently superior validity compared with the other, since the validity of either flows to an equal degree from the validity of the science that postulates a linkage between the two. But, process and outcome do have, on the whole, some different properties that make them more or less suitable objects of measurement for given purposes. Information about technical care is readily available in the medical record, and it is available in a timely manner, so that prompt action to correct deficiencies can be taken. By contrast, many outcomes, by their nature, are delayed, and if they occur after care is completed, information about them is not easy to obtain. Outcomes do have, however, the advantage of reflecting all contributions to care, including those of the patient. But this advantage is also a handicap, since it is not possible to say precisely what went wrong unless the antecedent process is scrutinized.

This brief exposition of strengths and weaknesses should lead to the conclusion that in selecting an approach to assessment one needs to be guided by the precise characteristics of the elements chosen. Beyond causal validity, which is the essential requirement, one is guided by attributes such as relevance to the objectives of care, sensitivity, specificity, timeliness, and costliness (Donabedian, 1980, pp. 100–118). As a general rule, it is best to include in any system of assessment, elements of structure, process, and outcome. This allows supplementation of weakness in one approach by strength in another; it helps one interpret the findings; and if the findings do not seem to make sense, it leads to a reassessment of study design and a questioning of the accuracy of the data themselves.

Before we leave the subject of approaches to assessment, it may be useful to say a few words about patient satisfaction as a measure of the quality of care. Patient satisfaction may be considered to be one of the desired outcomes of care, even an element in health status itself. An expression of satisfaction or dissatisfaction is also the patient's judgment on the quality of care in all its aspects, but particularly as concerns the interpersonal process. By questioning patients, one can obtain information about overall satisfaction and also about satisfaction with specific attributes of the interpersonal relationship, specific components of technical care, and the outcomes of care. In doing so, it should be remembered that, unless special precautions are taken, patients may be reluctant to reveal their opinions for fear of alienating their medical attendants. Therefore, to add to the evidence at hand, information can also be sought about behaviors that indirectly suggest dissatisfaction. These include, in addition to complaints registered, premature termination of care, other forms of noncompliance, termination of membership in a health plan, and seeking care outside the plan.

It is futile to argue about the validity of patient satisfaction as a measure of quality. Whatever its strengths and limitations as an **indicator** of quality, information about patient satisfaction should be as indispensable to assessments of quality as to the design and management of health-care systems.

SAMPLING

If one wishes to obtain a true view of care as it is actually provided, it is necessary to draw a proportionally representative sample of cases, using either simple or stratified random sampling. Because cases are primarily classified by diagnosis, this is the most frequently used attribute for stratification. But, one could use other attributes as well: site of care, specialty, demographic and socioeconomic characteristics of patients, and so on.

There is some argument as to whether patients are to be classified by discharge diagnosis, admission diagnosis, or presenting complaint. Classification by presenting complaint (for example, headache or abdominal pain) offers an opportunity to assess both success and failure in diagnosis. If discharge diagnoses are used, one can tell if the diagnosis is justified by the evidence; the failure to diagnose is revealed only if one has an opportunity to find cases misclassified under other diagnostic headings.

A step below strictly proportional sampling, one finds methods designed to provide an illustrative rather than a representative view of quality. For example, patients may be first classified according to some scheme that represents important subdivisions of the realm of health care in general, or important components in the activities and responsibilities of a clinical department or program in particular. Then, one purposively selects, within each class, one or more categories of patients, identified by diagnosis or otherwise, whose management can be assumed to typify clinical performance for that class.

This is the *tracer method* proposed by Kessner and coworkers (Kessner, Kalk, & James, 1973; Rhee, Donabedian, & Burney, 1987). The validity of the assumption that the cases selected for assessment represent all cases in their class has not been established.

Most often, those who assess quality are not interested in obtaining a representative, or even an illustrative, picture of care as a whole. Their purposes are more managerial, namely, to identify and correct the most serious failures in care and, by doing so, to create an environment of watchful concern that motivates everyone to perform better. Consequently, diagnostic categories are selected according to importance, perhaps using Williamson's principle of "maximum achievable benefit," meaning that the diagnosis is frequent, deficiencies in care are common and serious, and the deficiencies are correctable.

Still another approach to sampling for managerial or reformist purposes is to begin with cases that have suffered an adverse outcome and study the process of care that has led to it. If the outcome is infrequent and disastrous (a maternal or perinatal death, for example), every case might be reviewed. Otherwise, a sample of adverse outcomes, with or without prior stratification, could be studied (Kohl, 1955; New York Academy of Medicine, 1933; Rutstein, Berenberg, Chalmers, Child, Fishman, & Perrin, 1976). There is some evidence that, under certain circumstances, this approach will identify a very high proportion of serious deficiencies in the process of care, but not of deficiencies that are less serious (Mushlin & Appel, 1980).

MEASUREMENT

The progression of steps in quality assessment that I have described so far brings us, at last, to the critical issue of measurement. To measure quality, our concepts of what quality consists in must be translated to more concrete representations that are capable of some degree of quantification — at least on an ordinal scale, but one hopes better. These representations are the criteria and standards of structure, process, and outcome (Donabedian, 1982, 1986).

Ideally, the criteria and standards should derive, as I have already implied, from a sound, scientifically validated fund of knowledge. Failing that, they should represent the best informed, most authoritative opinion available on any particular subject. Criteria and standards can also be inferred from the practice of eminent practitioners in a community. Accordingly, the criteria and standards vary in validity, authoritativeness, and rigor.

The criteria and standards of assessment can also be either *implicit* or *explicit.* Implicit, unspoken criteria are used when an expert practitioner is given information about a case and asked to use personal knowledge and experience to judge the goodness of the process of care or of its outcome. By contrast, explicit criteria and standards for each category of cases are developed and specified in advance, often in considerable detail, usually by a panel of experts, before the assessment of individual cases begins. These are the two extremes in specification; there are intermediate variants and combinations as well.

The advantage in using implicit criteria is that they allow assessment of representative samples of cases and are adaptable to the precise characteristics of each case, making possible the highly individualized assessments that the conceptual formulation of quality envisaged. The method is, however, extremely costly and rather imprecise, the imprecision arising from inattentiveness or limitations in knowledge on the part of the reviewer and the lack of precise guidelines for quantification.

By comparison, explicit criteria are costly to develop, but they can be used subsequently to produce precise assessments at low cost, although only cases for which explicit criteria are available can be used in assessment. Moreover, explicit criteria are usually developed for categories of cases and, therefore, cannot be adapted readily to the variability among cases within a category. Still another problem is the difficulty in developing a scoring system that represents the degree to which the deficiencies in care revealed by the criteria influence the outcome of care.

Taking into account the strengths and limitations of implicit and explicit criteria, it may be best to use both in sequence or in combination. One frequently used procedure is to begin with rather abridged explicit criteria to separate cases into those likely to have received good care and those not. All the latter, as well as a sample of the former, are then assessed in greater detail using implicit criteria, perhaps supplemented by more detailed explicit criteria.

At the same time, explicit criteria themselves are being improved. As their use expands, more diagnostic categories have been included. Algorithmic criteria have been developed that are much more adaptable to the clinical characteristics of individual patients than are the more usual criteria lists (Greenfield, Cretin, Worthman, Dorey, Solomon, & Goldberg, 1981; Greenfield, Lewis, Kaplan, & Davidson, 1975). Methods for weighting the criteria have also been proposed, although we still do not have a method of weighting that is demonstrably related to degree of impact on health status (Lyons & Payne, 1975).

When outcomes are used to assess the quality of antecedent care, there is the corresponding problem of specifying the several states of dysfunction and of weighting them in importance relative to each other using some system of preferences. It is possible, of course, to identify specific outcomes, for example, reductions in fatality or blood pressure, and to measure the likelihood of attaining them. It is also possible to construct hierarchical scales of physical function so that any position on the scale tells us what functions can be performed and what functions are lost (Stewart, Ware, & Brook, 1981). The greatest difficulty arises when one attempts to represent as a single quantity various aspects of functional capacity over a life span. Though several methods of valuation and aggregation are available, there is still much controversy about the validity of the values and, in fact, about their ethical implications (Fanshel & Bush, 1970; Patrick, Bush, & Chen, 1973). Nevertheless, such measures, sometimes called *measures of quality-adjusted life*, are being used to assess technological innovations in health care and, as a consequence, play a role in defining what good technical care is (Weinstein & Stason, 1977; Willems, Sanders, Riddiough, & Bell, 1980).

INFORMATION

All the activities of assessment that I have described depend, of course, on the availability of suitable, accurate information.

The key source of information about the process of care and its immediate outcome is, no doubt, the medical record. But we know that the medical record is often incomplete in what it documents, frequently omitting significant elements of technical care and including next to nothing about the interpersonal process. Furthermore, some of the information recorded is inaccurate because of errors in diagnostic testing, in clinical observation, in clinical assessment, in recording, and in coding. Another handicap is that any given set of records usually covers only a limited segment of care, while in the hospital, for example, providing no information about what comes before or after. Appropriate and accurate recording, supplemented by an ability to collate records from various sites, is a fundamental necessity to accurate, complete quality assessment.

The current weakness of the record can be rectified to some extent by independent verification of the accuracy of some of the data it contains, for example, by reexamination of pathological specimens, x-ray films, and electrocardiographic tracings and by recoding diagnostic categorization. The information in the record can also be supplemented by interviews with, or questionnaires to, practitioners and patients — information from patients being indispensable if compliance, satisfaction, and some long-term outcomes are to be assessed. Sometimes, if more precise information on outcomes is needed, patients may have to be called back for reexamination. And for some purposes, especially when medical records are very deficient, videotaping or direct observation by a colleague have been used, even though being observed might itself elicit an improvement in practice (Peterson, Andrews, Spain, & Greenberg, 1956; *What Sort of Doctor*, 1985).

CONCLUSION

In the preceding account, I have detailed, although rather sketchily, the steps to be taken in endeavoring to assess the quality of medical care. I hope it is clear that there is a way, a path worn rather smooth by many who have gone before us. I trust it is equally clear that we have, as yet, much more to learn. We need to know a great deal more about the course of illness with and without alternative methods of care. To compare the consequences of these methods, we need to have more precise measures of the quantity and quality of life. We need to understand more profoundly the nature of the interpersonal exchange between patient and practitioner, to learn how to identify and quantify its attributes, and to determine in what ways these contribute to the patient's health and welfare. Our information about the process and outcome of care needs to be more complete and more accurate. Our criteria and standards need to be more flexibly adaptable to the finer clinical peculiarities of each case. In particular, we need to learn how to accurately elicit the preferences of patients to arrive at truly individualized assessments of quality. All this has to go on against the background of the most profound analysis of the responsibilities of the health-care professions to the individual and to society.

REFERENCES

Donabedian, A. (1966). Evaluating the quality of medical care. *Milbank Quarterly, 44,* 166–203.

Donabedian, A. (1972). Models for organizing the delivery of health services and criteria for evaluating them. *Milbank Quarterly, 50,* 103–154.

Donabedian, A. (1980). *The definition of quality and approaches to its management, volume 1: Explorations in quality assessment and monitoring.* Ann Arbor, MI: Health Administration Press.

Donabedian, A. (1982). *The criteria and standards of quality, volume 2: Explorations in quality assessment and monitoring.* Ann Arbor, MI: Health Administration Press.

Donabedian, A. (1983). Quality, cost, and clinical decisions. *Annals of American Academy of Political and Social Science, 468,* 196–204.

Donabedian, A. (1985). The epidemiology of quality. *Inquiry, 22,* 282–292.

Donabedian, A. (1986). Criteria and standards for quality assessment and monitoring. *Quality Review Bulletin, 12,* 99–108.

Donabedian, A., Wheeler, J. R. C., & Wyszewianski, L. (1982). Quality, cost, and health: An integrative model. *Medical Care, 20,* 975–992.

Eraker, S., & Politser, P. (1982). How decisions are reached: Physician and patient. *Annals of Internal Medicine, 97,* 262–268.

Fanshel, S., & Bush, J. W. (1970). A health status index and its application to health service outcomes. *Operations Research, 18,* 1021–1060.

Greenfield, S., Cretin, S., Worthman, L., Dorey, F. J., Solomon, N. E., & Goldberg, G. A. (1981). Comparison of a criteria map to a criteria list in quality-of-care assessment for patients with chest pain: The relation of each to the outcome. *Medical Care, 19,* 255–272.

Greenfield, S., Lewis, C. E., Kaplan, S. H., & Davidson, M. B. (1975). *Peer review by criteria mapping: Criteria for diabetes mellitus.* The use of decision-making in chart audit. *Annals of Internal Medicine, 83,* 761–770.

Kessner, D. M., Kalk, C. E., & James, S. (1973). Assessing health quality — The case for tracers. *New England Journal of Medicine, 288,* 189–194.

Kohl, S. G. (1955). *Perinatal mortality in New York City: Responsible factors.* Cambridge, MA: Harvard University Press.

Lyons, T. F., & Payne, B. C. (1975). The use of item weights in assessing physician performance with predetermined criteria indices. *Medical Care, 13,* 432–439.

McNeil, B. J., Pauker, S. G., Sox, H. C., Jr., & Tversky, A. (1982). On the elicitation of preferences for alternative therapies. *New England Journal of Medicine, 306,* 1259–1262.

McNeil, B. J., Weichselbaum, R., & Pauker, S. G. (1978). Fallacy of the five-year survival in lung cancer. *New England Journal of Medicine, 299,* 1397–1401.

McNeil, B. J., Weichselbaum, R., & Pauker, S. G. (1981). Tradeoffs between quality and quantity of life in laryngeal cancer. *New England Journal of Medicine, 305,* 982–987.

Mushlin, A. I., & Appel, F. A. (1980). Testing an outcome-based quality assurance strategy in primary care. *Medical Care, 18,* 1–100.

New York Academy of Medicine, Committee on Public Health Relations. (1933). *Maternal mortality in New York City: A study of all puerperal deaths 1930–1932.* New York: Oxford University Press, Inc.

Palmer, R. H., & Reilly, M. C. (1979). Individual and institutional variables which may serve as indicators of quality of medical care. *Medical Care, 17,* 693–717.

Patrick, D. I., Bush, J. W., & Chen, M. M. (1973). Methods for measuring levels of well-being for a health status index. *Health Services Research, 8,* 228–245.

Peterson, O. L., Andrews, L. P., Spain, R. A., & Greenberg, B. G. (1956). An analytical study of North Carolina general practice, 1953–1954. *Journal of Medical Education, 31,* 1–165.

Rhee, K. J., Donabedian, A., & Burney, R. E. (1987). Assessing the quality of care in a hospital emergency unit: A framework and its application. *Quality Review Bulletin, 13,* 4–16.

Rutstein, D. B., Berenberg, W., Chalmers, T. C., Child, C. G., 3rd, Fishman, A. P., & Perrin, E. B. (1976). Measuring quality of medical care: A clinical method. *New England Journal of Medicine, 294,* 582–588.

Stewart, A. L., Ware, J. E., Jr., & Brook, R. H. (1981). Advances in the measurement of functional states: Construction of aggregate indexes. *Medical Care, 19,* 473–488.

Torrance, G. W. (1986). Measurement of health status utilities for economic appraisal: A review. *Journal of Health Economics, 5,* 1–30.

Weinstein, M. C., & Stason, W. B. (1977). Foundations of cost-effectiveness analysis for health and medical practices. *New England Journal of Medicine, 296,* 716–721.

What sort of doctor? Assessing quality of care in general practice. (1985). London: Royal College of General Practitioners.

Willems, J. S., Sanders, C. R., Riddiough, M. A., & Bell, J. C. (1980). Cost-effectiveness of vaccination against pneumococcal pneumonia. *New England Journal of Medicine, 303,* 553–559.

Williamson, J. W. (1978). Formulating priorities for quality assurance activity: Description of a method and its application. *Journal of American Medical Association, 239,* 631–637.

ADDITIONAL READING

Developing a patient measurement system for the future: An interview with Eugene C. Nelson, DSc, MPH. (1993). *Journal on Quality Improvement, 19*(9), 368–373.

Donabedian, A. (1985). Twenty years of research on the quality of medical care 1964–1984. *Evaluation and the Health Professions, 8*(3), 243–265.

Hodges, L. C., Icenhour, M. L., & Tate, S. (1994). Measuring quality. In J. McCloskey & H. K. Grace (Eds.), *Current issues in nursing* (4th ed.). St. Louis, MO: Mosby.

O'Leary, D. (1993). The measurement mandate: Report card day is coming. *Journal on Quality Improvement, 19*(11), 487–491.

Papps, E. (1994). How do we assess "good nursing care"? *International Journal for Quality in Health Care, 6*(1), 59–60.

Redfern, S. J., Norman, I. J., Tomalin, D. A., & Oliver, S. (1994). Assessing quality of nursing care. *Quality in Health Care, 2*(2), 124–128.

G. Ross Baker
Sherril B. Gelmon

CHAPTER 5

Total Quality Management in Health Care

INTRODUCTION

Total Quality Management (TQM) and similar organization–wide quality improvement strategies developed in industry have been attracting increasing attention from health-care leaders. Over 50 percent of hospitals in recent surveys indicate that they are involved in developing TQM applications (Baker, Barnsley, & Murray, 1993; Eubanks, 1992). The Joint Commission on the Accreditation of Healthcare Organizations in the United States and the Canadian Council on Health Facilities Accreditation have adopted new **standards** that encourage managers to study quality-improvement strategies. Continued financial pressures and a growing recognition of the inadequacy of current approaches to assessing and improving the **quality** of health-care services have reinforced this trend.

Many providers and managers have sought "quick fixes" through partial application of the ideas and methods of quality improvement. Experience from industry suggests, however, that such limited attempts are likely to fail. Successful implementation of TQM requires that managers and providers develop a thorough knowledge of the core ideas of quality improvement and actively work to lead others in learning and applying these ideas.

This chapter outlines the historical development and key principles of the TQM approach, from the origin of TQM principles in manufacturing industries in the United States and Japan to the application of these principles to health-care organizations in the United States and Canada. The achievements of some of the leading organizations that have applied TQM to health care are also discussed. Finally, information regarding changes in the accreditation process and organizational supports for health-care organizations that seek to apply TQM is provided.

BACKGROUND AND HISTORICAL PERSPECTIVE

In his book *Managing Quality: The Strategic and Competitive Edge*, David Garvin (1988) traces the evolution of modern approaches to quality in industry. Garvin distinguishes four separate eras: inspection, statistical quality control, company-wide quality improvement (which he labels "quality assurance," a term with a somewhat different meaning in health care), and strategic quality management. The inspection era refers to early efforts in industry to monitor quality based on the after–the–fact review of manufactured goods and the development of methods to ensure the standardization of products produced by different workers. This approach was well suited to the manufacturing industry when work was done in small shops where managers and inspectors could monitor production.

Statistical Quality Control

Statistical techniques developed in the 1930s allowed managers to select samples of production (rather than testing the entire output) and to distinguish acceptable variation in products from the fluctuations that signaled problems. Walter Shewhart (1980 [1931]), an engineer at Bell Laboratories, recognized that whereas some variation resulted from small, "normal" changes in the production process, other variation resulted from "abnormal" causes such as machine malfunction or worker error. Shewhart's techniques formed the basis for a body of knowledge referred to as *Statistical Quality Control (SQC)*. Statistical Quality Control provided a powerful new tool called the **control chart**. This tool provided a graphical display of data on work performance. The control chart permitted managers and workers to determine whether interventions were required to correct work defects.

These SQC techniques received increasing attention during World War II in response to the need to ensure that large quantities of arms and munitions could be procured from multiple suppliers at consistently acceptable levels of quality. Manufacturing and engineering departments hired quality professionals to apply SQC techniques. Responsibility for quality control thus became the purview of technical specialists rather than of managers, and managers often ignored quality issues. With the end of World War II, the pent-up demand for consumer products fueled an economic boom for North American industry. With little competition for their products, managers in North American manufacturing industries felt no pressure to assess and improve quality. Although the 1950s saw advances in the measurement of quality, and quality experts such as Armand Feigenbaum and Joseph Juran argued that responsibility for quality needed to be everyone's job, these experts found little receptivity to their message in America (Feigenbaum, 1961; Juran, 1993; Walton, 1986).

The concept of company–wide quality improvement was received quite differently in Japan. Japanese industrial leaders in the postwar era faced the need to rebuild their industries and improve living standards. They saw improvement in product quality as an important strategy in enabling Japan to increase exports and, consequently, increase earnings from abroad. A concensus gradually developed among Japanese leaders that quality improvement would provide the means to achieve their goals, and they supported new national organizations and large-scale training programs to support this initiative (Cole, 1991).

W. Edwards Deming

Ironically, much of the knowledge regarding quality issues and many of the associated techniques adapted and developed by the Japanese were originally conceived and taught by Americans in the 1950s. Among these Americans was W. Edwards Deming, a statistician and consultant who was invited by the Union of Japanese Scientists and Engineers (JUSE) to teach quality-improvement principles in Japan. Deming's message was primarily statistical, but he also emphasized the importance of adopting a systematic approach to problem solving to ensure that the results of statistical quality control led to changes in how things were done (Garvin, 1988). This approach, which Deming derived from Shewhart, was called the *Plan–Do–Check–Act* cycle. The concept suggests that managers should encourage continuous improvement in work processes and, equally important, that these improvements should be designed to meet customer needs (Ishikawa, 1985).

Deming also recognized that statistical methods alone were insufficient to ensure quality improvement. What was required was an explicit management philosophy that supported the use of these methods. Deming's philosophy is captured in his "Fourteen Points" (Walton, 1986). These fourteen principles outline what Deming believed were the crucial issues for management in transforming organizations. Deming initially formulated this list for his lectures in Japan, and has amended and added to it over the years, using these principles to instruct managers on how to build quality into their organizations. Deming's fourteen principles are:

1. Create constancy of purpose toward improvement of product and service.
2. Adopt the new philosophy.
3. Cease dependence on inspection to achieve quality.
4. End the practice of awarding busliness on the basis of price tag.
5. Improve constantly and forever the system of production and service.
6. Institute training on the job.
7. Institute leadership.
8. Drive out fear so that everyone may work effectively.
9. Break down barriers between departments.
10. Eliminate slogans, exhortations, and targets for the workforce asking for zero defects and new levels of productivity.
11. Eliminate work standards (quotas) and management by objective.
12. Remove barriers to pride of workmanship.
13. Institute a vigorous program of education and self–improvement.
14. Put everybody in the organization to work to accomplish the transformation. (1986, pp. 23–24)

Joseph Juran

Another American, Joseph Juran (1988, 1989), also taught large numbers of Japanese executives about quality principles. Juran's work emphasized the importance of planning and of management's responsibility for quality. Juran stressed the need to set quality goals and to be concerned about organizational issues in achieving these goals. He helped Japanese industrial leaders to recognize that success in quality required more than just statistical quality control; it required a systematic approach led by management and the involvement of all of the organization's employees.

Juran defined quality as fitness for use, meaning that those who use a product or service should be assured that the product or service will meet or exceed their needs. Juran identified two dimensions of quality: freedom from deficiencies (including, in addition to reduced deficiencies, reduced rework, reduced need for inspection, and reduced customer dissatisfaction) and quality that comes from an increased number of product features (products more appealing to customers, increased competitiveness and sales, and potentially increased costs) (Juran, 1989). To achieve quality, Juran advised managers to develop quality activities in three areas: quality planning, quality control, and quality improvement. A summary of the Juran quality trilogy follows:

- *quality planning* — determining who the customers are and their needs, developing product features to meet those needs, developing processes to produce these products, and transferring these plans into action
- *quality control* — evaluating actual performance, comparing performance to goals, and taking action on these differences
- *quality improvement* — establishing the necessary infrastructure, identifying specific improvement projects, establishing a team for each project, and providing the resources and support to determine causes, stimulate remedies, and establish controls to hold the gains (1989, pp. 14–27)

Each area involves other members of the organization; together, they provide a strategy for ensuring organization–wide quality improvement.

The Contributions of the Japanese

The influence of Deming, Juran, and other Americans in the development of what the Japanese refer to as *Total Quality Control (TQC)* has led some observers to minimize the important contributions of the Japanese in developing this new approach to quality. Although American experts argued for company–wide quality control, it was the Japanese who developed Quality Control circles (QC circles), which provided the means for employees to become involved in quality. Quality Control circles (or quality circles, as they have become known in the United States) originated as study groups for employees to learn about statistical control methods. Groups practiced the new methods by problem solving. Over time, such groups became a major element in the success of Japanese quality efforts. Quality Control circles take responsibility for using quality-improvement tools and a problem–solving method to analyze quality problems and improve products and services (Garvin, 1988). Quality Control circles are widespread in Japan, and members present the results of their work at many conferences. Other Japanese innovations, such as the **cause–and–effect diagram**, developed by Kaoru Ishikawa, have been spurred by the need for tools and techniques to support the work of QC circles (Ishikawa, 1985).

The Japanese Challenge

Support and involvement by top Japanese business leaders for company–wide quality control, coupled with strong research and training efforts coordinated by JUSE and the development of a system of national standards, helped ensure the success of the Japanese quality movement (Garvin, 1988). As a result of their focus on quality, by the late 1970s Japanese manufacturers had begun to present a formidable challenge to traditional United States market leaders, particularly in the electronics and automobile industries. Xerox, for example, which developed the xerography process for copying documents and held 96 percent of United States copier revenue in 1970, discovered by 1980 that the Japanese were making more reliable and less expensive machines. Indeed, the Japanese were able to sell their machines for less than it cost Xerox to manufacture theirs. Xerox and other United States companies in similiar situations faced an enormous challenge: to change the ways they produced goods and services or quit the business (Kearns & Nadler, 1992).

United States Companies Fight Back

Xerox, Hewlett–Packard, Motorola, Ford Motor Company, and other major United States industrial corporations took up this challenge. In the past decade they have invested considerable resources in developing new quality approaches to improve work processes, reduce costs, diminish the time needed to bring new products to the market, and ensure that new products meet existing or emerging customer needs. They have developed a variety of new techniques that adapt and extend the quality improvement processes and tools developed by Japanese corporations. By the late 1980s, use of such techniques had become standard practice among a wide spectrum of North American companies, from large manufacturing firms, which were early innovators, to smaller organizations and service companies.

The Malcolm Baldrige Quality Award

One measure of the extent of the TQM movement on United States companies has been the wide circulation of the **Malcolm Baldrige National Quality Award** criteria. Begun in 1988, the Baldrige award recognizes United States companies that excel in **Quality Management (QM)** and quality achievement. Although only a relatively small number of companies have applied for the award, hundreds of thousands of copies of the award criteria have been provided to organizations that use them as a basis for internal assessment and improvement (Garvin, 1991). There are seven categories of award criteria: leadership, information and analysis, strategic quality planning, human resource development and management, management of process quality, quality and operational results, and customer focus and satisfaction (United States Department of Commerce, 1993).

The Health-Care Industry Takes Notice

Health-care leaders noticed the growing interest of United States companies in quality management and recognized the potential for these methods in their own organizations. Increasing criticisms of traditional approaches to defining and improving health-care quality (Berwick, 1989; Laffel & Blumenthal, 1989) and, in particular, dissatisfaction with hospital **Quality Assurance (QA)** programs, led to the development of the National Demonstration Project (NDP) in 1987. The purpose of the project was to test the applicability and effectiveness of industrial QM approaches in health-care organizations. The NDP was headed by Donald Berwick, a pediatrician and health-services researcher at Harvard Community Health Plan; Paul Batalden, also a pediatrician and head of the Quality Resources Group at the Hospital Corporation of America; and A. Blanton Godfrey, vice president of the Juran Institute. Berwick, Batalden, and Godfrey raised foundation money and recruited twenty–one health-care organizations to work with QM experts from industry and universities. Each organization was asked to identify a pilot project and to use QM tools and a standardized quality improvement method on that project. Eight months later, the organizations reconvened to review their results. Nearly all of the projects showed successful results, indicating the potential for these methods in health care (Berwick, Godfrey, & Roessner, 1990).

The success of the NDP led to the development of TQM initiatives in many health-care organizations. Interest in TQM within the health-care industry has grown steadily in the years following the NDP pilot projects. One measure of this growing interest is the steadily increasing number of conferences and courses on quality improvement in health care. The annual conference held by the NDP (now the Institute for Healthcare Improvement), which discusses current issues and presents the results of quality improvement projects, has grown in attendance from 300 in 1988 to over 1,700 in 1993. In a few short years, industrial quality improvement ideas have advanced from trials in a few innovative organizations to a major new managerial framework adopted by significant numbers of health-care organizations.

KEY PRINCIPLES OF QUALITY MANAGEMENT

Although organizations vary in the emphasis they place on specific aspects of QM, certain key elements underpin and integrate the theoretical orientations to TQM developed in industry and now used in health care. These elements derive from the core principles identified by Deming, Juran, Ishikawa, and others (see Table 5-1).

Table 5-1 • **KEY QUALITY PRINCIPLES**

- Customer Focus
- Process Improvement
- Variation
- Leadership
- Employee Involvement
- Scientific Method
- Benchmarking

Customer Focus

Total Quality Management defines customers as those individuals or groups who receive what is produced. This notion of the **customer** is central; quality is defined in terms of the ability of the organization to meet the needs and expectations of its customers. There are two types of customers: **external customers** and **internal customers**. In health care, external customers include patients and families, payers, and communities — all those who benefit from or are affected by the services health-care organizations provide. Many professionals who are accustomed to referring to people in their care as patients, residents, or clients are uncomfortable with the term customer. The term is useful, however, since it does not connote the dependence or passivity associated with the term *patient* (Laffel, 1991). Deming notes that organizations exist to serve customers; efforts toward improvement must be focused on identifying and serving those customers (Deming, 1986).

A health-care organization's internal customers include staff, physicians, and others in the organization who depend on each other to provide information, materials, patient referrals, and whatever else they need to be able to do their work. Internal customers are part of a chain of customer–supplier relationships linking work units. Nurses, physicians, pharmacists, lab technicians, admitting clerks, and others take turns being customers and suppliers. For example, nurses are customers of physicians, who provide them with patients and information on the patients' medical status. Physicians are customers of lab technicians, who provide them with test results, and nurses, who provide them with reports on patients' conditions. Nurses, physicians, and lab technicians are customers of porters who transport specimens and results to and from the laboratory. Each of these relationships is defined not in terms of authority, but in the way the work of the organization is structured. In each step of a work process, one group or individual supplies someone or something necessary for the next step in the process (see Figure 5-1).

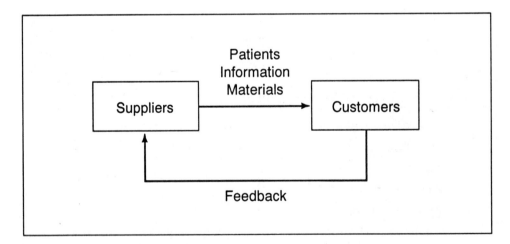

Figure 5-1 *Customer-Supplier Relationships*

Because quality is defined in terms of the needs and expectations of customers, identifying customers and meeting their requirements is a prerequisite for quality improvement (Leebov & Ersoz, 1991; Marszalek-Gaucher & Coffey, 1990). The more clearly and completely the customer can define these needs and expectations, the better able the supplier will be to plan and deliver products that meet them. Suppliers need to have in place methods to acquire knowledge about customers, and need to be able to adapt their processes in response to this information. Knowledge about external customers may come from suggestions and complaints, or may be elicited by focus groups or surveys. Information about the needs of internal customers can be obtained by similar data collection activities, perhaps as part of the work of quality improvement teams and other cross-functional groups. Focusing on customers and their needs is essential. Otherwise, improvements may be made in areas that turn out not to have been important to customers.

Process Improvement

Improving quality requires understanding and improving work processes linking customers and suppliers. Modern health-care organizations are very complex workplaces, involving many individuals with different skills who have responsibilities for a wide variety of activities. Routine, yet important, work processes may have thirty or forty steps, involving people from five or six different departments and clinical disciplines. Such processes are rarely designed; rather, they evolve over time. Because no one individual knows the entire **process**, there are often redundant or unnecessary steps. Waste in each process adds cost and reduces effectiveness. Because health-care organizations have hundreds of major processes, there is an enormous potential for improvement.

In most health-care organizations, changing a process, such as admitting a patient or ordering and processing a lab test, requires negotiation and coordination between managers of different departments. This often leads to conflict over resources and authority. Organizational incentives encourage managers and workers to optimize the work of individuals or departments without considering what impact changes may have on the organization as a whole. Suggested changes often focus on requests for more staff or more equipment instead of on ideas for using existing resources more effectively. These changes are likely to focus on improving the work environment and productivity of departmental employees; they are less likely to begin by considering the needs of patients, families, or others in the organization who depend upon the department.

Quality improvement offers a different approach to addressing work problems — an approach that can overcome turf battles between departments by focusing on the work itself, not on the preferences of those doing the work. Frontline employees are taught to use a problem–solving method and a variety of analytical tools to gain an understanding of their work processes. The problem–solving method becomes a road map to help the team understand and improve the process. Team members gather data to identify the root causes of problems, and then together they design and carry out small-scale experiments to improve this work.

Quality-improvement teams use a variety of quality improvement tools. These tools include **flow charts** and cause–and–effect diagrams, which can be used to describe work processes and identify potential root causes. Other tools, such as **run** (trend) **charts, histograms,** and **Pareto charts,** use basic descriptive statistics to analyze data. More sophisticated tools, such as control charts, provide additional insights. (See Chapter 24 for a detailed discussion of the most commonly used quality-improvement tools.)

Quality-improvement teams using quality-improvement tools are capable of identifying ways to improve processes, often entailing little or no additional cost, by removing unnecessary steps, eliminating duplication, and clarifying responsibilities. Health-care organizations that have invested resources in understanding and improving key processes have shown convincing results. For example, a quality-improvement team at Rush–Presbyterian–St. Luke's Hospital in Chicago worked on improving the process for admitting patients into the hospital. Information gathered by the team in September 1987 showed that the waiting time for scheduled admissions averaged 120 minutes. An average of seventy–five complaints per month were received from patients unhappy with these waits, and hospital staff had to deal with angry patients, families, and physicians. To address these problems, the hospital asked the team to reduce the amount of time spent by scheduled patients waiting in the admission lounge. The team collected data, analyzed the root causes of the process problems, and instituted several improvements. By August 1988, the average waiting time had decreased to twenty–four minutes, and by 1991 to ten minutes or less than 10 percent of the average in 1987. Complaints dropped to three per month, and the quality of work life improved dramatically for admitting clerks. One of the changes was to consolidate preadmission review, admitting, and patient accounts, resulting in a reduction of annual expenses by $213,000, a savings of 13 percent (Melum & Sinioris, 1992).

Variation

One of the crucial characteristics of processes is *variation.* Variation refers to the inevitable differences between individual outputs of a process. Health-care processes, like those in other areas of work, produce variable results. For example, the length of stay for pneumonia patients varies from patient to patient, the percentage of tests done prior to admission varies from month to month, and the number of surgical-wound infections varies from doctor to doctor. Such variation is often seen as positive or negative in relation to previous experiences or external standards. However, such standards are usually arbitrary, rather than empirically derived, and it is often unclear whether action is needed to change the results. For example, when the number of hospital–acquired infections increases from fifteen to twenty cases in a month, does this change indicate a problem, or is it simply the high point in a relatively stable pattern? Paul Plsek has noted that it is common sense that any set of data contains one point that is the highest. Yet many managers often act upon such data without knowing if the results are truly different (Plsek, 1992).

Quality management has developed knowledge about variation which permits managers to assess when changes in results require action. Using data from the process, variation can be classified into two types: **common cause variation** derives from the random, expected differences in results generated by any complex biological or production process; **special cause variation** is outside of what is expected and derives from identifiable changes in the people, machines, materials, methods, or measurements involved in a process (Batalden & Nolan, 1994; Berwick, 1991).

Knowing whether variation comes from special or common causes is important, because improving quality requires a different response in each case. When variation is the result of special causes, such as people doing new tasks, machines needing recalibration, or changes in the way data are collected, workers or managers must engage in problem solving to identify what is different and then take appropriate action. Removing special causes improves results and reduces variation, making the results more predictable. When variation results from common causes, reflecting the normal distribution of results inherent in complex work, however, managers and workers must first decide whether they find these results satisfactory. If so, then they should do nothing, because the seemingly unusual "high" or "low" result is attributable to random variation and future data are likely to be better. Alternatively, if the pattern of results is deemed unsatisfactory, the process needs to be carefully studied (for example, by a quality-improvement team) to determine ways to improve it and create better outcomes.

Responding to common cause variation as if it were special cause variation creates false alarms. The search for the reasons that things are different often leads to blaming individuals for poor results. Follow-up investigations waste resources, create resentment, and may increase variation as people seek to change behaviors that (if they are the product of random variation) were likely to change anyway. For example, internal reports used for quality often select out departments, units, or individuals who score the highest on a particular measure without knowing if these scores are significantly higher than other results. Reacting to data points as if they resulted from special cause when they are just varying in a random fashion is called *tampering* because it leads to unnecessary adjustments in a work process. Tampering can actually increase variation and is demoralizing to people who work on the process (Plsek, 1992). Responding to special cause variation as if it were common cause variation creates other problems. For example, a quality-improvement team may be created to investigate and improve a process when the source of the problem stemmed from the use of a new tool, or the failure to train replacement staff — both special causes. In this case there is no need to redesign processes or create new policies, but only to find out why existing processes and policies failed. Special causes are often easily remedied; more intensive responses waste resources.

A graphical tool, the control chart, has been developed to distinguish between common cause and special cause variation. Data from a process are plotted on a chart. Mathematically derived "control limits" are calculated and placed on the chart (see Figure 5-2). When all the results of a process fall between two lines, the upper and lower control limits, the process is said to be "in control" and any variation to be common cause. However, when one or more points falls outside the upper or lower control limit (UCL and LCL), the process is said to be "out of control," and managers or providers need to seek out the special causes that led to those results. (See Plsek, 1992, for a useful discussion on the construction and interpretation of control charts.)

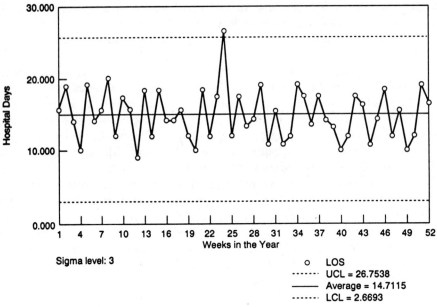

Sigma level: 3

○   LOS
‐‐‐‐‐‐‐ UCL = 26.7538
—————— Average = 14.7115
‐‐‐‐‐‐‐ LCL = 2.6693

Note: Each point represents the average length of stay for a sample of 10 patients discharged from the hospital with a principal diagnosis of pneumonia during a specified week.

Figure 5-2 *Control Chart: Length of Stay (LOS) of Pneumonia Patients by Week*

Leadership

Leadership is central to the success of the quality-improvement process. Leadership has two essential components (Joint Commission, 1991). The first is knowledge and understanding of the concepts and techniques of quality improvement. Leaders must be familiar with the concepts, understand the statistical techniques and tools, and be knowledgeable about processes and systems in their organization and how to improve them. The second component is personal involvement. Leaders must not only ensure that there are people to perform the various tasks and functions of quality improvement; they must also participate in the quality-improvement efforts by helping to set priorities, reviewing reports, participating in interpretation of data, formulating and/or approving actions, and monitoring and reevaluating priorities for action. Senior managers can also serve as excellent role models by identifying the core processes in their own work and using quality-improvement methods and tools to improve them.

Essential roles and responsibilities of management leadership in TQM include being personally committed, serving as a role model, developing a vision statement and other components of the TQM plan, training others, providing resources, aligning management systems with the TQM process, giving recognition, regularly reviewing progress, managing resistance, and empowering others (Melum &

Sinioris, 1992). These roles have several implications: management must change its own behavior before expecting others to do so, TQM must become a basic function of management, and management must make an investment in TQM.

Employee Involvement

The successful implementation of quality improvement cannot be dictated or conducted by the CEO or senior management; it requires the active participation of employees from all parts of the organization and cooperation across departmental and professional lines. Achieving such participation and cooperation requires intensive efforts by managers and strong support for employees in learning and adopting new roles and behaviors.

Employees are encouraged to participate when training in quality-improvement principles, methods, and tools is widespread. Organizations such as St. Joseph's Health Centre in London, Ontario, have stressed the need for a broad-scale educational strategy in implementing their quality initiatives. At St. Joseph's, the Education Department was expanded and reorganized to provide courses on quality improvement. Senior and middle managers took part in these courses and then became teachers, helping to teach other managers and frontline staff (Hassen, 1993). Leaders and facilitators working with quality-improvement teams have also received additional training in quality-improvement tools and group facilitation skills.

Quality-improvement teams provide an important vehicle for employee participation in quality efforts. The membership of these teams is selected to represent staff familiar with various steps of a specific process (for example, taking and processing blood specimens). Initial quality-improvement teams often include frontline staff who have never participated in any interdepartmental groups. Although relatively few staff may participate in the initial projects, these experiences provide firsthand evidence that quality improvement requires participative management practices that allow and encourage staff to become involved in change efforts.

Training and team participation alone, however, are insufficient to support the fundamental changes required to initiate quality improvement in health-care organizations. Studies in other industries show that effective participation requires pushing power, information, knowledge, and rewards to all levels of the organization (Lawler, 1986). Health-care organizations implementing quality improvement must examine their human resources practices, alter information systems, and empower workers and teams to make decisions. These changes are difficult in any organization; they present even greater obstacles in health-care organizations where professional leadership, individual responsibility, and clinical autonomy are accepted work norms. Implementation of quality improvement requires that managers reshape organizational cultures, support top and middle managers in altering their roles, and work to ensure that a broad range of professionals and staff are given opportunities to contribute to work decisions (McLaughlin & Kaluzny, 1990).

Organizations successful in TQM have involved and empowered their employees, who are a major source of knowledge about the organization and of creativity in pursuing enhanced quality and performance. Empowerment includes enhancing employees' decision-making authority and involving them actively in searching for improved methods of delivering patient care and other services (Gaucher & Coffey, 1993).

Scientific Method

Traditional management approaches to improving work are based largely on trial and error — the implementation of solutions often with little study of underlying causes and just as little evaluation of results. Not surprisingly, these trial–and–error approaches frequently either fail to improve outcomes or result in small improvements and greatly increased costs. Many times the changes made have unintended results, and today's solutions become tomorrow's problems. Such problem solving creates an expanding spiral of problems, and managers are caught in unending circles of "fire–fighting," continually addressing symptoms without ever understanding the root causes of the problems that led to those symptoms.

In quality improvement, the search for root causes builds upon a through–going understanding of complex work processes. This knowledge must be based on relevant and representative data, not on assumptions or "gut facts." The emphasis of quality improvement on fact–based management is reinforced by the use of an explicit quality-improvement method and the widespread teaching and use of simple statistical tools such as run charts, **scatter diagrams**, and Pareto charts (Plsek, 1990; Plsek & Onnias, 1988).

Quality management requires ongoing and systematic experimentation to test new ways of doing work. Continual small-scale experimentation permits the organization to improve its efficiency by testing new ideas. This approach requires changes in behaviors (trying new ways rather than maintaining old ones); more fundamentally, it demands a change in attitudes. Risk taking, instead of being frowned upon, is supported. Work teams are encouraged to experiment, and to learn from failures as well as successes.

To be effective in teams with diverse membership, methods need to be both systematic and capable of being understood by all work group members. One approach, called FOCUS–PDCA, provides a method for designing, carrying out, and evaluating changes in work processes. Unlike many descriptions of experimental design written for experts, the straightforward step–by–step method of FOCUS–PDCA encourages the democratization of such studies, permitting team members to share insights and jointly decide where to focus their improvement efforts. This method is also useful for individual problem solving (see Table 5-2) (Batalden, 1991).

Benchmarking and Best Practices

Benchmarking, the identification and adaptation of best practices, is a powerful tool developed originally by Xerox (Camp, 1989), and widely used to improve work processes. Simply put, benchmarking requires careful study of work processes in other organizations, and use of this knowledge to improve processes in one's own organization. Effective benchmarking involves identifying key measures (such as turnaround time) of a production or service process, comparing this process in different organizations, seeking the best example, and then using that knowledge to design new processes or improve existing ones.

Although managers and clinicians often examine health-care programs developed in other settings, they are only beginning to use the detailed and systematic

Table 5-2 • FOCUS–PDCA

- Find a process to improve
- Organize a team that knows the process
- Clarify current knowledge of the process
- Understand sources of process variation
- Select the process improvement
- Plan the improvement and continued data collection
- Do the improvement, data collection, and analysis
- Check and study the results
- Act to hold the gains and continue to improve the process

Reprinted with permission of Hospital Corporation of America from Quality Resources Group, Hospital Corporation of America, A Brief History of Hospitalwide Quality Improvement at HCA, copyright 1992.

methods of benchmarking to improve care. In many health-care organizations, the benchmarking process begins with attending national meetings, talking to colleagues, and reviewing the literature to identify key organizations. (Key organizations are not limited to health care, but may even be other industries [Marszalek–Gaucher & Coffey, 1990].) Teams then visit the key organizations to study and discuss their methods and determine how the lessons of the key organizations can be applied in their own organization. This sharing of knowledge allows the team to improve their own performance.

Baxter Healthcare has developed a benchmarking model which has been used by a number of hospitals to improve clinical processes and reduce the costs of care. Presbyterian Hospital in New York City, for example, used the Baxter model to reduce the costs of coronary artery bypass graft (CABG) surgery while maintaining quality of care. Prior to their investigation, Presbyterian Hospital had much higher costs compared with comparable hospitals. Study of practices in other hospitals helped identify unnecessary lab testing, encouraged efforts to reduce lengths of stay, and led to changes in operating room procedures. These results generated considerable cost savings, improved patient satisfaction, and increased cooperation among staff (Lenz, Myers, Nordlund, Sullivan, & Vasista, 1994).

APPLICATION TO PRACTICE

Organizations have initiated the quality-improvement process in a variety of ways. Some have made major resource commitments to training staff in quality-improvement philosophy and methods. Following training, these organizations commission large numbers of teams and provide skilled facilitators to coach the teams. They recruit or develop experts to provide ongoing coaching and consultation to senior management on strategic directions for these quality-improvement efforts. Other organizations have begun more slowly. In these cases, senior managers and clinicians often take one to two years developing knowledge about this new management approach, then gradually initiate training and pilot projects within the organization. Either approach can be successful, as long as senior leadership remains focused on quality improvement and does not delegate these activities to staff.

Hospital–Wide Quality Improvement

Paul Batalden and the Quality Resource Group at the Hospital Corporation of America have developed an explicit guideline for implementing quality improvement, which they have used with a number of HCA and other hospitals. This guideline, which they call the *Roadmap for Change*, is a step–by–step approach to organizational transformation (Quality Resource Group, 1992). The roadmap starts with the curiosity of the CEO and stresses the involvement of the organization's top leadership in learning, practice, commitment, and organizational follow–through for **Continuous Quality Improvement (CQI)**. Although the members of the Quality Resource Group stress that their roadmap is a guide, rather than a set of requirements, their experience has reinforced the need for senior leaders to invest efforts in learning and practicing quality improvement before initiating a wide–scale involvement of other levels of the organization (P. B. Batalden, 1992). The Quality Resource Group (1992) notes that the transformation to a quality organization "requires thoughtful and anticipatory leadership. Starting simple, practicing often, and seeking deeper knowledge will build a strong quality culture" (p. 4).

West Paces Medical Center, an HCA hospital in Atlanta, Georgia, was one of the first HCA hospitals to adopt quality improvement as a management approach. Chip Caldwell, the CEO, has taken an active role in orienting all existing and new employees in the quality principles used at the hospital. After training senior managers, physicians, and many employees, the hospital initiated twenty–two quality-improvement teams. These teams initiated many improvements: they reduced the turnaround time between patients in the operating rooms, decreased the waste in intravenous medications by 45 percent, and lowered the number of caesarean sections performed (Walton, 1990). Caldwell believes that their success with quality-improvement rests on two critical components: first, the adoption of a standard quality-improvement model based on the FOCUS–PDCA approach coupled with a strong emphasis on measuring key processes within the organization; and, second, the establishment of an organizational culture supportive of quality improvement. The cultural transformation requires establishing TQM vision and policy, deploying this policy to all parts of the organization, and maintaining the momentum for change by celebrating achievements and reviewing progress at regular intervals (Caldwell, 1993).[1]

---

[1]The merger of HCA with Columbia Healthcare in 1993 led to the dismantling of the HCA Quality Resource Group, and a decreased emphasis on quality-improvement efforts in hospitals such as West Paces Medical Center. The knowledge gained from these activities, however, continues to be applied in other settings.

Clinical Quality Improvement

Most hospitals have focused their initial quality-improvement efforts on improving administrative processes (such as billing) or processes supporting clinical care (such as dispensing medications or discharging patients). Because these issues are often quite visible to the senior managers initiating the quality-improvement efforts, this emphasis is natural. Such experiences, however, have engendered some fears that physicians, nurses, and other clinicians may resist involvement in quality-improvement efforts, or that quality improvement has little potential for improving the processes of direct-patient care. There is considerable evidence, however, that clinicians find quality improvement useful, and that the results of clinical quality improvement can improve both patient outcomes and satisfaction with care.

At Intermountain Health Care, an integrated health-care system located in Utah and two adjoining states, Brent James, a physician and quality expert, has developed a clinical quality-improvement model that links a computerized clinical information system with quality tools and methods. Data on clinical processes and outcomes are analyzed to identify ways to improve care delivery. Five initial teams studied quality improvement in five clinical areas: transurethral prostatectomy (TURP), CABG, pneumonia, gall bladder, and total hip replacement. Over 160 other teams focusing on both clinical and support processes have been created at Intermountain. These teams have implemented a number of improvements in patient care. For example, a team studying renal failure following cardiac catheterization discovered that patients were inadequately hydrated before the catheter was inserted. The new treatment protocols recommended by the team have eliminated renal failure in these patients. Another team, studying postoperative deep-wound infections at one of the hospitals, discovered that better timing of the delivery of prophylactic antibiotics could decrease the incidence of infections by 50 percent (GOAL/QPC, 1992). Clinical quality improvement at Intermountain Healthcare and other organizations has demonstrated the potency of quality-improvement methods for improving patient outcomes.

Community–Based Quality Improvement Efforts

Many of the health-care organizations that were early leaders in quality improvement have been teaching hospitals or members of multi–institutional health-care systems that have the resources to devote to training staff, supporting quality improvement teams, and measuring results. Smaller hospitals, health maintenance organizations (HMOs), and community agencies, although they often have more limited resources, can also develop effective quality-improvement efforts. Smaller size may mean fewer cross–disciplinary barriers to overcome in improving systems of care. Such agencies have an additional advantage in that their sizes and roles may help them develop stronger linkages with other agencies, and together the agencies can generate a strategy for improving the health of their communities.

Magic Valley Regional Hospital in Twin Falls, Idaho, recognized early in its examination of TQM that the hospital needed to work with other health-care agencies (including a competing hospital), local businesses and government, the junior college, and other groups to create a community–wide effort to improve the health of local citizens. The TQM efforts at Magic Valley have both helped to build more effective working relationships within the hospital and strengthened efforts to improve community health. Among early efforts at Magic Valley have been the development of a free prostate screening clinic, a program to reduce motor vehicle accidents through education, and the improvement of perinatal outcomes by ensuring better coordination between hospital and community care for newborns. The work at Magic Valley has provided a model for other groups seeking to use quality-improvement methods to improve the health of their communities (Joint Commission, 1992). The Institute of Healthcare Improvement launched a demonstration project on community–based quality-improvement projects to support such efforts.

HEALTH-CARE SYSTEM ISSUES

The successes achieved by these organizations (and many others) in applying industrial quality-improvement methods has influenced changes in accreditation standards for health-care organizations. These changes encourage the use of quality improvement methods. Other supports have emerged to facilitate quality-improvement efforts and to transfer lessons learned between leaders and organizations. New organizations and networks are supporting health-care organizations in learning about and adopting the quality-improvement philosophy and methods.

Health Care Accreditation

The Joint Commission on Accreditation of Healthcare Organizations (Joint Commission) is an organization that fosters improvement in the delivery of health care through its peer review program of United States health-care organizations. In 1987, it initiated its "Agenda for Change" to make the accreditation process more effective by revising the standards with which organizations were reviewed and developing a set of quality **indicators** to measure performance (Joint Commission, 1991). The Joint Commission considers quality improvement as a means to the end of improved performance. It recognizes that quality must be adopted as a priority by individual organizations and cannot be imposed through external regulation. The Joint Commission has therefore adopted a philosophy of improvement oriented to the achievement of improved performance, which includes leadership commitment, communication, and performance measurement (O'Leary, 1991).

The 1994 Joint Commission standards for accreditation incorporate principles and techniques of CQI. The standards encourage leadership responsibility for quality improvement, the use of specific techniques, education and training, communication and collaboration, and the evaluation of the effectiveness of the quality-improvement activities. This initiative is meant to encourage and assist health-care organizations in implementing quality improvement. (See Chapter 17 for an in–depth discussion of the Joint Commission and organizational performance.)

The Canadian Council on Health Facilities Accreditation (CCHFA), the Canadian counterpart of the Joint Commission, has also adopted new standards based, in part, on the principles of quality improvement. These new standards integrate concepts of vision, leadership, teamwork, and employee empowerment. They emphasize the improvement of patient care and support processes, and look for evidence that organizations seek out and incorporate information based on the needs of patients, families, and others who benefit from their work. (See Chapter 15 for a discussion of quality in the Canadian health-care system.)

Institute for Healthcare Improvement

The Institute for Healthcare Improvement (IHI) was created to succeed the National Demonstration Project on Quality Improvement in Health Care. It aims to help the United States and Canadian health-care systems continually increase their quality and value (Institute for Heathcare Improvement, 1993). The measures of this improvement include better clinical outcomes, improved health status, improved access to care, greater ease of use, lower cost, and higher satisfaction for those who receive care and for their communities.

The IHI has adopted four key strategies: (1) to build knowledge about quality improvement in health care, (2) to augment the capacity of organizations and health-care systems to improve, (3) to facilitate the demonstration of successful improvements, and (4) to support collaborative change. To achieve these goals, the IHI emphasizes increasing the impact of efforts by cooperating, rather than competing, with others; encouraging the building of knowledge through scientific study of improvement efforts; and focusing on improvement at the community and health-care system levels, as well as the organizational level.

The IHI sponsors an annual National Forum on Quality Improvement in Health Care, continuing education courses on quality philosophy and methods, and special initiatives dealing with such issues as regulation, research, professional education, and support to transformational managers. The IHI has been a major driving force in fostering knowledge about quality-improvement applications in health care and disseminating shared experiences and lessons learned to a wide audience. In addition to the courses and conferences it offers, the IHI has sponsored leadership councils and networks to facilitate linkages among professionals across the country.

Networks

All health-care organizations face similar challenges in their quality-improvement efforts. To accelerate the development of organization–wide quality-improvement initiatives and reduce duplication, a variety of quality-improvement networks have developed to exchange information about education, quality-improvement projects, and systems alignment. These networks decrease the need for separate efforts in each organization. The best known of these networks is the Quality Management Network (QMN), which links over thirty health-care organizations from across the United States. Network members participate in regular meetings at which they interact with leading experts, share their experiences, and identify key needs and strategies. Other networks, such as the Quality Improvement Networks (QINs) sponsored by Healthcare Forum, the GOAL/QPC Health Care Application Research Committee, and the Ontario Network for Continuous Quality Improvement, also disseminate information and provide support to member organizations that are seeking to learn and apply quality-improvement principles and methods (Baker, 1992).

CONCLUSION

Total Quality Management has attracted a number of vocal critics who view it as a passing management fad unlikely to have a sustained impact on the effectiveness of organizations. However, TQM ideas are not new; they build upon a knowledge base that has developed over sixty years. Although experience with quality-improvement methods is still at early stages in health-care organizations, many companies in Japan and North America have achieved notable successes using TQM.

Initiating quality improvement is neither quick nor easy. Many experts suggest that organizations require five to eight years to incorporate these new approaches. Although immediate benefits from quality-improvement teams will be evident in early stages, full deployment requires changing organizational cultures and the ways managers, clinicians, and staff work. Many organizations will fail in their TQM efforts because their senior leaders see TQM as a quick fix rather than a framework for enduring change; because they delegate responsibilities for quality to staff rather than assuming leadership; and because they fail to integrate their quality efforts into the strategic direction and daily operation of their organizations. Some studies suggest that as many as two–thirds of the organizations initiating quality improvement will abandon these efforts when they perceive only limited returns for their efforts. One study has suggested that many of these failures result from an inability or unwillingness to focus quality-improvement efforts on issues important to customers ("Business: The Cracks in Quality," 1992).

There is no one best way to initiate quality-improvement efforts in health-care organizations. It is important, however, that these efforts be based on careful study and thorough understanding of the key principles of quality improvement. And, although many initial improvement projects may focus on administrative and clinical-support processes, it is crucial that quality improvement involve clinicians, and that quality-improvement projects focus on improving health outcomes by improving the care delivered to patients.

The successful TQM organizations are likely to be those whose senior leaders continue to pursue an understanding of how to employ TQM methods to improve their organizations. They will seek out and remove barriers to improving work, and help others in the organization learn to adopt new roles and new behaviors. Rather than becoming tied to particular ideas or methods, they will search for new ways to improve. As they develop greater understanding, they will abandon labeling certain activities as quality improvement; instead, quality methods and efforts will be integrated into the day–to–day operations and the very fabric of the organization.

REFERENCES

Baker, G. R. (1992). Networks for continuous quality improvement in health care. *Canadian Journal of Quality in Health Care, 9*(4), 3–8.

Baker, G. R., Barnsley, J., & Murray, M. (1993). The development of quality improvement in Canadian health care organizations. *Leadership in Health Services, 2*(5), 18–23.

Batalden, P. B. (1991). Organization-wide quality improvement in health care. *Topics in Health Records Management, 11*(3), 1–12.

Batalden, P. B., & Nolan, T. W. (1994). Knowledge for the leadership of continual improvement in healthcare. In R. Taylor & S. Taylor (Eds.), *The AUPHA manual of health services management* (pp. 60–72). Rockville, MD: Aspen.

Berwick, D. (1989). Continuous improvement as an ideal in health care. *New England Journal of Medicine, 320*(1), 53–56.

Berwick, D., Godfrey, A. B., & Roessner, J. (1990). *Curing health care: New strategies for quality improvement.* San Francisco: Jossey–Bass.

Berwick, D. M. (1991). Controlling variation in health care: A consultation from Walter Shewhart. *Medical Care, 29*(12), 1212–1225.

Business: The cracks in quality. (1992). *Economist, 7755*(323), 67–68.

Caldwell, C. (1993). Accelerators and inhibitors to organizational change in a hospital. *Quality Review Bulletin, 19*(2), 42–46.

Camp, R. C. (1989). *Benchmarking.* Milwaukee, WI: American Society for Quality Control.

Cole, R. (1991). Large scale change and the quality revolution. In A. Mohrman et al. (Eds.), *Large scale organizational change* (pp. 229–254). San Francisco: Jossey–Bass.

Deming, W. E. (1986). *Out of the crisis.* Cambridge, MA: Massachusetts Institute of Technology.

Eubanks, P. (1992). The CEO experience: TQM/CQI. *Hospitals, 66*(11), 24–36.

Feigenbaum, A. (1961). *Total Quality Control.* New York: McGraw–Hill.

Garvin, D. (1988). *Managing quality: The strategic and competitive edge.* New York: The Free Press.

Garvin, D. (1991). How the Baldrige Award really works. *Harvard Business Review, 69*(6), 80–93.

Gaucher, E. J., & Coffey, R. J. (1993). *Total quality in health care.* San Francisco: Jossey–Bass.

GOAL/QPC. (1992). *Putting the "T" in health care TQM. A model for integrated TQM: Clinical care and operations.* Meuthen, MA: Author.

Hassen, P. (1993). *Rx for hospitals: New hope for Medicare in the nineties.* Toronto, Canada: Stoddart.

Institute for Healthcare Improvement. (1993). *Mission and principles for the work of the IHI.* Boston: Author.

Ishikawa, K. (1985). *What is Total Quality Control? The Japanese way.* Englewood Cliffs, NJ: Prentice–Hall.

Joint Commission on Accreditation of Healthcare Organizations. (1991). *The transition from QA to CQI: An introduction to quality improvement in health care.* Oakbrook Terrace, IL: Author.

Joint Commission on Accreditation of Healthcare Organizations. (1992). *Striving for improvement: Six hospitals in search of quality.* Oakbrook Terrace, IL: Author.

Juran, J. M. (1988). *Juran on planning for quality.* New York: The Free Press.

Juran, J. M. (1989). *Juran on leadership for quality.* New York: The Free Press.

Juran, J. M. (1993). Made in U.S.A.: A renaissance in quality. *Harvard Business Review, 71*(4), 42–50.

Kearns, D. T., & Nadler, D. A. (1992). *Prophets in the dark: How Xerox reinvented itself and beat back the Japanese.* New York: Harper Business.

Laffel, G. (1991). Education: Total Quality Management in health care — The need and the opportunity. *Current Surgery, 48*(9), 617–625.

Laffel, G., & Blumenthal, D. (1989). The case for using industrial quality management sciences in health care organizations. *New England Journal of Medicine, 262*(20), 2869–2873.

Lawler, E. E., III. (1986). *High–involvement management: Participative strategies for improving organizational performance.* San Francisco: Jossey–Bass.

Leebov, W., & Ersoz, C. J. (1991). *The health care manager's guide to Continuous Quality Improvement.* Chicago: American Hospital.

Lenz, S., Myers, S., Nordlund, S., Sullivan, D., & Vasista, V. (1994). Benchmarking: Finding ways to improve. *Joint Commission Journal on Quality Improvement, 20*(5), 250–259.

Marszalek-Gaucher, E., & Coffey, R. J. (1990). *Transforming healthcare organizations: How to achieve and sustain organizational excellence.* San Francisco: Jossey-Bass.

McLaughlin, C. P., & Kaluzny, A. D. (1990). Total Quality Management in health: Making it work. *Health Care Management Review, 15*(3), 7–14.

Melum, M. M., & Sinioris, M. K. (1992). *Total Quality Management: The health care pioneers.* Chicago: American Hospital.

O'Leary, D. S. (1991, November). Moving healthcare toward CQI: The Joint Commission's plans for the future. *The Quality Letter, 3*(9), 12–16.

Plsek, P. E. (1990). Resource B: A primer on quality improvement tools. In D. Berwick, A. B. Godfrey, & J. Roessner, *Curing health care: New strategies for quality improvement* (pp. 177–219). San Francisco: Jossey–Bass.

Plsek, P. E. (1992). Tutorial: Introduction to control charts. *Quality Management in Health Care, 1*(1), 65–74.

Plsek, P. E., & Onnias, A. (1988). *Quality improvement tools.* Wilton, CT: Juran Institute.

Quality Resource Group, Hospital Corporation of America. (1992). *A brief history of hospital-wide quality improvement at HCA.* Nashville, TN: Author.

Shewhart, W. A. (1980 [1931]). *Economic control of quality of manufactured product.* Milwaukee, WI: American Society of Quality Control.

United States Department of Commerce. (1993). *Malcolm Baldrige National Quality Award 1994 award criteria.* Gaithersburg, MD: National Institute of Standards and Technology.

Walton, M. (1986). *The Deming management method.* New York: Perigee Books.

Walton, M. (1990). *Deming management at work.* New York: G. P. Putnam's Sons.

ADDITIONAL READING

Batalden, P. B., & Buchanan, E. D. (1989). Industrial models of quality improvement. In N. Goldfield & D. B. Nash (Eds.), *Providing quality care: The challenge to clinicians* (pp. 133–159). Philadelphia, PA: American College of Physicians.

Batalden, P. B., & Stoltz, P. K. (1993). A framework for the continual improvement of health care: Building and applying professional knowledge to test changes in daily work. *Joint Commission Journal on Quality Improvement, 19*(10): 424–447.

Berwick, D. M. (1989). Sounding board: Continuous improvement as an ideal in health care. *New England Journal of Medicine, 320*(1), 53–56.

Crosby, P. B. (1989). *Quality without tears: The art of hassle free management*. New York: The Free Press.

James, B. C. (1993). Seeking health care quality: The implications of medical practice guidelines. *Frontiers of Health Services Management, 10*(1), 3–37.

Joiner, B. L. (1994). *Fourth generation management: The new business consciousness*. New York: McGraw–Hill.

Langley, G. J., Nolan, K. M., & Nolan, T. W. (1994). The foundations of improvement. *Quality Progress, 27*(6), 81–86.

McLaughlin, C. P., & Kaluzny, A. D. (1994). *Continuous improvement in health care: Theory, implications and applications*. Gaithersburg, MD: Aspen.

Sahney, V. K., & Warden, G. L. (1991). The quest for quality and productivity in health services. *Frontiers of Health Services Management, 7*(4), 2–40.

Avedis Donabedian

CHAPTER **6**

Models of Quality Assurance

INTRODUCTION

Our notions of how the quality of health care can be assessed and improved are now being scrutinized and reshaped. There seems to be, as it were, a contest between two models of **Quality Assurance (QA)** — one indigenous to our field and the other a newcomer to it. The traditional I shall call the "health-care model" and the new the "industrial model." Neither of these two terms stands for anything entirely homogeneous or precise. Each offers a variety of concepts and methods. Nevertheless, two families are distinguishable, and it is only familial features that I shall compare. Moreover, I shall be dealing not with actual everyday examples of each, but with the intended, idealized forms of the models.

I shall try in this chapter to examine the main features of the two models hoping to identify and understand their similarities and differences. The first, and potentially most fundamental of these features, is the meaning assigned in each model to **quality** itself.

THE NATURE OF QUALITY

A distinctive characteristic of the industrial model is its overwhelming emphasis on the consumer as the final arbiter of quality. Whether one offers a service or a product, it is ultimately the consumers who say whether or not these meet their needs

---

Note: This chapter is adapted from "Continuity and Change in the Quest for Quality" in *Clinical Performance and Quality Health Care,* *1*(1), 9–16, Jan., Feb., March, 1993. It is a revised version of an address to the Ninth World Congress of the International Society for Quality Assurance in Health Care, Mexico City, May 1992.

and expectations. Hence, the aim is not only to merit consumer satisfaction but also, if possible, by exceeding expectations, to elicit joy, enthusiasm, and continuing loyalty.

In the industrial model there is, accordingly, continuing preoccupation with eliciting consumer requirements and translating these into product characteristics. In one influential formulation, the consumer becomes, in fact, part of the production line, because by using a product or experiencing a service, the consumer tests its quality and generates information conducive to its improvement. It also is recognized, of course, that scientific and technological progress can create products or services judged by their producers to be of superior quality. Still, only eventual consumer approval can validate that judgment.

In the industrial model, cost enters the definition of quality because, in the customer's mind, price and quality are linked. Consequently, cost control by producers is needed to ensure consumer satisfaction, to generate sales, and to confer market advantage, eventuating in financial success and growth.

If we now turn to the health-care model, we find both remarkable similarities and significant differences. We are similar in our obligation to merit consumer satisfaction by providing care in ways convenient, congenial, and pleasant to patients. Moreover, in a manner even more fundamental than postulated by the industrial model, we hold that the preferences of the informed patient, as to both **outcomes** and means, are ingredients essential to any definition of quality in health care.

But the health-care model is also different, because it needs to accommodate a much more complex set of responsibilities toward individual consumers and society in the definition of quality. This adds both richness and inner tension to the definition of quality in health care. I shall comment briefly on these distinctions under three headings: responsibilities toward individuals, responsibilities toward society, and responsibilities for managing the cost/quality relationship.

Responsibilities toward Individuals

Regarding individuals, we are not simply purveyors of satisfaction. Perhaps because patients are often very ill equipped to distinguish good care from bad, we, in common with other professionals, have been assigned a fiduciary responsibility: that of acting on behalf of patients, to serve their best interests as we judge these to be. It is true that this can lead to paternalism, authoritarianism, and even arrogance — dangers to be avoided at all costs. But the moral imperative remains: to guard the patient's best interests, even against the patient's own wishes.

Furthermore, because health care touches upon such profoundly intimate, sensitive, and threatening aspects of life, our concepts of how the interpersonal relationship should be conducted are infinitely more complex than the more superficial supplier/customer exchanges of the business world. And, finally, health care is so dominantly a product of the joint efforts of practitioners and patients that the **customer** is more intimately part of the production line than even the industrial model has envisaged. The ability to capacitate patients to participate in the production of health care is a correspondingly more salient attribute of quality in health care.

Responsibilities toward Society

The health-care professions function under a social contract very different from that governing business or industry. On the one hand, we are responsible for the welfare of individuals, and on the other hand, for social welfare. Our social responsibilities take many forms that I shall not stop to consider in detail. I need only mention the compelling need to achieve equity in the distribution of the benefits of health care and, a related matter, the greater centrality of the cost/quality relationship, as I shall immediately show.

Responsibilities for Managing the Cost/Quality Relationship

The two models are in agreement on the central importance of efficiency as an ingredient either inherent to quality or closely linked to it. But because the industrial model is more subject to the influence of relatively free markets, efficiency has a more determining role in it.

The industrial model also has a somewhat different view of the cost/quality relationship. It is recognized, although not sufficiently emphasized, that improvements in design can add to cost. But it is usually affirmed that these added costs are more than offset by efficiencies in production and larger sales. Quality, in the industrial model, not only is free, it actually pays. Thus, happily, the potential conflict between higher quality and lower costs is eliminated. This ability of the industrial model to harmonize seeming opposites is one manifestation of its fundamentally optimistic nature, even its utopianism. And it is responsible, in no small measure, for the model's powerful appeal.

In contrast, the health-care model is much more cognizant of the added cost of added quality, primarily in expenditures for care, and secondarily in the contribution to a longevity that some would regard as unproductive, if not downright wasteful. Hence, our model is much more concerned with the balance of costs and benefits than is the industrial model. This is only partly attributable to the diminishing returns of health to added care, and the consequences of longevity as a product. It is also because we function in a context less responsive to market forces and more obedient to ethical and social imperatives.

The balance of costs and benefits also creates a severe perturbation within the definition of quality itself, robbing us, irrevocably, of the harmoniousness that the industrial model so seductively offers. This is because health care is not only a private good, but a public good as well. It is financed to a large degree by the public, and the benefits of its goodness, as well as the harmfulness of its badness, spill beyond the individual. The harmonization of the individual and social preferences and interests becomes, therefore, a knotty problem in the health-care model of quality.

These differences, I hasten to say, are more often matters of degree than absolute divergence. The industrial model could easily accommodate the cost/benefit exchange in estimating the salability of services and products; increasingly, it needs to account for social consequences such as resource depletion and environmental pollution. The more one compares social policy in different fields, the more one is impressed, not so much by apparent disparities as by the constant recurrence of common themes.

THE SCOPE OF QUALITY

The industrial model prides itself on being all-inclusive — total. *Total quality* is the banner under which it marches. So we must ask in what ways may quality, or the concern for it, be total. The architects of the industrial model have three answers.

First, quality may be total by expansions in the definition of quality itself. In the development of the industrial model, this has meant a progression from initial preoccupation with meeting engineering specifications to a virtual deification of consumer wishes and expectations, followed by smaller steps to the inclusion of costs and, possibly, the production of the precisely correct quantities as well.

Second, quality may be total by embracing the entire set of structural units, processes, and persons involved in the conceptualization, design, resource use, production, sales, and consumption of any product or service. This encompasses all extrainstitutional as well as intrainstitutional participants in the sequence.

Third, quality may be total by pervasiveness of involvement in quality planning and improvement of everyone in an organization, at all levels, in all units, and vertically down a hierarchy, as well as horizontally across all of its subdivisions.

How is the health-care model similar or different in these respects?

It is easy to find, in theoretical formulations of the health-care model, crystal-clear advocacy for successive expansions in the definition of quality accompanied by corresponding expansions in the objects of **Quality Assessment and Improvement (QA&I)**: for example, from preoccupation with technical care to inclusion of the interpersonal relationship as well; from preoccupation with effectiveness to inclusion of efficiency first, and then of optimality as well; and from preoccupation with individual welfare to inclusion of the welfare of the collectivity as well.

Our conceptual formulations also have emphasized the need to take a more embracive view in assessments of quality, so that one includes not simply the contributions of physicians to care, but the contribution of all caregivers; not simply the contributions of professional caregivers but the contributions of patients and of their families as well; and not simply the care provided at any one site in isolation, but the care given at any site for any given episode of illness, and eventually, care given during successive episodes as well.

The health-care model, no less than the industrial model, requires that concern for quality pervade the institution as a whole. But there is a fundamental distinction. The health-care model has concerned itself almost exclusively with the properties of clinical care and the functions closely related to that care, irrespective of whether the care has been given by professional personnel, by technical personnel, or by patients and family members. But attention is not uniformly accorded to all segments of this spectrum. There is an explicit or implicit set of priorities that focus attention — priorities guided by consequentiality, relevance, scope of responsibility, and capacity to influence. As a result, the technical care provided by physicians to individual patients has generally emerged as the predominant preoccupation. And it is this preoccupation that our critics have justifiably condemned as "narrow." It is a deficiency we should be ready to acknowledge and quick to remedy.

Yet there is also a danger in defining quality too broadly, by including the efficiency and effectiveness of all products and services supportive to clinical care, no matter how remote. The danger is one of goal displacement, from clinical care to marginal operations, often accompanied by disproportionate concern for cost savings. If this widening of scope is accompanied by a relative neglect of clinical care, we could justly call it not *total quality*, but *peripheral quality*. And if we wished to be exceptionally charitable, we would call it *contextual quality*, at best. We must ask ourselves if the word *quality* could lose its distinctive meaning and we, our distinctive function, if the term is applied almost indiscriminately to too many things.

THE NATURE OF "THE QUALITY PROBLEM"

At the heart of the industrial model is a set of postulates that constitutes what variously has been called "the new philosophy," or in a more radical vein, "a thought revolution." These postulates include the total view of quality I have just described. There are also postulates about the nature of what we might call "the quality problem" and of the strategies appropriate to dealing with it.

As to the quality problem (which devotees of "right-speak" prefer to call the quality "challenge" or "opportunity"), we can perceive it in terms of goals and causes.

Regarding goals, the dominant theme is a "constancy of purpose" in placing "quality first," and on defining quality as congruence with consumer requirements. A failure to embrace these goals is regarded, of course, as the root cause for deficiencies in quality. But, in a more immediate sense, deficiencies in quality are held to arise only infrequently from the unskillfulness of individual workers, and even less often from their being insufficiently motivated to do well. The dominant causes, rather, are held to be deficiencies in the systems and processes that are responsible for the design and production of goods and services. Each complex of system, process, and product characteristics has necessarily associated with it an inherent capacity to produce goods and services of definable quality. To the extent that individual workers are, themselves, part of a system or **process**, their own characteristics contribute to the inherent capacity for quality that I have described. But workers cannot by their own efforts make a system perform better than it is programmed, almost predestined, to perform. Therefore, such systems tend to fall into a steady state characterized by an average level of quality, accompanied, necessarily, by random-seeming variations around that average. These variations are attributed to what has been called *common causes* inherent to the system or process itself.

Superimposed on these, from time to time, are unaccustomed variations produced by intercurrent events called *special causes* that perturb, to a greater or lesser degree, the steady state. These special causes can be perceived, identified, localized, and corrected as they occur. But the underlying steady state cannot be altered without fundamental changes in the system itself. And because workers, by their unaided efforts, usually cannot bring about such fundamental change, the greater responsibility for the programmmed deficiencies in quality must rest squarely on those responsible for the design and management of systems, processes, and products.

How does the health-care model stand relative to these formulations? Regarding goals, it has been, from time immemorial, our highest purpose to put quality first. In this respect, we have nothing to learn from the industrial model, except perhaps a reaffirmation that can vivify the constancy of purpose that we also need. One must wonder at the irony in seeing the industrial model adopt values we have long held, while powerful forces all around us are pushing us to abandon these in favor of putting cost first!

As to the causes of deficiencies in quality, the health-care model has affirmed without question that the fundamental determinants of quality are inherent to the design of systems and processes, which, in our vocabulary, we have called **structure**. The activity by which performance is kept under constant review we regard primarily as a source of information that helps us adjust quality by appropriate modifications in system design. In all these respects, despite differences in vocabulary, the two models are essentially congruent.

There is, however, a significant difference as well. In the health-care model there is a predominant emphasis on the contribution of professional workers to excellence or the lack of it. This is not an unreasonable stance, given the nature of our science and of our work; it is a stance well supported by empirical evidence. Serious failures in quality have been demonstrably attributable, in a large percentage of cases, to defects in professional judgment and skill. Our attention to modifying professional behavior is consequently well justified. But our model specifies, as does the industrial model, that worker qualifications are an integral part of the system of production. Therefore, the two models differ not so much in whether deficiencies in quality arise in system properties or individual performance, but in which parts of a system are most likely to fail. Our model, I believe quite justifiably, places more emphasis on the human components of a system. Still, we could learn from the industrial model to take account of a larger range of system properties in our search for the causes of variations in quality, and to be much slower to assign blame to individuals. The theoretical formulations that underlie the distinction between **common cause variation** and **special cause variation** could help us in this respect.

STRATEGIES OF QUALITY ASSURANCE AND IMPROVEMENT

The strategies advocated by the industrial model to protect and enhance quality flow partly from its postulates concerning the determinants of quality. To an equal, if not greater, degree, they flow from an almost utopian view of human nature and of formal organizations as social systems. In another of its grand harmonizations, the industrial model affirms a fundamental congruity of goals and interests between production workers and management. This congruity it proposes to cultivate and reinforce through a carefully crafted set of ideological and instrumental manipulations.

The centerpiece of these efforts is a redefinition of authority and responsibility that harnesses production workers to the quality promotion enterprise, without in any way diminishing management's ultimate accountability for it. To some extent, this realignment simply recognizes the strategic location of production workers, at the point where the many cognitive and material resources of an organization are converted to products or services. Production workers are the agents of this transformation, have detailed knowledge of its properties, obtain early intimations of any abnormalities it might suffer, and are in a position to take early corrective action. But awareness of this instrumentally critical location would count for little were it not accompanied by a radical reassessment of human potential and motivation. At its most metaphysical, this reassessment views humans as essentially good rather than perverse. More proximately, it recognizes in them both a capacity and an urge for knowledge, self-actualization, and social integration. It intends, therefore, to give scope to these powerful impulses in the workplace. By granting workers the opportunity and the means to monitor and adjust their own work, it restores individual pride in workmanship; by providing continuous opportunities for group activities designed to identify and solve problems shared by coworkers, it adds the force of social approval to its arsenal of motivators.

The industrial model promotes social cohesion even further by fostering a sense of responsibility, at each stage in the sequence of production, for the needs and requirements of the next stage. By perceiving each stage in this sequence as a "customer" of the stage before and a "supplier" to the stage that follows, it does not merely affirm an instrumental reality, it sets up a chain of obligational relationships that pulls together the entire enterprise.

The foregoing reformulation of the capacities, motivations, roles, and responsibilities of production workers carries with it, necessarily, a radical reformulation of the nature of management as well. Now management must lead rather than dictate; it must motivate rather than intimidate; it must educate rather than direct; and it must be ready to listen and learn, rather than merely to instruct. And even the structure of an organization must now change: it becomes less hierarchical, less layered, with many more cross-departmental linkages as well as closer linkages between those who produce and those who plan and manage.

How does the health-care model stand in these respects? In remarkably familiar territory. For what the industrial model purports to accomplish for production workers is a well-established reality in our professional values, our professional privileges and responsibilities, and our professional forms of governance. Quite emphatically, what the industrial model stands for is not the industrialization of professional work, but the professionalization of industrial work. Rather than question or contradict us, it reaffirms the soundness of our own established traditions. It only urges us to be truer to these traditions in practice than perhaps, heretofore, we sometimes have been.

But we also have some lessons to learn. One lesson is that we have to pay greater attention to what we have called *continuity and coordination*, the clear analogues to the supplier/customer chains envisaged by the industrial model. More importantly, those of us who already enjoy the privileges of a profession, while we carry its burdens, should be willing, if the industrial model is valid, to permit analogous opportunities and responsibilities to others involved in the health-care enterprise. They should have the same opportunities to serve quality in their own respective spheres, and to derive satisfaction and pride from doing so, that we have had for so long in our own domain. Perhaps more difficult still, because patient care is almost always **multidisciplinary**, we should not only be willing to adopt a multidisciplinary approach to quality assurance, but insist on it.

There is another kind of redeployment of responsibility and opportunity that one may infer from comparing the industrial model with ours. If in business and industry there has been overwhelming concentration of power in the managerial directorate, there has been in some health-care systems a contrary imbalance: an overconcentration of power in the hands of a key production worker, the physician. Because it is characteristic of the industrial model to seek a harmonious balance between management and production, I could venture to suggest that, in some cases, a flow of some power and responsibility from physicians to management could be beneficial to the performance of the health-care enterprise as a whole.

METHODS OF QUALITY ASSURANCE AND IMPROVEMENT

The industrial model offers us a set of methods for protecting and enhancing quality in line with the basic goals, orientations, and assumptions I have described. I shall comment only on a few methods, in each case touching on only the most obvious implications for the health-care model.

In the industrial model, the effort in support of quality has a number of mutually reinforcing components. First, there is a set of activities whose purpose is to introduce fundamental improvement in product development, so the products, by initial design, are more conforming to customer requirements and less vulnerable to inexpert use. Then comes the design of the processes that are efficient, effective, and more resistant to human error. And finally, the processes of production are subjected to continuing oversight, to make certain that they function as designed. This oversight takes two forms; one is *concurrent*, meaning that the workers themselves check what they produce, or otherwise assess their performance, during the course of production, supplemented by occasional checks by their supervisors. The purpose of concurrent monitoring is early intervention to forestall or remedy deficiencies. Still another component we could call *terminal* inspection of products, the purpose being to reject products that do not meet standards before these go to the customer.

In the health-care field, the function of product development is largely assigned to technology assessment, and we are unable to recall a service once it has been received, although we can prevent it from being given if we are informed early enough of the intent to give it. As to the rest, the components of the industrial model are even more congruent with ours.

As in ours, the entire system is governed mainly by internally generated **standards** subject to periodic review. As in ours, continuous self-monitoring by the production worker on the production line is the key to keeping processes in line. As in ours, the outcomes of these processes are used to warn of possible errors that need to be rectified. It is simply not true that the industrial model ignores outcomes, has abandoned standards, and rejects inspection. It merely says that assessment of outcomes is insufficient to improve quality; that externally imposed standards are often insufficient or irrelevant; and that terminal, exlusionary inspection of products is costly to implement on a large scale, comes too late, and is wasteful. With all this, the health-care model concurs.

The industrial model is also similar to the health-care model in conceptualizing quality improvement as a continuous cycle of activities. In its vocabulary, this is variously designated the *Shewhart Cycle*, the *Deming Cycle*, or the *PDCA Cycle*, the acronym standing for *Plan, Do, Check, Act*. Unfortunately, our own quite analogous cycles have not had the advantage of snappy acronyms or august affiliations, but they are no less powerful and are perhaps better suited to our circumstances.

The quality improvement cycle, by its very nature, envisages continuous readjustments of quality that are likely to be small, especially if much of the readjustment is in the hands of production workers whose abilities to make radical changes are limited. In one formulation of the industrial model, this gradualism has been elevated, I believe quite unnecessarily, to the status of an ideology. It seems to me immaterial whether quality improves painfully, in little steps, or exuberantly, in leaps, as long as it improves. It is categorically untrue that the health-care model aims to stabilize quality rather than improve it. Even if this were our avowed purpose, the continuous progress in our science and technology and rising social expectations would make it impossible for us to adhere to it.

Another important feature of the industrial model is a recommended, even prescribed, road map for identifying and solving problems of quality, accompanied by a set of analytic tools for doing so. Some of the processes, methods, and tools are designed to guide group interaction in pursuit of problem identification and consensus. Others are meant to guide data collection; localize aberrant phenomena in time, place, and person; assign priority, mainly on grounds of relative frequency; and map the several causal factors that are likely to have played a role in any given situation. None of these procedures, methods, and tools can be regarded as proprietary to the industrial model. And even those that seem to be, bear such a strong resemblance to the epidemiological concepts and methods characteristic of our field, that ours could easily be substituted for theirs, perhaps with a gain rather than a loss.

What is more characteristic of the industrial model is not the methods and tools in themselves, but the insistence that everyone in the organization, and especially workers on the production line, understand and use at least the simpler tools, almost daily, to scrutinize performance. Loosely speaking, the aim is to "statisticize" the entire enterprise, from its highest reaches to its lowest. At the very top is the statistical leader, at the right hand of the chief executive, able to participate and intervene in most fundamental decisions and processes. In descending order of competence and location are others in each department and in supervisory posts at the production line. And, most importantly, each worker is made to internalize and implement the principles and methods of data collection and analysis pertinent to the assessment and improvement of performance. A massive, intensive, continuous educational effort is undertaken to accomplish these ends.

The architects of our own health-care model have proposed, at least in theory, a similar restructuring and reform in our system, except that epidemiology, rather than industrial statistics, has been proposed as the more relevant analytic discipline. Accordingly, the properly qualified "clinical performance epidemiologist" is envisaged as the leader who embodies the function at the highest levels of the organization. We have failed, however, to implement this model. And, in particular, our production workers, who are most critically our health-care professionals, have been woefully unprepared to perceive, understand, and analyze the aggregate manifestations of quality in groups of people. They continue to focus on discrete, clinical events in individual patients, taken one at a time. We need to learn, from whatever success the industrial model has had, to implement what at least some of us, for a long time, have thought to be necessary.

There remains a particular set of theory and methods that seem distinctive of the industrial model. I refer to the discipline of statistical control. True enough, there have been examples of statistical control applied to our field, intentionally or unintentionally, fully or partially. A wider applicability of the method has been occasionally proposed. And, in essence, statistical control is not that different from the methods of epidemiological surveillance quite firmly established in our field. Still, one wonders why statistical control has not been more widely adopted as an instrument of quality control and improvement. Some reasons might include the scarcity, until recently, of a continuous flow of data on procedural and outcome events; the difficulty of precise stratification, without which such data are misleading, if not meaningless; and the unwillingness to wait for the manifestation of an established adverse pattern of outcomes to emerge. But perhaps, most fundamentally, we have been unwilling to accept the notion that, within bracketing limits, variability is not only to be expected, but can be tolerable. Our clinical training has led us to focus on each individual variation from expectation, impelling us to explain and eliminate the deviation. We sorely need an epidemiological perspective to supplement our clinical preoccupations.

THE OVEREMPHASIS ON VOCABULARY

As is true of any specialized field of endeavor, the industrial model is characterized by a vocabulary that reflects its science, its context, its history, and its ideological perspectives. Those who have attempted to apply the industrial model to our own field have seen, in unquestioning conformity to this vocabulary, assurance of orthodoxy, proof of distinctiveness, and evidence of progress. Even when this vocabulary threatens to do violence to our own traditions and usages, they insist upon it. They fail to see, or perhaps wish to exploit, the penumbral connotations that are perhaps more telling features of language, precisely because they are more subliminal.

For example, is your spouse your "customer"? And are you your spouse's? And what of your child? Am I God's customer? Is God mine? And why should the quality-improvement cycle carry a particular name to make it acceptable or efficacious? I shall spare you more examples to make the point.

It is also not true that terms we have long used are no longer acceptable to the industrial model as applied to our own field. In fact, the industrial model uses and assigns distinctive roles, not only to "quality improvement," but also to "quality assurance," and even to "quality control." "Quality Assurance," the words by which our activity is named, occupies a particularly central position in the industrial model.

It is time we abandon our preoccupation with right-speak in favor of a more fundamental concern for "right-think."

LESSONS WE COULD LEARN

There are a number of lessons we can learn from the industrial model, not so much because they are new but because they reinforce beliefs and practices we have had ourselves. Perhaps the most important of these is insistence on undivided commitment to quality throughout an organization, sustained by the personal devotion and participation of its top leadership. Only second in importance is the necessity to harness every worker in an organization to the quality-improvement effort through opportunities for self-actualization and pride in workmanship.

For workers to participate effectively it is important not only to provide scope and opportunity, but also to undertake the intensive, sustained educational effort needed to create sensitivity to quality issues and competence to deal with them. I have suggested that this requires, in our case, acquisition of an epidemiological perspective and of the corresponding descriptive and analytic tools.

And finally, without paying less attention to the contributions of professional skill and judgment to the achievement of quality, we ought to pay more attention to reforming the processes of work and of the contexts within which they are conducted. These structural features, and the incentives they embody, should facilitate and encourage good performance, rather than pose obstacles to it. In particular, the temptation to scapegoat and punish, so heavy-handedly encouraged by government regulation, should yield to our worthier professional traditions of self-examination and continuous learning.

These conclusions and other relevant inferences and recommendations are detailed, together with a comparison of the two models, in Table 6-1.

Table 6-1 • **MODELS OF QUALITY ASSURANCE: A TABULAR SUMMARY**

I. Are There Two Models?

The *health-care model* and the *industrial model* are two distinguishable "families," with similarities and also differences between the two.

II. Some Ways in which the Models Can Be Compared

A. The nature of quality
B. The scope of quality
C. The nature of "the quality problem"
D. The strategies of quality assurance and improvement
E. The methods of quality monitoring

Industrial Model	Health-Care Model
A. The Nature of Quality	
Quality is whatever consumers desire, endorse, buy.	Quality is what is good for consumers, as defined jointly by consumers themselves and their health-care advisors, subject to societal guidelines.
The customer-seller interaction is less prominent as a component of quality.	The patient-practitioner relationship is very complex, and its management is an integral part of quality.
The consumer is, by competence in use, a coproducer of quality.	The consumer (patient) is even more intimately and decisively a definer and coproducer of quality.

Table 6-1 • MODELS OF QUALITY ASSURANCE: A TABULAR SUMMARY
(continued)

Industrial Model	Health-Care Model
Low cost is a component of quality. The added cost of added quality can often be counterbalanced by efficiency of production and more sales. ("Quality is free!")	Low cost is less emphasized as a component of quality. The added cost of added quality is not so easily counterbalanced by efficiencies in production or higher sales; and it is added to by longevity. ("Quality costs money!")
Optimality and equity are less important issues.	Optimality and equity are important issues of policy and implementation.

B. The Scope of Quality

Emphasis on "total quality" includes: (1) lowering cost as well as meeting consumer requirements; (2) focusing on all steps in the process of designing, producing, selling, and servicing; and (3) involving everyone in an organization, at all levels, in all units.	Emphasis is primarily on the performance of professional personnel, and primarily in technical care; but with expansions to include the patient-practitioner interaction, the patient's contribution to care, and social issues of access and equity.
When applied to health care there is a danger of paying less attention to clinical care, and more attention to supportive activities, with preponderant emphasis on cost saving.	The danger is preponderant attention to the technical performance of physicians, with less attention to other professionals, and no attention to others.
Can be criticized as "marginal" or "peripheral."	Can be criticized as "partial" or "less than total."

C. The Nature of the "Quality Problem"

Most problems of quality arise from defects in the design of systems, products, and processes of production. They arise less often from failures of production workers to perform their duties.	The contributions of structural characteristics are recognized, but the competence of health-care professionals is a major structural characteristic, and variability in their performance an important problem.

D. The Strategies of Quality Assurance and Improvement

Emphasis is on changing structural characteristics, but includes worker retraining or reassignment.	Emphasis is on influencing professional performance more directly by education, retraining, supervision, encouragement, or censure.

Table 6-1 • **MODELS OF QUALITY ASSURANCE: A TABULAR SUMMARY**
    (continued)

Industrial Model	**Health-Care Model**
Management maintains ultimate responsibility but empowers production workers to monitor their own work by delegation of responsibility, education and training in methods of monitoring, and offering financial and nonfinancial rewards for improvements in quality. The organization is altered to become less hierarchical, more participatory.	What the industrial model advocates is already an established tradition in the self-monitoring and self-governance of physicians. But the two models would be even more similar if: (1) similar privileges were extended to other professionals and nonprofessionals, (2) physicians and others received more training in methods of Quality Assurance, and (3) the role of management in Quality Assurance was strengthened.

E. The Methods of Quality Monitoring

There is monitoring of production, using process and outcome measures, compared to relevant standards. This takes two forms: (1) concurrent monitoring, during the production process, by workers and supervisors, aiming for speedy detection of significant deviations and their correction; and (2) terminal monitoring of samples of finished product, aiming to prevent sale of defective lots, and learning how to prevent defects in the future.	There are corresponding forms of monitoring process and outcome, using analogous standards, except that services given cannot be recalled. However, services planned can be countermanded; care can be monitored while it is being given; and care can be assessed after it is completed, so as to learn from past success and failure, and make appropriate adjustments.
Monitoring is seen as a continuous cycle of activities meant to verify performance, determine the reasons for unsatisfactory performance, take appropriate action, and check the effects of such action.	Monitoring is seen in similar terms: as a cyclical activity, with an analogous succession of steps.
The aim is continuous improvement of performance.	The aim is continuous improvement of performance.
A rather specific set of methods is advanced for problem identification, consensus development, description of performance, determination of causation, etc. Statistical control methods are highly developed and widely used.	Similar methods are available, especially in the armamentarium of descriptive and analytic epidemiology; but clinical case review is the dominant method, and statistical control concepts and methods have not been widely used.

Table 6-1 • **MODELS OF QUALITY ASSURANCE: A TABULAR SUMMARY**
   (continued)

III. Some Conclusions

A. Despite differences in vocabulary, there are remarkable similarities between the two models; and many of the differences that remain are justifiable.

B. The industrial model, rather than being a negation of the health-care model (i.e., an "industrialization" of professional work), is a "professionalization" of industrial work.

C. The main dangers of applying the industrial model to health care are: (1) adoption of an oversimplified definition of quality, and (2) deflection of attention from clinical effectiveness to the efficiency of supportive activities.

D. The main lessons we can learn from the industrial model are:
   1. A new appreciation for the fundamental soundness of our traditions

   2. The need for even greater attention to consumer requirements, values, and expectations

   3. The need for even greater attention to the design of systems and processes as a means to Quality Assurance

   4. A greater appreciation for the interrelatedness of different segments in the health-care system (and of the human-welfare system that complements it) in assuring quality in health care

   5. A greater appreciation for the relevance of overall organizational effectiveness and efficiency to the quality of the clinical-care function

   6. The need to extend the self-monitoring, self-governing tradition of physicians to others in the organization

   7. The need to assess and assure the quality of care from a multi/**interdisciplinary** perspective

   8. The need for a greater role on the part of management in assuring the quality of clinical care (and, perhaps, on the part of health-care professionals in contributing to the effectiveness and efficiency of managerial activities)

   9. The need to develop and apply appropriate statistical control methods to health-care monitoring

   10. The need for greater education and training in quality monitoring and assurance for all concerned

LONG-RANGE DEVELOPMENTS

All our models of Quality Assurance, irrespective of their origins or affiliations, cry for more rigorous scientific investigation. As a beginning, it would help us to locate whatever approaches we propose within the broader theories of organizational behavior and organizational effectiveness. This should help us develop a more systematically differentiated set of models as a first step to empirical exploration of their performance. Empirical testing will, of course, take two forms: one observations, using epidemiological tools, and the other experimental, using the armamentarium of field tools. Thus, through model building and empirical testing we establish a distinctive endeavor: the comparative study of quality-assurance systems.

Some of the more specific issues that we need to address soon include the following:

- how professionals function in general and in formal organizations; what motivates them; how they make clinical decisions; how professional and managerial roles and functions are intertwined

- how to design formal organizations so as to achieve the proper balance between general managerial concerns and more particularistic professional concerns; how to motivate and channel professional activity in the service of legitimate organizational goals; and how to make the organization responsive to legitimate professional aspirations

- how to design and manage the process of professional work to minimize the occurrence and consequences of human error and elicit high levels of performance

- how to design quality-assurance activities as a system, rather than an assemblage of unrelated parts; how to relate that system to the organization as a whole, and to the larger, societal nexus

- what roles to assign in a quality-assurance system to the several health-care professionals and to managers; how to balance managerial responsibilities and contributions to Quality Assurance with the corresponding contributions and responsibilities of production workers, professional and other

- how to include client perspectives, concerns, and judgments in any system of Quality Assurance

- how to relate internal quality assurance activities to the corresponding activities of external agencies

I do not expect that, as a result of the studies I have proposed, we shall find how best to organize or conduct the quality-assurance enterprise. I hope, rather, that we shall learn what kinds of quality-assurance models will work better or worse, in what circumstances, and why. We shall be a mature discipline only when we are well on our way to framing and finding the answers to such questions.

CONCLUSION

I believe it is reasonable to conclude that what I have called "the industrial model" has many affinities to ours: in its emphasis on service to the consumer; in its recognition of the worthiness, dignity, devotion, and skill of all workers; in its refusal to blame individuals for inherent deficiencies of systems and processes; in its reliance on education rather than punishment; in its reliance on leadership rather than dictation; and in its emphasis on internal self-amelioration rather than external regulation.

The industrial model offers, in effect, a powerful antidote to the excesses of governmental regulation and its coercive, punitive approach; its readiness to censure, and reluctance to help; its fixation on error, divorced from recognition and celebration of the good. In all this, the industrial model, correctly understood, is an ally we can embrace without fear.

In exploring the pathways and byways of the industrial model, we do not end up in a different country. We discover, perhaps with an added sense of appreciation and wonder that, by a circuitous route, we have arrived home. But that is only so if we have remained true to ourselves. If we have lost our moorings, we may have gone fearfully astray.

The industrial model comes to us with flags and streamers, bugles and bells, speaking in a strange tongue, replete with homely aphorisms and vivid slogans. It is often misrepresented and exploited out of ignorance or greed. But, despite these carnival accoutrements, it is, in essence, true, sober, sincere. It says: "Care for quality. First, give your hearts to it. Set your minds upon it, and the rest will follow." And with all that is sacred within us we agree. Yes, above all to care; the tools are easy.

ADDITIONAL READING

Berwick, D. (1989). Continuous improvement as an ideal in health care. *The New England Journal of Medicine, 320*(1), 53–56.

Berwick, D. M. (1993). Do we really need a framework in order to improve? *Journal on Quality Improvement, 19*(10), 449–450.

Betalden, P. B., & Stoltz, P. K. (1993). A framework for the continual improvement of health care: Building and applying professional and improvement knowledge to test changes in daily work. *Journal on Quality Improvement, 19*(10), 424–447.

Camp, R. C., & Tweet, A. G. (1994). Benchmarking applied to health care. *Journal on Quality Improvement, 20*(5), 229–238.

Cesta, T. G. (1993). The link between continuous quality and case management. *Journal of Nursing Administration, 2*(6), 55–61.

Donabedian, A. (1993). Avedis Donabedian: An interview [Interview by Richard Baker]. *Quality in Health Care, 2*(1), 40–46.

Laffel, G., & Blumenthal, D. (1989). The case for using industrial quality management science in health care organizations. *Journal of the American Medical Association, 262*(20), 2869–2873.

McLaughlin, C., & Kaluzny, A. (1994). *Continuous quality improvement in health care: Theory, implementation, and applications.* Gaithersburg, MD: Aspen.

Sheila Taylor Myers

CHAPTER 7

Program Evaluation as an Endeavor:
Value Oriented Yet Scientifically Based

INTRODUCTION

In the information age, increasingly diffuse information sources abound and competition for limited resources broadens. **Program Evaluation (PE)** is a means to hone the competitive edge by optimizing use of time and resources. Managers who make informed decisions with justification drawn from cogent findings are in a position to cross disciplines and share departmental assets. Findings from PE studies are useful in making decisions about setting priorities and program directions, as well as future operations.

Program Evaluation is a generic process that crosses multiple disciplines. This **multidisciplinary** aspect of PE is a strength at a time when diverse groups of people must work together to conduct health programs. Yet ambiguities are created by discipline-specific variations in terminology. Such vagueness led Newman, Jatulis, and Carpinello (1990) to document the confusing array of purposes and associated activities that decision makers in community health settings considered under the rubric of PE. This confusion can be reduced by thinking of PE as the overriding framework that has spawned such enterprises as **accreditation**, **Quality Assurance (QA)**, **Continuous Quality Improvement (CQI)**, and, more recently, **Total Quality Management (TQM)**.

The process of PE involves using scientific methods to understand a situation and the effects of some action directed toward changing that situation. Thus, PE includes both *formative* issues, reviewing program objectives and plans for activities being conducted, and *summative* evaluation, dealing with program outcomes. In the broad sense, PE can encompass issues that activate solutions to major social problems and the politics of policy change. More narrowly, PE is limited to the review of a specific program in a specific geographic location within a specific department. Discussion here will take the more circumspect route, directed toward programs within a single department, institution, or community.

This chapter offers an overview of PE, starting with a general history. Special emphasis is given to the evolution of ideas grounding present thought. The process used in PE and associated types of investigation are then introduced with illustrations from a clinical application that links concretely to the practice setting. Evaluator roles are summarized so the reader can better collaborate with professional evaluators to use project findings in health-care settings.

Throughout the discussion, terms and processes used in PE are compared with those used in research. The reader is assumed to have a knowledge of general research methods. Highlighting these similarities reduces the amount of new thinking undertaken and, thus, flattens the learning curve.

The intent is to highlight the common process of thought used across disciplines, intentionally bypassing discipline-specific technicalities. Decision makers can then identify the complexity of information needed, select the PE activities that can be undertaken in-house, and recognize when assistance of a professional evaluator will be required.

HISTORY OF PROGRAM EVALUATION

Program Evaluation is a commonsense idea that asks both what a program is doing and "so what?" — that is, what difference does it make that the program exists? Some might argue that PE is a product of our goal-directed society, spawned by technological expansion. However, the basic thinking is not new and has been traced through many societies. Berk and Rossi (1990) theorize that remnants of PE formulation existed in ancient Roman tax policies, which set taxation rates in direct valuative response to strategically observed shifts in revenue. Another account of PE thinking is found in the often-told story of the British naval requirement that stores of limes be carried for crew consumption, based on observations of differences in the incidence of scurvy between British crews and crews routinely sailing with such stores.

The Work of Florence Nightingale

The need for sanitation practices on the battlefield was documented in an evaluation conducted by Florence Nightingale (Woodham-Smith, 1951). She defined the scope of the problem by contrasting Army deaths with the lower death rates of the general civilian British population. When some complained that this was hardly a fair comparison, she explicitly emphasized the import of her findings. The general population included elderly and infants whereas the British Army population consisted of young, strong men who had undergone medical examinations to guarantee their physical fitness before marching off to duty. To pinpoint the hospitals, rather than enemy forces, as culprit, she then compared morbidity and mortality figures, showing higher death from disease within army hospitals than from injury or disease either on the battlefield or in the civilian population. The concluding statement of her evaluation, "Our soldiers enlist to death in the barracks" (Woodham-Smith, 1951, p. 204), served as a summary of her findings and as a political battle cry.

As part of this work, Nightingale calculated the impact of a sanitation program by outlining changes instituted in the hospital at Scutari and comparing death figures before and after the changes were implemented. Her PE was the basis for reorganizing the British War Office. Sanitation measures became part of army regulations for the first time in British history.

The Emphasis on Measurement

With the increase in mechanization following World War I, PE efforts were focused on measurement. Time and motion studies documented worker activities, and production output units were calculated. During this period the productivity of Western Electric workers was measured and the term *Hawthorne effect* was thus added to research terminology signifying changes influenced simply by subjects' awareness that they are special participants in a study. In education, increased ability to test intelligence led to evaluation of education programs focused on describing arrays of student test scores.

With the advent of technological development in the space race of the 1950s and expansion of social programs with large-scale governmental funding in the 1960s, concern for **accountability** increased the use of PE approaches. These efforts were designed to obtain information useful in making judgments about programs. By the late 1960s, demonstration of need was often required before a program could be instituted. Measurable goals and objectives leading to performance effectiveness were prerequisites for continued program funding. Thus PE became a growth industry.

What was originally the commonsense element of PE matured into a field based in action science (Argyris, Putnam, & Smith, 1985; Patton, 1978). From this base, program complexity was seen within a context of social value. Program Evaluation, as an overall process of thinking, became synonymous with evaluation research, drawing from all fields of social and behavioral sciences. Contributions ranged widely and included ethnographic methods, survey research, randomized experiments, and benefit-cost analysis. Computer technology made possible the use of sophisticated methods with the ability to examine large numbers of variables simultaneously. Thus, evaluation strategies formed an "eclectic repertoire" (Berk & Rossi, 1990).

The Evolution of Program Evaluation

Guba and Lincoln (1989) view PE as four generations of evaluation emphasizing an intentional maturation. The first generation focused simply on measuring, to such an extent that *measure* was often synonymous with *evaluate*. In a sense, regulatory requirements and enforcement typify the activity of this generation. The second generation focused on patterns of program strengths and weaknesses from the perspective of program objectives. Thus, first and second generation evaluation, firmly based in the reductionistic inquiry, centered on objective reality separate from experiences, beliefs, or values.

As demands increased to fund one program over another, the focus of the third generation shifted to making judgments about program strengths and weaknesses based on some standard comparison. Accreditation activities required in both academe and health care are typical of third generation evaluation. Still entrenched in objective reality, empirical evidence was generated as a base for judgment.

The advent of the fourth generation brought recognition of multiple realities. Divergent interests and political and social values clearly impacted programs. This fourth generation of PE is based in relativism or naturalistic inquiry. Appropriately, triangulation of multiple methods or perspectives and other responsive approaches are used to generate information and understanding that reflect this plurality of views. Thus, the thinking in PE has evolved into a very complex field of investigative questioning.

Guba and Lincoln's description of generations implies an evolutionary direction in which past approaches are left behind. It is productive, however, to think of each generation as making specific contributions to the conduct of PE. Each generation has added approaches and strategies that serve to strengthen the potential for conducting change. The most recent contribution is an open recognition of the value context of PE, tempering, if not negating, the existence of a value-neutral scientific stance.

DEFINING PROGRAM EVALUATION IN A CONTEXT OF VALUING

The meaning of the term *Program Evaluation* is hazy, perhaps because of its eclectic and evolutionary development. Various models have been posed which are not only discipline specific (Guba & Lincoln, 1985; Provus, 1971; Scriven, 1973; Stake, 1967; Stufflebeam, 1971; Tyler, 1950) but are also oriented toward specific intents consistent with Guba and Lincoln's classification of the four PE generations (Sarnecky, 1990). Recent definitions of PE show movement to fourth-generational ideas. For instance, in 1984 Wolf defined PE as a process necessary to collect and use information to make decisions about programs. Three years later Shortell and Richardson (1987) included the idea of valuing when defining PE as a set of methodologies that can be used to make a value judgment about a program with a view to modification. Similarly, Billue and Clayton (1988) defined PE as "a process that arrives at an assessment of worth or merit based on evidence collected and that contributes to decision-making" (p. 8) and Puetz (1988) focused on this valuing aspect when she defined PE as being "undertaken primarily to assess the worth and value of . . . programs and processes" (p. 64). Common among these definitions is the idea of a process by which one gains information that contributes to programmatic decision making within a context of values.

Thus, Program Evaluation must be discussed within the context of its linguistic root: the old French *valoir*, meaning "to be worth" or *value* (Soukhanov, 1984). Establishing worthiness, or valuing, or evaluating, involves technically measuring and rating in relation to some **standard**. In so doing, components are described to convey similarities or differences to an equivalent. This description is often in numerical terms requiring a judgment call in order to assign a quantifiable value and negotiate a suitable equivalent. Thus, to **evaluate** is to determine a relative state between things. Whether those things are as tangible as establishing the cash value of a material item or as intangible as the worth of an idea, the act of evaluating requires contrast between two or more elements using a standard for contrast.

The choice of which standards to use for making judgments in an evaluation is drawn from the values held. Values, whether or not acknowledged, drive the conduct of an evaluation and determine its usefulness in decision making about program conduct (see Figure 7-1).

Recognition and examination of driving values will only strengthen an evaluation and its consequent use.

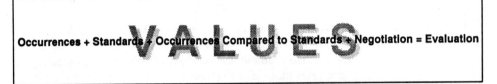

Occurrences + Standards + Occurrences Compared to Standards + Negotiation = Evaluation

Figure 7-1 *Program Evaluation Occurs in a Context of Valuing. (Reprinted with permission. Copyright 1995 by Sheila Taylor Myers.)*

Program Evaluation Terminology

The pervasive influence of valuing is highlighted in two terms critical to technical PE literature: policy space and **stakeholder.** *Policy space* refers to the area of general attention that surrounds specific concerns. Often this attention is generated when there is a conflict in values or when a value is gaining ascendancy. The "lime light" encompassing such issues is the policy space. Thus programs or policies that fall within the lime light will be candidates for evaluation because information is required to guide or support decisions that must be made.

Sensitivity to the policy space increases the likelihood of accurately predicting areas for productive evaluation. Those evaluations energized by critical policy space have greater opportunity to gather required support. Conversely, it is unlikely that one can harness the energies necessary to generate support for an evaluation of an area that is of no particular interest.

As identifying policy space defines the area of interest, identifying the *stakeholders* defines the players. Everyone with something "at stake" in the program or its evaluation is considered a stakeholder. They have a vested interest. Certainly those who have invested money, time, or interest in a program are major stakeholders. They may influence decisions about such critical elements as the parameters and the defining characteristics of an evaluation. Those who oppose a program or the evaluation because of possible repercussions are also stakeholders and may contribute to the evaluation effort by blocking or redirecting efforts. Those who are targets of a program, those who are affected on the periphery of the program, and those who conduct a program, all may be stakeholders and may impact decision making. Recognizing the policy space in which a PE is initiated and conducted and the stakeholders who influence that conduct are tangible evidence of the value function in program evaluation.

Valuing and Problem Identification

Problems for evaluation are socially constructed as attention is drawn to an unsettling situation. Social values define people's sensitivity and make the situation troubling.

This determines their construction of the problem. Thus, we begin to build problems by the very act of focusing attention on specific conditions. Conditions are *chosen* to be indicative of problems because of the interest they generate. Attention may be driven by cost concerns, by larger social change issues, or by administrative directive — all components of the policy space surrounding the problem.

For instance, the readmission rate of premature infants within two weeks of discharge from a particular hospital may be unsettling. Yet, the rate is not the problem; the rate is simply the condition or behavior *indicating* a problem exists. The problem is the driving force allied with the rate. In causal terms the problem is the situation that causes the rate to be at a certain level. This situation is the problem waiting for a solution. For instance, is it the expectation that *no* infants will return? Or is there a certain group of infants that have raised the alarm? If the focus is turned toward physiologically normal, low-birth-weight infants, the problem is different than if the focus is on infants with birth conditions that require continuing treatment. Both concerns are reasonable; they are neither "right" nor "wrong." It is simply a matter of defining clearly where the focus is directed. How **indicators** are set and the problem is conceived will determine which solutions seem feasible to change the problem and which solutions seem irrelevant and are screened out of consideration.

This defining sets the parameters of the problem. The first definition of the problem area might raise questions about the parents' ability to read infant cues and master the feeding skills necessary to care for such a small infant. Programs developed to solve the readmission problem of low-birth-weight infants might focus on early parent-infant contact to maintain and reinforce parent attachment and sensitivity to cues, as well as on increasing efforts to teach feeding skills and time regulation. With the second definition of the problem area, the birth condition may be highlighted, thus raising questions regarding the parents' knowledge of the given disability. Parents' ability to care for the child and to recognize early signs of change in physiological condition may also be questioned. Programs developed to solve this problem might focus on teaching parents about the disability and corresponding medical treatment, possible changes in the infant's condition, and management skills.

Problem identification is not a skill limited to program evaluators, and the responsibility should not be shouldered by evaluators alone. The major burden of defining the problem lies with those who are experiencing it, because they must endure the solutions imbedded within the problem. Discussing the consistency between the administrative charge and how the problem is defined will guide thought toward the consequences of any definition adopted. Different definitions will imply differing substantive and methodological elements. Thus, identifying and focusing problems for evaluation is an interactive process among evaluator, relevant decision makers, and information users. If the question answered is *not* the question really asked, the project will not have made any difference. It is critical to clearly identify the problem entertained before launching any investigation.

Valuing in the Use of Findings

Whether or not PE findings are actually used is a controversial criterion of study worth. Berk and Rossi (1990) describe systematic PE with a "third generation" focus on the ability to make cogent judgments. They recognize evaluation research as a political and managerial activity that can influence policy decisions and allocations. However, the authors still maintain that the use of evaluation findings is not necessarily a reflection of the rigor or quality of the research. This position succinctly divorces the act of evaluating from the act of using findings. On the other hand, those with an orientation toward action research focused on organizational change maintain that evaluation is value linked — a "fourth generation" stance. From this perspective if evaluation findings are not used for change, the investigation has not spoken directly or practically enough to the values at play and the efforts were not worth anything. This harsh criterion emphasizes the critical role of evaluators.

If PE findings are to be used upon completion, it is essential to recognize the social construction of problems in the concerns of primary users. To increase the possibility of using PE findings, Patton (1978) recommends that the solution to the problem should be: (1) unknown but necessary, (2) wanted internally rather than arising solely from external sources, and (3) relevant for future action.

When stakeholders are personally involved in building consensus, their intimate investment increases a commitment to change and ensures use of the evaluation. Findings often are shared in a case study, which allows description of the group consensus building and increases personal identification of stakeholders. Yet this fact remains: although the evaluator contributes to people's thinking, the evaluator is not the decision maker. Final direction of the project does not rest with the evaluator, and the ultimate decision to use the findings is beyond the scope of the evaluator.

It is obvious from the preceding discussion that PE is conducted within a context of values. This context permeates even the classification of PE approaches, because the purpose imbedded in the initial questioning of a PE study is the factor that determines the type of study.

TYPES OF EVALUATION

Earlier, PE was defined as a process in which the thinking is intentional, purposive, and progressive. Overall, PE can serve three major purposes: (1) to plan the conceptualization and design of a program, (2) to describe implementation of a new program or monitor an ongoing program, or (3) to test the utility or impact of a program.

These purposes are associated with specific types of investigations, all subsumed under the rubric of PE. *Planning studies* or *needs assessments,* the latter being a more limited idea, are used to denote evaluation studies directed toward gaining enough information about problems to conceptualize and design innovative programs. *Implementation* or *accountability* and *monitoring studies* describe program implementation while *outcome impact* or *utility studies* evaluate the effectiveness and the efficiency of a program. A fourth type of study, the *comprehensive evaluation,* is actually a study encompassing all three purposes of design, monitor, and impact. Evaluation questions are consistent with the purpose of the evaluation and direct the methodological strategies used.

Classifying types of evaluation approaches by purpose will seem familiar to the reader who has a background in research methods. Recall that specific research designs can be classified by the purposes of exploration, description, or testing.

Similarities between PE methods and previous experiences with organization of research methods can be taken a bit further (see Table 7-1). In some sense, it is useful to think of planning a program as similar to exploratory research, while monitoring an ongoing program depicts existing program components. Assessing the impact of a program is similar to the causal thinking at work in experimental and quasi-experimental designs set up to purposefully test the effect of an independent variable.

Table 7-1 • **COMMON PURPOSES SHARED BY RESEARCH AND PE DESIGN CLASSIFICATIONS**

Design Classifications	Planning or Needs Assessment	Implementation, Accountability, and Monitoring	Impact
Exploratory	Inquire		
Descriptive		Depict	
Experimental			Test

Source: Sheila Taylor Myers, copyright 1995.

Thus, just as in other research situations, the ability to cluster evaluation approaches helps organize thinking and increases the ability to logically manage several types of evaluation questions.

Design progression suggests that stages of PE are generated by specific questioning. Again, the similarity with other research learning is the principle of consistency between question and design. Various evaluation approaches can be seen as a sequence of questions forming a path that leads through the process of PE. This path of questions outlines an evolutionary process of thinking. The questions are not unlike those posed in other problem-solving processes such as the nursing process (i.e., the process of diagnosis and treatment) and the research process. In following sections questions are traced and investigations consistent with the questions are outlined. A clinical application will be used as an illustration.

Planning Study or Needs Assessment

How extensive is the problem, what are the defining characteristics, and how widely does the problem exist? Who are the players and how are they involved? These questions drive any planning study or needs assessment. Three objectives are inherent in these questions: (1) to identify why the problem exists, (2) to determine factors that contribute to the problem's existence, and (3) to determine the extent of the problem (i.e., how big or widespread is the problem, and who is experiencing the problem).

Planning studies usually provide rationale for a program's creation. They are also useful in documenting a persistent need when challenges are launched against continuing an ongoing program. To design a program and forecast costs appropriate to a given problem requires sound data about problem size, density, and scope. Throughout a planning study, as with any PE investigation, the accuracy, reliability, and validity of data must be guarded. Needless to say, data must be strong enough to warrant program development entailing commitment of resources necessary for the project.

Information sought during the planning and development stage will have a familiar ring to the reader experienced in health care. The planning study is similar in purpose to an assessment or diagnostic workup that precedes the nursing or medical diagnosis; it is an effort to make succinct statements about the parameters of the problem. Terms are similar to epidemiological terms. For instance, we must identify people presently experiencing the problem (population at need) and those who have a significant chance of developing the problem (population at risk). We want to know also how many people are experiencing the problem at a specified time and in a particular area (prevalence) and how many of those have just developed the problem (incidence). In addition, data describing the dynamics of the institution, such as structure, philosophy, and institutional reward systems to support change, will locate the problem contextually.

The common purpose of the planning stage of a PE and descriptive research designs necessary for scientific knowledge development is to carefully and accurately describe the parameters of the problem. Planning studies are similar to descriptive designs in their layout and analysis. Planning studies also use methods similar to those used in descriptive designs. Searching for a description of the problem itself, the "how high" and "how wide," is similar to univariate analysis. When we ask how the problem exists and what factors impinge on the problem condition, the description is of relationships. Asking what factors correlate with the problem indicator questions the problem's complexity.

Theoretical knowledge and experience guide choices of what data will be collected in the needs assessment or planning study. As in any descriptive investigation, the more we know about a problem, the more focused the approach. Conversely, the more uncertain we are, the broader the search.

Data may exist that will inform about the size of a problem, or at least begin to outline the density. For instance, city, state, and national statistics may be available to help understand an agency's rate in comparison with the rates of other agencies. Demographic factors can give a general picture of distribution patterns and can be compared with similar hospital statistics. Within an institution, those departments steering **Quality Management (QM)** are a source of data that identifies organizational distribution of the problem with reliable depiction of service availability and extent.

Various data-gathering strategies may be used that will help reveal how the problem is perceived by those actually living with it. Asking "experts," whether they be caregivers or parents, is a quick way of getting a thumbnail sketch of the complexity of the situation.

Implicit in any type of program whether innovation or ongoing, is a theory of what causes the problem. What are the leverage points to create change, and what can be done to intervene? These ideas may be made explicit in an intervention model built at the culmination of the planning study. Such a model forces careful thinking to specify the essential program elements and to delineate the dynamics expected.

INTERVENTION OR IMPACT MODEL

Program elements are linked explicitly to outcome effects in an *intervention* or *impact model.* This thinking guides subsequent development and testing of solutions that are effective and efficient in changing a problem. The model is built on information from the needs assessment and previous research findings, as well as from personal observation and experience. To create a viable intervention, it is necessary to describe factors that contribute to the problem's existence and identify leverage points for change.

Without an intervention model, findings of the needs assessment may not be linked carefully, and may not be linked at all, with the development of an innovative program, thus, the effort expended in the needs assessment is wasted. Too often programs are developed on general assumptions or untested practice without deliberately explaining the intervention. When thought and time are expended to plot an intervention model, measurable objectives are created that guide the program to impact the original problem indicator.

If the program is already in place, an inventory of existing information is required to construct an intervention model. It is important to identify the history of the program, how the problem was identified, and the cause of the problem that originally sparked creation of the program. It is necessary to know what was thought to cause the problem and why the program elements were expected to change the problem. Well designed program goals and objectives that offer this information may exist. However, as changes occur over time, informal goals often replace original goals and the program focus may shift from one causative factor to another. To design a useful intervention model for an ongoing program, any shifts in thinking must be uncovered and defined.

An intervention model can be expressed in measurable statements about expected relationships between the program and its goal. Thus, the model takes the form of a testable theory. Rossi and Freeman (1985) describe the model as composed of three types of hypotheses: causal, intervention, and action. When these statements are carefully joined, strategies for linking goals with the program, or solution, become obvious.

The *causal hypothesis* answers the question, "Why does the problem exist?" Such a question draws heavily on factors uncovered in the needs assessment. Reports in the literature of factors consistently correlated with the problem indicator will be useful. In other words, information from the needs assessment, from literature, and from practice and experience of both program personnel and program evaluator help name the independent variable in the PE.

Returning to the example of the readmission problem with physiologically normal premature babies, several contributing factors were identified during the needs assessment. Babies were readmitted because they did not eat well enough at home to maintain the growth rate seen in the Neonatal Intensive Care Unit (NICU). They were usually dehydrated and lethargic. Readmission rate was associated with low to moderate socioeconomic status of the parents, as well as with parents who were isolated and without family support systems nearby. Limited parent-support systems especially helped explain readmission of babies from homes where each parent was developing a professional career.

Parents usually blamed each other and themselves for readmission. Even before a baby was discharged from the NICU, however, the parents often said they were sure that such a small baby would not be able to stay out of the hospital. Parents were noticeably clumsy in feeding, diapering, and holding the infant. They consistently voiced fatigue, moderate depression, and fear of failure. In interviews, parents described themselves as doing "only passably" as parents, because they did not really feel like the parents of the baby and "didn't know how" to care for it. Nurses were fairly accurate in predicting which infants would return by listening to the mother's anxious "worryings" in the unit and watching mothers touch their babies as they dressed them to go home.

In an effort to answer the question posed in the needs assessment, i.e., "Why are physiologically normal but premature infants readmitted after discharge from the NICU?," several factors were identified. The list included limited parenting skills, low social and economic resources, inability to read baby cues, limited knowledge of infant capabilities, high parent fatigue, and depression. All of these items impacted readmission rate, yet only a select few could be addressed. Changing the economic status or social support resources of parents was not within the service scope of this acute-care hospital. However, increasing parents' ability to read infant cues, to appreciate the infant's capabilities, and to handle the baby's caretaking needs were feasible. Factors began to group themselves into recognizable patterns useful in creating causal hypotheses to test a theory of prematurity and hospital readmission.

Separation and disruptions in the attachment process between parents and babies might account for readmission of premature infants to the hospital, because parenting after separation is difficult. The hypothesis must be phrased in measurable terms in order to be tested; it must be operationalized. So, the evaluator could state the causal hypothesis as:

> Readmission of physiologically normal premature infants to the
> hospital within two weeks of NICU discharge is most likely among
> those parents who have had less touch contact with their infants or
> have participated less in infant care while the baby was in the NICU.

Separation could mean the length of time the parents held the baby at birth or the number of visits parents made to the NICU during initial hospitalization; participation could be measured by class attendance or watching a skill demonstration. The important point is that readmission, separation from infant, and participation in care must be stated in measurable terms consistent with the original intent of the program innovation. (It should also be understood that separation and level of participation are not the only variables that might be used in stating the causal hypothesis. Whether or not the infant was seen for "failure to thrive" syndrome or admission of the infant to the emergency department or physician's office could also be incorporated into a causal hypothesis.)

Intervention hypotheses from which to develop a new program can now be constructed. If separation between mother and baby is seen as the culprit variable, the intervention posed would decrease or change separation presently existing. *Kangaroo Care (KC)* is an intervention that gives parents, especially mothers, the opportunity to hold the infant closely in skin-to-skin contact for an extended period of time as soon as the baby is physiologically stable. While the parent is holding the baby, awareness of baby cues and infant handling increase, as does participation in care. Thus the intervention hypotheses become:

- The more time spent by the mother in KC with her infant during NICU hospitalization, the more likely she is to increase her spontaneous touch contact with the infant at other times.

- The more time spent by the mother in KC with her infant during NICU hospitalization, the more likely she is to increase her activities in feeding and diapering activities for her infant.

The two pieces of this hypothesis can now be combined to establish the *action hypothesis* of the model.

> Time in KC will be positively related to amount of time spent in touch contact between mother and infant, positively related to mother's participation in care activities, and negatively related to infant readmission within two weeks of NICU discharge.

Now that the cause, intervention, and action hypotheses have been established, the intervention model can be constructed. The diagrammed model helps illuminate both elements to be measured and anticipated relationships to be tested in subsequent investigations (see Figure 7-2). Goals for a program of KC can be stated succinctly. Direction and strength of program elements can be tested and the program refined by differentiating elements affecting readmission independently from those that are covariate and affect readmission in a more complex way.

In order for the model to be evaluated, it must be both *measurable* and *feasible.* Before the advent of high technology now available in the NICU, if infant physiological response to KC had been included in the model, measuring response items, such as oxygen saturation, could not have been accomplished.

It is important to note that even if causal hypotheses can be measured, it may not be feasible to address certain hypotheses in particular agency settings. Some

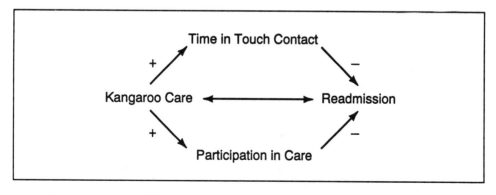

Figure 7-2 *Intervention Model for a Kangaroo Care Program. (Reprinted with permission. Copyright 1995 by Sheila Taylor Myers.)*

interventions, that are otherwise appropriate, may not be practical. They may be politically at risk, clients may not be willing to use them, or they may be administratively impossible. Traditionally, the emphasis of treatment in the NICU has been to create an artificial womb in the isolette. While these ideas are in their ascendancy, testing a program of KC, that takes the baby out of the isolette, is not feasible because paradigm conflict and consequent ethical dilemmas reduce stakeholder support. Further, policy space will not be conducive to investigation until cost of high-technology care is an issue.

It is essential to include the practice setting when considering health behavior scientifically. In the past, scientists have devalued PE as a reputable source for advancing knowledge because of the intricacies found in the health-care setting. Constructing an intervention or impact model illustrates explicitly how PE contributes to understanding a problem in health-care delivery. Once the model is outlined, the questions and focus shift to detailing the program description.

Implementation or Accountability and Monitoring Study

What can be done to change the problem situation? An *implementation* or *accountability and monitoring study* explicitly identifies the components of a program expected to change a given problem. Whether the study will be used to implement a new program or monitor one already in existence, the focus turns to documenting two areas: (1) the existence or conduct of the program (i.e., how the care is delivered), and (2) the identity of the participants who are being served.

To monitor a program, parameters must be established. Establishing parameters helps define which activities and people are within the program and which are without. Specific program elements must be enumerated and tracked. Generally, program elements include personnel (both program participants and program staff), specific services, time use, and cost. Each is a separate element.

Because the purpose of an implementation or accountability and monitoring study is to describe what is happening, it is appropriate to use descriptive research methodology. Record review, chart audit, and budgetary expenditures document past performance, while interviews and nonparticipant observations describe present function. With regard to the readmission problem, simply watching and recording the KC being given and comparing observations of what is taking place with what was planned to take place is one method of conducting an observational study of the program.

Documenting program participation turns attention from program existence to program use. Two areas are of major concern: coverage and bias. *Coverage* is the extent to which a program serves those for whom it is intended, directing attention to the target population as a whole. *Bias* is the difference in participation levels among subgroups.

Inappropriate coverage can be costly, so managers are concerned with both undercoverage and overcoverage. *Undercoverage* is the proportion of the target population *not* being reached. This proportion is calculated as those who are eligible but not participating in the program in relation to the total who are eligible for participation.

$$\frac{\text{eligible not participating}}{\text{total eligible}}$$

Undercoverage helps one judge whether the program is underserving the people for whom it was designed.

Accurately estimating undercoverage is problematic because it hinges on the ability to identify the number of people who are eligible but not participating — essentially counting people who are not there. An estimate of the target size may have been produced in a needs assessment used for program planning. If the program has strenuous eligibility **criteria**, the task of identifying the eligible group size is much easier than if the criteria are very broad and indistinct. In the readmission example, eligibility is limited to physiologically stable infants hospitalized in the NICU.

Calculating program *overcoverage* is usually easier to determine than undercoverage because the focus is on actual participants. The overcoverage rate helps determine whether eligibility standards are met. Overcoverage is the proportion of the number of ineligible users in relation to all program users.

$$\frac{\text{ineligible users}}{\text{total users}}$$

Rossi and Freeman (1985) suggest calculating another usage statistic, *Coverage Efficiency*, as:

$$100 \times \left[\left(\frac{\text{\# eligible served}}{\text{\# eligible}}\right) - \left(\frac{\text{\# ineligible served}}{\text{\# served}}\right)\right]$$

This formula yields a score between +100 and -100; this score serves as a standard score with which to compare similar programs when making administrative decisions. For instance, in the readmission example, a program manager faced with a dropping coverage efficiency score might impose additional exclusion criteria in an effort to reduce the time nurses are spending with larger babies who are not at such high risk. Another approach would be to question why small babies, who do meet criteria, are not being included.

Questioning participation differences turns the focus to program bias. *Bias* comes from two sources — participants are excluded either by program action or by participant choice. For instance, mothers who travel long distances to the hospital may not be able to participate, and, so, are underserved.

When a coverage or bias problem is documented, identifying explanatory factors facilitates program refinement. *Why is it that some who are eligible do not use the program? Why do some groups use the program more than others?* Issues of accessibility, acceptability, and accountability may contribute to participation of the target population. Overcoverage in the KC program, for example, might be occurring among certain groups, such as infants whose mothers are teenagers or whose mothers are not married. This may occur because staff think these groups of people need more support. Because of their bias, staff are selectively choosing to initiate care among some babies who are actually ineligible over other eligible babies. On the other hand, mothers in KC are asked to stay with their babies for an extended period of time and to come to the hospital every day. Transportation, support systems for children at home, and employment may all contribute to the explanation of why certain groups are or are not participating.

In comparing programs, participation bias is as important a consideration as is coverage efficiency. It is essential that participation elements be similar between programs contrasted. If one program has a preponderance of participants whose problems can be changed easily, this program will appear more successful because change will come more quickly than in a program where participant change scores are slower to respond. Similarly, if program participants come into a program with very low scores, the program will appear more effective, because the size of change between entrance and exit will be great.

Outcome Impact or Utility Study

How does the intervention affect the change expected — and was it worth it? In an *outcome impact* or *utility study* the focus is on program effectiveness — identifying what difference the program makes. Typically an impact study is undertaken either to test a new or refined program or to review outcomes of an ongoing program. Did the program produce the effect predicted? Are the goals being accomplished? Is the program changing the initial problem indicator such that the problem is solved?

There are two major requirements for conducting an impact study. First, the program must have goals and objectives stated clearly enough to identify measures of goal attainment. If goals do not exist or have not been outlined adequately, the evaluator may be able to establish reasonable objectives from what is known about the program's history and description. It is these program goals and objectives, outlining the intent of the program, that direct the impact study. The goals must be stated clearly enough to guide decisions about measuring outcomes and declaring success. Second, evidence of program delivery to the target population is essential because the program is considered the independent element that causes the program outcome.

To undertake an impact study without measurable program goals or without adequately implementing the program is a waste of time and money. As demands for outcome evaluation increase, undue emphasis is placed on measuring only program outcome. Progam Evaluation is not served well by this practice. It makes no sense to measure consequences without demonstrating existence of the program and ability to deliver the program to the people for whom it was designed. In other words, to make an accurate logical statement of causation, the independent variable (the program) *as well as* the dependent variable (the outcome or effect of that program) must be documented. Because monitoring the conduct of a program and documenting its impact are so closely linked, these two types of studies (implementation and impact) may be combined in a PE.

In designing an impact study, the reasoning is the same as that underlying experimental and quasi-experimental designs to establish causality. Campbell and Stanley (1967) describe sources of internal and external validity threat for various design types. These ideas can be used directly to construct impact studies.

Experiments are the design of choice to establish causal inference. However, this requires manipulation of the experimental treatment or program, as well as random assignment of participants to treatments — often particularly difficult to achieve in an ongoing program or care situation. If some clients are suddenly excluded from available services because of randomizing treatment, ethical and political questions may arise. Quasi-experimental designs are useful in such circumstances. Here, the strongest control of internal validity should be maintained. The static-group comparison is recommended with after-only outcomes measures. In this design only the treatment of the program group is documented, and then the outcome measures of the program are compared, simultaneously, to similarly measured outcomes of equivalent comparative groups after the tested program has been instituted. A somewhat weaker strategy would be to compare intervention outcomes of a program with established norms for the target population or to use expert judgments of administrators and participants about typical changes expected.

New programs are usually thought to be the strongest candidates for true experimental designs. Because client intake is just being initiated and benefits of the program have not yet been tested, both randomization of clients to one or another group for treatment, and manipulation of program elements within those treatments is reasonable. Thus, both methodological and ethical problems are reduced.

There is yet another way to use experimental designs in testing ongoing, as well as new, programs in a manner that addresses methodological and ethical concerns. If changes in an ongoing program can be conducted simultaneously with the present program delivery method, using present tested knowledge as well as newer elements to be tested, then it may be possible to make random assignment of clients to a program, old or new. The reasoning here is that the old program is the control group and does not deprive clients of present treatment, while the new program changes are built on the older tested knowledge but offer additional elements for testing. Thus all clients are receiving the present minimal level of program and no one is deprived because outcome of the newer elements is, until testing is completed, unknown.

The impact study should determine not only whether or not a change has been effected, but also the magnitude of that effect. But how big is big? Knowing if the change is a success is possible only if the acceptable size of change is set. Ideally this definition of success is negotiated early among program managers, constituents, and other stakeholders so that this decision is separated at the outset from the conduct of the study. When the goal of the KC program was operationalized, stakeholders defined "reduce" and, consequently, determined the interpretation of whether the change in readmission rate was large enough to call the program a success.

Defining success is often a difficult task precisely because it requires value judgments. For instance, if the KC program can prevent one baby a year from returning to the hospital, is it successful? How important is it to prevent the return of just one baby a year, or even one baby a month? If parents are setting the success level, the level may be different from that set by administrators. These are value judgments that enter into defining success in an impact study.

Program efficiency may also be part of success measured in an impact study. Data of the program effect, or outcome, can be converted to cost factors and so expand the definition of success to contribute to decision making. Efficiency is of particular concern when resource allocation decisions are made.

Calculating program costs as part of a PE is more complex than are traditional accounting practices that track expenditures. For instance, program accounting shows certain funds spent for personnel. Numbers and qualifications of personnel may be consistent with the original program plan; but, accounting methods will not question if personnel are used in the way outlined in the program definition. Further, traditional accounting approaches do not consider lost opportunity. That is, if the money is spent for one program, it cannot be used elsewhere. The cost of lost opportunity is not reflected in typical accounting analyses. Thus, calculating program costs to include information about benefits gained from a program in relation to costs of conducting the program is a complex technical field and may require consultation with specialists.

Usually the most practical way to define efficiency is to calculate program expenditures required per unit of output or benefit. This is called a *cost effectiveness analysis*. In the KC program with its goal of lowered readmission, cost effectiveness might be calculated as the proportionate program cost required for each readmission prevented. Cost effectiveness analysis uses usual accounting procedures to calculate monetary expenditures required to furnish the program, such as salaries, equipment, supplies, and space rental. However, benefits are expressed in terms of some unit of interest rather than in monetary terms.

In the KC program the outcome benefit sought is lowered readmission, so the efficiency of attaining the program goal is expressed in terms of cost per prevented readmission. The program also may affect patient satisfaction scores. Knowing that satisfaction scores correlate with continued use of this hospital over others, it may be helpful to know that KC has increased the NICU family satisfaction score an average of 25 points at a cost of $100 per family. The cost effectiveness of isolette care could be calculated in a similar way and the efficiency of the two programs compared. For instance, KC requires more intensive nursing time than isolette care and would have a higher per-day personnel cost. Yet, if the baby grows more quickly, is discharged earlier, and increases parents' satisfaction with hospital service, the cost per family can be compared for each of these benefit units when making program decisions of support or extension.

Two cautions are offered regarding comparing programs. First, the character of the programs must be similar. If one population served is easier to change than another, even though they are identical programs, the benefits and costs will not be comparable. Secondly, in comparing program costs the same unit of benefit must be considered. It is not comparable to use the cost of patient satisfaction change in one program as a contrast with lowered readmission in another program. The contrast must be based in the same benefit unit.

Analyses of program costs and benefits can be conducted from various perspectives — from the view of the individual participant or target, the funding agency, or a section of the community or society. Using these various viewpoints, costs and benefits must be calculated consistently with the analysis focus. Target costs and benefits will not be the same as community costs and benefits and must not be mixed.

The *cost-benefit analysis* is another more stringent, less practical, approach to assessing program efficiency. This analysis attempts to compute *all* the program benefits, tangible and intangible, and compare them to *all* the program costs, direct and indirect. For instance, what is the *extended* cost of a readmission? The hospital bill reflects some of the cost; but what of other elements? If the hospital admission rate is decreased, what is the cost of displaced personnel; the cost of requiring mothers to be with their babies during the NICU stay rather than returning to work; the cost of family separation? On the other hand, what are the benefits of increased attachment between mother and infant; of increased sensitivity to the baby's cues for caretaking; of gain in immediate growth and development milestones; of extensive long-term community consequences? Such analyses are intricate, if not impossible.

It is obvious that cost analyses are ex post facto analyses and, without knowing the program benefits, it is impossible to evaluate program cost. Therefore, a cost analysis is considered an extension of, rather than an alternative to, an impact study for programs that exhibit net benefits. A futuristic projection, or ex ante analysis, is sometimes used to predict program costs when planning an intervention. Although this method is a legitimate effort to estimate future costs, its usefulness is limited. Further, if an initial impact study revealed an ineffective program, it would seem a waste of resources to conduct a cost analysis.

Moving to a cost-efficiency study hastens assignment of dollar values to program elements and benefits that may be impacted by that assignment. Examining costs has a political component. Although information from a cost analysis can strengthen the decision making required in resource management, the temptation may be to reduce all elements to dollars and cents and act as though the common denominator has been identified with no further considerations weighed in the decision formulae. The very act of setting monetary values may increase attention or reduce concern about a program's benefit. Also critical is which stakeholder assigns the value settings. Decisions involving ascription of value to human life experiences have ethical and political components and are not limited to economics.

ROLES IN EVALUATION

The preceding overview of PE was meant to make the reader aware of questions asked in the course of progressive evaluation. This awareness is necessary to recognize functional roles played by those conducting evaluations.

The role of the evaluator is contingent upon a number of things, including the intent of the PE (i.e., measurement, description, judgment, or negotiation of values) as consistent with the four generations of evaluation (Guba & Lincoln, 1989). Sarnecky (1990) outlines evaluator roles from each generation as cumulative. If the intent of the evaluation is simply to measure activities performed, the role of the evaluator is as a technician requiring skills of testing and measurement. However, if the valuative intent is an objectives-oriented description, the evaluator adopts the additional role of describer to identify patterns within the program measurements, as well as strengths and weaknesses related to program goals. With the need to differentiate between programs, the evaluator assumes the role of judge, using the measures and pattern descriptions generated. In this role the evaluator may be expected to culminate an evaluation report with major recommendations about program changes to enhance congruity among goals and outcomes.

More recently, when confronted with organizational complexity, the evaluator takes on the role of negotiator. In this role the evaluator strives to affirm existence of the plurality of values at work and negotiate a framework that considers a variety of perspectives, rather than judging the merit of any one to the exclusion of others. Guba and Lincoln (1989) describe this fourth generation evaluator as playing a very complex role. Evaluators facilitate problem identification and share stakeholder ideas across groups to shape reality and mediate change. As such they may act as technician, describer, judge, collaborator, teacher, learner, stage manager, reality shaper, change agent, negotiator, collaborator, and mediator. Patton (1975) describes this evaluator stance as "active-reactive-adaptive."

It is worth noting that none of these role labels designate the evaluator as decision maker or implementer. In order to facilitate an evaluation and encourage contribution from all players, the evaluator stance must be maintained from a relatively neutral position. Similar to those in staff rather than line positions, the authority of the evaluator arises informally, rather than formally.

CONCLUSION

The intent of this chapter was to encourage collaboration among health-system decision makers and professional evaluators, thereby increasing the use of evaluation findings in health-care settings. Linkages between values and PE underscore the complexity of program realities and reinforce the recognition that PE is conducted in an ever-changing milieu. One component of these realities is the role of the evaluator, which will change with the intent of the evaluation. Values imbedded in the policy space and stakeholder expectations have a critical influence in problem identification and consequent conduct of a PE.

As part of this overview, three points were emphasized. First, evaluation is scientifically based and so must consider *both* process and outcome of a program for meaningful results. Today's push for "outcomes assessment" may cloud this issue and must not be misinterpreted. Recognizing outcomes without accounting for the process by which the outcomes are achieved wastes efforts and resources. Second, today PE is essential for managing program resources. According to Puetz (1988), "despite economic and other constraints, not conducting . . . evaluation studies is not an option" (p. 64). And, finally, if PE is to be serviceable in health-care delivery, it must link directly and meaningfully with changing milieu, and it must be used to bring about change. Efforts expended in program evaluations that are not used are worthless.

REFERENCES

Argyris, C., Putnam, R., & Smith, D. Mc. (1985). *Action science.* San Francisco: Jossey-Bass.

Berk, R. A., & Rossi, P. H. (1990). *Thinking about program evaluation.* Newbury Park, CA: Sage.

Billue, J. S., & Clayton, B. M. (1988). Views on research: Program evaluation. *Nurse Educator, 13*(6), 8–9, 33.

Campbell, D. T., & Stanley, J. (1967). *Experimental and quasi-experimental designs for research.* Chicago: Rand McNally.

Guba, E. G., & Lincoln, Y. S. (1985). *Naturalistic inquiry.* Beverly Hills, CA: Sage.

Guba, E. G., & Lincoln, Y. S. (1989). *Fourth generation evaluation.* Newbury Park, CA: Sage.

Newman, D. L., Jatulis, L. L., & Carpinello, S. E. (1990). What is evaluation: Nurse decision-makers' perceptions of program evaluation. *Journal of the New York State Nurses Association, 21*(3), 10–14.

Patton, M. Q. (1978). *Utilization-focused evaluation.* Beverly Hills, CA: Sage.

Provus, M. (1971). *Discrepancy evaluation.* Berkeley, CA: McCutchan.

Puetz, B. (1988). Editorial: Evaluation and quality assurance in nursing care. *Rehabilitation Nursing, 13*(2), 64.

Rossi, P. H., & Freeman, H. E. (1985). *Evaluation: A systematic approach.* Beverly Hills, CA: Sage.

Sarnecky, M. T. (1990). Program evaluation part 1: Four generations of theory. *Nurse Educator, 15*(5), 25–28.

Scriven, M. (1973). Goal-free evaluation. In E. R. House (Ed.), *School evaluation: The politics and process.* Berkeley, CA: McCutchan.

Shortell, S. M., & Richardson, W. C. (1987). *Health program evaluation.* St. Louis, MO: C. V. Mosby.

Soukhanov, A. H. (Ed.). (1984). *Webster's II new Riverside University dictionary.* Boston: Houghton-Mifflin.

Stake, R. E. (1967). The countenance of educational evaluation. *Teachers College Record, 68*(7), 523–540.

Stufflebeam, D. L. (1971). *Educational evaluation and decision-making.* Itasca, IL: Peacock.

Tyler, R. W. (1950). *Basic principles of curriculum and instruction.* Chicago: University of Chicago Press.

Wolf, R. M. (1984). *Evaluation in education: Foundations of competency assessment and program review.* New York: Praeger Special Studies.

Woodham-Smith, C. (1951). *Florence Nightingale: 1820-1910.* New York: McGraw-Hill.

ADDITIONAL READING

Brooten, D., Brown, L. P., Munro, B. H., York, R., Cohn, S. M., Roncoli, M., & Hollingsworth, A. (1988). Early discharge and specialist transitional care. *Image: Journal of Nursing Scholarship, 20*(2), 64–68.

Brooten, D., Gennaro, S., Knapp, H., Jovene, N., Brown, L., & York, R. (1991). Functions of the CNS in early discharge and home follow-up of very-low-birth-weight infants. *Clinical Nurse Specialist, 5*(4), 196–201.

Brooten, D., Kumar, S., Brown, L. P., Butts, P., Finkler, S. A., Bakewell-Sachs, S., Gibbons, A., & Delivoria-Papadopoulos, M. (1986). A randomized clinical trial of early hospital discharge and home follow-up of very-low-birth-weight infants. *The New England Journal of Medicine, 315*(15), 934–939.

Brown, L. P., York, R., Jacobsen, B., Gennaro, S., & Brooten, D. (1989). Very-low-birth-weight infants: Parental visiting and telephoning during initial infant hospitalization. *Nursing Research, 38*(4), 233–236.

del Bueno, D. J. (1990). Evaluation: Myths, mystiques, and obsessions. *Journal of Nursing Administration, 20*(11), 4–7.

Love, A. J. (1991). *Internal evaluation: Building organizations from within.* Newbury Park, CA: Sage.

Martin, K. S., Scheet, N. J., & Stegman, M. R. (1993). Home health clients: Characteristics, outcomes of care, and nursing interventions. *American Journal of Public Health, 83*(12), 1730–1734.

Munro, B. H. (1983). A useful model for program evaluation. *Nurse Educator, 8*(1), 35–38.

Muraskin, L. D. (1993). *Understanding evaluation: The way to better prevention programs* (USGPO: 1993-349-449). Washington, DC: U. S. Department of Education.

Paine-Andrews, A., Francisco, V. T., & Fawcett, S. B. (1994). Assessing community health concerns and implementing a microgrant program for self-help initiatives. *American Journal of Public Health, 84*(2), 316–318.

J. W. Mold
K. R. Knapp

CHAPTER *8*

Interdisciplinary Teamwork

INTRODUCTION

The nature of health and health care have changed substantially over the past fifty years. Improvements in public health, sanitation, and prenatal and perinatal care, and the development of immunizations and antibiotics in concert with a variety of sociodemographic events have resulted in an aging population. The predominant health problems are no longer acute infectious diseases, but chronic disabling ones. Many of these diseases are the byproducts of a technological society: overnutrition, stress-related disorders, and diseases caused or exacerbated by environmental pollutants, sedentary lifestyles, and addictions to tobacco, alcohol, and a variety of illicit drugs. Others could be considered diseases of medical progress: iatrogenesis; loss of confidence in and dissatisfaction with health; polypharmacy; and induced disability (learned helplessness).

The capabilities of the health-care system continue to increase rapidly through the general advancement of science, and in response to a better educated and more demanding populace. It is now possible to detect many diseases long before symptoms appear. A number of diseases can be prevented, and with further advances in genetic engineering, the potential for doing so seems almost unlimited. Improvements in diagnostic testing, curative therapies, rehabilitative techniques, and information technology for clinical decision making have been equally impressive.

The health-care system has responded to this explosion of information and technologies by producing an increasing number of health-care professionals with focused areas of expertise. Medicine, nursing, and dentistry, for instance, have become partitioned into an array of specialties and subspecialties. In addition, a variety of completely new *allied-health* disciplines have emerged (Mold, 1991).

As the variety of health-care professionals has expanded, so have the settings in which health care is delivered. Unfortunately, health-care services have expanded more rapidly than the systems required for their coordination. Individual clients often become lost in the shuffle of admission and discharge summaries, consultation requests, and insurance forms.

The escalation of the national debate on health-care reform has underscored two of the current health-care-delivery system's most serious shortcomings — insufficient coordination and integration of services (Starfield, 1992). The emergence and growing acceptance among key public policy figures of concepts such as managed care and managed competition signal a renewed interest in placing the patient/client in the center of a system that improves the probability of positive outcomes, including patient satisfaction (Blandon, Knox, Brodie, Benson, & Chervinsky, 1994). This will require more effective and efficient interdisciplinary teamwork, and it will demand fundamental changes in the way that health and health care are defined, taught, practiced, measured, and managed (Banta, 1990).

BACKGROUND AND HISTORICAL PERSPECTIVE OF HEALTH CARE

The biomedical model upon which our current health-care system is based began to take firm root in the early nineteenth century following Gregor Mendel's discoveries in the area of genetics and his subsequent systematic classification of plants. Physicians, taking a similar approach, began to classify diseases according to their manifestations. Autopsy methods, improvements in the microscope, germ theory, and rapid advancements in scientific methods reinforced the notion first espoused by Sir Francis Bacon two centuries earlier that man, through the pursuit of science, was destined ultimately to be in complete control of his environment.

The Evolution of Medicine

Physicians became identified with the evolving science of medicine and, particularly since the Flexner Report (1910), received an education grounded in the basic biomedical sciences. The practice of medicine, thus, came to be viewed as an applied science. As diagnostic testing methodologies improved, the number of classifiable diseases increased. This resulted in an increasing array of subspecialties, each concentrating on a subset of these diseases. Pharmacy and dentistry, which also have long historical roots, developed along similar lines, and dentistry, particularly, has become increasingly subspecialized.

The Role of Nurses

In 1855, during the Crimean War, Florence Nightingale introduced hygienic standards into military hospitals. Largely as a result of her efforts, nursing became firmly established as a vital health-care profession (Friedman, 1990). Nurses have always viewed their role as unique; however, they have traditionally viewed themselves as being complementary and subservient to physicians. In the past twenty-five years, the nursing profession has more fully developed its own identity separate from medicine (Stein, Watts, & Howell, 1990) and has itself begun to develop multiple areas of subspecialization within the discipline.

The New Disciplines

Since World War II, a number of new disciplines have emerged to fill perceived gaps in the health-care system. Examples include occupational therapy, physical therapy, speech pathology and the expressive therapies, recreational therapy, clinical dietetics, and orthotics. Initially regulated by medical licensure boards, many of these disciplines are now trying to develop their own separate professional identities. As the concept of health has expanded to encompass social and psychological problems, social work, chaplaincy, and a variety of mental-health professions have become more closely affiliated with the health-care system.

The Biomedical Paradigm

Two fundamental assumptions serve as the basis for the current biomedical paradigm. First is the conceptualization of health as the absence of disease; second is the unstated belief that all diseases can, should be, and will eventually be understood and eradicated through the application of science. These assumptions have placed physicians in a firm position of authority among the health-care disciplines. As the most highly trained biomedical scientists, they are considered to be in the best position to direct efforts toward the identification, classification, and eradication of disease. The other professions must either fill supporting roles or develop new paradigms. In fact, it seems clear that new paradigms are emerging.

Tracing Interdisciplinary Teamwork

The history of interdisciplinary teamwork in health-care is somewhat difficult to trace. Certainly physicians and nurses have worked closely together for over a century. Surgical operating room teams represent an early example of teamwork. Rehabilitation teams have become the standard of rehabilitative care.

The application of interdisciplinary teamwork to primary-health-care delivery may have first occurred in this country in the late 1940s at Montefiore Hospital in New York City. It sprung from the belief that the provision of comprehensive, coordinated health-care services to families could only be provided effectively by a team of health professionals, because no single professional had all of the requisite skills. Subsequent federal funding priorities in the 1960s led to a number of similar initiatives around the country. Research to demonstrate the benefits of this approach was, unfortunately, not accomplished. With reductions in federal funding, many of these projects had to be discontinued.

In the past approximately ten years, there has been a revival of interest in interdisciplinary teamwork, as more and more health professionals recognize that health care has become too complex to be practiced in a fragmented, unidisciplinary mode. Clinical trials conducted in a variety of settings have documented the benefits of teamwork when practiced well and applied appropriately (Campbell & Whitenack, 1983; Halstead, 1976; McLaughlin, Altemeier, Christensen, Sherrod, Dietrich, & Stern, 1992; Rubenstein, Stuck, Siu, & Wieland, 1991; Williams, Williams, Zimmer, Hall, & Podgorski, 1987). It is both ironic and unfortunate that the very complexity which suggests the need for teamwork has created a system full of obstacles to its implementation.

THEORETICAL/CONCEPTUAL ORIENTATION OF TEAMWORK

Rothberg (1981) defined a health-care team as "a group of persons, each possessing particular expertise, who have a common purpose and goal" (p. 408). Health-care teams come in a variety of shapes and sizes depending on their setting, purpose, and administration. **Intradisciplinary** teams consist of two or more members of the same discipline. **Multidisciplinary** teams are made up of professionals from two or more different disciplines who carry out discipline-specific activities and are primarily responsible to their own departmental supervisors and to the client. Members of multidisciplinary teams are expected to know and apply the knowledge and skills of their own disciplines to the care of the client. Communication is generally written but may be more direct. Rarely do more than two team members, however, interact at the same time. **Interdisciplinary** teams are those in which members of two or more disciplines have agreed to work *together* toward common goals. Although members work within their own areas of competence, an attempt is made to avoid excessive duplication of efforts. Allegiance is primarily to the team and to the client, rather than to members' departments. Communication is generally direct and includes regular team meetings. Interdisciplinarity requires that members have and use skills for effective group interaction and synergism (Rothberg, 1981). The term *transdisciplinary* has been used to describe an interdisciplinary strategy in which members function outside their usual areas of expertise to complement and reinforce each others' efforts. For example, a rehabilitation team might agree that each member would use the communication methods prescribed by the speech therapist during every encounter with an aphasiac client.

Benefits and Drawbacks

Conventional wisdom holds that two heads are generally better than one. The more information and perspectives included in making a decision, the better the probability for a successful outcome. An appropriately constructed and functioning team can maximize the diversity of knowledge and skills required to complete a task effectively. Coordination of effort, and, therefore, reduced duplication and fragmentation, is more attainable in a team setting. And the empowerment of the team's members to creatively problem solve, individually and corporately, is strengthened because of shared ownership in the decisions reached as a team. Experience has shown, however, that there is no foolproof formula for establishing a team of the right size or composition — and that performance is never guaranteed. Furthermore, there can be a point of diminishing returns.

The Importance of Interdependence

A highly functioning team is generally one which has discovered how to balance its members' roles with their respective areas of expertise, interest levels, motivations, energy, and availability (Pfeiffer, 1991). Moving the team's members away from dependence and independence toward interdependence is an important early goal.

Dependence is the paradigm of "you and you take care of me; you came through for me; you didn't come through for me; and I blame you for the results." *Independence* is the paradigm of "I and I can do it; I am responsible; I am self-reliant; and I can choose." *Interdependence* is the paradigm of "we and we can do it; we can cooperate; we can combine our talents and abilities and create something greater together." Interdependent people combine their efforts with the efforts of others to achieve their greatest success (Covey, 1989).

Defining Quality

Quality in health care has been somewhat difficult to define despite a variety of well-organized approaches to assure it. An assumption is generally made that quality of care can be determined by examining outcomes, particularly undesirable ones, or by assessing certain elements of the process of care, such as the completeness of the evaluation or the appropriateness of the ordered tests. Steffen (1988) proposes that quality health care be defined as care that has the capacity to achieve legitimate health-related goals, such goals to be developed through a collaborative process involving the client and the health-care provider. By this definition, any evaluation of **outcomes** must take into account the goals of the individual client and health-care professionals. **Indicators** related to the **process** of care would have to be viewed within a similar context.

The Implications of a Goal-Oriented Approach

Acknowledging the importance of goals to the concept of quality challenges the basic tenets of the problem-oriented biomedical model. If health is defined as the absence of disease and discomfort; and clients are expected to desire health; and methods that most effectively and efficiently eliminate disease and discomfort have been determined, then there is really very little need for goal setting. The goals and appropriate strategies are considered to be self-evident.

In contrast, a goal-oriented approach to health care assumes that health encompasses more than the absence of disease and discomfort, that the concept of health and the desire for it can be different for different individuals, and that the goals of health care for each individual should, therefore, be based not only on science, but also on that individual's values, preferences, needs, and resources (Mold, Blake, & Becker, 1991; Mold, 1995). This view seems to be gaining in popularity, particularly among primary-health-care providers and health-care consumers. It opens up several cans of worms, however, for health-care professionals. This view both lengthens and blurs the boundary that had previously been so carefully drawn around the concept of health. Thus, it is less clear where health ends and where psychological growth and development, satisfaction with social relationships, spirituality, and even financial security begin. This opens the door for nonphysician health professionals to take a larger, more important role in health care. It also renders current assessment methods inadequate and suggests the need for better approaches to goal setting. It clearly diminishes the power and control of all health-care professionals by empowering clients to take a greater role in their health care, and it reveals the need for better integration at a practical level of the expertise and services of health professionals.

CHALLENGES OF APPLYING TEAMWORK TO PRACTICE

Interdisciplinary teamwork can, in theory at least, improve the quality of health care. There are, however, some potential obstacles to teamwork. For instance, because frequent, direct communication among the various team members is needed, a substantial amount of time is required on a regular basis for team meetings; scheduling can be a major obstacle. Further complicating this problem is the fact that team members may, of necessity, be based in different locations (e.g., dentists, pharmacists, physical therapists). And it is often difficult to involve clients in team discussions. On the other hand, it could be argued that the time saved by coordinating efforts and avoiding duplication might outweigh the time required to do so. It has, unfortunately, been difficult to calculate the amount of time and money wasted because of poor communication and coordination among health professionals.

When several individuals are involved in such a complex decision-making enterprise, there is a potential for conflict and frustration, for diffusion of responsibility, and for greater rather than less coercion of clients (Rae-Grant & Marcuse, 1968). That the views of various health professionals often differ is neither unexpected nor unhealthy. For these differences to be resolved in the interests of quality care, they must be recognized. In a fragmented health-care system, they occur at least as frequently but are less often acknowledged and discussed.

Interdisciplinarity raises several ethical (Pellegrino, 1977) and legal issues. An issue of particular concern to physicians is liability. Will the physician continue to accept a disproportionate amount of liability for untoward outcomes? If so, what incentives will there be for the physician to relinquish any part of the decision-making role and participate in the team, either as its leader or as a member?

Some of the other commonly witnessed barriers to cooperation and team formation involve funding and organizational politics. This is particularly true in health care, where reimbursement can so often dictate who is involved, for how much time, doing what to whom and why. Organizational politics is more than turf and territorial protection; it can include unpredictable variables like personal egos and professional recognition needs, ownership of ideas, corporate climate for risk taking, and attitudes about the value of team decision making. Any of these, singly or in combination with each other, can, and most often do, influence the development and effectiveness of interdisciplinary teams.

Overcoming Obstacles

It is generally not enough to merely bring a diverse group together and expect its output to somehow transcend what the individual members might have achieved on their own. The whole may *not* be greater than the sum of its parts if left solely to spontaneous generation. In order for positive outcomes to outweigh potential *inefficiencies*, it is critical that the team's members learn how to function as one, both as effective team members and as team leaders, with clearly defined roles and expectations for themselves and each other (Scholtes, 1988).

Health professionals receive little training in teamwork. In fact, as students they rarely interact with students in other disciplines. This is not because their teachers are unaware of the importance of interdisciplinary instruction, but is apparently more related to the organizational structure of educational institutions (Mold & Holt, 1993).

As the individual disciplines have struggled to define turf, they have strayed to varying degrees from the traditional conceptual model of health and health care. This creates difficulties for members of these disciplines when they try to function on an interdisciplinary team (Clark, Spence, & Sheehan, 1987). In fact, they are often unaware of the extent to which the perspectives of other team members vary from their own, assuming, instead, that everyone is operating from a similar frame of reference. Until a common conceptual model can be developed, this will likely remain a significant obstacle.

Communication and coordination of effort are critical elements of an effective team. Language is only an effective means of communication if the receiver hears what is intended by the sender. The same word or phrase used in clinical documentation by members of different disciplines may carry very different meanings for each of them, respectively. And it can be especially difficult to effectively coordinate efforts if the team members are, in essence, speaking different languages. Something as simple as a common glossary of terms can contribute significantly to the effectiveness of a team.

Most people simply rely on naturally developed interpersonal skills to survive the team experience. Because so few people are aware of any rules or guidelines, many teams are inefficient — and can remain that way indefinitely — unless their dynamics improve with practice or the team members take it upon themselves to become more familiar with how to be more effective in their respective roles on the team. Perhaps the best single source of information on building effective teams is Peter Scholtes' *The Team Handbook: How to Use Teams to Improve Quality* (1988). It provides all the necessary tools and background for those interested in elevating their proficiency in teamwork.

While it is critical that team members be primarily responsible to the client and the team, in most health-care settings health professionals are primarily responsible to their individual department heads. Brill (1976) has stated that a departmental organizational structure and interdisciplinary teamwork are like oil and water. For interdisciplinarity to flourish, new organizational models must be developed within health-care systems.

ISSUES AND TRENDS

All across America, organizations big and small have been rediscovering an axiom of effective leadership — *empowerment.* Corporations are finding that people are most productive when opportunities are created that strengthen their personal stakes in the outcomes of the organization. This new focus on empowering people means that individuals who have traditionally had very little to say about the direction of an organization are beginning to actively participate in planning strategies, implementing new programs and services, monitoring progress, and sharing in corporate success.

In Georgetown, Kentucky, every employee at the Toyota Motors Assembly Plant receives extensive initial and ongoing training in team concepts, including measurement techniques for identifying quality improvement opportunities. At Connaught Laboratories, a pharmaceutical firm, a janitor who learned to function as part of a problem-solving team contributed recommendations that resulted in improved safety for personnel. The improved safety achieved a 40 percent reduction in waste. The firm credits its increased profitability to commitment to training at all levels (Paton, 1993).

Occurring simultaneously to the trend toward empowerment in business and industry is a mounting interest in quality among both manufacturers and service industries, and especially among health-care and human-service providers. The terms **Quality Assurance (QA)**, *Infection Control, Risk Management,* and *Product Inspection* are increasingly being replaced by **Continuous Quality Improvement (CQI), Total Quality Management (TQM),** and **Kaizan.** Notably central to the description of each of these promising approaches to achieving quality is the concept of *team* (Scholtes, 1992).

Starting with W. Edwards Deming and his *Fourteen Points* (Walton, 1990), and followed by a steady stream of popular authors who have studied the methods of the world's most successful corporations, management literature has inundated with one account after another illustrating the importance of structuring traditional hierarchical organizations. Collectively, these authors have built a compelling argument for how essential teamwork is as an ingredient for effective, lasting empowerment to occur (Walton, 1986).

Organizations that have been slow to investigate the advantages of teamwork, empowerment, and *self-directed work groups* often invoke what Peter Block (1987) describes as the *Franco Rationale.* Francisco Franco, dictator of Spain, claimed for many years that he would just love to hold popular elections, but that the people of Spain were not ready for them. The same argument is often used by people at every level of traditional organizations, especially hierarchical health-care organizations. "We say we would like people to be more participative . . . to take more responsibility for themselves . . . to create autonomous work teams . . . but people right now are not ready for this" (Block, 1987, p. 31).

Dr. William Byham (1993) describes the American health-care delivery system as the next frontier of the empowerment movement. He contends that greater empowerment of health-care employees — job identification and ownership — can lead to better patient care, greater job satisfaction, and lower health-care costs. Empowerment energizes the people "who are closest to the patient and the technology to continuously look for ways to provide high-quality patient care and improve processes" (pp. VII–X). The accumulation of ideas from many people can consistently result in better patient care and operational efficiencies.

Driven by the ever-increasing costs of the health-care system, efforts to improve its efficiency and effectiveness can be expected to continue for some time to come. There is, unfortunately, no limit to the amount of money that can be expended in the quest for perfect health when health is defined as the absence of problems and when the range of normalcy keeps getting narrower. Despite remarkable advances in diagnostic and therapeutic technologies, however, more and more people seem to be dissatisfied with their health care and with the health-care system. Many have already turned to *alternative health-care providers* such as naturopaths, homeopaths, chiropractors, and rolfers. At the same time there is increasing pressure from nursing and the allied-health disciplines for physicians to take a more holistic view of health. These forces can be expected to lead eventually to the paradigm shift that must occur before true reform will be possible.

Models of health care in which a known population of people are provided with services designed to meet their unique needs are likely to become more common. Such models have been called *managed care* and *community-oriented primary care.* Interdisciplinary teamwork has generally been an important feature of such models. In the foreseeable future, primary-care services are likely to be provided from moderately sized group practices with a centralized base clinic and multiple satellite clinics. Key members of the primary-care team will likely be nurses and nurse practitioners, physician assistants, physicians, and social workers and counselors. Support staff will include radiology and laboratory technicians and medical assistants. Dieticians, pharmacists, dentists, and dental hygienists may also be housed within the base clinics. These primary-care teams will coordinate the entire health-care system, requesting specific services, when needed, from secondary and tertiary providers while maintaining longitudinal interdisciplinary records, and taking primary responsibility for outcomes.

The aging of the population and the increase in the prevalence of chronic diseases and disabilities will also contribute to the anticipated paradigm shift and will require an even greater emphasis upon rehabilitative approaches. Although interdisciplinary teamwork is already considered to be an essential feature of rehabilitation, rehabilitation teams are frequently more multidisciplinary than interdisciplinary. Physicians tend to dominate decision making, records are rarely integrated, and goals are often compiled from lists written separately by each discipline based upon the problems identified by that discipline. This unquestionably will change.

Long-term care settings, including nursing homes, home care, and same-day hospital/therapeutic day-care programs have made tremendous strides toward interdisciplinarity, largely because of federal Medicare guidelines. Decision making is, however, still problem oriented, records are multidisciplinary rather than interdisciplinary, and physicians rarely participate in care planning. Advances in health-care teamwork are likely, however, to be seen earliest in these settings.

Hospitals have more to learn about interdisciplinarity than do most other health-care institutions. The generally strong departmental organizational structure encouraged by tradition, turf issues, and accreditation guidelines; the apparent effectiveness of the biomedical model in this setting; the strength of subspecialty physician involvement; and the somewhat greater potential liability involved have all served to inhibit change in this setting. As less care is rendered in the hospital, and as primary care takes a more dominant position in the health-care system, substantial changes can be expected to take place in both the organization and process of care delivery for seriously ill patients.

The concept of CQI has attracted widespread interest among health-care administrators and professionals. A critical step in this approach to **Quality Management (QM)** is the formation of a team that understands the processes involved (Walton, 1990). A literature of examples of interdisciplinary CQI initiatives is building. The experience gained by the participants in these projects may inspire them to learn more about other disciplines and about interdisciplinarity. As a result, it may increase the number of health professionals striving to develop new conceptual models, organizational patterns, and delivery systems that are more compatible with interdisciplinary collaboration. Likewise, quality-improvement efforts should be much more effective as a result of teamwork.

Interdisciplinary cooperation and understanding, commitment to training, empowerment of the team, remaining client-centered — all are important components of the successful and productive team. But in today's world (and, more importantly, in tomorrow's world), the effective support of technology will help distinguish one organization from its competitors. What do the Toyota plant, American Express, and McDonald's have in common? They all match a people orientation with a systems emphasis, blending people with each other as well as with technology. This emphasis will be an essential ingredient of highly effective teams and their organizations in the years ahead (Peters, 1987).

Communication technologies will be extremely important. Videoteleconferencing will facilitate team meetings with members at different sites. Computer networks that allow multiple users to communicate through modems may also be used for this purpose. The development of fully integrated, computerized record systems that allow team members to contribute to a unified database should result in less duplication of effort and more consistent communication of information.

Electronic storage of large amounts of patient data will enable organizations to base quality improvement decisions on better, more current information than previously possible. It will also make it much more possible for researchers to study patient-outcome predictors, to compare and test caregiver models, and to perform research in a variety of settings traditionally limited to the hospital. Effective strategic planning at both the micro and macro levels will be significantly enhanced, as well, by the availability of more information. Finally, public health data and vital statistics will be more comprehensive, with more sources for specific information that could be useful to policymakers and health officials.

The relatively recent trend toward interdisciplinarity in research and the development of a variety of multidisciplinary centers on health-science campuses, by enhancing collegiality among faculty and providing an administrative home, should result in more effective interdisciplinary teaching efforts. Efforts are being made in several parts of the country to accelerate this trend. In Louisville, Kentucky, an interdisciplinary training consortium called LIFE SPAN has been formed. This consortium enables health-and-human-service students to experience teamwork firsthand in geriatric settings. Six area institutions of higher learning, four long-term care organizations, and an acute-care hospital cooperate to provide students from nine disciplines the opportunity to learn about and work with one another before entering their respective fields of practice (Roberts, Wright, Thibault, Stewart, & Knapp, 1993).

CONCLUSION

Interdisciplinarity in health care is essential to improving its quality. When successfully implemented it very likely improves coordination and efficiency, encourages excellence, amplifies creativity, and improves health outcomes. Seemingly formidable obstacles to its implementation still exist, however. A variety of simultaneous trends are making conditions much more favorable for its growth, but until a new health-care paradigm emerges, true interdisciplinary teamwork will continue to be difficult and frustrating. The authors propose that the organizing principle of the new paradigm be goal setting rather than problem solving, because a goal-oriented model would be expected to be more holistic, client-centered, and compatible with interdisciplinary collaboration. As organizational structures develop around this new paradigm, educational institutions begin to teach in accordance with it, and technologies are applied to its implementation, interdisciplinarity will probably become the accepted mode of health-care delivery.

REFERENCES

Banta, H. D. (1990). What is health care? In A. R. Kovner & S. Jonas (Eds.), *Health care delivery in the United States* (pp. 8–30). New York: Springer.

Blandon, R. J., Knox, R. A., Brodie, M., Benson, J. M., & Chervinsky, G. (1994). Americans compare managed care, Medicare and fee-for-service. *Journal of American Health Policy, 4*(3), 42–47.

Block, P. (1987). *The empowered manager: Positive politic skills at work.* San Francisco: Jossey-Bass.

Brill, N. I. (1976). *Teamwork: Working together in the human services.* Philadelphia: J. B. Lippincott.

Byham, W. C. (1993). *Zapp: Empowerment in health care.* New York: Ballantine Books.

Campbell, L. S., & Whitenack, D. C. (1983). An interdisciplinary approach for consultation on multiproblem patients. *North Carolina Medical Journal, 44*(2), 81–87.

Clark, P. G., Spence, D. L., & Sheehan, J. L. (1987). Challenges and barriers to interdisciplinary gerontological team training in the academic setting. *Gerontology and Geriatrics Education, 7*(3/4), 93–110.

Covey, S. R. (1989). *The seven habits of highly effective people.* New York: Simon and Schuster.

Flexner, A., & Carnegie Foundation. (1910). *Medical education in the United States and Canada: A report to the Carnegie Foundation for the Advancement of Teaching.* Washington, DC: Science and Health Publications.

Friedman, E. (1990). Troubled past of the "invisible" profession. *Journal of the American Medical Association, 264*(22), 2851–2858.

Halstead, L. S. (1976). Team care in chronic illness: A critical review of the literature of the past 25 years. *Archives of Physical Medicine and Rehabilitation, 57*(11), 507–511.

McLaughlin, F., Altemeier, W., Christensen, M., Sherrod, K., Dietrich, M. S., & Stern, D. T. (1992). Randomized trial of comprehensive prenatal care for low-income women: Effect on infant birth weight. *Pediatrics, 89*(1), 128–132.

Mold, J. W. (1991). The health care system. In M. B. Mengel (Ed.), *Principles of clinical practice* (pp. 267–296). New York: Plenum Medical Book Co.

Mold, J. W. (1995). An alternative conceptualization of health and health care: Its implications for geriatrics and gerontology. *Journal of Educational Gerontology, 21*, 85–101.

Mold, J. W., Blake, G. H., & Becker, L. A. (1991). Goal-oriented medical care. *Family Medicine, 23*(1), 46–51.

Mold, J. W., & Holt, R. (1993). A survey of faculty opinions regarding interdisciplinary education in a health sciences center. *Journal of Gerontology and Geriatrics Education, 13*(4), 65–73.

Paton, S. M. (1993). Quiet janitor becomes team's "waste guru." *Quality Digest, 13*(5), 12.

Pellegrino, E. D. (1977, May 9–10). The ethics of team care: Some notes on the morality of collective decision-making. *American Cancer Society Inc. Proceedings, 2nd National Conference on Cancer Nursing,* American Cancer Society.

Peters, T. (1987). *Thriving on chaos: Handbook for a management revolution.* New York: Harper and Row.

Pfeiffer, J. W. (Ed.). (1991). *The encyclopedia of team-development activities.* San Diego: Pfeiffer and Company.

Rae-Grant, Q. A. F., & Marcuse, D. J. (1968). The hazards of teamwork. *American Journal of Orthopsychiatry, 38*(1), 4–8.

Roberts, K. T., Wright, J. C., Thibault, J. M., Stewart, A. V., & Knapp, K. R. (1993). Geriatric partnerships in health care: The LIFE SPAN model. *Educational Gerontology, 20*(2), 115–128.

Rothberg, J. S. (1981). The rehabilitation team: Future direction. *Archives of Physical Medicine and Rehabilitation, 62*(8), 407–410.

Rubenstein, L. Z., Stuck, A. E., Siu, A. L., & Wieland, D. (1991). Impacts of geriatric evaluation and management programs on defined outcomes: Overview of the evidence. *Journal of the American Geriatrics Society, 39*(Suppl. no. 395), 8S–16S.

Scholtes, P. R. (1988). *The team handbook: How to use teams to improve quality.* Madison, WI: Joiner Associates.

Starfield, B. (1992). *Primary care: Concept, evaluation, and policy.* New York: Oxford University Press.

Steffen, G. E. (1988). Quality medical care: A definition. *Journal of the American Medical Association, 260*(1), 56–61.

Stein, L. I., Watts, D. T., & Howell, T. (1990). The doctor-nurse game revisited. *The New England Journal of Medicine, 322*(8), 546–549.

Walton, M. (1986). *The Deming management method.* New York: Perigee Books.

Walton, M. (1990). *Deming management at work.* New York: Perigee Books.

Williams, M. E., Williams, F. W., Zimmer, J. G., Hall, W. J., & Podgorski, C. A. (1987). How does the team approach to outpatient geriatric evaluation compare with traditional care: A report of a randomized controlled trial. *Journal of the American Geriatrics Society, 35*(12), 1071–1078.

ADDITIONAL READING

Brill, N. I. (1976). *Teamwork: In working together in the human services.* Philadelphia, PA: J. B. Lippincott.

Carcuff, R. R. (1983). *The art of helping.* Amherst, MA: Human Resource Development Press.

Clark, P. G., & Grinka, T. J. K. (Guest Eds.). (1994). Conceptual foundations for interdisciplinary education in gerontology and geriatrics. *Educational Gerontology, 20*(1).

Ducanis, A. J., & Golin, A. K. (1979). *The interdisciplinary health care team: A handbook.* Germantown, MD: Aspen Systems.

McEwen, M. (1994). Promoting interdisciplinary collaboration. *Nursing and Health Care, 15*(6), 304–307.

Miller, P. A., & Toner, J. A. (1991). The making of a geriatric team. In W. Meyers (Ed.), *New techniques in the psychotherapy of older patients* (pp. 203–291). Washington, DC: American Psychiatric Press Inc.

Qualls, S. H., & Czirr, R. (1988). Geriatric health teams: Classifying models of professional and team functioning. *The Gerontologist, 28*(3), 372–376.

Rubin, I. M., Fry, R. E., & Plovnick, M. S. (1978). Making health teams work: An educational program. In J. Medalie (Ed.), *Family medicine: Principles and application* (pp. 316–328). Baltimore: Williams and Wilkins.

Schmitt, M. H., Farrell, M. P., & Heinemann, G. D. (1988). Conceptual and methodological problems in studying the effects of interdisciplinary teams. *The Gerontologist, 28*(6), 753–764.

Sundrom, E., De Meuse, K. P., & Futrell, D. (1990). Work teams: Applications and effectiveness. *American Psychologist, 45*(2), 120–133.

White House Domestic Policy Council (1993). *The president's health security plan: The Clinton blueprint.* New York: Times Book.

PART II

QUALITY MANAGEMENT: NATIONAL PERSPECTIVES

Margaret J. Bull

CHAPTER *9*

Past and Present Perspectives on Quality of Care in the United States

INTRODUCTION

Quality — what is it? Who defines it? What does it mean with respect to health care? What does it mean with respect to nursing care? Quality is an elusive concept, and the way in which it has been defined throughout our history reflects the values and societal forces prevailing at specific points in time. These changing values and societal forces provided an impetus for a shift in paradigms, or ways of viewing quality care. Recognizing these changes and our heritage in providing quality care is essential in charting the future of health care in the United States. This chapter provides a description of the paradigm shifts, a historical perspective on the evaluation of quality health care in the United States, and a discussion of directions for the future.

Central to a discussion of perspectives on quality of health care is the issue of how one measures quality. Measurement can be based on **structure** criteria, such as educational preparation or staffing; **process** criteria, which focus on activities performed in delivering care; or **outcome** criteria, which focus on the end result of care or a measurable change in the client's health (American Nurses Association [ANA], 1976). The values prevailing at different times in our history influenced the selection of structure, process, or outcome criteria. Political, economic, and professional factors also influenced the **criteria** selected as well as the ways in which quality is defined and **evaluated**. Figure 9-1 illustrates the major societal factors that have influenced developments in **Quality Assurance (QA)**.

Although the role played by each factor has shifted over time, and QA has given way to **Continuous Quality Improvement (CQI)**, these forces continue to shape the directions of health care and quality care.

SHIFTING PARADIGMS OF QUALITY

A paradigm is a model or way of viewing things. Paradigms reflect values and beliefs, and influence the ways in which a person acts toward the world. For

141

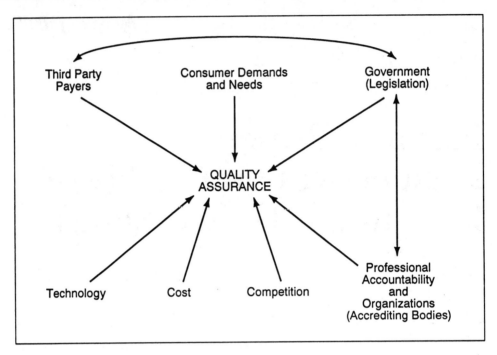

Figure 9-1 *Societal Forces Influencing Quality Assurance. (Reprinted from Bull, M.J., "Quality Assurance: Professional Accountability via Continuous Quality Improvement," in* Improving Quality: A Guide to Effective Programs, *C. Meisenheimer, Ed., p. 4, with permission of Aspen Publishers, Inc., copyright 1992.)*

example, initial efforts in QA reflected professional values, focused on inspection and identifying deficiencies rather than on continuous improvement and preventing problems. In the 1980s and 1990s increased concern about costs led to a focus on entire patient-care episodes and how to recognize how systems influence quality outcomes. It also brought a shift in perspective — from reacting to deficiencies to proacting to prevent problems. Consumer input is the driving force in the new paradigm. The shift from QA to CQI also meant moving from competition to cooperation; from meeting an acceptable level of quality to continuous improvement; from placing blame (usually on the worker) to problem solving, with managers assuming responsibility for quality; from a department- or unit-based approach to a system-wide approach; and from a philosophy of cost *versus* quality to a philosphy of cost *and* quality (Crosby, 1984; Deming, 1984; Gillem, 1988).

EVALUATING QUALITY OF HEALTH CARE: HISTORICAL PERSPECTIVE

Today's emphasis on evaluating the quality of health care can best be understood in light of history. The following section describes the forces that influenced quality care and its measurement at different points in time.

The Early Years: The Focus on Structure

In the 1860s most nursing care in hospitals was disorganized. Following the Civil War, Dr. Valentine Seamon initiated the first comprehensive educational program for nurses in North America (Kalisch & Kalisch, 1978). During the same period Sister Helen, a graduate of the Nightingale School, came from England to serve as superintendent of New York's Bellevue Hospital School of Nursing (Nightingale, 1911). The goal was to improve nursing care by improving the educational preparation of nurses.

During the early twentieth century health-care professionals provided the major impetus for assuring quality care. Efforts focused on the development of structural **standards**, although there is some evidence that client outcomes were also considered. It was during this period that the first state nurses' associations organized to work for legislation requiring licensure to practice nursing. The four components included in licensure laws were:

1. preliminary education

2. professional training

3. licensing examinations

4. registry (Bull, 1992)

However, states varied on the specific criteria for each component. For instance, by 1912 six states required nurses to complete high school; four states required one year of high school; and three required only completion of grammar school. Requirements for professional training also varied: twenty-one states mandated completion of a two-year nursing program; nine states mandated completion of a three-year program; and two states did not have any requirements. Although all states required nurses to take an examination, persons who were licensed in one state could obtain a waiver to practice in another state (Goodrich, 1912).

The development of structure standards was also apparent in the criteria for community-health nurses proposed by the Joint Committee for Consideration of the Standardization of Visiting Nurses in 1912. These first standards required that the nurse:

1. be at least 25 years of age

2. be a graduate of a recognized general hospital of not less than fifty beds, giving a course of training of not less than two years, including obstetrics

3. be a graduate of a hospital acceptable to the state board of registration, where state registration applies (Wald, 1912)

In addition, this Committee urged organizations that employed visiting nurses to pay salaries that would secure and retain visiting nurses of the highest grade (Wald, 1912).

During this period physicians also developed standards. The American Medical Association (AMA) pushed for reforms in medical education and obtained assistance from the Carnegie Foundation, which conducted a national survey of medical schools. The results were published in the Flexner Report (1910), which condemned the standards of proprietary colleges and revealed that many physicians were poorly educated. Foundation grants were given to colleges that met the standards proposed in the Flexner Report and as these standards were instituted, many medical schools closed (Fee, 1982). The Flexner reforms emphasized education and **licensure** requirements rather than how medicine was practiced. It was assumed that changes in education would improve practice.

In 1914 Dr. Ernest Codman, a surgeon affiliated with Massachusetts General Hospital, proposed a patient follow-up system that emphasized outcome-oriented medical audits. Dr. Codman examined all of his patients one year after surgery to determine whether the operation had alleviated symptoms and whether there were any iatrogenic effects (Codman, 1914). His efforts led the American College of Surgeons to develop standards for hospitals in 1918.

The health-care reforms of this period corresponded with other social reforms. The growth of cities was accompanied by disease, high death rates, and social disorganization. Corruption in city government provided an impetus for municipal reforms emphasizing efficiency and honest accounting in public administration. City-manager forms of government and regular, independent audits of city accounts tended to bring local government into a more manageable compass (Glaab & Brown, 1983). During this era, consumers did not question the quality of health care. A poor outcome was accepted as something beyond human control rather than the fault of an individual practitioner.

1920 to 1940: A Limited Focus on Quality

Work in the area of quality care was limited during the period of 1920 to 1940. A study conducted by the Committee on the Grading of Nursing Schools, however, demonstrates early efforts to obtain consumers' perspectives on quality (Burgess, 1928). The purpose of the study was to identify the type, quality, and number of nurses needed to provide adequate care for patients; to determine patient satisfaction with nursing care; and to determine physician satisfaction with nurses and nursing care. Questionnaires were mailed to all members of the American Medical Association and to a national sample of hospitalized patients. Forty-four percent of the patients (N=1,892) and approximately 25 percent of the physicians (N=23,500) returned the questionnaire. The findings indicated that the majority of the patients (86 percent) were satisfied with their nurses and expressed a desire to have the same nurses again. Patients felt that a major problem was in getting the "right" nurse; however, 54 percent of the patients stated that paying the nurse was the most difficult problem. Patients associated the following characteristics with good nursing care: patience, adaptability, gentleness, and loyalty to the family and physician. Patients' most frequent complaint about hospital nursing care was that they were awakened at 5:00 or 6:00 A.M. for morning care. They stated that sick people need all the rest they can get. Other common complaints were that they were given dirty bedpans, there were too few nurses to care for the patient, and nurses were not receptive to suggestions from patients. Patients stated that if a nurse felt she knew best she should still be willing to discuss a subject with a patient, rather than acting omnipotent (Burgess, 1928).

In contrast, physicians wanted nurses to meet the following criteria: take care in following medical orders, possess skill in observing and reporting symptoms, be skilled in giving general care and making the patient comfortable, and have an attractive personality. Ninety percent of the physicians reported that they were satisfied with the nursing care the patients received. The findings from this study also indicated that there was a shortage of hospital nurses and that more nurses with preparation in community health were needed (Burgess, 1928).

Societal issues during this time focused on recovery from World War I and the collapse of the economy. With the Depression, access to health care became a key issue. Although several bills for national health insurance were introduced in Congress during the 1930s, none was enacted. Special-interest groups such as the AMA and the American Federation of Labor opposed the national plans. However, the AMA endorsed voluntary hospital insurance as long as physician services were not included, and further proposed that local medical societies develop insurance plans to cover physician services. Consequently, the 1930s witnessed the evolution of voluntary health insurance programs to meet hospitals' needs for payment (Kingsbury, 1939).

1940 to 1960: The Focus on Process

During the period of 1940 to 1960 managers of American business focused on improving quality of their operations by restructuring work systems to improve worker motivation (Dienemann, 1992). Their strategies concentrated on processes such as worker participation and job enrichment. Perhaps as a carryover from business, and, possibly, as a result of increased education of the public, consumers developed greater interest in the planning, organization, and evaluation of health care. Increased demand for access to health care led to the Hill-Burton Act of 1946, which provided funds for the expansion of hospitals. The major impetus for evaluating the quality of care, however, continued to come from the professional sector.

During the 1950s three landmark studies, which focused on the process of medical care, were published. The first study, conducted by Dr. O. L. Peterson (Peterson, Andrews, Spain, & Greenberg, 1956), examined the care provided by general practice physicians. He evaluated medical practice on the basis of the adequacy of the history, physical exam, therapy, and amount of follow-up care. The second study, conducted by Dr. Morehead (1958), evaluated the ambulatory care provided by a prepaid group practice in New York. Data were obtained by talking with physicians and reviewing the patients' records. The third study, conducted by Dr. Payne in Michigan, examined the medical care provided in a select group of general hospitals in Michigan. Information documented in medical records was compared with disease-specific criteria developed by a group of physicians (Fitzpatrick, Reidel, & Payne, 1962). All three of these studies reported major deficiencies in the medical care provided (Brook & Avery, 1975).

Nursing studies during this period focused primarily on the process of care. For instance, Reiter and Kakosh (1963) developed an observation guide to evaluate the nursing care in hospitals. The criteria for the guide were derived from actual nursing-care situations that were observed and described by practicing nurses, and included nursing activities such as observing, teaching, and communicating (cited in Abdellah, 1970, p. 12). In contrast, a study by Wandelt (1954) compared differences in hospitalized patients' outcomes when planned instruction versus incidental instruction was used. The findings indicated that patients had a better understanding of their diseases when planned instruction was used. In addition, nurses continued to develop structure standards. The ANA published its *Functions, Standards, and Qualifications for Practice* (1963), and the National League for Nursing published *What People Can Expect of a Modern Nursing Service* (1959).

The Joint Commission on Accreditation of Hospitals (JCAH), which was formed in 1952, was one of the best known proponents of structure criteria. The JCAH sent teams of experts to hospitals to evaluate their quality against a checklist of minimum standards. For instance, hospitals were required to post signs where oxygen was used. Both professionals and health-care organizations assumed that meeting structure and process standards would automatically result in quality care (Bull, 1992).

The 1960s: Stretching Beyond Process

Societal influences during the 1960s included concern for consumer protection, human rights, and health care as a right. In response to the view of health care as a right, the decade witnessed the enactment of federal legislation to improve access to care for the poor and the elderly. The 1965 amendments to the Social Security Act created Medicare and Medicaid. Requirements for utilization review accompanied the Medicare and Medicaid programs in an effort to assure accountability and quality care in acute-care hospitals and nursing homes.

The Comprehensive Health Planning Act was passed in 1966 in order to link spending to better planning and foster the setting of priorities for federal and state funding. This legislation was followed by the Regional Medical Program Act, which provided funds for research and development. Emphasis was on improving service by applying knowledge (Taft & Levine, 1977). In Wisconsin, the Regional Medical Program appointed a committee to delineate the needs of nursing (Hinsvark, 1976). The nursing committee concentrated on mechanisms to improve the delivery of nursing care to patients, families, and communities. Their efforts resulted in several nursing projects, including a Film Script for Quality Assurance developed by J. Lund, and studies of nurse utilization and patient outcome (Hinsvark, 1976).

Also during this period Donabedian (1966) proposed a model for evaluating quality of care that advocated for comprehensive assessments including structure, process, and outcome. Still, little attention was given to outcomes. Nationally, nurses' efforts in the area of QA concentrated on developing measures to assess the process of care. The process audit developed by Maria Phaneuf (1964) was based on the following legal functions of professional nursing:

1. execution of physician's orders

2. observation of signs and symptoms

3. supervision of the patient

4. supervision of others who contribute to the care of patients (except for physicians)

5. reporting and recording

6. application and execution of nursing procedures and techniques

7. promotion of physical and emotional health by directing and teaching patients (Phaneuf, 1976)

The Phaneuf audit was designed to evaluate nursing care in community-health agencies, nursing homes, and hospitals through retrospective review of the patient record. It was one of the few instruments of this period that had been tested for validity and reliability (Phaneuf, 1972). Another process audit, developed by Eleanor Lambertson (1965), consisted of six basic standards with substandards. The substandards could be adapted to each specific service. The advantage was that it allowed nurses who worked in different specialties to develop their own measures for the substandards.

Although the major focus of quality assessment was process, Aydelotte and Tener (1960) conducted a study that exemplified an early effort to link structure, process, and outcome. They examined the effect of increasing registered nurse staff on a medical-surgical unit on patterns of medication administration and subsequent outcomes. The outcomes of care included length of hospital stay, number of fever days, and patient's physical and mental status. They found that the relationship between nursing activity and patient outcomes was not statistically significant. In summary, the impetus for evaluating the quality of health care continued to come primarily from professionals and professional organizations. The predominant focus was on processes of care.

The 1970s — Rapid Growth of Quality Assurance

Quality was the buzzword of the 1970s. *Quality Assurance* became common terminology in health care. The decade was marked by rapid growth in the literature on quality care and increased public concern about the rising costs of care. Although articles that discussed quality-care issues outnumbered actual studies of care (Oliver, 1979), the work during this decade evidenced nurses' concern for patients' perspectives and needs. For example, Kraegel, Schmidt, Shukla, and Goldsmith (1972) proposed a system of care based on patient needs. Kirchhoff (1976) conducted a study of pulmonary-intensive-care-unit (ICU) patients' perceptions, and advocated for patient input in evaluating nursing care. Other researchers examined the relationship between structure, process, and outcome criteria (Atwood & Hinshaw, 1977; Given, Given, & Simoni, 1979; Haussmann, Hegyvary, & Newman, 1976). Articles and monographs proliferated on the development of process criteria and outcome criteria for specific patient populations, often based on medical diagnosis (Jelinek, Haussmann, Hegyvary, & Newman, 1974; Zimmer, Lang, & Miller, 1974). An innovative approach to generating outcome criteria sensitive to the impact of nursing care was developed by Horn and Swain (1976). Instead of using medical diagnoses, they focused on four dimensions of health status, namely physiology, knowledge, performance, and affect.

Two process instruments also were published during this decade: The Slater Nursing Competencies Rating Scale and the Quality Patient Care Scale (QUALPACS). The Slater Scale had six subsections and included psychosocial care of individuals and groups, physical care, communication, general care, and professional implications. The Slater Scale used observation and required nurses to rate the care given by peers (Wandelt & Stewart, 1975). The QUALPACS focused on the individual patient as recipient of care and the level of care received, rather than on the care provider. In other words, the same criteria were used to evaluate care whether the care provider was a registered nurse, licensed practical nurse, or nurse aide. The standard was set at the level of care provided by any first-level registered nurse (Wandelt & Ager, 1974).

The federal government also was concerned about rising health-care costs and, particularly, about the expenditures incurred for the Medicare and Medicaid programs enacted during the 1960s. These concerns led Congress to enact two laws that addressed cost and quality with respect to federal programs. In 1972, the Bennett Amendment established Professional Standards Review Organizations (PSROs) to determine that services rendered were medically necessary and that the quality of those services met professionally recognized standards of health care. Review, however, was limited to care delivered to persons enrolled in federally financed programs and to care provided in hospitals and nursing homes (Office of Professional Standards Review, 1974). Because a number of established interests felt threatened, reaction to PSROs was mixed. Hospital administrators were placed in the position of bystanders; physicians thought PSROs might attempt to control their practices; the Joint Commission viewed PSROs as competitors; and nurses were not even mentioned in the legislation (Bull, 1992). In 1974, however, the federal government did award a contract to the ANA to develop criteria to evaluate the quality of nursing care and to develop guidelines for nurse participation in the PSRO review processes (Lang, 1976). It was not until 1982, however, that Norma Lang became the first nurse appointed to the board of the Professional Standards Review Council (ANA, 1982).

In 1974, the National Health Planning and Resource Development Act (PL93-641) was enacted. The intent of this legislation was to correct the maldistribution of health-care facilities and manpower by freeing decision making about allocation of resources from provider control. Under the law, Health Systems Agencies (HSAs) were created to correct problems with allocation and distribution of resources. Although consumer representation on HSAs was mandated, the law did not give the HSAs the authority to carry out their mission.

During this period, nurses, working through the ANA, continued to develop standards of practice for maternal-child health, community health, and oncology. As noted in Figure 9-2, the ANA adopted a QA model developed by Norma Lang to assist nurses in evaluating patient care (ANA, 1976).

The components of the model are:

- *identify values* (as professional, societal, scientific, and consumer values change, the characteristics of quality change)
- *identify standards and criteria* in terms of structure, process, and outcomes of nursing care
- *secure measurements* to determine the current level of practice
- *interpret* the findings (examining both strengths and weaknesses of practice)
- identify possible *courses of action*
- choose a *course of action*
- *take action*

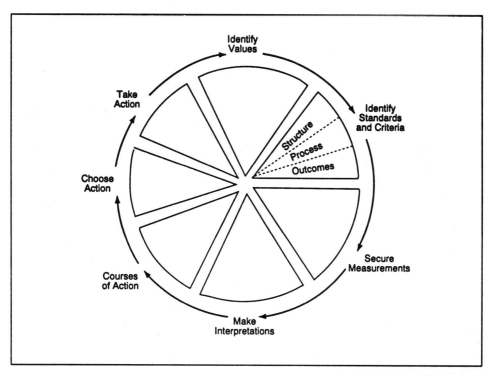

Figure 9-2 *Quality Assurance Model. (Reprinted from* American Nurses Association Quality Assurance Workbook *with permission of American Nurses Association, copyright 1976.)*

One strength of the model is that it suggests ongoing evaluation. The arrows around the circle indicate that the process is continuous, with subsequent evaluations incorporating previous findings as well as changes in values. In addition, the model encourages nurses to examine the interrelationships among structure, process, and outcome criteria. This model has stood the test of time and remains viable today.

During the 1970s the JCAH introduced retrospective process and outcome audits. If an outcome audit identified a deficiency or problem with nursing care, then the process audit might be employed to acquire a better understanding of the problem (Jacobs & Jacobs, 1974).

Also during this time, the American Public Health Association conducted a survey of QA activities in public health agencies and reported that supervisory and record audits were the most common mechanisms used to assess quality of care (Januska, Engle, & Wood, 1976). Few community-health agencies reported using outcome criteria. Also during this period, the National League for Nursing's criteria for accrediting community-health nursing services emphasized structure standards.

A number of political, social, and economic factors contributed to the growth of QA during the 1970s, yet much of the activity stemmed from health-care professionals, who developed standards and criteria that reflected their values. Consumer input was limited.

The 1980s and 1990s: A Shift in Philosophy

Health-care issues of the 1980s and 1990s reflected changing values and advances in technology. Efforts to contain health-care costs predominated early in the 1980s and appeared to take precedence over issues of quality care. Yet the latter 1980s and early 1990s were marked by renewed interest in quality of health care. The belief that cost containment results in poor quality care was dispelled by the diffusion of the business philosophy of Crosby, Deming, and Juran to health-care organizations (Crosby, 1984; Deming, 1984; Gillem, 1988). Deming postulated that improvement in quality attracts new customers, and yields gains in efficiency and productivity that translate to lower costs (Deming, 1984). Consequently the philosophy shifted during the late 1980s, from cost *versus* quality to cost *and* quality. In fact, nationally, outcomes of health care were emphasized, with particular interest in developing uniform standards and data-collection mechanisms. The laws enacted during the 1970s were ineffective in curtailing costs and resolving problems of resource allocation, thereby providing an additional impetus for taking a different approach.

The dramatic shift from focusing exclusively on cost, to focusing on cost and quality, becomes apparent when contrasting laws enacted during the early 1980s with those enacted later in the decade. In the early 1980s Congress responded to rising health-care costs with legislation that introduced further regulations. In 1982 Congress passed the Tax Equity and Fiscal Responsibility Act (TEFRA), which placed a cap on Medicare reimbursement for hospital services. TEFRA was followed by the 1983 Social Security Amendments, which mandated Medicare's prospective payment system based on diagnosis-related groups (DRGs). Regardless of a patient's length of stay, hospitals were paid a set rate for each case within a specified DRG. Linking payment to diagnosis was thought to more accurately reflect the product purchased and, thereby, establish the government as a prudent buyer of services. As noted in "Medicare Program" (1984), the intent was to curtail Medicare expenditures by providing hospitals with incentives to contain costs.

The 1983 Social Security Amendments also replaced PSROs with *Professional Review Organizations (PROs)*. Hospitals were required to contract with a PRO for utilization review. If the PRO found the hospital had questionable admission practices, they could take corrective action. Such action might range from a more intensive review of hospital admissions to punitive steps, such as monetary fines ("Federal Health Insurance," 1983). The PROs differed from PSROs in the following ways:

1. PROs could monitor either for-profit or non-profit organizations. Their scope extended beyond acute-care hospitals to organizations such as extended-care facilities and home-health agencies. PSROs concentrated their efforts on acute-care hospitals that processed Medicare or Medicaid reimbursement.

2. Inclusion of physicians was optional for PROs; in contrast, PSROs were required to include at least 25 percent of the physicians in their area in the membership.

3. PROs were required to develop operational objectives; PSROs were not.

4. PROs were required to consult with nurses and other nonphysician providers about PRO responsibilities for reviewing the professional activities of nurses (and other health-care providers). (Bull, 1992)

(See Chapter 27 for a detailed discussion of utilization management.)

Later in the decade, the Omnibus Reconciliation Act of 1987 mandated development of patient-outcome measures that could be used throughout the country. Two years later the Omnibus Reconciliation Act created the **Agency for Health Care Policy and Research (AHCPR)** to explore the appropriateness and effectiveness of health-care services (Cummings, 1992). A number of efforts to develop instruments to measure the care provided followed. In fact, the AHCPR funded ninety-four Medical Treatment Effectiveness Program research grants and contracts in fiscal year 1991 (Cummings, 1992). The United States Department of Health and Human Services, Health Care Financing Administration (USDHHS, HCFA) developed a Uniform Needs Assessment for Posthospital Care (UNAI). The intent of the UNAI was to evaluate patients' needs for nursing-home care, rehabilitation services, or home care following hospitalization U.S. Department of Health and Human Services [USDHHS, HCFA, 1992]. Also during this period Werley and Lang (1988) developed a nursing minimum data set (NMDS) to establish uniform standards for collecting essential nursing data. The essential nursing-care elements in the NMDS included nursing diagnosis, interventions, outcomes, and intensity of nursing care.

The AHCPR increased the emphasis on processes of care through its Office of the Forum for Quality and Effectiveness in Health Care. The primary responsibility of the Forum was to facilitate the development, periodic review, and update of practice guidelines that assist practitioners in managing clinical conditions (USDHHS, 1994). Between 1992 and 1994 a number of clinical-practice guidelines were developed and disseminated. Each set of guidelines is intended for interdisciplinary use and usually contains three documents: (1) patient guidelines, (2) clinical guidelines, and (3) a quick reference. (These documents are available free of charge from the AHCPR Publications Clearinghouse, P.O. Box 8547, Silver Springs, MD 20907, 1-800-358-9295.) Examples of these clinical-practice guidelines relate to the following clinical conditions:

- acute pain management
- cancer pain
- angina
- congestive heart failure
- urinary incontinence
- benign prostatic hypeplasia
- pressure ulcers
- depression
- cataract
- sickle-cell disease
- mammography
- HIV infection
- low-back pain in adults

It is projected that additional guidelines will be forthcoming for other clinical conditions. At the current time, there is increasing emphasis on the evaluation of the effects of implementation of these guidelines.

During the late 1980s and early 1990s, hospitals and home-care organizations also emphasized process criteria in developing critical pathways and caremaps (Goodwin, 1992; Graybeal, Gheen, & McKenna, 1993). Although the focus of these efforts was primarily on standardizing practice or plans of care for specific populations, a few hospitals integrated patient outcomes in their plans (Woodyard & Sheetz, 1993; Zander, 1992).

An emphasis on outcomes was evident in nursing studies conducted during the later part of the 1980s and early 1990s. Martin and Scheet (1992) and Martin, Scheet, and Crews (1986) worked with the Visiting Nurse Association of Omaha to develop a patient classification system for community-health nursing. As part of the Omaha project, outcomes were classified in categories of knowledge, behavior, or status. Rinke (1988) also developed a classification of outcomes for home-health care. Rinke's outcomes were categorized as physical, behavioral, psychosocial, knowledge, and functional. Another project addressing outcomes for home-health care was conducted by Lalonde (1986). The outcomes measured in this project included general symptom distress, taking prescribed medications, discharge status, caregiver strain, functional status, physiologic indicators, and knowledge of major diagnosis and health problems. The emphasis on patient-outcomes research also was evidenced by the National Center for Nursing Research Conference, which examined the effectiveness of nursing practice as well as funding priorities (National Institutes of Health, 1992).

During the 1980s hospitals also faced new standards imposed by the JCAH. The new standards stipulated that QA activities must be integrated in a comprehensive, hospital-wide program focusing on problems related to patient care. In the late 1980s, as part of its Agenda for Change, the JCAH changed its name to the Joint Commission on Accreditation of Healthcare Organizations or Joint Commission. The new Agenda emphasized the concept of CQI and required input from the health-care consumer in evaluating care. At the present time, Joint Commission emphasis is toward the improvement of organizational performance (Joint Commission on Accreditation of Healthcare Organizations [Joint Commission], 1994). (See Chapter 17 for a detailed discussion of current Joint Commission **accreditation** requirements.)

Prompted by the Joint Commission's new standards and the acceptance of cost and quality as compatible concepts, CQI began replacing QA in health-care organizations. Several models for **Total Quality Management (TQM)** and CQI appeared in the literature. Those proposed by Deming, Juran, and Crosby are among the better known. Although these three leaders differ on some elements of CQI, they agree that the key to improving quality is commitment by top management to removing organizational barriers to quality (Crosby, 1984; Deming, 1984). Though CQI models differ, a theme central to each of them is a commitment to the principles of **Quality Management (QM)**. These key principles include:

1. defining the work process

2. meeting the needs of customers (e.g., patients/clients, payers, professionals)

3. recognizing workers as key resources to improve the process

4. using scientific methods to get to the root of problems and make decisions

5. assuring effective leadership (Plsek, 1993)

(See Chapter 5 for a detailed discussion of TQM.)

THE CHALLENGE OF APPLYING QUALITY PRINCIPLES TO PRACTICE

In health care, the development of practice guidelines might be viewed as one mechanism for defining the work process and assuring quality care. However, implementation of practice guidelines presents a major challenge. Even within the same geographic area, hospitals and other health-care organizations frequently work within the confines of their own organizations to develop guidelines. Sharing guidelines with other institutions often is impeded by an organization's need to maintain a competitive edge in the marketplace. Yet providing quality care demands going beyond integration and communication among providers on a particular unit or in a specific setting. It is vital that health-care providers step out of their institutional or organizational boundaries and collaborate to provide quality care across settings. Also, questions as to whether measures of quality used for acute-care are applicable to long-term care can be addressed more readily when providers collaborate across institutional boundaries.

CONCLUSION

Models of CQI challenge health-care professionals to use scientific methods. This necessitates knowledge of not only content, but also design and methods. Improving quality of care requires individuals who possess these skills, as well as the ability to work effectively in teams.

It is also vital to remember that consumer needs provide the driving force for CQI. Although consumers include payers, professionals, and patients/clients, previous standards and criteria for quality have been dictated largely by third-party payers and health-care professionals. Limited attention has been given to systematically obtaining clients' perspectives on quality, and incorporating their values in establishing criteria for quality care (Bull, 1994). Patient-satisfaction questionnaires have been used as one measure of client input. Campen, Friele, and Kerssens (1992) note, however, that the concept of patient satisfaction has not been defined and that there is a lack of consensus among researchers as to what they are assessing in studies of patient satisfaction. This lack of definition makes it impossible to establish validity of patient-satisfaction instruments. Consequently, the future challenges us to develop valid, reliable instruments to assess quality of care and to identify consumers' values and perspectives regarding quality of care. Integrating the perspectives of consumers in the standards and criteria developed is essential if we are to give more than lip service to the CQI paradigm. A focus on the perspectives of clients is not new for nursing. Within the CQI paradigm, however, clients are just one of the consumers. How can we maximize our potential to meet the needs of the greatest number of consumers? Will it be a utilitarian approach — the greatest good for the greatest number — that dictates our actions? When the needs of third-party payers and professionals conflict with those of clients, whose needs will we choose to serve? Will nurses risk their professional accountability to clients in an effort to meet the needs of other consumers of health-care services? The future indeed challenges us to examine our values and decide what collective action we need to take to shape the future of quality in health care.

REFERENCES

Abdellah, F. (1970). Overview of nursing research 1955–1968: Part I. *Nursing Research, 19*(1), 12.

American Nurses Association. (1963). *Functions, standards, and qualifications for practice.* Kansas City, MO: Author.

American Nurses Association. (1976). *Quality assurance workbook.* Kansas City, MO: Author.

American Nurses Association. (1982). Norma Lang named to Standards Council, 1st nurse appointed. *American Nurse, 14*(4), 32.

Atwood, J., & Hinshaw, A. (1977). Multiple indicators of nurse and patient outcomes as a method for evaluating change staffing patterns. *Communicating Nursing Research, 10*(5), 235–255.

Aydelotte, M., & Tener, M. (1960). *An investigation of the relation between nursing activity and patient welfare.* Ames, IA: State University of Iowa.

Brook, R., & Avery, A. (1975). *Quality assurance mechanisms in the United States: From there to where?* Santa Monica, CA: Rand.

Bull, M. J. (1992). Quality assurance: Professional accountability via continuous quality improvement. In C. Meisenheimger (Ed.), *Improving quality: A guide to effective programs.* Gaithersburg, MD: Aspen.

Bull, M. J. (1994). Patients' and professionals' perceptions of quality in discharge planning. *Journal of Nursing Care Quality, 8*(2), 47–61.

Burgess, M. A. (1928). *Nurses, patients, and pocketbooks.* New York: Committee on the Grading at Nursing Schools.

Campen, C., Friele, R., & Kerssens, J. (1992). *Methods for assessing patient satisfaction with primary care.* Utrecht, The Netherlands: NIVEL.

Codman, E. (1914). The product of a hospital. *Surgical Gynecology Obstetrics, 18*, 491–494.

Crosby, P. (1984). *Quality without tears: The art of hassle-free management.* New York: McGraw-Hill.

Cummings, M. (1992). Patient outcomes research-nursing, an important component. *Journal of Professional Nursing, 8*(6), 318.

Deming, W. E. (1984). *Quality, productivity, and competitive position.* Cambridge, MA: Massachusetts Institute of Technology.

Dienemann, J. (1992). Approaches to quality management. In J. Dienemann (Ed.), *CQI — Continuous Quality Improvement in nursing.* Washington, DC: American Nurses Association.

Donabedian, A. (1966). Evaluating the quality of medical care. *Milbank Memorial Fund Quarterly, 44*, 194–196.

Federal health insurance for the aged and disabled. (1983, September 1). *Federal Register, 48*, (No. 171): p. 39807.

Fee, E. (1982). A historical perspective on quality assurance and cost containment. In J. Williamson Assoc. (Eds.), *Teaching quality assurance and cost containment in health care.* San Francisco: Jossey-Bass.

Fitzpatrick, T., Reidel, D., & Payne, B. (1962). Character and effectiveness of hospital use. In W. J. McNermy (Ed.), *Project 2, Hospital and medical economics* (pp. 361–592). Chicago, IL: Hospital Research and Educational Trust.

Flexner, A. (1910, reproduced in 1960). *Medical education in the United States and Canada.* Washington, DC: Science and Health Publications.

Gillem, T. R. (1988). Deming's 14 points and hospital quality: Responding to the consumer's demand for the best value health care. *Journal of Nursing Quality Assurance, 2*(3), 70–78.

Given, B., Given, C. W., & Simoni, L. (1979). Relationships of processes of care to patient outcomes. *Nursing Research, 28*(2), 85–93.

Glaab, C., & Brown, A. T. (1983). *A history of urban America.* New York: Macmillan.

Goodrich, A. (1912). A general presentation of the statutory requirements of the different states. *American Journal of Nursing, 12*, 1001–1005.

Goodwin, D. R. (1992). Critical pathways in home health care. *Journal of Nursing Administration, 22*(2), 35–40.

Graybeal, K. B., Gheen, M., & McKenna, B. (1993). Clinical pathways development: The Overlake model. *Nursing Management, 24*(4), 42–45.

Haussmann, R. K., Hegyvary, S., & Newman, J. (1976). *Monitoring quality of care part II.* Bethesda, MD: U. S. Department of Health, Education, and Welfare.

Hinsvark, I. (1976). *And the winds of change blew: A report of the Nursing Committee of the Wisconsin Regional Medical Program.* Milwaukee: Wisconsin Regional Medical Program.

Horn, B., & Swain, M. (1976). An approach to development of criterion measures for quality patient care. In *Issues in Evaluation Research* (ANA Publication No. G-124 2M9/76) (pp. 74–82). Kansas City, MO: American Nurses Association.

Jacobs, N., & Jacobs, C. (1974). *The PEP primer.* Chicago: Joint Commission on Accreditation of Hospitals.

Januska, C., Engle, J., & Wood, J. (1976). *Status of quality assurance in public health nursing.* New York: American Public Health Association.

Jelinek, R., Haussman, R., Hegyvary, S., & Newman, J. (1974). *A methodology for monitoring quality of nursing care.* Bethesda, MD: U. S. Department of Health, Education, and Welfare.

Joint Commission on Accreditation of Healthcare Organizations. (1994). *The accreditation manual for hospitals.* Chicago: Author.

Kalisch, P., & Kalisch, B. (1978). *The advance of American nursing.* Boston: Little, Brown, and Company.

Kingsbury, J. (1939). *Health in handcuffs.* New York: Modern Age Books.

Kirchhoff, K. (1976). Let's ask the patient — Consumer input can improve patient care. *Journal of Nursing Administration, 6*, 36–39.

Kraegel, J., Schmidt, V., Shukla, R., & Goldsmith, C. (1972). A system of patient care based on patient needs. *Nursing Outlook, 20,* 257–264.

Lalonde, B. (1986). *Quality assurance manual for the Home Care Association of Washington.* Edmonds, WA: The Home Care Association of Washington.

Lambertsen, E. (1965). Evaluating the quality of nursing care. *Hospitals, 39,* 61–66.

Lang, N. (1976). Issues in quality assurance in nursing. In American Nurses Association (Ed.), *Issues in evaluation research.* Kansas City, MO: American Nurses Association.

Martin, K., & Scheet, N. (1992). *The Omaha system.* St. Louis, MO: Mosby.

Martin, K., Scheet, N., & Crews, C. (1986). Client management information system for community health nursing agencies: An implementation manual (NTIS No. HRP-0907023). Rockville, MD: U. S. Department of Health and Human Services.

Medicare program: Changes in the inpatient hospital prospective payment system. (1984, July 3). *Federal Register, 49*(129), p. 27422.

Morehead, M. (1958). *Quality of medical care provided by family physicians as related to their education, training, and methods of practice.* New York: Health Insurance Plan of Greater New York.

National Institutes of Health. (1992). *Patient outcomes research: Examining the effectiveness of nursing practice* (NIH Publication No. 93-3411). Bethesda, MD: U. S. Department of Health and Human Services.

Nightingale, F. (1911). Editorial. *American Journal of Nursing, 11*(5), 331–338.

Office of Professional Standards Review. (1974). *PSRO program manual.* Rockville, MD: U. S. Department of Health, Education, and Welfare.

Oliver, N. R. (1979). Diffusion of knowledge in a scientific community: The growth of quality assurance in nursing literature. Unpublished master's thesis, University of Wisconsin, Milwaukee.

Peterson, O., Andrews, L., Spain, R., & Greenberg, B. (1956). An analytical study of North Carolina general practice 1953–1954. *Journal of Medical Education, 31,* 1–165.

Phaneuf, M. (1964). A nursing audit method. *Nursing Outlook, 12,* 67.

Phaneuf, M. (1972). *The nursing audit: Profile for excellence.* New York: Appleton-Century-Crofts.

Phaneuf, M. (1976). *The nursing audit: Self-regulation in nursing practice.* New York: Appleton-Century-Crofts.

Plsek, P. (1993). Tutorial: Quality improvement project models. *Quality Management in Health Care, 1*(2), 69–81.

PRO regulations issued by HCFA. (1984). *Capital Update, 2*(3), 7.

Reiter, F., & Kakosh, M. (1963). *Quality of nursing care: A report of a field study to establish criteria 1950–1954.* New York: New York Medical College, Graduate School of Nursing.

Rinke, L. (1988). *Outcome measures in home care: State of the art: Volume 3.* New York: National League for Nursing.

Taft, C., & Levine, S. (1977). Problems of federal policies and strategies to influence the quality of health care. In R. Egdahl & P. Gertman (Eds.), *Quality assurance in health care.* Gaithersburg, MD: Aspen.

U. S. Department of Health and Human Services, Health Care Financing Administration. (1992). *Report of the Secretary's Advisory Panel on the development of uniform needs assessment instrument(s).* Washington, DC: U. S. Government Printing Office.

U. S. Department of Health and Human Services. (1994). *Unstable angina: Diagnosis and management* (AHCPR Publication No. 94-0602). Rockville, MD: Author.

Wald, L. (1912). Report of the Joint Committee Appointed for Consideration of the Standardization of Visiting Nurses. *American Journal of Nursing, 12,* 894–897.

Wandelt, M. (1954). Planned versus incidental instruction for patients in tuberculosis therapy. *Nursing Research, 3,* 52–59.

Wandelt, M. A., & Ager, J. (1974). *Quality of patient care scale.* New York: Appleton-Century-Crofts.

Wandelt, M. A., & Stewart, D. S. (1975). *Slater nursing competencies rating scale.* New York: Appleton-Century-Crofts.

Werley, H. H., & Lang, N. (1988). The consensually derived nursing minimum data set: Elements and definitions. In H. Werley and N. Lang (Eds.), *Identification of the nursing minimum data set.* New York: Springer.

Woodyard, L., & Sheetz, J. (1993). Critical pathway patient outcomes: The missing standard. *Journal of Nursing Care Quality, 8*(1), 51–57.

Zander, K. (1992). Focusing on patient outcome: Case management in the 90s. *Dimensions of Critical Care Nursing, 11*(3), 127–129.

Zimmer, M., Lang, N., & Miller, D. (1974). *Development of sets of patients health outcome criteria by panels of nurse experts.* Milwaukee, WI: Wisconsin Regional Medical Program.

ADDITIONAL READING

Dienemann, J. (Ed.). (1992). *C.Q.I. — Continuous Quality Improvement in nursing.* Washington, DC: American Nurses Association.

Frederick, B., Sharp, J., & Atkins, N. (1988). Quality of patient care: Whose decision? *Journal of Nursing Quality Assurance, 2*(3), 1–10.

Hirshfield, D. (1970). *The lost reform: The campaign for compulsory health insurance in the United States from 1932 to 1943.* Cambridge, MA: Harvard University Press.

Lang, N., Kraegel, J., Rantz, M., & Krejci, J. (1990). *Quality of health care for older people in America.* Kansas City, MO: American Nurses Association.

Lang, N., & Marek, K. (1990). The classification of patient outcomes. *Journal of Professional Nursing, 6*(3), 158–163.

New JCAHO data spotlights quality problems. (1990). *American Journal of Nursing, 90,* 18.

U. S. Department of Health and Human Services. (1992). *Urinary incontinence in adults* (AHCPR Publication No. 92-0038). Rockville, MD: Author.

U. S. Department of Health and Human Services. (1993). Sickle cell disease: Screening, diagnosis, management, and counseling in newborns and infants (AHCPR Publication No. 93-0562). Rockville, MD: Author.

Michael Lummis

CHAPTER *10*

The Quality Improvement Movement:
An Epidemiologist's Viewpoint

INTRODUCTION

Given the current popularity of the **Continuous Quality Improvement (CQI)** movement in America, any examination of the relationship between epidemiology and systemic, organized efforts to improve the quality of health care might logically be expected to approach the topic from an *external* perspective. For purposes of this chapter, however, both *internal* and *external* perspectives offer significant insights into an examination of quality in health care from the perspective of epidemiology.

The science of epidemiology predates CQI by several centuries, providing the basic foundation of contemporary health-care delivery. Valanis (1986) provides a useful working definition: "Epidemiology is the study of the distribution of states of health and of the determinants of deviations from health in human populations" (p. 7). Epidemiology is generally considered a branch of the basic sciences that deals with three components of disease; the *host*, the *agent*, and the *environment*. Within this context, three major factors are given consideration in this chapter:

- the independent evolution of quality-improvement methodologies within the health-care field, and the degree of integration, or lack thereof, between epidemiology and quality improvement

- the impact of external forces, notably America's belated romance with CQI and **Total Quality Management (TQM)**

- the quality improvement benefits that might result from adoption/integration of proven epidemiologic principles

QUALITY IMPROVEMENT IN HEALTH CARE: AN EPIDEMIOLOGIC HISTORY

The history of medicine is replete with examples of improvement in the quality of health care. Valanis (1986) wrote an excellent epidemiology text that charts improvements in health-care quality, from the pre-Christian-era isolation of persons with leprosy and other infectious diseases to James Lind's experiments that identified the cause and cure of scurvy. Also cited is John Snow's investigation of cholera in the 1850s, which led to significant quality improvement long before Koch's isolation of a specific causal organism in 1883.

As evidenced in Valanis, the history of medicine, the rise of the nursing and allied-health professions, and the exponential growth of the biotechnical knowledge base combine to provide a proud history of accomplishment. Unfortunately, the topic of **quality**, notably systematic improvements in the quality of health care, is often regarded as a late development. This position is apparent in a review of the current quality literature. Reeves and Bednar (1993) state, "In spite of increasing pressure from the government and other payers to increase quality and decrease costs, the health care industry has been slow to adopt quality principles" (p. 42). This viewpoint, while prevalent in the current literature, is worthy of further review. Careful examination of nearly 2,500 years of health-care history clearly identifies the fact that quality improvement has *always* been a primary focus.

The Triumph over Puerperal Fever

One of the triumphs of medicine provides insight into a classic quality-improvement "project." Puerperal fever, or childbirth fever, took the lives of thousands of new mothers from the dawn of history. Puerperal fever was the name given to septicemia resulting from an infection (probably caused by a streptococcus) of the mucous membrane of the parturient canal during the postpartum period. A detailed history of this disease (Graham, 1951) includes a case summary of the death of Thasus, wife of Philinus, recorded by Hippocrates in the early fifth century B.C. This disease could truly be described as the "mother of all epidemics," with more than 200 outbreaks of epidemic proportion recorded between 1750 and 1850 in Europe alone.

Modern efforts to improve health-care quality through control of puerperal fever began with Charles White, an English physician who believed the disease was caused by "matter" which was absorbed into the body (Graham, 1951). In 1772 White proposed a revolutionary quality-improvement strategy. First, he recommended that women should bathe regularly during pregnancy and lactation. He also advocated exposure to copious quantities of "fresh and sweet air." Each of these suggestions came at a time when baths and fresh air were widely accepted as *causes* of disease. White also invented and advocated the use of a bed that maintained the occupant in an early version of Fowler's position. Finally, he recommended that midwives and other attendants be absolutely clean, especially their hands. Implicit in his approach was the concept of a contagious disease, with identification of measures that were remarkably successful for their time. Not unlike twentieth-century proponents of **Quality Assurance (QA)** or quality improvement, the work of Charles White was largely ignored.

Nearly seventy-five years passed before Oliver Wendell Holmes (Professor of Anatomy and Physiology at Harvard University, 1847–1882) took up the cause in 1843 stating that "the disease known as puerperal fever is so far contagious as to be frequently carried from patient to patient by physicians and nurses" (Graham, 1951, p. 167). Holmes was one of the first to suggest a causal relationship for puerperal fever. With little regard for personal reputation, his research linked excessively high mortality rates to physicians who autopsied victims of the disease immediately before attending women in labor. Utilizing methods not unlike those used by contemporary infection-control or QA practitioners, he also developed data that compared mortality rates between various doctors, clinics, and hospitals.

Holmes' views were aggressively attacked by the obstetrical establishment. Opponents took particular umbrage at the suggestion that any eminent physician (or gentleman) could have unclean hands. While Holmes did see some change in the behavior of his colleagues, he enviously lauded the success of a physician he called "Senderin," who had significantly decreased the incidence and severity of puerperal fever in Austria.

Holmes' Austrian colleague was actually Ignaz Philip Semmelweis, a Hungarian who practiced medicine and taught at the Vienna Lying In Hospital. In 1847, Semmelweis began requiring his students and attendants to scrub their hands in a chloride of lime solution before touching any patient. Within a short period of time, the mortality rate from puerperal fever dropped from 11.4 percent to 1.27 percent. This quality-improvement effort illustrates the benefits that result when basic epidemiology (in this case, a comparison of simple incidence rates) is applied to quality-improvement activities.

The Rise of Nursing and Evaluation of Quality

The middle years of the nineteenth century also witnessed two dramatic changes in health care. The first was the rise of nursing as a profession, and the second was the development of planned, systematic attempts to **evaluate** and improve quality. Bull (1992) provides an extensive review of the history of quality and its improvement. One such effort to improve quality in health care occurred in 1854, during the Crimean War, when Florence Nightingale utilized data to substantiate that the addition of nurses to the staff of British field hospitals resulted in a reduction in the mortality rate from approximately 32 percent to less than 2 percent within six months. In Great Britain, this seminal work by Ms. Nightingale led to adoption of the Audit Department Act of 1866, the first effort by organized government to evaluate quality on an ongoing basis.

Internal Influences: The Evolution of the Joint Commission

During the balance of the nineteenth century, most organized efforts to improve health-care quality centered in Great Britain. American health care was also impacted, however. In the early twentieth century organized efforts to improve quality took the form of improvements in medical education, the continuing development and recognition of professional nursing, and the founding of the Joint Commission on Accreditation of Hospitals (JCAH). It is significant that each of these changes came about as a result of movements from *within* health care.

In 1910, research conducted by the Carnegie Foundation at the request of the American Medical Association (AMA) resulted in the Flexner report, which lead to significant improvements in medical education. Many schools closed, the standards of the remaining institutions were uniformly increased, and the medical profession increasingly focused on identification and elimination of inferior practitioners. Other examples of quality improvement were the continuing development of professional nursing associations, and the effort that organized nursing devoted to improvement of the educational process, standardization of licensing standards, and adoption of state **licensure** laws.

In addition to professional improvements, the early twentieth century saw the founding of the JCAH in response to the promulgation of minimum standards for hospitals by the American College of Surgeons in 1918. Since that time, the JCAH, now the Joint Commission on Accreditation of Health Care Organizations (Joint Commission), has actively pursued quality improvement through the steady development and improvement of the *Standards for Accreditation of Hospitals*.

During the 1960s, agencies created by the Comprehensive Health Planning Act of 1966 and the Regional Medical Planning Program Act of 1966 were heavily committed to quality improvement. The American Nurses Association and the Robert Wood Johnson Foundation also made significant contributions. Methods for evaluating quality in the 1960s primarily focused on *process*. This was particularly true in nursing, where specific tools for nursing process audits were developed and utilized with mixed results. Although his focus was primarily on evaluation of care provided by physicians, Donabedian (1966) defined three types of criteria for quality evaluation: (1) **structure**, (2) **process**, and (3) **outcome**.

PEER EVALUATION PROGRAM

Enabling legislation for regional medical programs and comprehensive health-planning agencies expired during the 1970s, clearing the way for the emergence of the Joint Commission as the major force promoting quality improvement in health care. Formalized, retrospective studies became a significant focus for **accreditation** and reaccreditation with the adoption of *Peer Evaluation Program (PEP)* audits in 1974. Although the intent of the PEP audits was to focus on outcomes, the net result was somewhat different. Under close scrutiny, flaws in the methodology become apparent.

Selection of Topic   While the intent was to focus on outcomes, topics for PEP audits were often identified intuitively or through convenience. Hospitals developed broad, general topics acceptable to the medical staff. All too often, this process coincided with notice of an impending JCAH site visit. Although some of the audit topics held promise, the suspicion remains that quality improvement that resulted from PEP audits was as attributable to serendipity as it was to planning.

It was also true that topic selection was often influenced by success. Successful PEP audits frequently reappeared at multiple hospitals. After "endorsing" a cholecystectomy audit, for example, most JCAH surveyors could anticipate spending the balance of the accreditation cycle reviewing similar studies.

Adoption of Criteria   Depending on the institution and the degree of cooperation which existed between the medical staff and hospital personnel, criteria were developed and/or approved by physicians. The Joint Commission surveyors were usually helpful, either sharing criteria or providing guidelines. Occasionally, criteria were adopted from the literature and/or emerging national standards. In many cases, criteria were passed collegially from hospital to hospital.

In many respects, the criteria development process was the most meaningful outcome of the PEP audits. As JCAH changed its approach from short-term PEP audits and evaluation, successful efforts often utilized **indicators** which bore strong resemblance to PEP audit criteria.

Data Management   PEP audits were generally conducted by nursing or medical-records personnel utilizing paper forms to retrospectively review completed medical records. Study duration of three to six months was common, and little or no consideration was given to the retention of denominator data. Instead, most audits were limited to an identification of cases (numerators) that "dropped out" by failing one or more criteria. A more valuable, epidemiologic approach would have identified both the exceptions (numerators) and the population at risk (denominators) in order to consider a valid comparison of *exception rates*. The simplest rates are expressed as percentages. For example, in a typical PEP audit, 100 surgical cases might have been studied (the denominator). If exceptions were found in 15 cases (the numerator), the rate of exception would be calculated by dividing the numerator by the denominator, resulting in an exception rate of 15 percent for the audit. Assuming that two surgeons were responsible for all the cases, with 50 cases each (surgeon-specific denominators), a valid comparison could be made of specific surgeon exception rates. With 5 exceptions in 50 cases, surgeon "A" would have an exception rate of 10 percent; with 10 exceptions in 50 cases the exception rate for surgeon "B" would be 20 percent.

Occasionally, through the intervention of an interested physician or the participation of trained personnel (e.g., infection-control personnel), some principles of epidemiology were utilized. even in those cases, unfortunately, little or no effort was directed to long-term retention or to aggregation of the data, denying any possibility of a long-term examination or comparison.

Corrective Action   Further action on cases which "dropped out" of the audit criteria was handled through a variety of methods, the method often being dependent on the size of the hospital. Final medical review of cases might be conducted by a medical director, department chair, committee, or, in smaller institutions, by the entire medical staff. During the late 1970s and early 1980s, a new subculture seemed to develop wherein chosen physicians, nurses, and administrators routinely met for breakfast on the third Thursday of each month to pronounce the mystical incantation "care deemed appropriate" over stacks of coffee-stained medical records.

In some cases, however, care was not deemed appropriate, and action was taken. Most often, an explanation was requested from the attending physician or, possibly, from nursing personnel. In rare cases, a letter of admonition might be placed in a physician's credentials file or a nurse's personnel file. No information is available to determine whether any modification or curtailment of physician privileges was ever contemplated as a result of information developed during a PEP audit. More likely, collegial pressure influenced the practice of an offending physician. Perhaps the best outcomes came in those hospitals where medical staffs maintained a working relationship between audit committees and the medical education function. This often led to the timely and appropriate selection of medical education topics.

PEP audits were time consuming, sometimes wasteful of resources, and of dubious value. But two important accomplishments remain. Even before the implementation of the JCAH Quality Assurance Standard, many hospitals developed committees, such as QA steering committees, to coordinate the work of quality review throughout the institution. These efforts provided a strong foundation for future quality-improvement activities. In most cases, these committees became accustomed to appropriate data utilization, preserving numerators and denominators, and utilizing simple rates to continuously review important quality concerns. Areas of focus included the rates of neonatal mortality, surgical wound infection, nosocomial infection, iatrogenic injury, unplanned returns to surgery, and myocardial infarction mortality. The best of these efforts yielded sophisticated data that provided valid comparative rates across time, medical-staff departments, and hospital units. In a surprising number of hospitals, data were sufficiently sophisticated to provide an evaluation of individual physician performance.

THE QUALITY ASSURANCE STANDARD

In 1979 the JCAH announced a new Quality Assurance Standard, to become mandatory in 1981. The watchwords for the 1980s thus became "monitoring and evaluation of quality and appropriateness." During a ten-year period, the scope of the Quality Assurance Standard was expanded and defined to include nursing and allied-health professionals, and a ten-step approach was developed and utilized for all QA activities.

With the adoption of the Quality Assurance Standard, the JCAH mandated broad general parameters for monitoring and evaluation, but left specific methodology up to individual health-care institutions. Emphasis was placed on anesthesia review, blood utilization review, emergency services, infection control, laboratory proficiency, medical records review, nursing process, licensure and staffing, special care units, and surgical case review. The results were disappointing. With two or more years of advance notice, a decade of experience, and the expenditure of millions of dollars, little progress seemed to made in the area of quality improvement, as measured by JCAH Quality Standards. Beginning in 1986, regular reports of hospitals placed on probation through conditional accreditation, or of hospitals receiving nonaccreditation began to appear in trade journals (*Modern Healthcare*, March 18, 1991). More startling, however, was the Joint Commission's 1991 release of *Hospital Accreditation Statistics 1986–1989.* In a brief analysis of this data, Koska (1991) notes *noncompliance* rates among more than 5,000 hospitals. Noncompliance rates included surgical and anesthesia services at 1.7 percent (26 hospitals), emergency services at 2.9 percent (147 hospitals), anesthesia services at 3.9 percent (125 hospitals), and special services at 4.9 percent (216 hospitals). Nursing and allied health fared much better. Noncompliance did not occur for laboratory proficiency, nursing licensure, and staffing, and was minimal for infection control (0.1 percent), nursing process (0.1 percent), and medical records (0.8 percent).

While total noncompliance seemed surprisingly high, an examination of more current data released by the Joint Commission revealed an even more startling trend. This data was based on the five-part evaluation found in the *Scoring Guidelines*, which accompany the *Accreditation Manual for Hospitals* (AMH) (Joint Commission, 1993a, b). The meaning of substantial compliance, the highest score, is self-evident. The other four scoring increments, in descending order, are: significant compliance, partial compliance, minimal compliance, and noncompliance. According to the *Scoring Guidelines*, compliance decisions were based on the degree to which a standard was met, and the length of time for which compliance was demonstrated. As a result, a determination of *significant compliance* was based on two factors:

> The organization meets most provisions of the standard
> The hospital will receive a score 2 (substantial compliance) if it
> can demonstrate that it has been in substantial compliance with
> the relevant standard(s) for at least 3 months. (Joint Commission,
> 1993a, pp. v, vi)

In some cases, the time requirement is as much as one year. In other words, with two years or more to prepare, a hospital was only required to demonstrate between three months and one year of compliance to meet a given standard. In general, substantial compliance provides accreditation without contingencies, and is a reasonable goal for most hospitals. Keeping these factors in mind, it is enlightening to take a deeper look at the data summarized in Table 10-1.

Table 10-1 • **COMPLIANCE WITH IMPORTANT JOINT COMMISSION STANDARDS**

Monitoring and Evaluation Focus	Percent Found in Substantial or Significant Compliance
Emergency Services	71.3
Surgical Case Review	48.7
Anesthesia Services	58.5
Special Services	50.3
Medical Staff/Department Care	43.7
Infection Control	93.0

Adapted from Hospital Accreditation Statistics 1986–1989, Chicago: Joint Commission, 1991.

At least four factors contributed to the disappointing results outlined in Table 10-1. The first related to the effort and resources that hospitals devoted to the task. In many cases, resource allocations were extremely limited. All too often, hospitals responded to the quality-improvement demands of the Joint Commission only when faced with an upcoming survey. The second factor was the failure of hospitals to utilize existing infection control and/or epidemiology professionals to cope with the demands of quality improvement. In response to the adoption of the JCAH Quality Assurance Standard in 1981, a new quality-assurance profession was established. The National Association of Quality Assurance Professionals, now known as the National Association for Healthcare Quality (NAHQ), was founded. By 1981, the membership had risen to 1300, and in 1994, more than 7,200 members participate. Quality Assurance/improvement professionals came from all walks of life, with no common background or training. In retrospect, NAHQ and its membership have made tremendous strides toward quality improvement; but it seems clear that early utilization of quality assurance personnel with a background in infection control, epidemiology, health-care administration, or biomedical research might have led to greater success in meeting the Joint Commission's Quality Standards. A third contributing factor was the attitude of medical staffs. In the case of a receptive medical staff, especially where a physician or physicians were willing to "mentor" QA personnel, a higher degree of success probably occurred. Finally, it would appear that responsibility for a significant portion of the overall failure to meet the Quality Standards resides with the Joint Commission. Much has been said and written about the quality of surveyors and the ability of the average surveyor to understand the basic principles incumbent with ongoing monitoring and evaluation of quality and appropriateness. Dennis O'Leary, M.D. (1990) acknowledged these concerns, and, in describing internal efforts to improve surveyor performance, dubbed 1991 as "The Year of The Surveyor" (p. 3). Despite this effort questions remain regarding the competence of some surveyors and the value of the survey process.

While compliance with the Joint Commission's Quality Standards is not the only measure of the success of the quality-improvement initiative in health care, the significance of these results should not be negated. The Joint Commission has adopted a new emphasis, designed to build upon the past, but it appears that significant momentum generated by the QA effort has been lost. In 1989, amid significant fanfare, the Joint Commission announced the Agenda for Change which states, "The Joint Commission's mission is to 'enhance the quality of health care provided to the public,' and the Agenda for Change is dedicated to finding better ways to carry out that mission" (Joint Commission, 1990, Appendix A, p. 3).

As a major component of this new agenda, the Joint Commission proposed to develop and implement:

> a national performance measurement database that will help to
> stimulate continual improvement . . . driven by our belief that
> health care quality improvement requires a standardized, universal,
> affordable, flexible and reliable data system which can provide risk-
> adjusted, comparative feedback to health care providers. (Joint
> Commission, 1990, Appendix A, p. 4)

The continuing evolution of the Joint Commission's approach has witnessed movement from quality assessment and improvement to improving organizational performance. Why have these dramatic changes in emphasis occurred? Perhaps the best answers are found outside the sphere of health care.

EXTERNAL INFLUENCES: TRAINING AND INTEGRATION WITH EPIDEMIOLOGY

In the face of a bewildering variety of entitlement programs inflicted on American health care over the past twenty-five years, the evolution of quality improvement methodologies within health care proceeded with little outside interference until American business and industry embraced quality improvement in the late 1980s. A brief review of the quality-improvement movement is helpful in understanding the impact of this external influence on health care.

The Influence of Continuous Quality Improvement

The **Continuous Quality Improvement (CQI)** movement is often attributed to Walter A. Shewhart, an engineer whose work was first published in the 1920s. James (1989) points out that the ideas formalized by Shewhart and other architects of CQI were not new, but, rather, were identical to those promulgated by medicine. In other words, one might argue that the seminal principles of the CQI movement were actually borrowed from methods that had existed in medicine and health care for centuries.

Whatever their source, Shewhart's ideas were modified and refined by W. Edwards Deming, who proposed a continual cycle characterized by the acronym *PDCA* (Plan-Do-Check-Act) (Walton, 1990). Deming also advocated heavy utilization of data, or statistics. As a result, statistical process control remains an important component of CQI. Others who contributed heavily to the CQI movement include J. M. Juran (1988), who advocated quality planning (processes designed to meet the needs of customers), quality control (comparison of actual results to goals with action on the results), and quality improvement (performance raised to "breakthrough levels" through improved infrastructure). Phillip B. Crosby provided further refinements by advocating "zero defects" and emphasizing the cost of "un-quality" (Crosby, 1979).

Continuous Quality Improvement was not an immediate success in America. Many of the methods espoused by Deming, Juran, Crosby, and other advocates found a place in management literature, but no broad undercurrent of support was obvious. This situation changed dramatically with the emergence of postwar Japan as an industrial power. In 1950, Deming went to Japan to introduce his methods; he was followed by Juran in 1954. King (1992) documents Japanese success in teaching CQI concepts, first to executives and engineers, and then to middle management. Finally, with the adoption of *total quality control (TQC)* in 1965, employees at every level of Japanese business and industry were included in the movement. Between 1960 and 1970, Hoshin Planning was developed to focus and transform organization and goals, and to involve all employees in the process. During the 1970s, seven management and planning tools were perfected and taught to all manufacturing employees. Eventually the use of these tools spread to service and administrative employees as well. The results of this uniform, national effort have been felt by all Americans, and are particularly well stated by Richard S. Johnson (1993):

> Certainly, all Americans must realize that we are suffering in the global marketplace. We are financing our current standard of living by borrowing money, much of it from foreign nations. The Japanese currently are the only manufacturer of many of the components for our high-tech military equipment. To make matters worse, they are buying into the high-tech industries of the Silicon Valley; we could see that technology migrating to Japan in the near future. What has happened?
>
> Somehow, quality escaped us for a period of time. Products, services, education, and quality of life itself all suffered while we became enamored with foreign products. (p. 48)

In other words, Japanese industry and business have been demoralizing American competitors, and **Quality Management (QM)** is believed to be a major component of the Japanese success. Based on this perception, Deming, Juran, Crosby, and other CQI gurus have suddenly assumed the status of favorite sons; and nearly fifty years after its inception, America has embraced the total-quality movement. Mimicking a similar award in Japan, the prestigious Malcolm Baldrige National Quality Award is pursued by thousands of corporations. The June 6, 1993, edition of *The Washington Post* included an article by staff writer Jay Mathews, who identified consulting firms that collect fees ranging from $25,000 to $1,800,000 for quality-improvement consultation. Faced with mounting criticism from a variety of sources, perhaps it was only natural that the Joint Commission would choose to follow this new trend in the quality movement.

An Epidemiologic Approach to Quality Improvement

At least two factors support a comprehensive approach to quality improvement that is soundly based in the principles and methodology of epidemiology:

- Continuous Quality Improvement came to health care as an *external* pressure. There is a paucity of evidence to suggest that any meaningful improvement in the quality of health care can be made by imposing this, or any other type of external methodology;

- The lessons of the past support a position that *internal*, epidemiologic solutions have promoted and will continue to promote significant improvements in the quality of health care.

Although it is clear that the CQI movement retains a great deal of momentum, all is not positive. Several major American corporations announced a total commitment to CQI, only to renounce the commitment at a later date. Even among those who have flourished during the resurgence of the movement, concern is apparent. In a recent editorial, Stratton (1993) bemoans the "easy money" realized by "TQM repairmen" who "create unsustainable processes and artificially raise expectations." Stratton also expresses concern that a leading newspaper has labeled the movement as a "fad." In point of fact, the Mathews article in *The Washington Post* appears under the title "Totaled Quality Management," followed by "Consultants Flourish Helping Firms Repair the Results of a Business Fad." Specific to health care, Sherer (1994) asks, " 'Can administrators of hospitals with TQM programs in place boast of cost savings?' " (p. 63). According to a recent consultant's analysis, the answer is likely "no." Negative attacks on a movement of this magnitude should not be unexpected. Perhaps it is more important to note, however, that Japan, with its record of stellar achievement and its position as the world leader, has not successfully applied quality improvement to health care. The best description available of Japanese efforts to improve the quality of health care comes from King (1992), who asks the rhetorical question, "What progress have Japanese hospitals made in total quality in health care?" and then succinctly provides the answer, "Not much!" (p. 375).

These arguments contribute to the growing suspicion that health care and CQI do not constitute a flawless match. Equally strong arguments support the position that no sustained effort to incorporate the principles and methods of epidemiology into quality improvement has occurred to date. Isolated success stories do exist, however. Hospitals that conducted monitoring and evaluation activities in an organized, epidemiologically sound manner seem to have fared well with the Joint Commission's Quality Standards. Why, then, has no widespread support for this approach to quality improvement been evident?

The most obvious answer resides with the rise of the health-care-quality profession. Previous discussion noted the wide spectrum of training and/or knowledge that characterizes the entry level of quality professionals. The NAHQ has promoted excellence through creation of Certified Professional in Healthcare Quality (CPHQ) designations for those who meet certain requirements, and by supporting development of uniform curriculum at both the undergraduate and graduate levels. The principles and methods of epidemiology, however, do not constitute a significant component of either the certification examination or the suggested curriculum.

A less obvious but more important answer comes from the perception, both within and outside health-care circles, that epidemiology constitutes a *macro* component of health care. In large part, definitions of epidemiology, such as the one quoted at the beginning of this chapter (Valanis, 1986), promote this macro view. While Valanis' definition is precise, it contributes to the popular notion of the epidemiologist as a nineteenth-century researcher working feverishly to overcome yellow fever; or of a modern specialist in infectious diseases, seeking a solution to human immunodeficiency viris (HIV). To understand the application to quality improvement, this and other definitions also must be examined from the *micro* view. In short, all those who seek health-care quality improvement are well served by epidemiology, regardless of whether the focus is on elimination of a virus that threatens the entire world population, or on improving the outcome of care for cerebrovascular-accident (CVA) patients in an isolated rural area with a limited population. The best example of a *micro* application of epidemiology is demonstrated by the success enjoyed by hospital infection-control programs.

Epidemiologic Principles/Methods

Earlier, three epidemiologic components, the *host*, the *agent*, and the *environment*, were identified. The traditional model assumes a single cause/single effect relationship, and is based on the premise that any change in a single component affects the frequency of the disease. Stallones' Axiom (1980) illustrates the central theme of modern epidemiology:

Axiom: Disease does not distribute randomly in human populations.

Corollary 1:   Nonrandom aggregations of human disease are manifested along axes of measurement of time, of space, of individual personal characteristics, and of certain community characteristics.

Corollary 2:   Variations in the frequency of human disease occur in response to variations in the intensity of exposure to etiologic agents or other more remote causes, or to variations in the susceptibility of individuals to the operation of those causes. (p. 8)

Valanis' (1986) commentary on this Axiom, with emphasis added and slight modification, clearly illustrates the applicability to health-care quality improvement:

> patterns of disease occurrence or *other alterations of states of health* in human communities are determined by *forces that can be identified and measured* and modification of these forces is the most effective way to [prevent disease]. (p. 7)

Epidemiology consists of three primary divisions, each involving a variety of methods. *Descriptive epidemiology* focuses on demographics, such as occurrence and distribution. *Analytic epidemiology* involves the conduct of retrospective, concurrent, prospective and cross-sectional studies. *Experimental epidemiology* focuses on the manipulation of and/or control of etiological factors in order to evaluate corrective measures. By way of comparison, Deming, Juran, Crosby, and other CQI founders stress the importance of accurate statistics. Implicit throughout their work is the premise that quality improvement requires quality control. Within that context, a catchall term, *statistical process control (SPC)*, is frequently used to describe data acquisition and evaluation. Similar but markedly superior statistical tools can be drawn from both descriptive and analytic epidemiology. Unlike SPC, which arose from industrial quality control and utilizes concepts such as "scrap" and "re-work," (which are hardly appropriate to health care), these tools offer data management for quality improvement that is specific to health care.

An important concept in epidemiology is the identification of *risk*, or the probability that an unfavorable event will occur. This concept is not unlike representative SPC methods, but *risk* is a concept specific to health care. *Attributable risk* refers to those unfavorable events with an identified causal factor. James (1989) utilizes the term *attributable variation* to describe the same concept. Another concept integral to the use of epidemiology in quality improvement is that of *rates*. According to Valanis (1986), "However when frequency is used as the numerator of a fraction that expresses a proportion with specification of a relevant time frame, it is of great value and is called a rate" (p. 59). Among rates available to quality improvement in health care, the rate of mortality is most frequently cited. This is evidenced by the Health Care Finance Administration's (HCFA) publication of comparative mortality rates for Medicare patients. Unfortunately, comparative mortality rates are of questionable value, particularly as promulgated by the HCFA. More appropriate are hospital-specific rates for such factors as neonatal mortality, nosocomial infection, surgical wound infection, nosocomial injury, and medication error. In many cases, these rates have been readily available from infection-control sources, but all too often, utilization of both infection-control data and epidemiologic methods has been lacking from quality-improvement efforts. In the *macro view*, crude and specific rates are frequently utilized for comparison. *Crude* refers to the total population and *specific* relates to a subpopulation. An example would be the comparison of the neonatal mortality rate for the entire United States (the crude rate) to the neonatal mortality rate for one state (the specific rate). Similarly, specific rates may be compared (i.e., among states) or a specific rate may be developed for a more limited subgroup, such as for black women in a designated city. In the *micro view*, rates may be calculated for the entire hospital population. An example would be the surgical wound infection rate (SWI). Through good data management, it is simple to compare the SWI across time (e.g., 1992–1993), between departments (specific — the SWI for the Department of Orthopedics and the SWI for the Department of Thoracic Surgery), or between surgeons (Dr. Jones and Dr. Smith). For purposes of extending quality improvement into performance-based credentialing, the rate of SWI for patients of Dr. Smith may be compared with the rate of SWI for Dr. Smith's department (Orthopedics) and, further, with the rate of SWI for all physicians on the medical staff who perform surgery.

Data management requires the careful preservation of both numerator and denominator data, and care must be taken to avoid invalid comparisons. For example, the rate of SWI (or any other rate for that matter) for an orthopedic surgeon who practices pediatric surgery might be expected to be lower than for a similarly trained surgeon who operates primarily on geriatric patients. A variety of epidemiologic methods exist for calculating *adjusted rates* to provide valid comparisons between dissimilar populations and/or subpopulations. Other methods to adjust rates exist, and other comparisons have much to offer. For example, those hospitals that utilize a severity scoring system have the ability to compare within severity levels, and to compare across severity levels in order to validate data for those physicians who take the position that, "My patients are sicker."

A New Conceptual Framework

Although the traditional components of epidemiology have been seen as the host, the agent, and the environment, and investigation has dealt primarily with interactions between these components, new approaches began to appear in the 1970s. Dever (1984) summarized these efforts by proposing a *health field concept:*

> As stated, an overall framework or conceptualization of health is
> needed for examining and studying the relationship between risk
> factors and states of health and disease. The ultimate purpose of
> such an exercise is to preserve and restore health. The underlying
> framework should force the investigator or analyst to consider all
> factors coming into play in the preservation and restoration of
> health. . . . The health field concept is such a framework, allowing
> the broad psychosociobiological analysis of any state of health or

> disease. It is a comprehensive structure that forces the equal
> examination of lifestyle, environmental, and biological elements
> as well as health care organization factors. (p. 76)

In essence, Dever proposes this conceptual approach to health-services management as a "new link." He goes on to characterize a new approach to quality improvement; "The dimensions of health — lifestyle, environment, biology, and the delivery system of care — and their application to the management of services must be considered if the health status of population and individuals is to continue to improve" (p. 84).

If Dever's conceptualization is familiar, perhaps it is because this approach to health planning has been largely implemented in the Canadian health-care system. Just as it has been widely applied to a national problem (the macro approach), so can it be applied to specific efforts to improve the quality of care within specific institutions (the micro approach). It is possible that additional conceptualization will be necessary to create a working model for the use of epidemiology to improve the quality of care in hospitals. Even if modification is required, it is clear that a sound, scientific approach within the framework of epidemiology is worthy of significant investigation. Because of the number of trained professionals available through hospital infection-control programs, staffed by and/or in consultation with trained epidemiologists, it behooves quality-improvement professionals to utilize these skilled professionals, and to become more conversant with the techniques involved.

CONCLUSION

A long and successful history of improvement in the quality of health care is demonstrated through the history of medicine and the development of epidemiology. During the last decade, under the influence of the Joint Commission, a new quality-improvement profession arose within health care, largely without consideration for or integration with infection control and/or epidemiology. In the face of mounting external pressures, largely based on Japanese success with CQI, health care, with a mandate from the Joint Commission, has actively embraced the CQI movement. Early results from this massive effort are unclear. Past and present health-care reform efforts have added significant new factors to the picture. It should be absolutely clear that health care, in general, and health-care professionals, in particular, are dedicated to quality improvement. Perhaps the time is ripe to look inward — for health care to rediscover epidemiology, merging new concepts with two thousand years of experience, in order to evaluate and improve the quality of care delivered by America's health-care system.

REFERENCES

10 hospitals placed on six month probation (1991, March 18). *Modern Healthcare, 21*(11), p. 6.

Bull, M. J. (1992). Quality assurance: Professional accountability via Continuous Quality Improvement. In C. G. Meisenheimer (Ed.), *Improving quality: A guide to effective programs.* Gaithersburg, MD: Aspen Systems.

Crosby, P. B. (1979). *Quality is free.* New York: McGraw-Hill.

Dever, G. E. A. (1984). *Epidemiology in health services management.* Rockville, MD: Aspen Systems Corp.

Donabedian, A. (1966). Evaluating the quality of medical care. *Milbank Memorial Fund Quarterly, 44*(3, Pt. 2), 166–206.

Graham, H. (1951). *Eternal eve: The history of gynecology and obstetrics.* Garden City, NY: Doubleday & Company.

James, B. C. (1989). *Quality management for health care delivery.* Chicago, IL: The Hospital Research and Educational Trust of the American Hospital Association.

Johnson, R. S. (1993, January–May). TQM: Leadership for the Quality Transformation. Printed in five parts in *Quality Progress, 26*(2–6).

Joint Commission on Accreditation of Health Care Organizations (1990). *Quality assurance data management — The next generation (QADM).* Chicago: Author.

Joint Commission on Accreditation of Health Care Organizations (1991). *Hospital accreditation statistics 1986–1989.* Chicago: Author.

Joint Commission on Accreditation of Health Care Organizations (1993a). *Accreditation manual for hospitals: Vol. I. Standards.* Chicago: Author.

Joint Commission on Accreditation of Health Care Organizations (1993b). *Accreditation manual for hospitals: Vol. II. Scoring guidelines.* Chicago: Author.

Juran, J. M. (1988). *Juran's quality control handbook.* New York: McGraw-Hill.

King, R. (1992). Implications of Japanese quality advances for U.S. health care quality. In M. M. Melum & M. K. Sinioris (Eds.), *Total Quality Management: The health care pioneers.* Chicago: American Hospital Publishing.

Koska, M. T. (1991, January 5). New JCAHO report assesses hospitals' standards compliance. *Hospitals, 65*(1), 32–33.

Mathews, J. (1993, June 6). Total Quality Management: Consultants flourish helping firms repair results of a business fad. *The Washington Post,* p. H1, col. 1.

O'Leary, D. S. (1990, May/June). President's Column. *Joint Commission Perspectives,* reprinted in *Quality Assurance Data Management — The Next Generation (QADM).* Chicago, IL: The Joint Commission on Accreditation of Health Care Organizations.

Reeves, C. A., & Bednar, D. A. (1993, April). What prevents TQM implementation in health care organizations? *Quality Progress, 26*(4), 41–44.

Sherer, J. L. (1994, April 5). Hospitals question the return on their TQM investment. *Hospitals and Health Networks, 68*(7), p. 63.

Stallones, R. A. (1980). To advance epidemiology. *Annual Review of Public Health (Vol. I),* pp. 69–82.

Stratton, B. (1993, August). Who ya gonna call? TQM repairman! (Editorial comment). *Quality Progress, 26*(8), p. 5.

Valanis, B. (1986). *Epidemiology in nursing and health care.* Norwalk, CT: Appleton-Century-Crofts.

Walton, M. (1990). *Deming management at work.* New York: G. P. Putnam's Sons.

ADDITIONAL READING

Brewer, J. H., & Gasser, C. S. (1993). The affinity between Continuous Quality Improvement and epidemic surveillance. *Infection Control and Hospital Epidemiology, 14*, 95–98.

Donabedian, A. (1985). The epidemiology of quality. *Inquiry, 22*(3), 282–292.

Evrett, W. D. (1993). An epidemiological approach to quality assurance in the hospital. *Health Care Management Review, 18*(1), 91–96.

Howland, R., & Decker, M. (1992). Continuous Quality Improvement and hospital epidemiology: Common themes. *Quality Management in Health Care, 1*(1), 9–12.

Edward N. Brandt, Jr.

CHAPTER *11*

The Health-Care Environment in the United States

INTRODUCTION

T he United States health-care environment is in a state of rapid change attributable to the rising costs of health care and the inability of many people to obtain health insurance because of job loss or existing illness. Major businesses, physicians, and others have led the way to change the existing system. As a consequence, reform of the health-care system became a major issue in the presidential election of 1992 and during the Clinton presidency. In reality, changes were already occurring at an accelerating rate prior to this era. This was due to the activities of major businesses, of hospitals, of insurance companies, and of physician organizations. In addition, the public was concerned about rising health-care costs and was demanding change. However, not all of the changes, even those that lowered the rate at which health-care costs increase, were viewed by the various **stakeholders** as beneficial. For example, some employers began to offer only one health-care plan, thereby restricting individual choice of physicians and hospitals. This chapter provides an overview of the health-care environment in the United States. Included are discussions of the history of health care, health-care reform, implications for quality, and predictions for the future.

HISTORY OF THE HEALTH-CARE SYSTEM

From the founding of the Republic until World War II, the federal government's role in the provision of health care was limited to providing care to active-duty military, eligible veterans, federally recognized Indian tribes, and merchant mariners. Care for the poor was assumed by religious groups, individual physicians and hospitals, and state and local governments. Individuals were expected to be responsible for their own health care. Indeed, in 1854 President Franklin Pierce vetoed a bill to set aside land for mental hospitals with the following comments:

> If the Congress has power to make provision for the indigent
> insane . . . the whole field of public beneficence is thrown open to
> the care and culture of the Federal government . . . I readily . . .
> acknowledge the duty incumbent on us all . . . to provide for those
> who in the mysterious order of providence are subject to want and
> to disease of body or mind, but I cannot find any authority in the
> Constitution that makes the Federal Government the great
> almoner of public charity throughout the United States. To do so
> would, in my judgment, be contrary to the letter and spirit of the
> Constitution . . . and be prejudicial rather than beneficial to the
> noble offices of charity. (Sharfstein & Koran, 1990, p. 214)

Prior to World War II, two events of significance to our current health-care system occurred. In 1929, Baylor University Hospital of Dallas introduced a health-care plan for school teachers. This led to the development of Blue Cross/Blue Shield plans. In the early 1930s in Elk City, Oklahoma, Dr. Shadid began a "medical cooperative" in which he provided total medical care for a fixed amount per year. This was the beginning of health maintenance organizations (HMOs) as they are known today.

During World War II, wage and price controls imposed by the government, coupled with the limited work force, led employers to offer incentives for employment including health insurance that was paid by the employer. This was acceptable to the government, which permitted a tax deduction for the premiums. Hence, through the tax code, the federal government began to underwrite the cost of delivering care.

In his State of the Union speech in 1948, President Harry Truman called for national health insurance, but that call was opposed vigorously by both medicine and business. Actually, President Roosevelt had considered the addition of health insurance to the Social Security legislation as early as 1935, but decided that such inclusion would generate too much opposition.

Relatively few changes occurred from 1948 until the presidential campaign of 1960. John F. Kennedy, the democratic nominee, argued for federal legislation to provide health care to the elderly and the poor. Upon his election, he attempted to pass such legislation; but to no avail. In 1961, the Kerr-Mills Act, which paid for health care for elderly poor who were receiving welfare benefits, was passed. Medicare and Medicaid legislation added Titles XVIII and XIX to the Social Security Act in 1965. This legislation led to health insurance for the elderly and permitted states to develop and implement programs for the poor using federal matching funds. Arizona was the only state that held to its determination not to participate in Medicaid until the early 1980s. Medicaid and Medicare resulted in additional access to health care for certain poor persons as well as the elderly and disabled. This was accomplished at significantly greater cost than was originally projected, however. The addition of preventive steps such as early periodic screenings, diagnosis, and treatment had a positive impact on the health of children. Unfortunately, for many years neither Medicaid nor Medicare provided funding for disease prevention or early detection (although some progress has been made in this direction in recent years).

During the remainder of the 1960s and the early 1970s, the federal government created a number of programs designed to provide access to care for underserved people. Among these programs were Community Health Centers and the National Health Service Corps. The remainder of the 1970s was characterized in large part by improving existing programs and correcting their deficiencies, including some onerous reporting requirements and the inability to combine programs to effect comprehensive care. (For example, Community Health Centers were not able to obtain funding for family planning.) It is important to note that during the latter part of the 1970s, health-care costs began to increase at a rate well above the overall rate of inflation.

The 1980s saw health-care costs continue to rise at a rate two to three times that of inflation. Businesses began to note that health-care costs were preventing them from both increasing wages and remaining competitive in a global economy. Factors responsible for these cost increases included the rapid introduction of new technology, increased population (especially of the elderly), and increased bureaucratic requirements imposed by insurance companies and federal and state governments. Several attempts were made by the federal government to contain costs, such as introduction into the Medicare program of the Prospective Payment System for hospital services. This system set the rates of payment based on "Diagnosis Related Groups" or DRGs. Other attempts included raising the co-payment for certain services and reducing the payments for indirect medical expenses.

THE CURRENT HEALTH-CARE SYSTEM

The United States health-care system is arguably the most complex system in the world. This system is based on an intricate arrangement of:

1. health insurance purchased in whole or in part by employers for their employees;

2. health insurance purchased by individuals;

3. copayments and deductibles paid "out of pocket" by individuals;

4. self-insurance by individuals such as those who are self-employed and choose to pay directly for health care rather than purchase health insurance;

5. Medicare payment provided by the federal government for eligible elderly; and

6. Medicaid payment provided by a combination of federal and state funds for certain categories of poor people.

In addition, the federal government provides care directly to active-duty and retired military and their dependents; eligible military veterans, through Veterans Affairs Medical Centers and clinics; and members of eligible Indian tribes and Alaskan natives, via the Indian Health Service. The federal government provides care indirectly to poor and underserved people via Community Health Centers and the National Health Service Corps. State governments provide care to persons through public health clinics and to those with mental illness. In some instances, states treat those with substance-abuse problems. Finally, it is widely believed, albeit with limited evidence, that there are some 37 million people who have no health insurance on any given day, with 10 million of those having been uninsured for 12 months or more. (It should be noted that some of the latter may be uninsured by choice [for example Christian Scientists].)

To complicate the situation further, health care is delivered in a variety of ways. The majority of Americans receive their health care from individual physicians practicing singly, in partnership with other physicians, or in group practices. The charges for physician and hospital services are paid, at least in part, by their insurance carrier on a fee-for-service basis. In some cases, employers negotiate fee-for-service arrangements that require their employees to obtain care from the physicians and hospitals involved in the negotiations (often referred to as Preferred Provider Organizations). Finally, some people obtain care through "managed care" or HMOs wherein individuals or their employers pay a fixed amount for their total care. Many HMOs, however, have instituted co-payments for services. Indeed, two methods for decreasing utilization of health-care services are *deductibles*, which require patients to pay an amount before the insurance plan pays, and *co-payments*, which require patients to pay a fixed amount in addition to the insurance payment for each service received. Both methods provide an incentive for people to avoid using the system for simple problems at the risk, perhaps, of waiting too long to seek care and, thereby, increasing costs and endangering their lives.

Also contributing to the complexity of the current United States health-care system is the indemnity basis of most health-insurance programs. Indemnity insurance provides "security against hurt, loss or damage" (Wolf, 1974, p. 584). Hence, insurance premiums are lowest for those groups with the least risk of health-care costs. This has led to exclusions for persons with illnesses that can lead to high costs — a practice known as *pre-existing condition clauses*. Furthermore, indemnity insurance traditionally does not pay for preventive services such as immunizations, pap smears, and mammographies. Another feature of the current health-care system is the fact that most Americans have health-care coverage through their employers who pay all or a large portion of the premiums. Hence, many people are unaware of their health-care costs, and, therefore, have no incentive to reduce those expenditures. Furthermore, changing employment can mean loss of coverage at least for a time. Also, health-insurance premiums paid by the employer are usually tax exempt, again providing no incentive to reduce utilization of services and expenditures.

Liability costs, both for professional services and medical products, are also a problem. For professional services alone, the most recent estimate is an expenditure of $34.9 billion per year. Most of this cost is for *defensive medicine*, or the ordering of diagnostic tests not necessarily indicated clinically, but intended to provide a defense against malpractice suits.

Sound data is, unfortunately, not available to estimate the total impact of product liability costs for such things as drugs, vaccines, and medical devices. Nevertheless, some manufacturers maintain that liability costs for vaccines and new drugs exceed the costs of production.

Finally, the large number of uninsured persons combined with the fact that Medicare and Medicaid payments often do not meet the costs of care have led to a practice known as *cost shifting*. Thus, insured persons pay more for their health care to make up for the losses incurred in caring for the uninsured and for the recipients of government-financed care.

HEALTH-CARE REFORM

The increasing costs of health care, the employer-based system, and decreasing access to primary care has led to public dissatisfaction with the current health-care system in the United States (Bass & Sprague, 1993). Companies see their health-care costs consuming a greater percentage of their profits, and employees see wage increases frozen because health-care costs have demanded changes in business practices. However, the public has thus far been unwilling to forego their choice of physician or hospital, decrease their access to specialized services, or pay higher taxes to help cover the uninsured. President Clinton made health-care reform a major part of his 1992 campaign for the presidency. In this way, Clinton followed the lead of his self-described hero, John F. Kennedy, who thirty years earlier had called for a more limited approach, namely government-sponsored health care for the elderly and those poor persons who were eligible for welfare. Interestly enough, business, which had opposed governmental changes in the health-care system during the 1930s and 1940s, was now in favor of it. The business community, however, was divided on how strong an influence government should have on the health-care system. The major goal of those companies providing health-care coverage to their employees was to avoid the cost shifting from the uninsured and from recipients of other government programs. They argued that they were, in effect, paying for the health care of these groups — a responsibility they saw as belonging to government.

A Shift in Values

It is interesting how the values of the country have changed over the past thirty years. For example, it was at one time considered moral and ethical to charge people according to their ability to pay. In other words, the more affluent paid more so that the poor could receive care — the practice now called *cost shifting*. By 1990, this practice was perceived as one of the evils of the health-care system. One of the major factors behind this value shift was the increase in health-care costs. This shift also reflects a change in the American attitude toward the role of government.

Some Agreement on Needed Changes

One aspect of the health-care system about which there is general agreement is that changes in the health-insurance system are needed. Four areas in particular have been targeted for change. The first of these is claim forms. Nearly all concerned agree on the need for the use of a single claim form to eliminate the literally thousands of such forms currently in use. The use of numerous forms has increased administrative costs both for providers and insurers. Elimination of the pre-existing condition exclusions is a second area of agreement. This would permit all people to be insured and would minimize, if not eliminate, "job lock," or the inability of individuals to change jobs because a member of their family has developed some condition that a new employer's insurer will not accept. It should be noted, however, that elimination of this exclusion will lead to inclusion in the insured pool of persons with expensive illnesses, thereby increasing the costs to all members of that pool. Third, is portability of insurance coverage. In essence, portability refers to the ability of individuals to maintain insurance coverage should they change jobs or insurance coverage. At present, many insurers require waiting periods of six months to one year before they will cover a new person. Finally, there is the issue of community rating. At present, the health-insurance premiums of a given group are based on the health-care expenditure experience of that group. In other words, groups that experience large expenditures in a given period will see dramatic increases in their premiums. This system is known as *experience rating*. Under a *community rating* system, a community such as a Standard Metropolitan Statistical Area would have its risks determined on the basis of its demography and health-risk-factor characteristics. For example, a community with a large number of elderly, a high prevalence of smoking and obesity, and other such characteristics would have a higher risk factor. This risk factor can be translated into potential health-care costs and, therefore, premiums. In a pure community rating system, every member of the community would pay the same premium. There are some advantages to such a system. For example, it spreads the risk over a larger number of people more than does a group experience rating system. Furthermore, it is simpler to compute than experience-based rates, which involve numerous groups. On the other hand, it also represents a cost shift. For example, there are far greater expenditures on health care for the elderly than for the young. Hence, with community rating, costs would be shifted from the old to the young, and from those with chronic illness to those who are healthy. This has raised some controversy, leading some to advocate an age-adjusted community rating wherein all persons in a younger age group, say twenty-one to forty, would pay the same premium, but those in age group sixty-five and over would pay a different premium.

Another topic about which there is general, although not universal, agreement is that Americans should have a standard minimum benefit package. Disagreement centers around what should be in that package; for example, should it include only basic benefits, or should it be comprehensive? Of particular debate is the issue of abortion coverage.

Health-Care Reform Proposals

A number of proposals were put forth in 1994 in response to the public demand for change in the health-care system. Included among these proposals were a single-payer system; the Clinton Plan; a pure managed-competition plan; a voluntary-purchasing cooperative plan; and a medical IRA plan. In addition, a number of legislators favor an incremental approach, which is, in effect, a "do what we know will work" plan. The aforementioned plans differed in the following ways:

- a mandate on businesses to provide health insurance for their employees versus a mandate on individuals to purchase health insurance, or both, or neither
- the rapidity with which the uninsured are covered by tax sources
- the use of managed-care systems versus fee-for-service plans
- the methods for funding of the uninsured
- the role of federal and state governments

Following are summaries and comparisons of some major health-care reform proposals that were advanced in 1994.

THE CLINTON PLAN

On September 22, 1993, President Clinton addressed a joint session of Congress to reveal a health-care proposal that had been developed by a task force of some 520 people (United States Department of Commerce, 1993). Based on the six principles shown in Table 11-1, his plan mandated employer-subsidized health insurance; the creation of insurance purchasing cooperatives called alliances; changes in health-insurance practices, specifically the use of a single claim form, elimination of pre-existing condition exclusions, and the use of community ratings; creation of a National Health Board with certain assigned duties (including definition of a standard benefits package); and some flexibility for state plans (e.g., states would be able to adopt a single-payer system if they so chose).

Under the Clinton plan, a set of preventive services would be included in the standard benefits package.

Table 11-1 • **PRINCIPLES OF THE CLINTON HEALTH PLAN**

---

1. *Security*

    a. health care that is always there

    b. health care that cannot be taken away

    c. health-care security card

2. *Simplicity*

    a. one standard insurance form to be used by all companies

    b. easing of regulatory burden on physicians

3. *Savings*

    a. plans must produce savings

    b. plans must compete on price and quality

    c. government regulation

4. *Choice*

    a. consumers can select health-care plan

5. *Quality*

    a. consumers will be provided quality information

6. *Responsibility*

    a. everyone must assume responsibility and not abuse system

---

Costs would be controlled both by the National Health Board, which would set the maximum premium that could be charged by each alliance, and by competition among the provider groups (called health plans) that contract with each alliance.

The unemployed poor would have their premiums subsidized by the government, and small businesses would receive a government subsidy for insurance costs exceeding 3.5 percent of their payrolls. The Clinton plan also provided negative incentives for choosing fee-for-service plans by requiring higher deductibles and co-payments *even if the premium for such a plan was less than that for other plans.* Hence, there would be financial incentives to select managed-care or preferred-provider organizations. Through the mechanisms of employer- and government-subsidized health coverage, every American would have health insurance and access to a health plan. In order to facilitate the creation of health plans, the Clinton plan offered some relief from antitrust laws; health-care providers would be permitted to negotiate with the purchasing cooperatives. Furthermore, limited tort reform was also proposed in an attempt to lower the costs of defensive medicine.

The voluminous Clinton plan contained other desirable features, such as financial incentives for practice in rural areas. There was also an emphasis on the education and training of primary-care providers and on a continuing commitment to medical research.

There was also minimal disagreement with the president's six principles, and, as described later, most other health-care plans also included them. However, the Clinton plan was criticized for mandating subsidization by businesses, especially small businesses; the extensive amount of government regulation at both federal and state levels; the absence of a financing mechanism without new taxes; and the potential for severe limitations on spending leading to rationing of expensive services. At the same time, the president's plan was praised for representing a concrete proposal to meet an important national problem.

THE CHAFEE PLAN

Another health-care reform plan was developed by a group of senators under the leadership of Senator Chafee of Rhode Island. It encompassed many of the features of the Clinton plan including the formation of purchasing cooperatives for individuals and small businesses. It differed in several important respects, however. First, there would be no mandated employer subsidization of health-insurance premiums. Instead, all individuals would be required to purchase health insurance. Second, membership in a purchasing cooperative would be voluntary rather than mandated as in the Clinton plan. This would permit mid-size or even small companies to negotiate their own arrangements for health insurance with either an insurance carrier or a group of health-care providers. Third, there would be a maximum cap on tax-exempt payments for health insurance. Any payment over that amount would be taxable. This maximum would be adjusted annually on the basis of the cost of a standard benefit package. Fourth, the tort-reform portion of the proposal called for a ceiling of $250,000 for noneconomic damages, and it included product-liability-insurance reforms for drugs and devices approved by the Food and Drug Administration (FDA). Although both plans called for mandatory non-binding arbitration, tort reform was not included in the Clinton plan. Fifth, the Chafee plan included a demonstration program which consisted of seven states, each with training consortia to experiment with methods of changing the physician specialty mix. Sixth, the benefit package, although less well defined, was similar to that of the

Clinton plan, and specifically called for preventive services and co-payments on all other services.

The major criticism of the Chafee plan was its lack of emphasis on control of costs. Critics maintained that the voluntary approach would not lead to the most efficient use of monies.

THE SINGLE-PAYER SYSTEM

The single-payer plan was based on the health-care system of Canada and some other countries. In essence, the government (federal and/or state) would be the single payer and negotiate fees and other payments with providers. Payments would be made from taxes collected either specifically for health care or from the general fund. The benefit package and other features were similar to the other two plans. The government would operate the system and determine all of its features. The claimed advantage of this approach was the savings in administrative costs, centralized cost-control mechanisms, and coverage of all Americans.

OTHER APPROACHES

The other health-care reform plans were based primarily on the concept of individuals being responsible for providing their own health-care coverage. The rationale was that if individuals must pay for their health care, they would "shop" for the best possible price. Furthermore, they would be prudent purchasers and seek health care only when they needed it. Proponents of such plans argued that if an employer or the government payed for health care, the incentive for prudence among individuals seeking health care was removed. They further maintained that government should play as small a role as possible in the operation of the health-care system.

The Political Process

The political processes involved in enacting legislation such as a health-care reform bill are indeed complex and time-consuming. After introduction of six proposals for reform, the debate in the Congress was underway. Each of the relevant committees in the House and Senate held hearings and examined the issues. The result was that five bills were voted out of Committee. These bills included one by the House Ways and Means Committee, two by the House Education and Labor Committee, one by the Senate Finance Committee, and one by the Senate Labor and Human Resources Committee. The bills from the Ways and Means Committee, the Labor Committee, and the Human Resources Committee were variations of the original Clinton plan. (The ways in which these bills differed from the original Clinton plan included the method of financing and the type of employer mandate.) The Education and Labor Committee voted two bills out of Committee, one being a single-payer plan and the second being yet another variation of the Clinton plan. The bill from the Finance Committee was more moderate relying more on voluntary participation by employers and the medical marketplace. All of the bills projected significant savings from Medicare and Medicaid, with such savings to be used to finance health care for the uninsured.

In July 1994, the democratic leadership of the House of Representatives and the Senate met with the president and his advisors to tell him that his proposal was not going to be enacted.

After further congressional debate on various proposals, the United States Congress determined in the fall of 1994 not to pursue changes in the health-care system. There were several apparent reasons for this decision. Polls indicated that the public had decided that crime and jobs were more important than health-care system changes. Furthermore, people found the proposals too complex and the cost implications too unclear. Finally, there was increasing cynicism about the ability of government to solve a problem as complex as health care. Indeed, most polls indicated that the majority of people were quite satisfied with their health care and feared that changes would disrupt that relationship.

The November 1994 elections, in which a majority of Republicans won seats in both the House of Representatives and the Senate, emphasized the public's concern with the role of government. What will happen to health-care system changes in this new Congress?

The Impact of Reform on Quality of Care

Clearly, it is desirable that the impact of any change in the health-care system be to enhance, or at least not diminish, the quality of care received by patients. The emphasis on cost control, however, cannot help but raise the possibility that care will be denied to save money. Indeed, managed care has been accused of under-utilization of services, and, in particular, the denial of needed specialist care. Although the evidence to support such charges is not overwhelming, accusations persist. It is vital that any changes putting special emphasis on cost control be monitored to ensure that quality of care is not sacrificed. If one considers the interdependent triad of volume, cost, and quality, cost reductions must result in a diminution of either volume or quality, or both.

Several of the reform plans emphasized the periodic measuring of quality and making such measurements public. These measurements would have been based on both patients' perceptions of their care and the outcomes of such care. Although patient perceptions are important, they do not necessarily indicate scientific quality (Vuori, 1991). That is, the best that scientific medicine has to offer may be given patients, but patients may still be dissatisfied because the care did not meet their expectations. For example, surveys have indicated that the most common complaint patients have regarding health care is having to wait to get an appointment and/or the physician being late for the appointment. Although it is important to address both of these complaints neither one has much to do with the scientific quality of the care rendered.

The measurement of outcomes of medical care is relatively new. Indeed, the theory underlying such measurements is still being developed. Nevertheless, it is possible to compare alternate therapeutic modalities and measure pathophysiologic and other variables to determine which is the more effective. If they are equally effective, other criteria, such as cost, duration of recovery, and recurrence rates, can be used to determine the more efficient treatment. Note that it is necessary to be able to define the outcome variables, which is often a subject of debate. Quality of life is one outcome variable that would be desirable to be able to measure, especially in chronic illness or incurable fatal diseases. Because it is the most difficult to define, however, related or indirect measurements such as activities of daily living

(ADL), pain control, and the ability to remain at home are used.

The Clinton administration has made a major commitment to enhanced funding for outcomes research, as well as to health-services research in general. New and more refined techniques will be of great value to quality monitoring.

CONCLUSION

It is difficult to predict the outcome of the health-care reform movement but it is the author's view that the entire system will not be overhauled. Rather, it is more likely that there will be changes in the insurance system which will (1) eliminate pre-existing condition exclusion clauses and (2) assure portability from one job to another. It is also possible that there will be an attempt to shift from "experience rating" to a community-based rating system. However, consideration must be given to an age-related, community-based system or the younger people will see a significant increase in premiums. Indeed, even eliminating the pre-existing condition exclusion willl raise premiums due to the inclusion of persons with expensive illnesses. Only time will tell what the outcome will be, but it is most unlikely that a major change in the health-care system will be attempted or prove successful.

REFERENCES

Bass, K., & Sprague, L. (1993). *Health care 101: The basics of reform.* Washington, DC: United States Chamber of Commerce.

Sharfstein, S. S., & Koran, L. M. (1990). *Mental health services.* In A. Kovner and S. Jonas (Eds.), *Health care delivery in the United States* (4th ed., pp. 209–239). New York: Springer.

U. S. Department of Commerce, National Technical Information Service. (1993). *The president's health security plan — Preliminary summary* (Report No. PB 93-234979). Springfield, VA: Author.

Vuori, H. (1991). Patient satisfaction: Does it matter? *Quality Assurance in Health Care, 3*(3), 183–189.

Wolf, H. B. (Ed.). (1974). *Webster's new collegiate dictionary.* Springfield, MA: G. & C. Merriam.

ADDITIONAL READING

Aaron, H. J., Altman, S., Enthoven, A. C., Singer, S. J., Fuchs, V., Hadley, J., Zuckerman, S., Newhouse, J. P., Pauly, M. V., Reinhardt, U. E., & Wilensky, G. R. (1994). Economic analysis of the Clinton plan. *Health Affairs, 13*(1), 56–191.

Angell, M. (1993). The beginning of health care reform: The Clinton plan. *New England Journal of Medicine, 329*(21), 1569–1570.

Epstein, A. M. (1993). The framework of health care reform. *New England Journal of Medicine, 329*(22), 1666–1676.

Fein, R. (1992). Prescription for change. *Modern Maturity, 35*(4), 22–35.

Feingold, E. (1994). Health care reform: More than cost containment and universal access. *American Journal of Public Health, 84*(5), 727–728.

Goldfield, N., Freeman, F., Bracken, B., Dorfman, G., Gitterman, B., Harris, C., Holt, M., Lundess, R., Siegel, D., & Smithline, W. (1993). Health reform principles for quality: Recommendation for the congressional debate. *Quality Review Bulletin, 19*(6), 174–181.

Healthcare Forum. (1993). *What creates health? Individuals and communities respond.* San Francisco: Author.

Iglehart, J. K. (1993). Health care reform: The labyrinth of Congress. *New England Journal of Medicine, 329*(21), 1593–1596.

Kovner, A. R. (Ed.). (1990). *Health care delivery in the United States* (4th ed.). New York: Springer.

Meador, A. C. (1993). The United States healthcare system and quality of care. In A. F. Al-Assaf & J. A. Schmele (Eds.), *Textbook of total quality in healthcare* (pp. 13–25). Delray Beach, FL: St. Lucie Press.

Relman, A. S. (1993). Medical practice under the Clinton reforms — Avoiding domination by business. *New England Journal of Medicine, 329*(21), 1574–1576.

Shortell, S. M., & Reinhardt, U. E. (1992). Creating and executing health policy in the 1990s. In S. M. Shortell & U. E. Reinhardt (Eds.), *Improving health policy and management* (pp. 3–36). Ann Arbor, MI: Health Administration Press.

Sinioris, M. E. (1994). QMHC interview: Stuart H. Altman, Ph.D., *Quality Management in Health Care, 2*(2), 82–88.

White House Domestic Policy Council. (1993). Health security: The president's report to the American people. Washington, DC: U. S. Government Printing Office.

Williamson, J. W. (1994). Issues and challenges in quality assurance of health. *International Journal for Quality in Health Care, 6*(1), 5–15.

PART III

QUALITY MANAGEMENT: INTERNATIONAL PERSPECTIVES

A. F. Al-Assaf

CHAPTER *12*

International Health Care and the Management of Quality

INTRODUCTION

The triad of *quality, access,* and *cost* has always been the center of much heated discussion and many important decisions in the United States. This same triad is equally important in health-care decisions made on the international scene. Health-care workers from different locations and nationalities are finding that the same issues affecting the delivery of health care in the United States are equally applicable in their countries. These issues continue to center around one important aspect of care — **quality**.

Availability, accessibility, and affordability of health care are all important components of the delivery of health-care services; but without the mechanisms to monitor, improve, and manage quality, targeted goals are not met. Managing care **outcomes** to improve the **structure** and **process** of health-care delivery is becoming a universal paradigm applicable in different settings and in different systems, both nationally and internationally. Without considering the quality of care delivered, and without assuming the effectiveness of services to improve patients' health outcomes, all efforts to increase access to care and to decrease health-care costs will fail. These efforts will fail not because health-care professionals are not doing a good job, but because the *right* issues are not being addressed. These issues relate to communication, **customers**, delivery systems, and care standards. Managing quality will improve communications efforts with the customer; managing quality will improve methods of health-care delivery; managing quality will continually improve standards of care; and managing quality will open further communications channels in order to share ideas and experiences to improve health care.

The problem of communication is prevalent both within a single country and between multiple countries. There is a problem with disseminating information and making information accessible for people to use and share. One of the main objectives of **Quality Management (QM)** is to improve communication. This improved communication will facilitate the ability to benchmark trends and practices within and between countries.

The world is certainly becoming smaller through advances in communication avenues and transportation linkages. There are, therefore, fewer barriers to sharing ideas and learning from one another. Further, QM and excellence in service are no longer being judged solely on a regional or even a national level; but it is becoming increasingly important for organizations to compete in these areas on an international level, as well. Quality of care and the management of care on a global level is, therefore, of particular interest and importance. Hence, one of the objectives of this chapter is to provide an overview of international health care and to compare the health care in the United States to that of other countries.

Also included in this chapter is a discussion of the history of international health care, the key players on the international scene, and the organizations that support those players. An overview of the international systems structure and a presentation of a world-health-systems model that is ultimately compared to the systems in the United States is also provided. The chapter concludes with synopses of the status of health care quality in selected countries and discussions of their strengths and weaknesses.

HISTORY OF HEALTH CARE ON THE INTERNATIONAL SCENE

According to Roemer (1985) the world has evolved gradually but continuously during the twentieth century along very specific socioeconomic development factors. He lists several factors that he attributes to world development. These factors are: science and technology, population growth, economics, crises and wars, socialism, liberation of colonies, migration and urbanization, mass education, dictatorships and repression, international organizations, growth of wealth, recognition of resource limits, and collective action. These factors can and have had a tremendous effect on the shaping and reorganization of a nation, a world region, or the world as a whole. Certainly change in societal organizational structure is normally followed or associated with change in the organization and hierarchy of health-care systems. Whatever the factor might be in assisting the development of a better world health care, it must be realized that, even on a global basis, one country is still dependent on others. Each country is part of a collection of other countries that share common characteristics, needs, and resources. Therefore, it is imperative to learn about development of health care from a global standpoint and try to see how this development affects individual systems development.

Pickett and Hanlon (1990) look at world health history as a continuum of improving conditions in sanitation, health, and disease prevention. They discuss world health history by starting with the primitive societies, where hygiene was derived from survival experiences. Rules and procedures were established for driving away the evil spirits (illness) according to previous experiences with success or luck. Pickett and Hanlon next focus on the classical cultures, starting with Minoans and Myceneans (around 1500 B.C.), and moving on to the Egyptian, Greek, and Roman civilizations. In these cultures several accepted procedures and practices were underway that could be considered early attempts to improve hygiene and control sanitation. Achievements in administration and engineering practices, such as personal cleanliness and environmental sanitation, enhanced improvement efforts in health and hygiene.

Pickett and Hanlon go on to discuss the Middle Ages (500–1600 A.D.). This period was highlighted by the collapse of the Roman Empire. People of this time period revolted against anything related to the Roman Empire. Unlike in the Roman and Greek societies, personal hygiene was considered immoral; in fact a new practice known as "mortification of the flesh" (wherein a negative attitude was taken toward personal cleanliness) became prevalent. Hence, sanitation and hygiene practice declined a great deal and were further impacted by the increase in mobility of people (and, especially, armies) across continents. This, of course, brought the spread of endemic diseases, resulting in widely know pandemics of diseases such as cholera, leprosy, and plague (black death). Other diseases, including small pox, diphtheria, typhoid, typhus, and great pox (syphilis), also started to become more prevalent and widespread. This era therefore proved a detriment to public health, with the only effective, although crude and inhumane, measure being quarantine.

Sanitary and hygenic conditions did not improve in the seventeenth and eighteenth centuries. Slavery and labor abuses were common practices. Ill-treated children were raised in dormitories with the poorest of sanitation, diet, and health conditions. They were required to work sixteen to eighteen hours a day with minimum breaks and food; and they often were chained to their machines. When they reached the age of apprenticeship (usually in their teenage years) they were sold to a "Master," who then continued to abuse them for his own benefit. Chadwick, in 1842, described these poor conditions, and noted that the average life expectancies of tradesmen and laborers were twenty-two years and sixteen years respectively.

In response to critical reviews such as Chadwick's and other reports on public health, England established a General Board of Health in 1848. This move triggered work in biology, epidemiology, and, later, microbiology. In 1850 John Snow concluded that cholera was caused by a microscopic living organism that lived in the human intestines and was spread through the community sewage. In 1867 Lister described antisepsis (materials against sepsis and germs); and in the 1870s Louis Pasteur discovered the reproduction of microorganisms and, thus, cleared the way for discovery of immunization. At the same time, pathology was described and Koch introduced epidemiology and pathogenesis. Similar achievements in science and health continued through the nineteenth and into the twentieth century. These accomplishments in public health also had a positive impact on the social environment. New legislation was passed to improve labor conditions, child welfare, and the care of the elderly and the mentally ill.

While advances in public health were being initiated in Europe, similar efforts were also underway in the United States. In 1850 Lemuel Shattuck wrote an extraordinary report on sanitary conditions in Massachusetts. He called for sanitary reforms based on analysis of vital statistics records. Even before Shattuck's report local health departments had begun to form throughout the country, first in Baltimore (1789), and later in Charleston, South Carolina (1815), and Philadelphia (1818). These departments were more concerned with specific sanitary conditions, such as crowded living conditions, public baths, and dirty streets, than with the causes of such conditions. Still, these concerns started to emerge, as did later concerns regarding epidemics and the wide spread of disease. The emphasis, however, was on quarantine.

With the formation of the American Public Health Association (APHA) in 1872, the scope of interest regarding public health was significantly broadened to include such things as sanitation, disease prevention, hygiene, and longevity (Pickett & Hanlon, 1990). As a result of a proposal by APHA, the National Board of Health was established in 1879. Although some APHA leadership was included in the administrative body of the Board, the Board was given only four years of authorization. Because of early and powerful opposition to its existence, the Board was not reinstated after this four-year period.

On the global front, the first International Sanitary Convention was held in Paris in 1851. A convention strategy was not adopted, however, until 1892 at which time the strategy was restricted to cholera. Another convention in 1897 dealt with plague. In 1902 the International Sanitary Bureau was formed in Washington, D.C. This body was renamed the Pan American Sanitary Bureau, and later the Pan American Organization. It was ultimately reorganized as the Pan American Health Organization (PAHO), which became the regional office of the World Health Organization (WHO) in the Americas.

Also in 1902, in an attempt to give further authority to and broaden the responsibilities of the United States Marine Hospital Services, the United States Congress renamed this organization the Public Health and Marine Hospital Services. In 1912, this agency became the United States Public Health Service. In 1907 another international body was established in Paris: L'Office International d'Hygiene Publique (OIHP). This was followed in 1919 by the establishment of the Health Organization of the League of Nations, which was "to take steps in matters of International concern for the prevention and control of disease" (WHO, 1990, p. 2). Other International Sanitary Conventions were later adopted to include smallpox and typhus in 1926 and regional communicable diseases in 1938. In 1946 WHO was founded. The World Health Organization adopted its first constitution on April 7, 1948 (later observed as "World Health Day" each year) during the first World Health Assembly in Geneva. Several regulations were adopted that replaced the earlier ones regarding such diseases as cholera, small pox, and yellow fever. Additional regulations included other diseases and health services. Annual World Health Assemblies followed, and new regulations were adopted. These included more aggressive and collaborative approaches to deal with issues such as immunization, sanitation, and health. The involvement and new role of WHO was further reinforced in 1977 during the thirtieth World Health Assembly in Alma Ata, which called for "Health for All by the Year 2000." The declaration for worldwide eradication of small pox followed in 1979. Further advancement in technology and science supported by collaboration with WHO and other regional organizations had a positive impact on public health conditions and the quality of health services. Other issues and diseases continued to be targeted for continuous improvement of health and health-care services.

It is evident from this discussion that improving health care is no longer a local or regional matter. Spread of disease and poor sanitary conditions have an impact not only on health, but also on economic and social structures. This socioeconomic and political impact has the tendency to spread to other countries and regions, which is the rationale for strong collaborative efforts between countries and through international agencies such as WHO.

MAJOR WORLD DEVELOPMENTS

A helpful synthesis is provided by Roemer's (1985) presentation of major historical developments and modern trends in health care. He describes the changes in focus which led to advances in health care. These advances relate to social and economic factors first, and to health status second. Dr. Roemer presents this summary as fifteen major world developments:

1. *Health manpower growth* surpassed the growth of population. Increasing needs for new skills, knowledge, and personnel for the provision of health-care services continued rising. These rising needs triggered further education and training, which produced more need for personnel.

2. *Specialization* and further subspecialization was an inevitable development stemming from the explosion of skills and knowledge.

3. The *establishment of local, national, and international organizations* became widespread, while sharing of information, personnel, and resources increased. Organizations encouraged teamwork to achieve increased levels of understanding of disease conditions and promote quality of health-care services.

4. *Geographic regionalization* was intended to reach rural communities and produce a better understanding of regional health issues through concentration of resources. This development came as a reaction to specialization and limited resources.

5. *Population control* followed. Widespread birth-control measures were adopted, and new methods of family planning were disseminated.

6. Emphasis on *geriatric services and rehabilitation* began to emerge. With the improvement of health care and longevity, the aging population kept increasing. New services and health-care delivery systems started to develop, and the focus of objectives shifted from curing diseases to rehabilitation and tertiary prevention.

7. *Environmental sanitation* was quickly needed as urbanization kept increasing. New methods of disposing of waste and modern methods for treating water started to develop, while sanitation measures to eliminate disease vectors started to be implemented.

8. *Health-care planning* came as a by-product of world "expansion." With the increased number of independent nations, new methods for planning socioeconomic structures included health-care planning. These planning efforts included the need for increased appropriations and the implementation of effective strategies to improve the provision of health-care services to the entire population.

9. Socialized health-care systems started to evolve with the organization and emergence of centralized government control of social and economic services. The function of delivering care shifted from the private sector to the government in an effort to increase access and to include all sectors and individuals of the population.

10. *Greater expenditures* in health care became evident as the wealth, as well as the per capita income, of nations started to rise. An increasing percentage of

the gross national product (GNP) was devoted toward health care. In the United States, this trend reached significantly higher levels than in any other nation on the globe, with over 13 percent of the GNP being spent on health care in 1992.

11. An increase in *collectivized financing* to fund health-care services started to emerge. Private entities started providing additional funding to finance increasing health-care expenditures. Also, it became an acceptable practice for the wealthy sector of the population to share some of their wealth or income with the government which was directed toward further improvement in health-care provisions and access. Taxes, charitable contributions, Medicaid, and the like are examples of such trends.

12. *Quality protection* became a sought-after provision as cost-sharing and cost-containment measures spread. It became rapidly evident that individual populations started asking not only for access to health-care services, but also for quality services from a quality structure (human and physical) and delivery process.

13. *Primary care and prevention* began to re-emerge as costs for specialized services became more expensive. As strategies for cost containment evolved, **gatekeepers**, or primary-care providers, enjoyed renewed levels of consumer confidence and importance as they "managed" the delivery of and access to health-care services by the general population.

14. *Medical humanism* and *service management* came into focus. The patient was finally treated as a customer with needs and expectations. Ombudsmen and patient representatives/advocates were appointed, while the participation of patients on various advisory committees increased.

15. *Internationalism* in health was realized. With the inception of WHO in 1946, and with the annual converging of the World Health Assembly, the concept of improving health status became an internationally shared effort. Heightened by the WHO's call of "Health for All by the Year 2000," health-care issues began receiving global attention almost simultaneously in different countries and world regions.

MAJOR INTERNATIONAL PLAYERS IN HEALTH CARE

According to the National Council for International Health (NCIH) (1990), there are numerous agencies, organizations, and associations involved on a regular basis in the improvement and policy making regarding international health. The one that many are familiar with, of course, is the United Nations (UN).

The United Nations

The UN was originally created as the League of Nations in 1919. The organizational structure of the UN systems is illustrated in Figure 12-1. The six principal organs of the UN system are the Secretariat, Security Council, Economic and Social Council, General Assembly, International Court of Justice, and Trusteeship Council. Each of the six organs was established to achieve goals on a global scale, and each has several other agencies related to its mission. The discussion following focuses on the agencies that have the most tangible impact on the improvement of international health and the quality of health-care services.

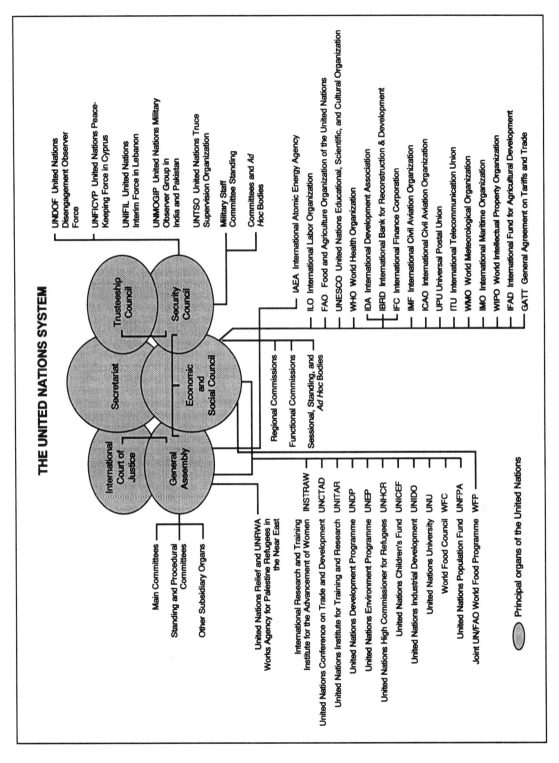

Figure 12-1 *The United Nations System*

THE WORLD HEALTH ORGANIZATION

The World Health Organization (WHO) reports directly to the Economic-and-Social-Council organ of the UN (Figure 12-1). Although created by the UN in 1946, WHO's constitution was not enforced until April 7, 1948. The WHO's main responsibility is to direct international health work. It has three administrative bodies: the Secretariat, Executive Board, and World Health Assembly. The latter body is responsible for policy making, preparing and administering WHO's budget, and appointing the Director General. This body has several other offices, which assist in formulating and enforcing policies, proposing and implementing resolutions, and fund-raising for conducting their business. The organizational structure of the secretariat branch of WHO is illustrated in Figure 12-2.

It becomes obvious when considering the organizational structure of WHO that this branch of the UN has a wide range of responsibilities and activities related to international health.

The PAHO is the organization that represents WHO in the Americas region. The PAHO has the same mission as does WHO, but for the Americas region. The other locations of WHO's regional offices are shown in Figure 12-3.

The WHO has been very successful in implementing new programs to improve the health status of certain communities. The WHO is currently working closely with the various countries to achieve the goal of "Health for All by the Year 2000." The WHO is also involved in such initiatives as the Extended Program on Immunization; the World Health Organization Action Program on Essential Drugs and Vaccines; the Acute Respiratory Illness Control Program; and World Health Day. The Global Program on AIDS (1986–1990), which had an annual budget of $100 million (United States currency), is another recent program in which WHO was involved. This program succeeded in involving more than 150 of the 166 WHO member countries to report AIDS cases and to develop national plans to control this disease (National Council for International Health [NCIH], 1990).

UNITED NATIONS CHILDREN'S FUND

The United Nations Children's Fund (UNICEF) reports directly to the General Assembly and the Economic and Social Council organs of the UN (see Figure 12-1). The United Nations Children's Fund, headquartered in New York City, was created by the UN in 1946 to address child-related problems in developing countries (NCIH, 1990). This mission is to be achieved through efforts of advocacy for children's issues, with direct involvement in project assistance; training; education; and providing necessary and appropriate technology, as well as other resources. Key projects have been mainly related to nutrition, education, and primary care, with a focus on reducing infant mortality rates. Other projects of UNICEF included the organization of a "World Summit for Children" in 1990. This provided a convention forum to deal with the rights of the child and the protection of children from environmental and other abuses.

UNITED NATIONS POPULATION FUND

The governing body of the United Nations Population Fund (UNFPA) reports to the same organs of the UN as does UNICEF (see Figure 12-1). The UNFPA, located in New York City, started operations in 1969 (NCIH, 1990). This agency was created by

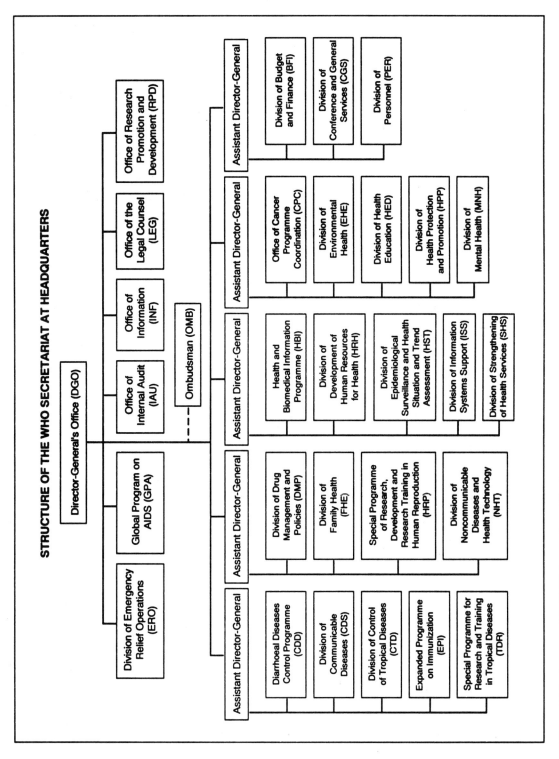

Figure 12-2 *Structure of the WHO Secretariat at Headquarters*

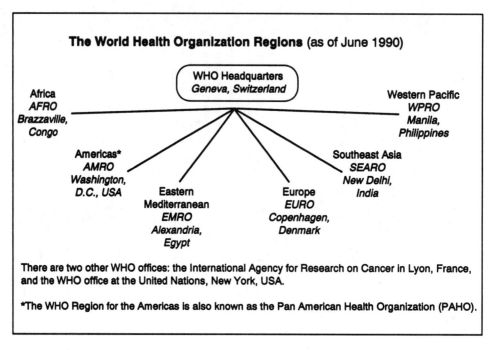

Figure 12-3 *The World Health Organization Regions*

the UN to provide funding, assistance, education, and advice in the area of population control, primarily in developing countries. Projects of UNFPA have included increasing women's education and involvement in human-development programs. Educational programs, as well as the promotion of population-control methods and strategies, are UNFPA's main objectives. Besides birth-control strategies, UNFPA is also involved in other related activities to control excessive population growth. Such projects include HIV/AIDS control, maternal and child health improvement projects, reduction of maternal mortality, and other family-planning efforts.

FOOD AND AGRICULTURE ORGANIZATION

Reporting to the Economic and Social Council, the largest UN specialized agency is the Food and Agriculture Organization (FAO), which was founded in 1945 to provide nutritional and agricultural technical assistance to countries in any area. According to NICH (1990), FAO's objectives are to prevent and correct malnutrition and hunger in the world. The agency provides expertise to enhance the production of food, and to improve crop production, fisheries, farms, and forests. It also provides capital for new projects and for training and education on methods and strategies that have a positive impact on the food supply of a country. Allocation of FAO funding resources is divided into thirds. One third is devoted to increasing and improving food production. Another third is allocated for the improvement of irrigation. The remaining third is expended on building fisheries, farms, and forests; cultivation of cash crops; livestock production; education and research; and other miscellaneous areas.

OTHER UNITED NATIONS AGENCIES

In addition to the previously mentioned agencies, the UN encompasses several other international agencies that have a direct or indirect impact on improving the health status of individuals. These agencies include the UN Development Programs (UNDP), UN Development Fund for Women (UNIPEM), the UN Relief and Work Agency for Palestine Refugees in the Near East (UNRWA), the World Food Program (WFP), the World Bank Group, the International Monetary Fund (IMF), the Organization for Economic Cooperation and Development (OECD), the Regional Development Bank, and numerous bilateral and multilateral Development Assistance Agencies. (Although these agencies are not discussed in this chapter, the reader is encouraged to seek additional information from the references listed at the end of this chapter.)

Additional Health-Care Organizations

The UN is certainly not alone in its devotion to concerns of international health. Many countries have a plethora of local and national agencies and organizations that have similar missions and responsibilities to those of the UN. For example, in the United States there are a number of Private Volunteer Organizations (PVOs) that have a wide variety of responsibilities and activities in improving health care. Three major areas are identified by these organizations as primary target areas for involvement and assistance: public health education, international health policy, and fund allocation. The National Council for International Health (1990) categorizes PVOs as either international PVOs or church-based PVOs. Examples of the former include such organizations as International Planned Parenthood Federation, International Committee of the Red Cross, Project Hope, and Helen Keller International. Other PVOs in the United States include the Population Institute, National Council for International Health, American Public Health Association, Bread for the World, Interaction, Institute for Food and Development, and World Neighbors. Examples of the church-based PVOs include Catholic Relief Services, MAP International Inc., Southern Baptist Foreign Mission Board, Christian Medical Commission, and World Vision.

Still other agencies in the United States include the Inter-America Foundation, which supports development activities in Latin American countries, and the Africa Development Foundation (ADF), which has development and improvement projects in twenty-five different countries. In addition, the United States Aids for International Development (USAID) and the Peace Corps provide skillful personnel and technical advice, as well as funds, to other countries when needed. The list would not be complete without mentioning those educational institutions that provide education and training in the area of international health, such as the Schools and Colleges of Public Health. It would also be negligent to omit United States philanthropic foundations such as the Carnegie Corporation, Ford Foundation, W. K. Kellogg Foundation, Rockefeller Foundation, and Robert Wood Johnson Foundation. These organizations and foundations commit a considerable amount of financing to a variety of different projects and programs in an effort to improve health-care access and services.

The preceding brief discussion highlighted the major international agencies involved in health care on a global level. The following few paragraphs contain a presentation of a world-health-systems model based on reimbursement and funding structure, which will provide a better understanding of world health-care systems at a country level. This model divides the world health-care system into four distinct systems, as described following.

WORLD HEALTH-CARE SYSTEMS

In discussing international health and its key players, it is useful to understand the basic organizational structures of the different health-care systems operating in the world. It is also important to realize that although the different systems can be divided into four major and distinct types of systems, some countries may have one or more system structures operating almost simultaneously. In such countries, duplication and overlap of services is somewhat inevitable as subsystems arise on their own or by the influence of the major systems operating in those countries (Saltman, 1988). This point is further explored in the following discussion of the four different world health-care systems.

There are several models for structuring the world health-care-delivery system. Whether they are based on political structure, cultural environment, or socioeconomic aspects, all systems tend to have broad and comprehensive health-care services. In this discussion an attempt has been made to classify the health-care systems of the world based on funding and access to care. This classification, as mentioned earlier, tends to be considerably more specific in demarcation, with the distinct features of each system thus making these four systems easier to study and understand. The four systems are *Free Enterprise, Social Insurance, Universal Service,* and *Public Assistance Systems.*

Free Enterprise Health-Care System

Prior to health-care reform, the health-care system in the United States has been recognized as the principle example in the world today of a predominately free enterprise fee-for-service type health-care system. (See Chapter 11 for a detailed discussion of the current health-care environment in the United States.) Private practitioners are paid fee for service either directly by the patient or through a third-party payer. Increasingly, however, those third parties, such as insurance companies and government, are emerging as purchasers of large amounts of care. As a result of the health-care reform initiatives, this fee-for-service structure may consolidate centrally through major health-care alliances that would include practitioners, providers, and insurers; these health-care alliances would then decide on service and expenditures. Government would also be playing a much more active role in health care, with increased emphasis on access, cost controls, and quality improvement.

In the free enterprise health-care system of the United States, providers operate fairly independently of government intervention, at least with regard to their structures and organizations. External review organizations that are backed by government, however, have enforced these providers to ensure and improve quality. Such organizations have promulgated specific standards and guidelines for health-care organizations to meet and follow to maintain quality of care. Also, with increased dependence on government-supported programs, health-care institutions have found themselves following those standards to gain participation in these programs. Additionally, education, research, and "other" care institutions (i.e., voluntary agencies) are currently receiving much subsidization. This trend may change as health-care reforms become reality.

Social Insurance Health-Care System

Australia, Canada, France, Germany, and the Scandinavian countries fit into the social insurance model. Japan has a similar model, but also has a major free-enterprise system, as well. In this type of system, the providers (physicians, practitioners, and hospitals) are reimbursed for their services, either directly or indirectly, through a specifically designated national fund. This compulsory, national health-insurance program provides the necessary funding for health-care services. These revenues are further subsidized by general tax revenues of the government. Providers enter into negotiations annually to structure payment schedules of services rendered. Institutional, "global" budgets are provided annually from monies collected in this "sickness" fund. The federal government in this system model plays a major role in administering the fund, sometimes at the provincial or state level. The government also provides **Quality Assurance (QA)** regarding appropriate services and care rendered by the provider. The government, in consultation with representative bodies of health professionals, formulates national health policies and regulations. Each resident in countries utilizing this system model is entitled to a comprehensive health-care plan with at least the provision of necessary health-care services. Therefore, rationing of care is controlled at the national or state/provincial level.

Although most of the physicians are in private practice, hospitals are usually government-owned and employ salaried professionals, including a considerable percentage of physicians. Still a small number of private insurance companies, hospitals, and other health-care institutions do exist, catering to those desiring "extra" services that they are willing to pay for.

Because government controls the "purse strings" in the service model, quality-improvement initiatives would appear to be inevitable. In reality, countries using this system model are in the beginning stages of an organized quality-improvement effort. In several of these countries (as discussed later in the chapter) quality initiatives did not start until the 1990s. Nevertheless, seemingly genuine efforts are underway in these countries to establish national, regional, and local guidelines to improve the quality of health care.

Universal-Service System

Russia, the United Kingdom, New Zealand, and China are examples of countries using a universal-service system. In this system model, health care is considered a public benefit for all and is financed through general tax revenues. In such a system all health personnel are salaried and all health-care institutions are government owned and operated. There are, however, a few exceptions, depending on the country being examined. In the United Kingdom, for example, there is a growing private industry in health care. Hospitals, practitioners, and a plethora of support services are being offered through private (usually for-profit) organizations and, indirectly, through private insurance companies. These "pockets" of private enterprise are growing in number but likely constitute no more than 2 to 5 percent of the total health-care industry. These organizations, however, have found that an increasing number of residents are willing to spend extra on their health care in order to receive a "perceived" higher quality of health care.

Health-care facilities in the universal-service model are reimbursed through allocated annual global budgets, while physicians are primarily salaried, full-time staff members of hospitals. In the United Kingdom and New Zealand the general practitioners, who are the gatekeepers to the health-care system and are actually the referring agents to the more expensive health-care services, are usually paid on a capitated basis. In China, however, the physician extenders like the "barefoot doctors" act as both gatekeepers and primary-care givers, especially in rural communities. These health-care personnel have had a positive impact on keeping health-care costs down.

Quality Initiatives in countries presently using the universal-service model are in their infancies. With the exception of the United Kingdom, these countries do not have a structured, well-followed, quality-improvement-and-assurance process. Sporadic, unit-by-unit QA programs do exist in some of these countries, but the concept of quality improvement is certainly far from being implemented.

Public-Assistance Systems

The public-assistance system is typical of many developing countries in Latin America, Asia, and Africa, where the majority of the population can afford neither private care nor social insurance. The government, through tax revenues and national income, provides health-care services without charge for most of the population under the auspice of hospitals and clinics. Almost all of these facilities are government owned, and most of the health-care professionals, including physicians, are salaried, full-time staff members of hospitals.

Residents of countries using this system receive comprehensive health care that is primarily for the treatment of diseases. Primary prevention, as well as tertiary prevention, is inadequate and, if provided, is done so in a disorganized manner and on a case-by-case basis. This system usually attracts the less wealthy residents of a country. The wealthy individuals, and those who can otherwise afford it, may seek care under a limited free enterprise subsystem, which also exists in most of these countries. Such a subsystem possesses all the characteristics of a free enterprise system, with the added characteristic of the lack or limited use of health insurance. Patients pay out-of-pocket for services received through this subsystem.

INTERNATIONAL QUALITY OF CARE

As the preceding discussion makes evident, reimbursement and access are the main factors in classifying the world health-care systems. Although in describing these models, reimbursement and access were emphasized in order to make distinctions, it should be noted that quality also plays a major role in shaping these systems. There are those who propose that access and cost (i.e., reimbursement) are key elements of quality. In fact, the patient satisfaction level in each of these systems is almost directly proportional to increased access and decreased expenditures for necessary services. It should also be emphasized that as quality is stressed and practiced, more cost savings are incurred and more services become available.

Of course, for certain countries, especially developing countries, other needed programs and changes take and receive priority over quality-improvement efforts. With the increasing emphasis on quality improvement that is surfacing in several countries, however, other countries are taking notice and starting to develop plans toward improvement.

Following are mini case studies of quality-management-and-improvement efforts in Italy and France. The purpose of these case studies is to increase awareness regarding QM efforts in other countries. It should be noted that an industrially advanced country should not be assumed to have an equally advanced QM system. (See Chapters 13, 14, and 15 for detailed discussions of QM efforts in other countries.)

CASE STUDY: *The Status of Health-Care Quality in Italy*

In 1987 discussion between the medical trade unions and the government lead to the idea, which later became a regulation, that physicians become actively involved in QA activities. Since that time three levels of participation: national, regional, and local have been set up. A national QA committee is in charge of oversight and accreditation of health-care institutions. At the regional level several twenty-two-person committees were established by a special office within the Office of Planning at the Ministry of Health. These committees are responsible for QA activities at each of the regions specified in the country. The three categories of committee responsibilities are:

1. education evaluation of health services in terms of appropriateness, adequacy, and necessity of services and personnel

2. promoting the dissemination of service improvement methods, training, and education

3. validation and evaluation of local committee activities and programs (Gardini, Tonell, Morosini, & Marsili, 1993)

At the local level a coordinator is appointed to facilitate the conducting of QA studies. Local committees are established according to priority needs and include such improvement opportunities as admissions practices, drug utilization, time studies, inpatient length of stay, resource utilization, management of bedsores, evaluation of nursing care modalities, distribution of health personnel, medical record quality, and nosocomial infection control.

Also part of the QM initiative in Italy are the inclusion of QA in regional plans and the establishment of the Society for Quality Assurance in Health Care. Among the activities of this society has been disseminating information and education related to QA in health care, publishing a bimonthly newsletter, organizing annual meetings, and publishing a quarterly journal on quality called the *Journal QA*. Other activities include providing advice and consulting services on quality-related issues to various committees.

Quality-improvement efforts in Italy appear to be continuously growing and maturing. Considering these new initiatives in quality improvement and the emphasis on quality at the national, regional, and local levels, the future of quality improvement in Italy appears to be positive.

CASE STUDY: *The Status of Health-Care Quality in France*

In France the term QA is not used liberally, as it is in other countries. The term *medical evaluation* is more commonly used because health-policy initiatives almost always involve physicians. It should also be noted that QA is not appealing to physicians in France, where the individual promotion and recognition systems are based entirely on clinical research and publication, rather than on the assurance or control of clinical applications. The concept of medical evaluations, therefore, is only slowly moving toward the direction of QM and process improvement (Raffel, 1984).

Medical evaluations and QA activities are voluntary in France. The government and policy-making bodies provide suggestions and a limited incentive package to implement QA efforts. It is never made compulsory or obligatory on any profession to engage in these activities. Also, with the relatively long history of government emphasis on cost containment, physicians, in particular, are skeptical about government-endorsed activities that attempt to assure quality only without an implied cost savings. With that in mind, the country is obviously lagging behind several other European countries in the area of health-care quality improvement. Nevertheless, initiatives in France date back fifteen years. In 1979–1980 a group of large hospitals started to import ideas on QA processes from the United States and began slowly to implement QA practices in their facilities. A number of "evaluation" committees were established in several hospitals around the country with the objective of conducting studies in QA. These studies quickly took the form of *medical audits* in such areas as admissions, use of drugs, and resource allocations. When the country elected its first socialist president in twenty-three years in 1981, however, the attention previously given to QA shifted toward other areas. In 1982, the fifty-hospital Council of Paris established the Committee for the Evaluation and

Diffusion of Technological Innovations. Composed of doctors and administrators, the committee's major emphasis was on assessment of technology and away from the evaluation of care practices.

In 1987, as a consequence of the 1986 International Symposium on Quality Assurance held in Paris, a QA unit was created by the Paris Hospital Council. This unit became responsible for promoting QA activities among member hospitals. However, the concept of QA was introduced as a cost-saving effort and, thus, received minimal responses from hospital administrators who clearly recognized that savings in one year's budget may curtail next year's budget.

The late 1980s brought about the concept of consensus conferences. Held by different organizing bodies periodically, these conferences focused on discussing issues related to improving clinical practice and the delivery of care. Other initiatives included the establishment of medical specialty societies for medical evaluation. Examples of such societies are those for surgery, intensive care, and obstetrics. In 1988 the Society for Quality Assurance and Technology Assessment was created. The mandate of this Society is to increase QA awareness among physicians and other health professionals.

In 1989, a government report on medical evaluations was published. In this report the Ministry of Health revived the National Committee for Medical Evaluation and gave it an enhanced role in shaping medical evaluations. Among the responsibilities of the revived committee are suggesting topics for study, overseeing evaluations and disseminating the results, and becoming an advisory body to the ministry on such topics. In response to this report, the National Agency for the Development of Medical Evaluations was created in 1990. Again this agency has a physician focus. Its activities have included the development, implementation, and dissemination of results of QA studies in health-care organizations and the provision of technical follow-up. The membership of this agency is very prestigious, comprising well-known and competent physicians from all of France. This agency has been received very positively by physicians and hospitals since its inception. It has organized several consensus conferences and has initiated a national hospital QA project to improve the delivery of care.

As mentioned earlier, although France is an industrially advanced European country, its health-care QM efforts are still in their infancies. It is the author's belief, however, that these efforts will continue to receive increasing acceptance from the health professionals in the country and that France's efforts in QM will continue to proceed in a positive direction.

CONCLUSION

When considering the global perspective of health-care quality, it is evident that health professionals in general are committed to delivering quality care. The question is, "How can the quality of care be improved internationally?" It is important to develop awareness of national quality movements and to compare QM efforts between different countries.

Priorities such as access to service, attainability of appropriate care, affordability of services, and acceptability are all important quality issues that need attention in every country. Developing countries, in particular, take the position that they must first tackle the issues of availability and access before addressing other quality issues. In those developed countries where problems of availability and access are nearly solved, however, the issues of affordability and cost containment are typically in the forefront. There are also several countries that are addressing all of the previously mentioned priorities with some success.

Whether global or country-specific QM efforts are studied, QM should not be directed only to the elite. Quality-management efforts can be as simple as meeting patients needs, developing teamwork, decreasing waste and rework, or simplifying processes and curtailing bureaucracies. Even these simple measures can have a positive and promising impact on access, affordability, and availability (Al-Assaf & Schmele, 1993).

This chapter presented an overview of the historical development of international health. A discussion of those elements that shaped the development of international health was provided in an attempt to rationalize the evolution of international health care. An attempt was also made to convey the notion that QM is a global initiative and that countries around the world are slowly embracing its concepts and principles (although under such disguised names as "quality assurance," "medical evaluation," and "audits"). It is therefore incumbent upon healthcare professionals to seek additional information and share experiences with others in the United States and other countries. The value of comparative, international-health-systems studies seems clear. The field of comparative international health, especially with regard to the improvement of quality, can be enhanced by increasing the availability of literature and information about other countries. This demands a continuation of efforts to share experiences internationally.

REFERENCES

Al-Assaf, A. F., & Schmele, J. (1993). *The textbook of total quality in healthcare.* Delray, FL: St. Lucie Press.

Gadini, A., Tonell, S., Morosini, P., & Marsili, M. (1993). Italy: Country report. *Proceedings of International Society for Quality Assurance in Health Care, 10,* 184–190.

National Council for International Health. (1990). *Key players in international health and population policy: History, dynamics, and U. S. policy formation.* Washington, DC: Author.

Pickett, G., & Hanlon, J. J. (1990). *Public health: Administration and practice* (9th ed.). St. Louis, MO: C. V. Mosby.

Raffel, M. W. (Ed.). (1985). *Comparative health systems: Descriptive analyses of fourteen national health systems.* Park, PA: Pennsylvania State University Press.

Roemer, M. I. (Ed.). (1985). *National strategies for health care organizations: A world overview.* Ann Arbor, MI: Health Administration Press.

Saltman, R. B. (1988). *The international handbook of health-care systems.* Westport, CT: Greenwood Press.

World Health Organization. (1990). *Facts about WHO*. Geneva: Author.

ADDITIONAL READING

Collado, C. B. (1992). Primary health care. *Nursing and Health Care, 13*(8), 408–413.

Giraud, A. (1993). Medical audit in France: Historical prospective. *Proceeding of International Society for Quality Assurance in Health Care, 10,* 75–78.

Holleran, C. A. (1994). What are the ethical issues from a worldwide perspective? In J. McCloskey & H. K. Grace (Eds.), *Current issues in nursing* (4th ed., pp. 763–767). St. Louis, MO: C. V. Mosby.

Karmi, G. (1993). Equity and health of ethnic minorities. *Quality in Health Care, 2*(2), 100–103.

Kinsey, D. (1992). The moral and professional role of the Russian nurse. *Nursing and Health Care, 13*(8), 426–431.

Nicholas, D. D., Heiby, J. R., & Hatzell, T. A. (1991). The quality assurance project: Introducing quality improvement to primary health care in less developed countries. *Quality Assurance in Health Care, 3*(3), 147–165.

Ponce de León, S., & Ponce de León, S. (1993). Quality of medical care in Latin America: Do it yourself versus caveat emptor. Is there really a choice? *Clinical Performance and Quality Health Care, 1*(1), 49–50.

Reerink, E. (1989). Quality assurance in health care of developing countries. *Quality Assurance in Health Care, 1*(4), 195–196.

Roemer, M. I., & Montoya-Aguilar, C. (1988). *Quality assessment and assurance in primary health care*. Geneva: World Health Organization.

Ruiz, U., Karmele, A., Buenaventura, R., Coll, J., Coronado, S., Rivero, A., & Rocillo, S. (1992). Implementing total quality management in the Spanish health care system. *Quality Assurance in Health Care, 4*(1), 43–59.

Vuori, H. (1993). Quality of care in Eastern Europe: The diagnosis is clear, the therapy is not. *Quality Assurance in Health Care, 5*(2), 99–101.

Johanna C. M. H. Diepeveen-Speekenbrink

CHAPTER *13*

An International Perspective of the Health-Care Environment:
The Netherlands as a Case Study of Quality Health Care

• ─── •

INTRODUCTION

*H*igh-quality health care implies both the highest possible level of availability, accessibility, and affordability for all, as well as the highest possible level of care actually provided. The Netherlands can take pride in its high-quality health-care system. Life expectancy for a newborn Dutch girl today is 80.1 years; for a newborn boy it is 73.8 years. A recent, in-depth study predicts that these figures will rise to 81.5 years for women and 75.0 years for men by the year 2010 (Ruwaard & Kramers, 1993). In 1991, infant mortality was 6.5 per thousand live births (Netherlands Central Bureau of Statistics [CBS], 1993a); approximately 13 percent (1.9 million) of the population was over age sixty-five. These figures clearly reflect the standards of health and the quality of health care in the Netherlands today.

As elsewhere in the Western world, rising health-care costs are a matter of grave concern. In the Netherlands these costs have risen from 5.1 percent of the gross national product (GNP) in 1970 to 7.8 percent in 1985, 7.9 percent in 1989, 8.0 percent in 1990, and 8.2 percent in 1991 (CBS, 1993b). In 1994 health-care expenditure is estimated to reach 58 billion Dutch guilders or 8.3 percent of the GNP (Ministerie van Welzijn, Volksgezonheid en Cultur [WVC], 1993). Changes are imminent, but the basic constitution-rooted principle that every citizen and resident is entitled to basic health care will remain.

Presenting Dutch health care as a case study, this chapter first addresses the concept of **quality**, then briefly discusses key health-care-related facts and figures as well as key historical facts, and proceeds to outlining the Dutch health-care system. Next, major health-care governing laws and principles are addressed, as well as changes taking place at present or those changes that will be implemented in the near future. The history and work of the National Cross Association and the birth of the National Association for Community Nursing and Home-Health Services are also briefly discussed, followed by examples illustrating the meaning of the services for clients. Finally, the chapter focuses on the gradual shift from "health-care-centered thinking" toward "health-centered thinking" and on the role of nursing in the Dutch health-care system.

THE NETHERLANDS

In order to understand the Dutch health-care system it is important to consider the country itself as well as other health-care-related facts and figures. Health-care costs are of paramount importance in considering the context for the health-care quality endeavors of any country.

The Country

The Netherlands is one of the world's most densely populated countries with, since the end of 1991, 15 million inhabitants (including over 700,000 foreigners) sharing 41.160 square kilometers (15,892 square miles) of land. The population density, thus, is approximately 431 persons per square kilometer (1,090 per square mile).

Health-Related Facts and Figures

In 1991 the number of persons employed within Dutch health care was 435,000. Of these, close to 325,000 worked within institutions, and 110,000 worked in community-health services. The total nurse population was 173,100, including 92,000 first-level nurses, 31,700 student first-level nurses, 36,000 second-level nurses, and 13,400 student second-level nurses. (A first-level nurse in the Netherlands is comparable to a professional nurse in the United States; a second-level nurse is comparable to a practical or technical nurse.)

The Netherlands has twenty-seven regions for residential (intramural) health care, while the number of residential hospital beds at present is 3.4 per 1,000 inhabitants. This figure includes intensive-care beds and beds for day care, but excludes the beds of the general hospitals, of psychiatric departments, and the cribs for healthy newborns. Also excluded are the beds in sanatoria, centers for epilepsy, and for asthma patients, as well as the beds in rehabilitation centers (WVC & National Hospital Association of the Netherlands, 1989). The latest, though not yet official, target number of hospital beds is 3.2, although the Dekker committee report of 1987 (to be discussed later) recommends 3.0 or even a lower number per 1,000 inhabitants. Table 13-1 provides an overview of Dutch residential health-care facilities in 1992.

Table 13-1 • **DUTCH RESIDENTIAL HEALTH-CARE FACILITIES — 1992**

Hospitals

University hospitals	9
General hospitals	115
Rehabilitation centers	25
Specialized hospitals	42
	191

Nursing homes

Somatic	112
Psycho-geriatric	77
Combined	135
	324

Homes for the disabled

Psychiatric institutions — **132**

Psychiatric general hospitals	44
Others:	
• Homes for children under medical supervision	12
• Medical day-care centers for children	36
• Addiction clinics	11
• Other specialized institutions	38
	141
Total	**788**

Source: NZF (Nationale Zorg Federatie [Federation of Health Care Organizations in the Netherlands]), 1992.

Health-Care Costs

During the past two decades rising health-care costs have gradually become a matter of grave concern in many countries of the Western world. Table 13-2 illustrates the collective Dutch expenditures between 1970 and 1990, and Figure 13-1 illustrates the total health-care expenditure as percentage of the GNP in ten Western European countries. The table and figure illustrate how Dutch health-care expenditure has risen just over 3 percent since 1970, while the figure shows that a similar trend can be identified in other Western European countries. Only Sweden and Germany have recently managed slight decreases in their health-care expenditures. France thus far leads the list, with health-care expenditure of close to 9 percent of its GNP in 1990.

A QUALITY HEALTH-CARE SYSTEM

In the section that follows quality will be discussed as it relates to history, governmental regulations, and private-sector initiatives. These considerations provide insights into the rationale for the need for important quality-related changes in the Dutch health-care system.

Table 13-2 • **COLLECTIVE DUTCH EXPENDITURE AS PERCENT OF GNP — 1970-1990**

	1970	1980	1985	1990
Defense	3.6	3.4	3.2	3.1
Education	6.3	7.0	5.7	5.2
Public administration	8.1	10.2	9.6	9.1
Infrastructure	3.1	2.2	1.9	1.6
Health care and social services	5.1	8.0	8.2	8.8
Social security	13.7	20.5	21.3	19.4
Subsidies	1.1	3.0	4.4	3.9
Transfer foreign countries	1.1	1.7	1.8	2.2
Net interest costs	2.3	2.5	4.7	5.1
Collective expenditure	44.4	58.5	60.6	58.4

Source: CPB (Centraal Planburau [Central Planning Bureau]), CPB Work document No. 28. Reprinted with permission of CPB.

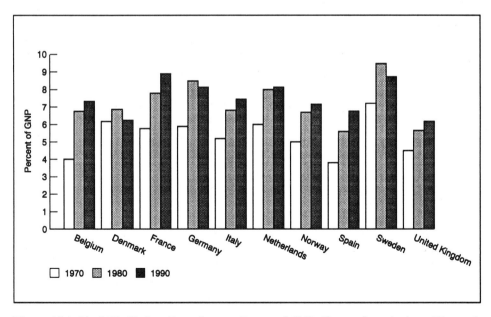

Figure 13-1 *Total Health-Care Expenditure as Percent of GNP. (Source: Organization of Economic Cooperation and Development, Paris. Reprinted with permission.)*

Quality

The concept of quality is very much linked with sociocultural and economic conditions and values, and may mean quite different things to different people living in very different or even in similar situations. Also, there are always higher levels of quality to aim for, and, pertaining to health care, there is the imperative to change goals of quality as new needs, resources, and values arise (Bergman, 1989). Quality health care is defined here as the appropriate application of health-care sciences and technology after careful consideration and balancing of all inherent hazards and expected outcomes for clients and patients (Diepeveen-Speekenbrink, 1993; Donabedian, 1980; Phaneuf, 1989). Taking into account both strong points and shortcomings the Netherlands today indeed has a high-quality health-care system. The following paragraphs discuss major elements in more depth.

Key Historical Facts

The Dutch health-care system is an interesting mix of elaborate government rules and regulations and private initiatives. It is not a socialized system, and there is no national health care such as in Great Britain and Canada. Of interest is that private initiatives were born where governing authorities failed. The following brief overview of key historical events highlights major milestones with the intention of providing some insight into the course of events leading to the present health-care structure, which has its roots in the nineteenth century (Rigter & Rigter, 1993).

LEGISLATION

As far back as the 1798 constitution, health care is mentioned as an important responsibility of governing officials. The first legislation relating to health care dates from 1804. After its failure, new legislation was passed in 1818, obliging the Minister of Internal Affairs to appoint provincial health-care committees. Communities, in turn, could appoint local committees. Both provincial and community committees, whose members were mainly physicians, were responsible for overseeing medical practice, for supervising the maintenance of rules and regulations pertaining to the health of the public, and for preparing measures to control communicable diseases. Governing officials unfortunately showed little interest in matters related to health care, and legislation again failed. This prompted local community physicians to start voicing their frustration over the lack of official support. Notwithstanding years of discussions about necessary improvement in the area of health care, it was not until 1865 and 1872 that new legislation was passed. Both of these attempts were, again, doomed to failure due to the mentality of the times and the diminishing interest of government officials in health-care matters. In 1865 the great nineteenth century Dutch statesman Thorbecke (1798–1872) attempted in vain to enforce, by law, community authorities to live up to their existing obligations and develop effective public-health policies. The 1872 law was an attempt to control communicable diseases after cholera, typhoid fever, and small pox had claimed thousands of victims. By the turn of the century tuberculosis had become the main cause of death, claiming approximately 10,000 victims annually. Combatting this disease later became a major target of both private organizations and government legislation

(Rigter & Rigter, 1993). To the nation's shame, however, official interest in controlling these devastating diseases vanished with the end of each epidemic.

Toward the end of the nineteenth century it was finally recognized that existing legislation needed urgent revision. This happened in 1901 with the establishment of the first Comprehensive Health Act (Gezondheidswet 1901), which was revised in 1919, 1956, and 1964. Passage of this act led to the post-World War II situation and the birth of the present health-insurance system, to be discussed later.

PRIVATE INITIATIVES

When goverment initiatives failed in the mid 1800s, private intiatives started to take over. In 1849 the Dutch physicians, as a result of their frustration over failed legislation, founded their professional organization called Nederlandsche Maatschappij tot Bevordering van de Geneeskunst, now called the Royal Dutch Medical Association. This organization has since had a strong influence on the developments of health care and legislation in the Netherlands.

Jacobus Penn (1821–1880) merits mentioning as one of the founding fathers, in 1875, of the first private Cross Association (the Provinciale Noordhollandsche Vereeniging Het Witte Kruis or Provincial North Holland Association, The White Cross). At the time Jacobus Penn was Inspector for the State Supervision of Health Care and Chairman of the Medical Board of the province of North Holland. The White Cross initially focused on combatting communicable diseases. Support of families in need due to illness was also an important objective. Penn's initiatives were soon followed by others, and the number of private Cross organizations gradually increased. Today an extensive network of services is available throughout the nation, providing care to approximately one million clients annually. Services range from prenatal care, to maternity care, to the care of the sick, including terminally ill patients who wish to die at home. (A later section discusses this important aspect of Dutch health care.)

Laws and Principles Governing Today's Health-Care System

Since 1983 the Dutch constitution entitles every citizen and resident to health care, which today is indeed available, accessible, and affordable for all. Legislation governing today's health care falls into the following main categories pertaining to:

- official advisory bodies
- the structure of care (available facilities)
- costs
- insurance
- quality
- the rights of clients and patients (still in a beginning phase) (WVC, 1987)

Under the current health-care-insurance system, approximately 95 percent of all health-care costs are covered by insurance premiums. The laws governing health-care insurance best illustrate availability and accessibility of health care and related facilities.

THE HEALTH INSURANCE ACT

The Health Insurance Act of 1964 (Ziekenfondswet) calls for compulsory insurance for all employees with a yearly income below an annually established level. In 1989 employees contributed 3.15 percent of their salaries toward this insurance, up to a set maximum. Employers contribute equally. At present approximately 60 percent of the Dutch working population is insured by means of the Health Insurance Act. Insurees are entitled to a range of services such as consultations from family physicians and specialists (excluding psychiatrists), limited dental care, medicines, and hospitalization for up to 365 days. In addition to compulsory insurance for employees, a number of specific groups also benefit from the same compulsory insurance. These groups include recipients of disability benefits and unemployment benefits, and people under the age of sixty-five who are entitled to social security. Unless they are wage earners, spouses and children under eighteen years of age are also insured free of charge.

STATUTORY HEALTH INSURANCE

A relatively small number of citizens, such as local and provincial servants, benefit from employment-specific statutory health-care insurance funds.

PRIVATE INSURANCE

Besides compulsory and statutory insurance approximately 32 percent of the population is privately insured. Premiums vary according to insurance packages and the personal risks insurees choose.

THE EXCEPTIONAL MEDICAL EXPENSES (COMPENSATION) ACT

The Exceptional Medical Expenses Act of 1967, or the Algemene Wet Bijzondere Ziektekosten (AWBZ), provides national insurance for all citizens and residents, regardless of income and irrespective of whether premiums have been paid. Traditionally this insurance covered exceptionally high medical costs, long-term illnesses, and serious disorders, the costs of which are so high that regular insurance is virtually impossible. Today the AWBZ covers hospitalization from the 365th day on. From the first day on, nursing-home care and care in homes for the mentally retarded are also covered, as are care in foster homes for the disabled, hospitalization in psychiatric institutions, psychiatric care, care provided in outpatient departments for mental-health care, and the services provided by Cross organizations, including community care and home nursing care. The AWBZ premiums are income dependent.

The Need for Change

During the past decades many well-known factors have made the expansion of health care (along with the inherent development of strengths and weaknesses and steadily rising costs) possible. Since 1974 a series of official government documents have addressed the problems and have suggested change varying from stronger government regulation to deregulation with more emphasis on individual responsibility. A 1988 government document analyzed the pros and cons of the present system as follows:

- pros
  - good quality care in terms of medical knowledge, technology, and treatment of patients;
  - even distribution and good accessibility of care facilities;
  - strong focus on prevention, health promotion, health protection, and inter-sectoral interaction within the health field;
- cons
  - barriers resulting from the complexity and diversity of the present financing and insurance system;
  - complexities and inefficiencies resulting from the partition of health insurance into social insurance and private insurance;
  - lack of incentives for health-insurance funds to improve efficiency and cost effectiveness;
  - cost-containment measures, as one of the main aims of present health-care policy, have not proved to be sufficiently effective and are no longer socially and politically acceptable. (WVC, 1988)

Some argue that one of the main reasons for lack of flexibility is the complex, pluralistic character of the country, which manifests with a highly institutionalized balance between government and private institutions (WVC, 1988).

AN EXTERNAL ADVISORY COMMITTEE
In recent years the shortcomings and rigidity of the present health-care system have become a challenge for change. This challenge led the Netherlands government, in August 1986, to install an external advisory committee with the assignment of reviewing the structure and financing of the Dutch health-care system. The Committee on Structure and Financing, better known as the Dekker committee (named after its chairman), was requested to:

- advise on strategies toward volume and cost containment against the background of an aging population
- preview the finance and insurance system
- advise on possibilities for deregulation and streamlining within the health-care system

In its report the committee focused on three central points:

1. *The integration of provisions for health and social care.* Under the current system, these provisions are very much separate entities. The committee attached great importance to removing existing barriers as a means of promoting coordination in health care and tailor-made care.

2. *Improvement of efficiency and flexibility.* The committee believed that application of market forces to the health-care system is an important means toward improving efficiency and flexibility. According to the committee the promotion of efficiency requires an increased financial responsibility on the part of clients, providers, and insurers. The principle of quality and equity cannot, however, be sacrificed to market forces.

3. *A shift of emphasis from government regulation to market regulation and self-regulation.* The role of the government should be facilitating rather than regulating. (WVC, 1988)

The committee's core recommendation called for fundamental restructuring of the present health-care-insurance system toward a single, highly simplified care-insurance system. The main elements proposed were: (1) compulsory basic insurance for every Dutch resident and (2) voluntary supplementary insurance.

According to the committee basic insurance should include:

- preventive care
- obstetric and maternity care (including well-baby clinics for babies from birth to one year old)
- nursing treatment and care of the chronically ill and others needing care and help (residential day and home care)
- rehabilitation including the disabled (residential and by means of district nursing)
- medical and surgical treatment and associated short-term nursing care
- psychosocial care
- nursing treatment and care of psychiatric patients
- nursing treatment and care of the physically disabled (residential, day, outpatient, and home care)
- nursing treatment and care of the mentally disabled (residential, day, and home care)
- care of the sensorially disabled
- dental care for insurees who are eighteen years of age or less

The main items covered by voluntary supplementary insurance would include:

- medicines
- artificial aids and appliances
- outpatient paramedical care (physiotherapy, speech therapy, remedial therapy)
- dental care for insurees over eighteen years of age
- well-toddler clinics (for toddlers from one to four years old)
- cosmetic plastic surgery
- in vitro fertilization
- abortion
- sterilization (WVC, 1987)

No in-depth explanations are needed to comprehend that the Dekker proposals evoked nationwide debate comprising both strong support and rejection. In March 1987 the Dutch government responded with an official policy document called Change Assured (*Verandering Verzekerd*), in which the main principles of the Dekker recommendations (for a compulsory basic insurance system, allowing market forces within health care, and the provision of custom-made or made-to-measure care) were accepted. The premiums for the basic insurance, covering 85 percent of all health-care costs, were to be means tested. The target date for phased introduction of the new system was January 1, 1992. Government decisions were, however, overruled when a government crisis regarding issues other than health care led to a subsequent change of government and a delay in the execution of the Change Assured policy (WVC, 1988). Much has happened since then, and a number of new policy documents have again caused nationwide deliberations.

Following national elections in mid 1994, the newly appointed government brought its own momentum to the transformation process. Changes in law require extensive legislation procedures, and every step toward changing the health-care system requires extensive political debate and consultations with all parties concerned. But the premise of a basic insurance package is generally accepted today. The main targets for change have remained strong and the Netherlands health-care system is gradually undergoing far-reaching alterations while upholding the constitutional right to health care for all.

FROM CROSS ASSOCIATION TO NATIONAL ASSOCIATION FOR COMMUNITY NURSING AND HOME-HELP SERVICES

Nursing and home services are exemplified in the work of the National Cross Association and the subsequent Home Help Services. This section describes the evolution of these organizations and by the presentation of Case Studies emphasizes the vital role of home care.

Cross Association

The first Cross Association, the White Cross (later the Green Cross) was established in 1875. This first private initiative was soon followed by others throughout the country. Regarding the name, White Cross, it is of interest to note that according to Querido (1973), the White Cross emblem was probably chosen because the founder, Jacobus Penn, saw the association's task as similar to (though a peace-time task version of) that of the Red Cross, which was founded by Henri Dunant in 1863. The Cross Association's initial main target was combatting communicable diseases. Supporting families in need due to illness was also an important goal (Rigter & Rigter, 1993). After a long period of religious segregation (the White-Yellow Cross was Roman Catholic, the Orange-Green Cross was Protestant, and the Green Cross was general) all existing Cross organizations fused in 1978 to become the National Cross Association. Today the Netherlands has approximately eighty local Cross units providing health-care services to Dutch communities (Landelijke Vereniging voor Thuiszorg [LVT], 1992). In line with other changes taking place within the Dutch health-care system, reorganization and integration are still in process as the local Cross Association units are gradually becoming part of one large national organization — the National Association for Community Nursing and Home-Help Services, formally established on April 2, 1990.

Another important organization, also originating in the nineteenth century and also gradually becoming part of the National Association for Community Nursing and Home-Help Services, is the Central Council for Family Care. Its original task was providing household assistance to families in case of illness, in particular, fitness of the mother. The greatest expansion of home care took place after World War II when many uprooted families experienced immense need. Although the value of this organization had long been recognized, the work received neither official status nor subsidy until the end of the 1940s. The Central Council for Family Care was not established formally until 1972. Today family-care services are rendered by a national network of approximately 200 centers. The National Association for Community Nursing and Home-Help Services is to be the overall organization for (1) services traditionally provided by the Cross Associations, (2) maternity care, and (3) family care (LVT, 1992).

Home-Care Services

In keeping with the Dutch National Advisory Council for Public Health concepts, Schrijvers (1993) defines home care as (in translation):

> the entirety of care, nursing, treatment, and support of the client
> in the home situation, performed by self-care, care given by the
> extended family and other non-professionals, volunteer's work,
> and/or additional professional care with the specific goal of
> enabling the client to maintain himself at home. (p. 96)

Close to 133,000 employees annually provide services for approximately one million clients. Services vary from household assistance, to specialized nursing care of the disabled or chronically ill, to care of the terminally ill patient who wishes to die at home. Services also include assistance at child birth and care of the well mother and newborn in the home. Services rendered by the Cross Association fall into three main categories:

- care for parent and child
- care for clients living at home, who are suffering from an illness or a disability
- health counseling, health education, and prevention

CARE FOR PARENT AND CHILD
This main category includes three subcategories: prenatal care, maternity care, and well-baby and well-toddler care (from birth to four years).

Prenatal Care   This category encompasses prenatal care (but excludes the physician or the midwife [see Case Studies, discussed later in this chapter]), maternity care within the home, and well-baby and well-toddler care in outpatient clinics for children from birth until the age of four. Prenatal care first offers prenatal gymnastics. Annually the local Cross Association units organize approximately 6,200 courses for approximately 80,000 clients. Secondly, in the case of a planned home delivery, the district nurse calls on the mother at home one or two months before the date of expected delivery to discuss the delivery procedure, oversee the home situation, and to advise on arrangements to be made. Last, the district nurses organize group counseling sessions for parents-to-be.

Maternity Care Of the 198,000 families in which a baby was born in 1990, approximately 80 percent received some kind of maternity home care. Services offered vary from: (1) care for mother and child, light housework, and care for other children during an average of eight hours per day for a period of seven to eight days; (2) two daily home visits to give care to mother and newborn; and (3) a combination of the two types of care mentioned in numbers (1) and (2). In addition every newborn is tested within the first ten days for phenylketonuria (PKU) and congenital hypothyroidism (CHT). The screening percentage is 95 percent.

Well-Baby and Well-Toddler Care Almost all Dutch parents with children between birth and four years of age make use of the services of well-baby and well-toddler clinics. In these clinics, growth and development of the child are overseen by teams composed of physicians and nurses; eyesight and hearing tests are routinely performed, counseling on feeding and nutrition is provided, and vaccinations are provided. Due to the very regular visits, any abnormality can be detected in an early stage, leading to referral to the family physician or a specialist.

CARE FOR CLIENTS LIVING AT HOME, WHO ARE SUFFERING FROM AN ILLNESS OR A DISABILITY

Care in this category includes nursing care; support of the family, including counseling related to the health situation of the client or patient; and assistance in choosing needed appliances. Appliances, such as anti-decubitus mattresses, high-low beds, wheelchairs, crutches, or even highly sophisticated technical aids, are available and can be borrowed or rented for a small fee. In addition, the Cross organizations offer group teaching sessions addressing topics such as nutrition, incontinence, dementia, and different illnesses and disabilities. For family members and others taking care of the sick at home, courses are offered to provide support and instructions.

HEALTH COUNSELING, HEALTH EDUCATION, AND PREVENTION

The main targets within this third category of services are preventing illness and disability as well as assisting clients in maintaining their independence as much and as long as possible. To achieve these goals the Cross Association units both provide individual counseling and organize a wide range of courses addressing illnesses and disabilities, appropriate use of medicines, stress management, and other important topics, as well as courses on healthy nutrition and how to stop smoking.

Financial Resources

The Cross Association's work is mainly financed by the AWBZ. Thus, Dutch residents contribute by compulsory means-tested contributions. Contributions by membership are an additional financial resource (approximately fifty guilders [ƒ] or ninety-five dollars per membership per year), while the government supplies a modest subsidy. In 1990 the total spending of the National Cross Association mounted to ƒ919 million (approximately $510 million), of which ƒ737 million were financed by the AWBZ and ƒ171 million by members' contributions. The government provided

the additional ƒ11 million in subsidies. This amount excludes the ƒ48 million provided separately by the AWBZ to perform the national vaccination programs. In addition, the total expenditure for maternity care was ƒ312 million, with the clients'
insurances as the main financial resource, supplemented with small, means-tested
contributions by clients (LVT, 1992).

THE CLIENT'S EXPERIENCE

The following three case studies illustrate how health care, including the insurance
system, functions for clients. The first two deal with care for parent and child; more
specifically the healthy mother, baby, and pre-school child.

CASE STUDY: *Normal Pregnancy, Healthy Baby*

This case demonstrates the experience of a young Dutch woman who had moved
to the United States for a few years shortly after her marriage. Her first child was
born in the hospital in the United States. Her second and third children were born
in the Netherlands, at home, with the assistance of a registered midwife using the
Cross Association's community prenatal care program and maternity-care services
in the home.

When she was expecting her third child, the mother-to-be was thirty-two years of
age. She turned to the midwife when three months pregnant. Her oldest child was
then four years and her second child three years old. Because both previous pregnancies had been healthy and all seemed perfectly well, she followed the normal routine of seeing the midwife at first once a month; then, later, every two weeks; and,
during the last month, once every week. Because she had already delivered once
before in the same house she knew the requirements for home delivery. These were
nevertheless reviewed with the midwife and found in order: provisions were fore-
seen to make a high bed, the house was warm enough, and there were sufficient
means for washing with running warm and cold water. The mother-to-be, by paying
the modest annual dues, was a member of the National Cross Association and had
already enrolled for a prenatal gymnastics course, which she took together with
other expectant mothers. A few weeks before the expected date of delivery the local
Cross unit's community nurse, who had been contacted by the mother-to-be, made
a house call to assess the home situation and to discuss the help needed. Because
there were already two young children, it was agreed that, if possible, a well-experi-
enced maternity assistant (comparable to a technical nurse specialized in maternity
care) would be made available. The maternity center was to be called at the very first
sign of pending birth so as to assure that the maternity assistant could be present in
time to assist the midwife with the delivery. As it happened, the delivery was so

uneventful and so quick that the assistant did not make it in time. As soon as she arrived, she took over care of the mother and her newborn for a daily average of eight hours. In reality this meant ten hours during the first two days, with the number of daily hours gradually lowering first from eight to six, and then to four. The schedule was kept flexible, so as to adapt to needs.

Having this type of assistance permitted the young mother to rest as much as necessary, to gradually take over the care of her baby, and to enjoy a very relaxed maternity period knowing that the meals were cooked, light household work was done, and the other children were taken care of.

During the eight-day period, the midwife paid two visits to assess whether all was well, and the family physician called to examine the baby. During the first six weeks after the baby's birth the district nurse also made two house calls. The purpose of these visits was to evaluate the entire situation of mother and baby and to prepare the mother for her first visit to the well-baby clinic. At this outpatient clinic healthy newborns are seen regularly during the first year for advice pertaining to feeding and nutrition, to assess growth and development, and to receive vaccinations (diptheria, whooping cough, tetanus, and poliomyelitis) at the third, fourth, fifth, and twelfth months. At the age of approximately eighteen months, the child will be referred to the well-toddler clinic where the then toddler will be seen at regular intervals until the age of four, when school health care will take over.

In this case, the costs of the midwife, the perinatal care in the home, and the house call by the family physician were covered by the client's private insurance. The costs for prenatal and postnatal gymnastics were covered by the AWBZ, with the exception of a modest personal contribution for postnatal gymnastics. All costs for the well-baby and well-toddler clinics were covered by the AWBZ.

Analysis

In summary, in the case of normal pregnancy and normal growth and development of the child, as described in this case, maternity and child care covers the period from early pregnancy (from the moment of the first visit to a professional) to the age of four. School health care covers the entire school period. After that, other insurance takes over. The mother discussed in this case is a professional nurse and a qualified maternal-child nurse-specialist in the United States. She would not have missed the experience of giving birth at home and enjoying maternity care at home for anything in the world. The fact that a midwife must refer to a specialist in case of a problem, and that in such a case delivery must take place in a hospital setting, is an assurance of high-quality care. In addition, the proximity of hospitals all over the country is a safeguard in case of unforeseen last minute complications.

CASE STUDY: *High-Risk Pregnancy*

This case bears many similarities to the previous case, although there are some distinct differences. The mother-to-be was thirty-one years of age and eight weeks pregnant when she first called on a midwife. Her wish to deliver at home was overruled in the fifth month of pregnancy because of a threatening miscarriage. This resulted in referral to an ostetrician, acute hospitalization with complete bedrest, medication, and constant supervision. Six weeks before the calculated date of delivery she was permitted to go home and gradually increase her daily activities. The delivery in the hospital was uneventful, though somewhat earlier than calculated. In the hospital she benefited from "day care," which in this case meant that after giving birth in the course of the evening, she stayed in the hospital overnight and returned home the next morning. When they arrived home, the maternity assistant was waiting to take over care of mother and baby. Because the mother was a member of the Cross Association (by way of paying the modest annual dues), she had made all the usual arrangements for obtaining at-home maternal and well-baby care with the coordinating district nurse ahead of time. Because of her first pregnancy's history and additional health problems, the second and third pregnancies also called for specialist care. In both cases she again delivered in a hospital , received day care, and returned home the morning after delivery to find the maternity assistant waiting for her.

Because of her relatively low income (from a part-time job) the mother-to-be in this case carried compulsory insurance according to the Health Insurance Act. Thus, all costs of her specialist's care, hospitalization, delivery in the hospital, and specialist follow-up were covered by this insurance, as well as all costs of the perinatal care at home (with the exception of a modest means-tested contribution). As far as the children were concerned, all three participated in the sequence of care in the home, well-baby and well-toddler clinics, and, eventually, school health care. All services were covered by the AWBZ insurance.

Analysis

In summary, the mother in this case study needed referral to a specialist in an early stage of her first pregnancy. Due to her condition, she could not make use of the Cross Association's services pertaining to prenatal gymnastics. She did, however, take the postnatal gymnastics course. For her second and third pregnancy she benefited from both prenatal and postnatal gymnastic courses, and for all three newborns she benefited from the services rendered by the Cross Association pertaining to well-mother and well-baby care in the home. All three children benefited from the Cross Association's services rendered by the well-baby and well-toddler clinics.

CASE STUDY: *Terminally Ill Patient*

This case discusses the care of a terminally ill male patient who passed away at home. Two years earlier the patient had undergone surgery for colon cancer. He was now suffering from liver metastasis and was bedridden most of the day. The patient was married, and he and his wife were in their sixties. There were no other family members living with them; thus, all care was initially provided by the wife alone. She was later assisted by two friends. As the illness progressed, the weakening patient needed twenty-four-hour attention and care. Professional help became a necessity. This led the wife to contact the local Cross Association. The key community nurse responded with a house call to assess the situation and discuss the help needed. Because the family was not yet a Cross Association member, membership dues covering two years needed to be paid, so as to ensure immediate assistance. From then on, the patient received nursing care first once and later twice daily. The nursing care consisted of daily body care (bathing and massage), help with making the bed, and other needed assistance. As much support and counseling as possible were given to the wife, who was suffering from the emotional strain of the impending separation by death. The physical strain of sleepless nights caused by the patient's restless nights also became quite an exhausting burden. Even with the two friends taking turns to stay in the house during nights in an attempt to offer the wife an opportunity to get some sleep, additional professional help became a necessity. The care given up to this point had been covered by the Cross Association membership. Additional professional help needed to be covered by the patient's insurance. Thus, it was necessary that the family physician or the community nurse write a formal recommendation. Because of the urgency of the situation, the community nurse was able to arrange all by telephone without delay, and a night nurse from a private organization took over the care during the patient's last nights. Because the insurance package of the patient did not cover more than a few hours of private nursing care per twenty-four hours, this meant additional costs for the couple. Other insurance companies offering different packages could have covered more hours of private nursing per day for a longer period of time. Regardless of the differences in insurance packages, most health insurances today cover terminal care in the home in addition to the care provided by the Cross Association. However, the number of hours and the length in terms of days (or weeks) may differ.

Analysis

In summary, in the case of this patient, his wish to die at home and the couple's clear wish to remain together until the end was fulfilled. This clearly demonstrates one of the most valuable aspects of the available health-care facilities of the National Association for Home-Care and its Cross Association's units. For the patient himself, staying at home in his own room and bed, surrounded and cared for by those who loved him most, meant as much peace as could be attained under the most difficult of circumstances. For the patient's spouse, it was most gratifying to take care of her husband until the very end, which would not have been possible without additional professional care. Having friends and neighbors willing and available to provide support was rewarding for all involved.

FROM HEALTH-CARE POLICY TO HEALTH POLICY

One might consider the Alma Ata Declaration of health for all by the year 2000 as the epitome of health-care policy development. This common health policy gave the Netherlands added impetus to continue their evolutionary journey to continued improvement of health services.

Health for All

In May 1977 the Thirtieth World Health Assembly resolved that "the main social target of governments and WHO in the coming decades should be the attainment by all citizens of the world by the year 2000 of a level of health that will permit them to lead a socially and economically productive life" (resolution WHA 30.43, World Health Organization (WHO), 1985, p. 1). The subsequent signing of the Alma Ata Declaration in 1978 was a true historical landmark toward the goal of "Health for All by the Year 2000." The urgency for the European Region was outlined as follows:

- the level of health in 1977 was still low despite the financial resources devoted to the health sector and despite the new drugs and medical technology then available;

- massive challenges of inequalities in health needed to be met despite the overall high level of development in the region and the scientific, economic, and educational level of most countries of the region.

These two basic facts formed the framework for the WHO European Region's first common health policy, agreed upon in 1980. The European Health for All (HFA) strategy defined four main areas of concern: "(1) lifestyles and health; (2) risk factors affecting health and the environment; (3) reorientation of the health care system itself and (4) the political, management, technological, manpower, research and other support necessary to bring about the desired changes" (WHO, 1985, p. 2). The strategy further urged that: (1) a much higher priority be given to health promotion and disease prevention; (2) all sectors with an impact on health should take positive steps to maintain and improve health; (3) the role of individuals, families, and communitites in health development be stressed; and (4) primary health care should be the major approach to bring about desired changes (WHO, 1985).

The Dutch Response to Health for All

All who are involved in developments pertaining to the WHO HFA strategy are well aware of the far-reaching impact of the 1978 Alma Ata Declaration on health-care thinking and policy developments. In the years following the declaration, many countries took initiatives to operationalize the WHO ideology. The Netherlands' formal response to the declaration, the 1986 Memorandum 2000 (Nota 2000), contains a detailed description of the population's health as well as expected developments until the year 2000 (WVC, 1986). Also included are most of the thirty-eight WHO targets. As of 1986 the Dutch administration publishes a health-policy document approximately every third year. These documents describe the population's past, present, and future health determinants. Both the Memorandum 2000 and the later policy documents demonstrate a shift from health-care services policy to a much broader policy encompassing prevention, health promotion, and health protection; or as van Maanen (1990) states, a shift from (in translation) "consumption to participation and shared responsibility requiring knowledge, insight, vision, involvement, and creativity" (p. 172). The major components of Dutch health policy today focus on (1) health per se, with a strong focus on prevention and (2) measures toward protecting and promoting public health in health-related areas such as environment, sanitation, housing, work, and education.

With the Memorandum 2000 as a starting point, the Netherlands at present uses the *scenario technique* as an instrument for developing long-term policies within the HFA framework (WVC, 1989). According to Makridakis and Wheelwright (1978):

> Scenario writing takes a well-defined set of assumptions, then develops an imaginative conception of what the future would be like if the assumptions were true. In this sense, scenarios are not future predictions by themselves. Rather they present a number of possible alternatives, each based on certain assumptions and conditions. (p. 496)

Scenarios sketch a potential future; the technique thus becomes an aid in planning and decision-making processes. The first issues to be addressed in the Netherlands, according to the scenario technique, were aging, cardiovascular diseases, and cancer. The long list of scenario reports now available demonstrates the many other important health and health-related topics that have since been studied and incorporated into clear policy recommendations and actions.

Another shift in Dutch thinking regarding health is toward the importance of home and community rather than intramural care, with a distinction between first-line health care and second-line health care. The first category encompasses services rendered by family physicians, midwives, Cross Associations, physiotherapists, and social workers. The second category refers to all intramural care, including hospitals and other institutions for health care.

NURSING'S ROLE

Earlier, a brief description summarized the establishment of the White Cross Association in 1875, noting that the organization was primarily geared toward combatting communicable diseases. Not yet mentioned was the importance of the White Cross with regard to nursing. The Cross initiative led to the start of the country's first nursing education programs in 1878. The two programs began in Amsterdam hospitals and were soon followed by programs in other hospitals (Diepeveen-Speekenbrink, 1992a), when it was recognized that improvement in health care needed to be paired with improved nursing care. The primary goal of the first programs was educating nurses for community nursing. Later, as more graduate nurses became available, modernizing nursing within the hospital setting became a next target (van der Kooij, 1990). Today, more than one century later, nurses are contributing their invaluable share to health care in a wide range of fields.

During past decades, much progress worth mentioning has been made in the development of the discipline of nursing. These more recent developments in the Netherlands, as well as the present-day struggle to receive the education needed to meet today's health-care challenges and to achieve the recognition the discipline deserves have been described by Diepeveen-Speekenbrink (1992a, 1992b, 1992c). For example, higher undergraduate education was first offered in 1972 and is offered today in nineteen schools for higher professional education. Additionally, the country's first nursing science program started at the University of Limburg in 1980; this was followed by programs at the universities of Utrecht and Groningen in 1990 (Diepeveen-Speekenbrink, 1992b, 1992c). Among the other positive developments associated with the nursing profession are the growing recognition of the importance of nursing research; an increasing number of nursing research publications in peer-reviewed nursing research journals; presentations at national and international nursing research conferences; increasing specialization; and increasing nursing QM. (See Chapter 14 for a detailed discussion of QM in nursing.)

Summarizing only the positive developments would not, however, do justice to the present vulnerable situation of nursing in the Netherlands. There is unfortunately reason for serious concern. Findings from a recent research project suggest that the many diverse changes in today's health care have weighty effects on the nursing profession. Advances in science, changing systems, and changing health-care needs are topics of particular significance. There is widespread discontent regarding the preparation nurses currently receive for nursing practice. Nurses often are not sufficiently equipped to meet today's health-care needs. There is also serious criticism regarding the continuation of apprenticeship education in nursing. The need for a body of scientific nursing knowledge demands expansion of graduate nursing education and nursing research. Finally, decision making is hampered by the lack of national consensus on potential solutions to these problems. This has a negative effect on policy making, resulting in a lack of adequate national policy decisions. Indeed, today's pressures on nursing require knowledge and skills not previously expected, which in turn require fundamental reappraisal of current Dutch systems pertaining to nursing education, nursing research, and the organization of nursing services. A vision, clear targets, belief in goals, and determination are essential for further progress and are needed to meet today's and tomorrow's nursing education and health-care needs (Diepeveen-Speekenbrink, 1992b, 1992c).

Widespread concern about nursing in the Netherlands led the Dutch government to install an official commission in September 1990 with the goal of examining existing problems pertaining to the professionalization of nursing and recognition of the nursing profession. The commission's report, published in June 1991, presents a clear analysis of the current serious problems, and offers twenty-one recommendations for urgent action. Many of the identified problems and recommendations correspond with the research findings mentioned previously, though the report covers a wider range of topics (WVC, 1991).

Also of significance is a recent extensive study titled "The Future of European Health Care" (Andersen Consulting & Burson-Marsteller, 1993), which focuses on health-care delivery methods and policies to be implemented during the next five years in ten Western European countries. The ninety-three page report contains a wealth of valuable information on health-care systems, costs, expected developments, and implementations for governments, insurers, providers, physicians, and clients. Nursing, however, is mentioned only once. This scant reference notes that all that doctors require of hospitals, relative to nursing, is that a high-quality nursing staff be provided. Notwithstanding the progress that has been made, nursing still has many problems and prejudices to overcome in order to attain and maintain the recognition the profession deserves.

CONCLUSION

The aim of this chapter was to provide an overview of the Dutch health-care system including historical and developmental aspects of the health-care insurance systems. The status and changes in major health-care governing laws were also addressed as were the history and work of the National Cross Association and the National Association for Community Nursing and Home-Health Services. It should be noted, however, that this overview in no way captures any aspect of the system in its entirety. The chapter also illustrated the quality of the health-care system, and included three case descriptions to promote better understanding. Because of their uniqueness, mother and child care and terminal care in the home received specific attention in the case studies. The gradual shift from "health-care-centered thinking" to "health-centered thinking" was mentioned, demonstrating the importance of prevention, health promotion, and health protection. Finally, nursing's role was outlined, including the present-day struggle for recognition and professional development. Not discussed was QM in nursing; this important topic is addressed in Chapter 14.

REFERENCES

Andersen Consulting & Burson-Marsteller. (1993). *The future of European health care.* London: Author.

Bergman, R. (1989). Towards Quality Assurance in community nursing. *Community Nursing, Proceedings of the International Conference on Community Nursing* (pp. 22–31). Utrecht, Netherlands: Netherlands Institute of Primary Health Care (NIVEL).

Diepeveen-Speekenbrink, J. C. M. H. (1992a). The developing discipline of nursing from a Dutch perspective. *International Journal of Nursing Studies, 29*(2), 99–111.

Diepeveen-Speekenbrink, J. C. M. H. (1992b). The need for graduate nursing education and nursing research in the Netherlands: An exploratory study. *International Journal of Nursing Studies, 29*(4), 393–410.

Diepeveen-Speekenbrink, J. C. M. H. (1992c). Nursing science in the Netherlands: The Utrecht contribution. *Journal of Advanced Nursing, 17,* 1361–1368.

Diepeveen-Speekenbrink, J. C. M. H. (1993). *Health care in the Netherlands — Available, affordable, and accessible for all.* Key note address for NEON (North East Organization for Nursing), Enfield, CT.

Donabedian, A. (1980). *Exploration in quality assessment and monitoring, Vol. I.* Ann Arbor, MI: Health Administration Press.

Kooij, C. H. van der. (1990). 1890–1990: De Vermaatschappelijking van de Zorg (1890–1990: The socialization of care). In A. H. M. van den Bergh-Braam, C. H. van der Kooij, & A. E. M. van de Pasch (Eds.), *Honderd jaar verpleging (One hundred years of nursing)* (pp. 13–64). Lochem, Netherlands: De Tijdstroom.

Landelijke Vereniging voor Thuiszorg (National Association for Community Nursing and Home Help Services in the Netherlands [LVI]). (1992). *125 jaar thuis in thuiszorg (125 years of home care).* Bunnik, Netherlands: Landelijke Vereniging voor Thuiszorg.

Maanen, J. M. Th. van. (1990). Health for all/Primary health care vanuit internationaal perspectief (Health for all/Primary health care from an international perspective). In A. H. M. van den Bergh-Braam, C. H. van der Kooij, & A. E. M. van de Pasch (Eds.), *Honderd jaar verplegen (One hundred years of nursing)* (pp. 171–186). Lochem, Netherlands: De Tijdstroom.

Makridakis, S., & Wheelwright, S. C. (1978). *Forecasting methods & applications.* Santa Barbara, CA: Wiley/Hamilton.

Ministerie van Welzijn, Volksgezondheid en Cultuur (Ministry of Welfare, Health, and Cultural Affairs [WVC]). (1986). *Nota 2000 (Memorandum 2000)* (Official Government Document, session 1985–1986, 19 500, nrs 1–2). Den Haag, Netherlands: Tweede Kamer der Staten Generaal.

Ministerie van Welzijn, Volksgezondheid en Cultuur (Ministry of Welfare, Health, and Cultural Affairs [WVC]). (1987). *Bereidheid tot verandering (Willingness to change).* Den Haag, Netherlands: Author.

Ministerie van Welzijn, Volksgezondheid en Cultuur (Ministry of Welfare, Health, and Cultural Affairs [WVC]). (1988). *Changing health care in the Netherlands.* Rijswijk, Netherlands: Author.

Ministerie van Welzijn, Volksgezondheid en Cultuur (Ministry of Welfare, Health, and Cultural Affairs [WVC]). (1989). *Highlights of Dutch HFA-policy.* Rijswijk, Netherlands: Author.

Ministerie van Welzijn, Volksgezondheid en Cultuur (Ministry of Welfare, Health, and Cultural Affairs [WVC]). (1991). *In hoger beroep: Een perspectief voor de verplegende en verzorgende beroepen (In higher appeal: A perspective for nursing and caring professions).* Rijswijk, Netherlands: Author.

Ministerie van Welzijn, Volksgezondheid en Cultuur (Ministry of Welfare, Health, and Cultural Affairs [WVC]). (1993). *Health care in the Netherlands. Factsheet.* Rijswijk, Netherlands: Author.

Ministerie van Welzijn, Volksgezondheid en Cultuur (Ministry of Welfare, Health, and Cultural Affairs [WVC]) & Nationale Ziekenhuisraad (National Hospital Association of the Netherlands). (1989). *Dutch health care system.* Utrecht, Netherlands: Nationale Ziekenhuisraad.

Netherlands Central Bureau of Statistics (CBS). (1993a). *Statistisch jaarboek 1993 (Statistical Yearbook 1993)*. The Hague: SDU/Uitgeverij.

Netherlands Central Bureau of Statistics (CBS). (1993b). *Vademecum of health statistics 1993*. The Hague, Netherlands: SDU/Uitgeverij.

Phaneuf, M. (1989). Quality assurance. In D. A. Gillies (Ed.), Nursing management: A systems approach (2nd ed., pp. 510–535). Philadelphia: W. B. Saunders.

Querido, A. (1973). *De Wit-Gele Vlam, Gedenkboek ter gelegenheid van het 50-jarig bestaan van de Nationale Federatie Het Wit-Gele Kruis 1923-1973 (The White-Yellow Flame, Memorial volume in honor of 50 years National Federation The White-Yellow Cross 1923–1973)*. Tilburg, Netherlands: Drukkerij Bergmans.

Rigter, H., & Rigter, R. B. M. (1993). Volksgezondheid: Een Assepoester in de Nederland se politiek (Public Health: A Cinderella in Dutch politics). *Gewina (Journal for History of Medicine, Natural Sciences, Mathematics, and Technology), 16*(1), 1–17.

Ruwaard, D., & Kramers, P. G. N. (Eds.). (1993). *Volksgezondheid Toekomst Verken-ning — De gezondheidstoestand van de Nederlandse bevolking in de periode 1950–2010 (Public Health Future Study - The health of the Dutch population from 1950–2010)*. The Hague, Netherlands: SDU/Uitgeverij. (Available only in Dutch.)

Schrijvers, A. J. P. (1993). *Een kathedraal van zorg: Een inleiding over het functioneren van de zorgverlening (A cathedral of care)*. Utrecht, Netherlands: De Tijdstroom.

World Health Organization (WHO). (1985). *Targets for Health for All*. Copenhagen, Denmark: WHO Regional Office for Europe.

ADDITIONAL READING

Mahler, J. (1981). The meaning of "Health for All by the Year 2000": *World Health Forum, 2*(1), 5–22.

Ministerie van Welzijn, Volksgezondheid en Cultuur (Ministry of Welfare, Health, and Cultural Affairs [WVC]). (1985). *Willingness to change*. Rijswijk, Netherlands: Author.

Ministerie van Welzijn, Volksgezondheid en Cultuur (Ministry of Welfare, Health, and Cultural Affairs [WVC]). (1991). *The quality of care in the Netherlands*. Rijswijk, Netherlands: Author.

Ministerie van Welzijn, Volksgezondheid en Cultuur (Ministry of Welfare, Health, and Cultural Affairs [WVC]). (1993). *Health care reform in the Netherlands*. Rijswijk, Netherlands: Author.

Ministerie van Welzijn, Volksgezondheid en Cultuur (Ministry of Welfare, Health, and Cultural Affairs [WVC]). (1994). *Care in the Netherlands 1994: A summary of the financial overview of the care sector, 1994*. Rijswijk, Netherlands: Author.

Nationale Zorgfederatie (Federation of Health Care Organizations in the Netherlands). (1992). (Information brochure). Utrecht, Netherlands: Author.

World Health Organization (WHO). (1979). *Formulating strategies for Health for All by the year 2000*. Geneva: WHO.

World Health Organization (WHO). (1986). *Targets for Health for All: Implications for nursing/midwifery*. Copenhagen: WHO.

CHAPTER *14*

Nursing Quality Assurance, Management, and Improvement in Western Europe

INTRODUCTION

During the late 1970s and early 1980s nurses in Europe became more and more interested in the **Quality Management (QM)** and **Quality Assurance (QA)** of their performance. This was a result of the World Health Organization (WHO) program "Health for All in the Year 1990" (later changed to "2000").

European professionals were inspired by the developments in the United States, where since the 1950s, nursing QA concepts were continually being developed. These initial QA efforts were followed by transitions to nursing QM and nursing quality improvement. Nurses in Europe began to develop their own systems for nursing QM, using systems for nursing QA. The main characteristic of the European nursing QA systems is that they integrate both an assessment and an improvement phase.

From 1985 on, a growing commitment on the part of European nurses to a dynamic approach for nursing QM and nursing QA has been noticeable (Andersen, 1992). The major characteristics of this approach are as follows:

1. the standards are owned and controlled by the practitioners who set them;

2. the standards are dynamic and must be evaluated;

3. the standards improve communication and specify actual practice. (Kitson & Giebing, 1990)

The quality-improvement system is decentralized at the unit level. It is coordinated in a manner, however, that ensures sharing of information on quality improvement and standards of care among each of the units within the health-care organization. On a countrywide basis, whenever possible, professional nursing organizations, national networks, or specially founded nursing councils are used for this purpose. The most important interactions in the European quality model take place within the organization between the organization level and the unit level. In other words, in each organization, interactions take place from the top down and from the bottom up. The interaction between local organizations (such as hospitals), units for primary health care, nursing homes, and national organizations (such as the Royal College of Nursing in the United Kingdom and the National Organization for Quality Assurance in the Netherlands) is also important (Kitson & Giebing, 1990).

The development of this dynamic approach was influenced by two European demonstration projects. First among these was the Royal College of Nursing Standards of Care project in the United Kingdom, which was started in 1985 under the leadership of Alison Kitson. During this project the Dynamic Standards Setting System, better known as DySSSy, was developed. With DySSSy, nurses develop their own standards for nursing care based on literature and research (Marr & Giebing, 1994). The second influential project was the Nursing Quality Assurance project of the Centraal Begeleidingsorgaan voor de Intercollegiale Toetsing (CBO) (the National Organization for Quality Assurance in Health Care), which was developed in the Netherlands from 1985 to 1987 (Giebing, 1987). During this project a dynamic approach to nursing QA was developed and became the start of the CBO Nursing Programme in 1988 (Giebing, 1994).

NURSING QUALITY MANAGEMENT AND QUALITY ASSURANCE IN WESTERN EUROPE

The section that follows describes the incentives for nursing QM and QA in Europe. The areas of discussion will include the need for nursing QM and QA, the role of the World Health Organization (WHO), the European Quality Assurance Network (EuroQuan), and, finally, the development of a European-wide research program (COMAC).

The Need for Nursing Quality Management and Quality Assurance

Kitson and Giebing (1990) give four main reasons why nursing QA needs to be part of nursing QM in Europe. First, there are the professional reasons so clearly put into words by Maria Phaneuf: "There is an irreducible minimum for the unique quality of practice for any profession, otherwise the quality will be controlled by another and becomes a technology" (Phaneuf & Wandelt, 1981, p. 2). Secondly, there are legal reasons. Until recently, nursing legislation in Europe has been more or less based on the extension of medical performance. Since the 1970s, however, there has been a growing movement toward professionalized nursing. Explicit quality standards make nurses aware of their practice and, at the same time, of the legal limitations of their practice. This both protects the public from unsafe practitioners and provides the profession with a more objective approach of measuring professional competencies. Thirdly, there are social reasons. Patients in Europe are becoming better informed and more aware of the **quality** of health care. Consequently, nurses need to demonstrate the quality of the services they are offering to the patient: the value-for-money principle. Lastly, there are political reasons. The cost of health care in most countries in Europe is increasing. Nursing staff in health-care organizations is expected to be cut considerably and the availability of nursing resources is threatened. Nursing QM and nursing QA can be used to prove the need for a sufficient and qualified number of nursing personnel. This need can then be translated into **standards**.

The World Health Organization and Nursing Quality Improvement in Europe

In 1980 the Nursing Unit of WHO's European Regional Office in Copenhagen arranged a meeting in Sundvollen in Norway to begin developing nursing QM and nursing QA. The aim was to establish a working group to define guidelines for nursing standards in Europe. Out of this meeting an English-speaking working group was founded. At four meetings held during the course of 1984 to 1988, the working group discussed concepts, procedures, and strategies for implementing of nursing QM and nursing QA in their respective countries. The WHO, in collaboration with its centers in Europe, subsequently started working groups, seminars, and pilot projects for nurses in French- and German-speaking countries (Andersen, 1992). Since these efforts, numerous approaches have been developed to implement systems for nursing QM. Of these approaches, systems for nursing QA are one of the most important.

Implementation of Nursing Quality Management

The level to which nursing QM and nursing QA are implemented in Europe differs depending on location, specifically with regard to linguistic region (Giebing, 1992). There are three main linguistic regions in Europe. First, there is the region where the majority of the nurses speak and understand the English language, such as the nordic countries (Denmark, Norway, Sweden, Iceland, Finland), the Netherlands, Flemish Belgium, Luxembourg, Greece, and, of course, Ireland, and the United Kingdom. Secondly, there is the German-speaking region. Most of the nurses in Germany, Austria, and the German-speaking part of Switzerland do not speak any foreign language. This is also often the case in the third region, which includes the countries where Latin-related languages are spoken, such as France, Spain, Italy, Portugal, French-speaking Belgium, and Switzerland.

Nurses familiar with the English language share an important characteristic; namely, they all have linguistic access to the Anglo-American professional literature. This literature includes numerous articles and books written on nursing QM and nursing QA, as well as a moderate amount of documentation on research in these fields. Because these nurses are familiar with the language, they are able to read these publications and research reports, and are, therefore, able to familiarize themselves with existing QM concepts in health care and, particularly, in nursing. As a result, nursing QM and nursing QA are better developed in the countries where nurses are familiar with the English language than in the other countries mentioned. Developments in QM and QA are, however, communicated to non-English speaking nurses (mostly by bi- and multilingual nurses) at international conferences, workshops, and seminars in Europe. Thus, nurses in the Western European countries are relatively familiar with the concepts of nursing QM, QA, and improvement.

THE EUROPEAN COMMUNITY

Twelve European countries are united in the European Community (EC). Since 1992 there has been a strong political and economical collaboration between these twelve countries. The challenge for the twenty-first century is to integrate the political and economic systems of each country into one European system. Accordingly, the borders of the twelve countries have been open to one another since 1992. The current buzzword in Europe is *integration.* Because of the existence of the EC free-labor market it is necessary to integrate nursing systems into one European system. Much work has yet to be done, however, before it can be said that a system for nursing QA as a part of nursing QM is implemented in each of the counties. Further, the establishment of one unified system is the ultimate goal in an integrated EC.

Before the goal of a unified system is attainable, a system for nursing QM and nursing QA must be implemented in each country in such a way as to fit the culture of that country. Despite differences in culture, nurses in most countries have chosen a dynamic approach for the implementation of QM and QA. In order for this model to be successfully implemented and adapted it must win acceptance in each country, first, within the nursing profession and, secondly, within the political and social realms. The next step will be the establishment of an integrated European model, where the systems developed in each country each have a place.

European Quality Assurance Network

In March 1992 an international network was launched with the goal of facilitating communication and collaboration between European nurses, especially with regard to QM and QA. This network is called the European Quality Assurance Network (EuroQuan) and is financed by the Foundation of Nursing Studies in the United Kingdom. The task of the members of EuroQuan is to translate and transfer the EuroQuan concepts into their respective languages and start a national network for nursing QM and nursing QA in their respecitve countries.

One nurse from each country in the EC is invited to join EuroQuan. (The nurse must be familiar with the English language.) According to the first EuroQuan Newsletter (1992), this European Network is one way of developing the collective confidence of nurses who, in turn, will feel better equipped to enter into collaborative QA projects with health-care colleagues. EuroQuan meets twice a year. Each participating country offers hospitality in turn. Sharing experiences, discussing progress, and, above all, learning from each other at these meetings offers the participants a great opportunity. Further, EuroQuan provides nurses the opportunity to work on nursing QM and nursing QA in an organized way. Nurses in less professionalized European countries feel strongly supported by the existence of EuroQuan, which itself does not provide support.

European Community Concerted Action Programme on Quality Assurance in Health Care

Since 1990 a concerted action program on QA in hospitals has been executed as part of the Fourth Medical and Health Research Programme of the European Community (EC). The project, in short COMAC/HSR/QA, started in January 1990 and lasted until July 1993. One of the aims of the COMAC project was to identify and encourage QA activities as a part of QM in hospitals at the country level. Two hundred sixty-two hospitals took part in this project. Of these hospitals, 108 were general hospitals, 95 were teaching hospitals, and 59 were university hospitals. In addition to the EC countries the Scandinavian countries, some Eastern European countries, and Israel also participated in the project. The project was coordinated by an international project management team, and each country that took part had its own country coordinator.

The starting point for the project was a dynamic approach to QA within the nursing and medical profession, wherein four topics were identified:

1. record keeping (the target group consisted of nurses and medical specialists in hospitals)
2. pre-operative assessment (the target group consisted of medical specialists in hospitals)
3. prophylactic antibiotic use in surgery (the target group consisted of medical specialists in hospitals)
4. prevention of bedsores (the target group consisted of nurses in hospitals)

The research project had three main phases: assessment, action, and evaluation. In the assessment phase, which was completed in 1991, the present status of existing QA activities was assessed. Each hospital taking part in the project was sent a questionnaire to assess: (1) the hospital context, (2) managerial organization, (3) medical and nursing organization, and (4) the existence of QA activities concerning the four topics. Among other findings, the assessment phase showed that 69 percent of the hospitals had a formally structured nursing staff. Of these hospitals 80 percent had a statutory nursing qualification, while 20 percent were students. Sixty-one percent of the hospitals had a written program for continuing nursing education. In 42 percent of the hospitals there was a Nursing Quality Assurance Committee at the hospital level and in 21 percent of the hospitals there was a Nursing Quality Assurance Committee at the ward level (Klazinga & Giebing, 1994).

The action phase started in 1991 and is now complete. During the action phase QA programs in the participating hospitals were started for the identified topics. Hospitals were asked to perform a QA study on two of the four topics in their own institutions. Packages were provided containing detailed background material on the methodology of QA studies, the four topics, and the introduction of change in hospital. One hundred fourteen hospitals chose prevention of bedsores as the specific nursing topic for a QA study.

The evaluation phase, the last phase, was completed in 1993 (Klazinga, 1993, 1994). During the evaluation phase the effects of the action phase were assessed, looking at the before and after situation in the hospitals concerning the chosen topics, the implementation strategies used, and the results of the local QA studies.

Nurses who participated in the COMAC project were, in most cases, also involved in EuroQuan activities. In this way, COMAC and EuroQuan were more or less linked to each other.

THE DUTCH MODEL: A CASE STUDY

In the early 1980s nursing departments, mainly in hospitals, confronted with a steady increase in workload, became interested in nursing QM and nursing QA

(Giebing, 1987). Also fueling this interest was the introduction in 1984 of a prospective budgeting system for health-care services, which was expected to result in considerable cutbacks of nursing staff.

The National Organization for Quality Assurance

To offer the nursing profession some assistance, nursing QA systems as part of nursing QM were introduced in 1985 by the National Organization for Quality Assurance in health care, better known as CBO. This independent organization was founded to develop QM and QA systems for professional performance in health care, and to assist and support professionals in applying these systems. Consequently, CBO does not investigate the quality of health care, but only assists and supports professional providers in applying systems for QM and QA. The CBO program is financed by Dutch legislation. Health-care organizations and providers voluntarily take part in the CBO program. The voluntary nature of QM and QA systems is one of the three premises for QM and QA development in the Netherlands. Another premise is the possibility for professional groups to turn to an independent organization (e.g., CBO) for help and support. The third premise is that government is not involved in legislating quality of care but, instead, provides the means for professional groups to develop and implement QM and QA systems (Reerink, 1990).

In 1985, because of the interest expressed by hospital-based nurses, CBO started a nursing program aimed at the target group of nursing departments in hospitals. As part of this program CBO offers nursing departments support in implementing of classic centralized systems such as Phaneuf's Nursing Audit (1972), developed in the United States; Goldstone's "Monitor" (Illsley & Goldstone, 1985), developed in the United Kingdom; and van Bergen and Holland's "Quality Profile" (van Bergen, Hollands, & Nijhuis, 1980), developed in the Netherlands.

Characteristics of these centralized systems are:

1. the nursing care is broadly evaluated;
2. the instruments used for assessment are often developed on a scientific level and reflect the designers' views on nursing care and its quality;
3. the assessment of quality is often done by "Quality Assurance nurses" from a "Quality Assurance department" in the organization;
4. nurse practitioners do not really participate in the assessments. (Marr & Giebing, 1994)

The Unit/Ward-Based Approach: Part of Nursing Quality Management

In addition to the more classical approaches, CBO also offers nurses support in implementing the Unit/Ward-based approach, which is a dynamic decentralized system for nursing QA. This approach was developed by CBO in response to the nursing structures in university and general hospitals in the Netherlands. The system also appeared to be applicable in other types of health-care organizations that provide nursing care. The explanation for the double name of the system (Unit/Ward) is found in the organizational structure of nursing in the Netherlands. Nursing units are only found in organizations for community nursing, while wards are only found in hospitals and nursing homes. The benefits of the Unit/Ward-based approach are that it is "owned" and controlled by the practitioners themselves, the practitioners are actively involved in nursing

QA and improvement as a part of nursing QM, and the practitioners have the opportunity to develop negotiation, facilitation, and evaluation skills. A main disadvantage of the system is the dependence on group motivation to carry out the program (Kitson & Giebing, 1990). In the Netherlands, the Unit/Ward-based approach is currently the preferred choice of nurses who want to undertake action in the field of nursing QA.

THE DIFFERENCE BETWEEN QUALITY ASSURANCE AND RESEARCH

In the Netherlands nursing research has been equated with nursing QA. Before the Unit/Ward-based approach could be further developed, the difference between scientific nursing research and QA needed to be sorted out. In order to clarify the relationship between research and QA, the CBO developed a framework using the 1974 analysis of John Williamson, M.D., professor at the Johns Hopkins University. Within this framework, professional care is divided into desirable (according to pre-set standards and criteria) and actual care (Donabedian, 1966). Desirable and actual care are further divided into attainable and not-attainable professional care (Williamson, 1978). When actual care is attainable but not attained according to the pre-set standards and criteria, then QA methods can be used to change the not-attained actual care into attained actual care. Sometimes the **outcome** of a QA assessment indicates the need for further scientific research. In most cases, however, the assessment is used to improve the actual care. If care is not-attainable because of professional limitation (e.g., because knowledge or proper methodologies are limited) then scientific research is the indicated way to try to solve the problem. One of the results of scientific research could be that not-attainable care becomes attainable through abolishment of the professional limitation. In this way the outcome of research occurs as attainable desirable/actual care within the scope of QA. An analysis of difference between QA and scientific research is illustrated in Figure 14-1.

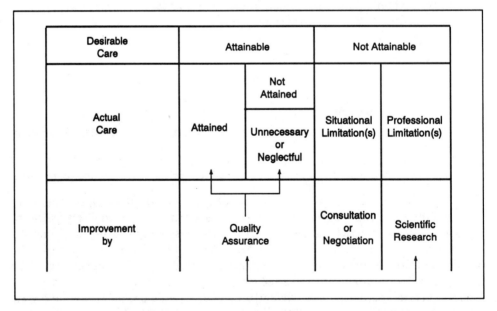

Figure 14-1 *Analysis of the Difference between Quality Assurance and Scientific Research. (Reprinted with permission of CBO, copyright 1990.)*

In short, QA activities are meant to improve quality of care according to pre-set standards and criteria, while scientific research is meant to add new knowledge and methodologies to the existing body of knowledge. Although they are related to each other, QA and scientific research are different activities, each having its own purpose.

THE ROOTS OF THE UNIT/WARD-BASED APPROACH

The Unit/Ward-based approach is an adaptation of Schroeder and Formella's (1982) unit-based approach developed in the United States (Giebing, 1994). In the 1970s, nursing QA activities stimulated the development of standard nursing care plans and outcome criteria in the United States. By the end of that decade, however, in Milwaukee's Saint Michael Hospital, nurses' dissatisfaction with the department's QA system had grown to the point that both staff nurses and nurse administrators considered the system irrelevant and impractical. Unit head nurses emphasized that staff nurses had special interest in QA and had identified priorities specific to their own units; staff nurses were eager to participate in QA activities pertinent to their daily work (Schroeder & Maibusch, 1984). In 1982, Schroeder and Formella, who at that time were both clinical nurse specialists in the Saint Michael Hospital, developed a method for nursing QA based on the participation of nurses in a unit. They called it the "unit-based approach to nursing quality assurance" (Schroeder & Formella, 1982).

Schroeder and Formella's unit-based approach was modified by CBO into a Unit/Ward-based approach, which better fit the Dutch situation. In the Netherlands a nursing department is divided into wards, each ward having its own group of patients. Most hospitals have two or more medical wards or surgical wards, which are independently organized. Nurses in the Netherlands are used to working with basic models. Because Schroeder and Formella's model appeared rather complex, CBO selected a model for nursing QA that was developed in the United States by Norma Lang (1976). Whereas the Schroeder and Formella model gives a detailed layout of the activities for each step, Lang's model gives only indications for each step in the QA process (Lang, 1976; Schroeder & Maibush, 1984). The CBO model does, however, maintain Schroeder and Formella's philosophy, which means that the nurses at unit or ward level are responsible for quality of care and QA.

THE CBO MODEL FOR THE UNIT/WARD-BASED APPROACH

The seven steps of the CBO model for the Unit/Ward-based approach are based on the assumption that all nurses in the unit or ward (the head nurse and nurse instructor included) are responsible for the quality of nursing performance and the assurance and improvement of quality in the unit or ward (Giebing, 1994). The main characteristics of the Unit/Ward-based approach are:

1. specific topics are identified and evaluated in programs;

2. criteria and standards are devised and modified by practitioners at the unit level;

3. the instruments used for assessing quality are applied to each topic individually;

4. quality assurance is part of the regular activities of the practitioners;

5. all nurse practitioners in the unit or ward are highly involved in the QA activities. (Marr & Giebing, 1994)

The CBO model is outlined in Figure 14-2.

There are seven steps in the CBO Model. Steps 1, 2, and 3 are highly affected by social values, professional values, and scientific knowledge. These factors are the source of the nursing values, which guide priority setting and provide the basis for standards and criteria.

Step 1. *Identify the nursing values.* The nursing values are the ethical-normative framework for nursing performance. Each nursing activity is based on those values. (Giebing, 1994)

Step 2. *Topic selection.* Often, more than one problem occurs; topic selection, therefore, often involves setting priorities. It is also possible to select topics in a systematic way, for example, starting with Topic A and ending with Topic Z.

Step 3. *Standards and criteria setting.* A standard is an agreed-upon level of nursing performance, and criteria are the measurable elements of the standard (Kitson & Giebing, 1990; Lang, 1976; WHO, 1987). Standards and criteria are formulated within Donabedian's tripartition: **structure, process,** and **outcome** (Donabedian, 1966; Kitson & Giebing, 1990). Standards and criteria formulated at the unit/ward level are to be confirmed by the nursing

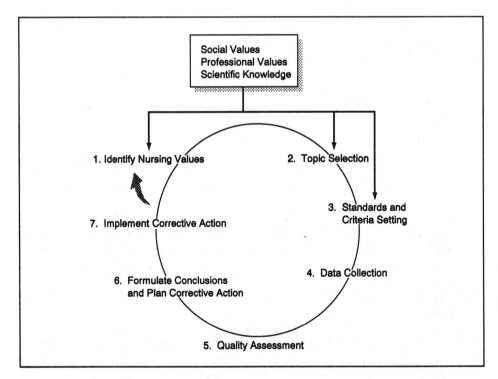

Figure 14-2 *CBO Model of the Unit/Ward-Based Approach. (Reprinted with permission of CBO, copyright 1990.)*

management of the organization. In this way, nursing QM comes within reach of nursing managers in the nursing department.

Step 4.   *Data collection.* An assessment tool is developed for each chosen topic. There are five main methods of data collection:
1. record audit or chart audit (both retrospective and concurrent)
2. use of questionnaires (for nurses, patients, and other health-care providers)
3. use of checklists
4. interviews (with nurses, patients, and other relevant persons)
5. direct observation

Step 5.   *Quality assessment.* During this step, standards and criteria (from Step 3) are compared to the collected data (from Step 4) to determine whether the standards and criteria meet the daily performance expectations.

Step 6.   *Formulate conclusions and a plan for corrective actions.*

Step 7.   *Implement corrective action.*
With the seventh step, all nurses of the ward should be involved in the presentation of the planned corrective action. It is important that the objectives are clear and that the time plan is known when this cycle is completed and another topic is selected. After some time, each topic will be reassessed to evaluate the effectiveness of the corrective action. For the second evaluation, the former standards can be raised through modification of the criteria. The QA cycle, put within the scope of nursing QM, results in the ongoing improvement of the quality of nursing care.

ORGANIZATIONAL MODEL FOR NURSING INVOLVEMENT

As part of the Unit/Ward-based approach an organizational body is established to ensure that all nurses in the unit or ward participate and apply the system on each unit or ward within a working group. In community-nursing organizations this body is called the Unit Quality Assurance Committee (UQAC); in hospitals it is called the Ward Quality Assurance Committee (WQAC). The UQAC or WQAC is composed of a head nurse or assistant head nurse, a senior staff nurse, a nurse instructor, and two or three junior staff nurses. In departments where patient stays are lengthy or patients return frequently, a patient may be invited to join the group. The UQAC or WQAC does the preliminary work for each step of the QA cycle. In consultation with all the nurses in the unit or ward, each step is accomplished before the next step is taken.

LOCAL ORGANIZATIONAL MODEL: QUALITY ASSURANCE COORDINATION COMMITTEE

To coordinate activities at the unit or ward level in each organization, a quality assurance coordination committee (QACC), composed of a nursing officer and the chairpersons of the working group, is established. If the organization has a department for nursing research or is working with clinical nurse specialists, the nurse researchers or clinical nurse specialists are asked to participate in the activities of the group. The QACC is charged with the following major tasks:

1. coordination of the QA activities on each unit or ward
2. critical inspection of the standards and criteria that have been formulated at the unit or ward level and the assessments that have been done by the UQAC or WQAC
3. formulation of organizational standards for nursing care through the use of the previously formulated unit or ward standards
4. effecting changes within available means, including those changes that go beyond the responsibilities and possibilities of the unit or ward due to their hospital-wide impact (Giebing, 1994)

It is important that a regular report be given to the Nursing Director regarding progress of the QA activities, outcomes of the assessment at the unit or ward level, and recently formulated organizational standards for nursing care. In this way, nursing QA becomes part of nursing QM at the organizational level. A facilitator, acting as an implementation-process supervisor, plays a major role in these activities. The facilitator is a nurse who works in the organization and has been educated and supported by CBO for this special task. This nurse facilitates the UQAC or WQAC and the QACC. The local organizational model of the Unit/Ward-based approach is illustrated in Figure 14-3.

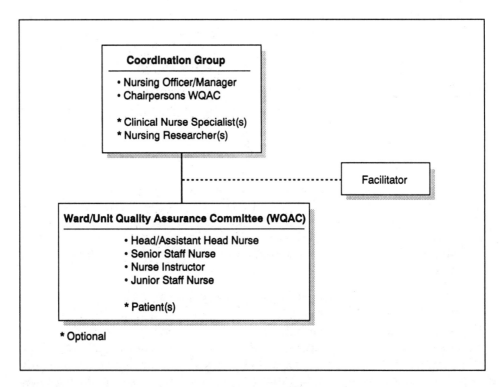

Figure 14-3 *Local Organizational Model of the Unit/Ward-Based Approach. (Reprinted with permission of CBO, copyright 1990.)*

Countrywide Organizational Model and the Nursing Quality Council

In addition to interfacing with locally organized nursing QM and QA, the Unit/Ward-based organizational model also allows for the possibility of countrywide nursing QM. In 1988 the Nursing Quality Council was started with the goal of achieving countrywide nursing QM. The council is active at CBO. Members of the council are delegates of professional nursing organizations and other relevant health-care organizations in the Netherlands. The Nursing Quality Council formulates, establishes, and publishes national standards of nursing care by using the standards established at the local level. The council publishes standards and guidelines for effective care. In case of controversies, the council is able to organize consensus meetings or delphi surveys. The main focus of the consensus meetings and delphi surveys is to attain consensus among professional nurses about a controversial topic. At the present, the guidelines and standards published by the council cover such topics as record keeping, vein-compression therapy, nursing care for delirious patients in hospitals, pain management, and preoperative nursing care. The work done by the Nursing Quality Council provides a means for countrywide nursing QM.

In summary, the CBO organization model for QA looks like a pyramid (see Figure 14-4). At the bottom of the triangle are the QA activities practiced by nurse practitioners at the unit or ward level, using the previously mentioned cycle. Nursing standards and criteria for the unit or ward are the outcomes of the activities on this level of the triangle. In the middle of the triangle are the activities that take place at the organizational level. The outcomes of activities on this level of the triangle are the organizationwide standards. At the top of the triangle are the activities of the Nursing Quality Council. The outcomes of these activities are the national standards

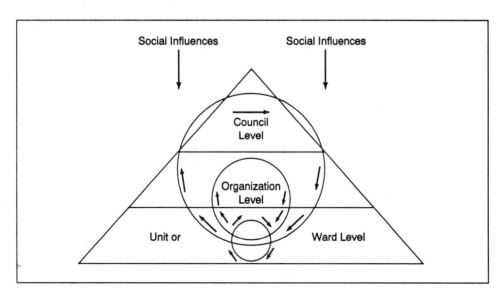

Figure 14-4 *CBO Organizational Model for Quality Assurance. (Reprinted with permission of CBO, copyright 1990.)*

for nursing care. The national standards can, in turn, be translated into organizational standards, which can then be turned into unit or ward standards and criteria. In this way, national standards become assessible at the unit or ward level, and nurse practitioners recognize these standards as part of their own standards. The cycle used at the unit or ward level becomes part of the higher levels. This is what makes the method dynamic. Within this system of ongoing feedback, changes in nursing practice change the organizational and national standards, and vice versa.

Standards and criteria formulated at the local level are at the disposal of CBO and the National Quality Council. The UQAC or WQAC and QACC send the standards and criteria to CBO when they have been locally accepted, and CBO then informs the Nursing Quality Council about those locally developed standards. These groups can, in turn, ask CBO to send them the standards and criteria developed elsewhere. In this way, there is opportunity for maximum use of the outcomes of each other's activities.

CONCLUSION

In 1993, approximately 20,000 to 25,000 of the 140,000 nurses in the Netherlands were applying systems for QA. These nurses worked in general hospitals, nursing homes, homes for the elderly, psychiatric hospitals, institutions for mentally handicapped persons, and primary health care. Their preferred choice for QA was the application of the Unit/Ward-based approach.

In 1994, it is expected that three new health-care laws will replace existing ones. The first law would make it obligatory for each professional in health care to apply a system for QA. A second law would make it obligatory for each health-care organization to apply a system for QM into which professional QA is integrated. The third law would integrate the first two laws and provide an overall framework for quality in health care. The establishment of standards and criteria for professional health care would still, however, be carried out by the professional groups themselves.

The next step expected in the development of QA in the Netherlands is research. Answers will be sought to questions such as, "What is the impact of the dynamic approach on direct patient care?" and "Is there visible quality improvement?" There is also a need to validate the locally developed standards and further analyze the costs and profits of QA, QM, and improvement. The relationship of general nurses and nursing managers to QA and QM is another possible topic for research. Without a strong relationship between nursing and research, QA activities are a nice and interesting way to spend time, but they are not very effective in enhancing the profession and increasing the quality of professional performance.

In the Netherlands, as in other countries, two major needs in the realm of nursing QM remain:

1. to persuade general nurses and nursing managers of the importance of nursing QA as a part of nursing QM

2. to determine how general nurses and nursing managers are able to incorporate outcomes into policies that improve the quality of nursing care in their organizations

Perhaps the recently developed concepts for **Total Quality Management (TQM)** will help satisfy these needs. It also is important to elicit the cooperation of managers; because without it, nursing QM will be no more than a concept on a piece of paper. Finally, it is nursing QA that gives perspective to Continuous Quality Improvement **(CQI)** in nursing, which is the ultimate goal of nursing QM and nursing QA in the Netherlands.

REFERENCES

Andersen, Y. (1992). Nursing standards in Europe. EuroQuan Newsletter. *Nursing Standard,* *6*(52), 5–7.

Donabedian, A. (1966). Evaluating the quality of medical care. *Milbank Memorial Fund Quarterly, 44*(3), 166–203.

EuroQuan Newsletter. (1992). *Nursing Standard, 6*(52).

Giebing, H. (1987). Unit-based approach for nursing Quality Assurance in the Netherlands: One year experience. *Australian Clinical Review, 7*(24), 28–31.

Giebing, H. (1992). *Quality Assurance in an integrated Europe.* Presentation at the RCN Autumn Conference: The Value of Nursing. Utrecht, Netherlands/London: CBO.

Giebing, H. (1994). Nursing Quality Management in the Netherlands. *International Nursing Review, 41*(313), nr 1, pp. 17–22.

Illsley, V. A., & Goldstone, L. A. (1985). *A guide to monitor for nursing staff.* Newcastle-upon-Tyne, United Kingdom: Polytechnic Products.

Kitson, A., & Giebing, H. (1990). *Nursing Quality Assurance in practice: A guide for practitioners using the dynamic approach to quality assurance.* Utrecht, Netherlands/London: CBO/RCN.

Klazinga, N. S. (1993). *Concerted action programme on Quality Assurance in hospitals: A multicentre comparative study on different Quality Assurance strategies and their effect on improvement of care; report on the evaluation phase.* Utrecht, Netherlands: CBO.

Klazinga, N. S. (Ed.). (1994). Concerted action programme on Quality Assurance in hospitals 1990–1993: Global results of the evaluation. In *International Journal for Quality in Health Care, 6*(3), 219–230.

Klazinga, N. S., & Giebing, H. (1994). Improving pressure sores prevention rates through Quality Assurance. *Wound Care, 3*(3), 141–144.

Lang, N. (1976). A model for Quality Assurance in nursing. In S. van Sell Davidson, *PSRO, utilization and audit in patient care* (pp. 20–26). St. Louis, MO: C. V. Mosby.

Marr, H., & Giebing, H. (1994). *Quality Assurance in nursing.* Edinburgh, Scotland: Campion Press.

Phaneuf, M. C. (1972). *The nursing audit: Profile for excellence.* New York: Appleton-Century-Crofts.

Phaneuf, M. C., & Wandelt, M. A. (1981). Obstacles to and potentials for nursing quality. *Quality Review Bulletin, 7*(4), 2–4.

Reerink, E. (1990). Improving the quality of hospital services in the Netherlands. *Quality Assurance in Health Care, 2*(1), 13–19.

Schroeder, P. S., & Formella, N. M. (1982). Unit-based approach to nursing Quality Assurance. *Quality Review Bulletin, 8*(3), 10–11.

Schroeder, P. S., & Maibusch, R. M. (Eds). (1984). *Nursing Quality Assurance: A unit-based approach.* Rockville, MD: Aspen.

Van Bergen, B., Hollands, L., & Nijhuis, H. (1980). *De ontwikkeling van een kwaliteitsprofiel.* Lochem, Netherlands: de Tijdstroom.

World Health Organization (WHO). (1987). *The consultant's role in Quality Assurance in nursing practice I.* Report on The Hague Meeting. Copenhagen: WHO-Regional Office.

Williamson, J. W. (1978). *Assessing and improving health care outcomes.* Cambridge, MA: Ballinger.

ADDITIONAL READING

Casparie, A. F. (1993). View from the Netherlands. *Quality in Health Care, 2*(2), 138–141.

Collado, C. B. (1992). Primary health care: A continuing challenge. *Nursing & Health Care, 13*(8), 408–413.

Giebing, H., & Westra, E. (1992). European quality: The Netherlands. EuroQuan Newsletter. *Nursing Standard, 6*(52), 11–12.

Reerink, E. (1991). Arcadia revisited: Quality assurance in hospitals in the Netherlands. *British Medical Journal, 302,* 1443–1445.

Vuori, H., & Roger, F. (1989). Issues in quality assurance. *Quality Assurance in Health Care, 1*(2/3), 125–135.

P. Susan Wagner

CHAPTER *15*

Quality Management Challenges in Canadian Health Care

INTRODUCTION

This chapter briefly describes the history and structure of the Canadian health-care system and the current pressures for reform in both effectiveness and efficiency. Six major trends that have developed in response to these pressures are also discussed: regionalization, community-based health care, partnerships in health care, role redefinition among health-care providers, the consumer-participation movement, and alternative medicine. Some of the Canadian organizations and initiatives that focus on the quality of health care are identified and explored. Finally, challenges and goals relating to **Quality Management (QM)** in health care are discussed. The challenges regarding QM in health care are different for **accreditation** bodies, governments, organizations, and professionals. Each group has a mandate and goals that must be rearticulated and resolved in cooperation with those of other **stakeholders**. The focus held in common is increasing the health status of clients, which is the ultimate indicator of **quality** health care. Emphasis on improving the quality of the Canadian health-care system is gathering momentum, and the future will be exciting.

MOMENTUM TOWARD QUALITY

A revolution is occurring in Canadian health care. The reform is not about the issue of insurance, as in the United States; the publicly funded universal insurance program has massive support (Deber, Hastings, & Thompson, 1991). Health reform in Canada is about the restructuring and reorientation of health-care delivery systems. The impetus for change is coming from governments, both federal and provincial; from health organizations, which are trying to provide the same or more care with fewer dollars; from professionals, who are attempting to maintain quality with fewer resources; and from consumers, who are becoming aware that the system is not addressing their needs. In cooperation with other sectors in the community, health-promotion activities regarding the determinants of health (such as income, housing, education, and healthy public policies) can have a positive impact on health status, particularly for poor, marginalized, and disabled populations. Jurisdictional responsibilities for health are being questioned as communities demand more control. The pressure for increased effectiveness and efficiency of health-care services has created a momentum toward quality in health care.

Jurisdictional Responsibilities

In contrast to the perception by other countries that all Canadian health services are publicly owned and delivered, the health-care system in Canada is a mixture of private and public providers reimbursed by public insurance. The provinces directly deliver a minority of health services, usually public health, mental health in large hospitals, and provincial programs such as cancer care, chiropody, children's dental care, and substance-abuse services. Most health services are delivered by non-government providers who are reimbursed by the public purse. Some providers are publicly owned hospitals or long-term care facilities overseen by independent layperson boards at arm's length from government. Private nonprofit and proprietary institutions receive large subsidies from provincial governments for the delivery of services. Private providers also include professionals such as physicians, chiropodists, physiotherapists, and chiropractors who bill the provincial health insurance plan for services provided to clients. Community services are a mixture of municipal, nonprofit, and proprietary organizations that attempt to gain as much income from provincial or federal grants as possible, but are also dependent on client fees and fund-raising efforts. An understanding of the evolution of universal health insurance is required to give a context for the discussion of QM issues in Canadian health care.

Within the confederation of Canada in 1867, the British North American Act gave the provinces control of the delivery of health-care services. The result was a country with twelve different systems, one in each of the ten provinces and two territories (Deber, Hastings, & Thompson, 1991). The federal government's role was primarily to establish policy and direction, but it had discretionary powers to spend in areas beyond its jurisdiction (Pineault, Lamarche, Champagne, Contandriopolis, & Denis, 1993). The federal government is responsible for health services for special groups such as the military, prisons, and Registered Indians.

During the 1950s and 1960s, quality health care was interpreted as access: more hospitals, more long-term care institutions, more physicians, and more technology. The major health-care debate in Canada was over who would pay for medical and hospital costs. Individuals had been paying for most services required, but that meant unequal access to services, uncertain quality of care in hospitals, and unpredictable income for physicians. The motivation for change was based on arguments for social equity and increased efficiency (Canadian Public Health Association, 1992). Legislation that enabled everyone to access physician and hospital services without paying directly was passed first in Saskatchewan. General tax revenues were used to support health services, thus avoiding any means testing prior to delivery of service. Equitable access was emphasized, and health professionals were trusted to ensure efficiency within the system.

In 1957, the Canadian Parliament implemented the Hospital Insurance and Diagnostic Services Act, through which the federal government shared the costs of provincial hospital insurance plans on a 50–50 basis, thereby providing public financing for hospital services for all residents. In 1968 the Medical Care Act was passed which extended universal access to physician services, and stated the five principles of 'Medicare': public administration, comprehensiveness, universality, portability, and accessibility. The federal government safeguarded these principles through the terms and conditions attached to the transfer payments to provinces. The national health-care system has been subject to periodic review, usually motivated by increasing costs. By the mid 1970s, the provinces were dissatisfied with the steering effect of the financial arrangements, which limited their ability to develop community-based, alternative health-care services. The federal government was concerned about the open-ended and unpredictable nature of the fiscal payments. Established Programs Financing came into being in 1977, in which the hospital and medical insurance programs already established "were de-linked from actual provincial expenditures, and paid in the form of a block fund transfer" (Ministers of Health and Finance, 1992, p. 5). An unconditional transfer for extended health-care services was also included, which enabled other services such as ambulatory programs, home care, and long-term-care facility care to be subsidized. Unfortunately, the change in financing made it much more difficult to monitor and enforce the five principles of Medicare. Increased instances of financial barriers to accessibility occurred, such as user fees and extra-billing, in which a physician would bill the client directly in addition to billing the government insurance plan for the service fee negotiated between the government and the provincial medical association (Ministers of Health and Finance, 1992). In 1984, after a Royal Commission report (Hall, 1980), the Canada Health Act was passed unanimously by Parliament, replacing the previous two health acts. This new act affirmed the five principles of Medicare, and specified sanctions for provinces that attempted to undermine them. No sanctions have been imposed since the Act was passed in 1984, but if a provinc was found to be in violation of the Act, the federal government would then deduct from the province's cash transfer payments an amount equal to the amount 'overbilled' to clients.

The five principles of Canadian Medicare (public administration, comprehensiveness, universality, portability, and accessibility) were rearticulated in the Canada Health Act of 1984. Public administration requires that "the health care insurance plan of a province be administered and operated on a non-profit basis by a public authority" (Canada Health Act, 1984, c.6, s.8). Comprehensiveness of services refers to the responsibility of provinces to insure and become the single payer for all medically necessary medical and hospital services, surgical dental procedures in hospitals, and selected other services that were provided to its citizens. Universality meant that the insurance program "must entitle one hundred percent of the insured persons to the insured health services on uniform terms and conditions" (Canada Health Act, 1984, c.6, s.10). Portability of benefits meant that provincial citizens would be insured under the same conditions for care received in other jurisdictions, until they had been resident there for over three months. For those Canadian residents who go to a different province or country, the provincial governments will reimburse costs of medical and hospital care up to the cost of the same services in the home province. Accessibility eliminated financial barriers to insured health services such as user fees or extra-billing by providers, although provinces were permitted to establish their own systems of payment for health services through legislation, either through taxes or annual premiums. People continued to choose their own physicians and the hospitals that they prefered. These five principles have shaped the expectations and confidence of Canadians in their health-care system, and have become an indicator of quality within the system.

The largest threat to maintaining the five principles of Medicare is the movement toward private, for-profit clinics which threaten the standard of accessibility. Clinics that provide specialized medical services such as hernia repair or cataract surgery may receive taxpayer money for the physician fee component of the procedure, but wish to charge clients a large facility fee to cover other costs and create a profit. The physicians may also choose to practice outside the provincial health plan entirely. The Minister of Health is currently investigating this privatization trend, and has informed provinces that a two-tiered health-care system, one for the rich and another for the poor, is unacceptable within the terms of the Canada Health Act. In the absence of a national definition of 'medically necessary,' the provinces have begun to de-insure medical procedures considered to be unessential, and, therefore, outside the jurisdiction of the Canada Health Act. Procedures such as optometric examinations or reversal of sterilization are being charged to the client, and provincial drug plans have been revised with higher deductibles. Portability of benefits does not cover the total costs of medical and hospital care received in another jurisdiction or the costs of some community services such as oxygen. Public nonprofit administration of the insurance plan is the only principle that has always been accepted, although the market for private health-insurance plans is growing as the provinces reduce their coverage of health services. It is expected that these five principles will be increasingly difficult to maintain and to monitor as the federal government contribution to provincial health-care expenditures relies more on personal and corporate tax points than on cash transfer payments.

Pressure for Increased Effectiveness of Health Care

Since the public health insurance bills were passed, health care has increased in cost but has not substantially affected the health status of Canadians (Canadian Public Health Association, 1992). In 1974, the Honorable Marc LaLonde, Minister of Health and Welfare, released a document calling for a reorientation of the treatment-based health-care system toward prevention of illness. He articulated four aspects to health: human biology, environment, lifestyle, and health-care system (LaLonde, 1974). It was one of the first admissions by a national government that the current system was not working effectively to meet health needs as defined by the World Health Organization (WHO), and that other factors also influenced health status. This report was endorsed more in Europe than in Canada, which maintained the status quo. Investment in institutional care and technology continued to rise, even without visible results, such as increased life expectancy or equalized distribution of illness across socioeconomic classes (Canadian Hospital Association, 1993). The Honorable Jake Epp, then Minister of Health, released another major document in 1986, *Achieving Health for All: A Framework for Health Promotion*. This document identified the health challenges in Canada as reducing inequities, increasing prevention, and enhancing coping. Self-care, mutual aid, and health environments were described as health-promotion mechanisms. Implementation strategies included fostering public participation, strengthening community-health services, and coordinating healthy public policy (Epp, 1986). Although federal health-research grants adopted the new priorities, provincial health-delivery systems did not.

Most stakeholders are beginning to recognize that the paradigm for health that supports the current system has weaknesses. The outdated conceptual model has four tenets, all of which have now been challenged.

1. We don't know what keeps people healthy or what makes them sick.

2. Medical and hospital care are the most important determinants of health.

3. Medicine is a science practiced with precision and devoid of discretion.

4. The necessity for medical care can be easily defined. (Canadian Public Health Association, 1992, p. 2)

Research and utilization data has demonstrated that none of these tenets is true today. Pressure for an effective health-care system is building as people become aware that medical science and technology have not solved their health problems, and may even have created new problems (Rachlis & Kushner, 1989). It is time for health-system reform because the goal of the system — better health for all Canadians — is not being met.

Pressure for Increased Efficiency of Health Care

The Canadian health-care system is also under scrutiny because of the economic status of the country (Chernomes & Sepehri, 1994). The federal and provincial governments in Canada are carrying almost insurmountable deficits. The total governmental debt for 1992–1993 is estimated at 87.5 percent of the Gross Domestic Product (Canadian Medical Association [CMA], 1993). The federal government's debt for 1992–1993 is estimated at 500 billion dollars, or $18,224 per capita (CMA, 1993). Gross debt interest charges are 35.6 percent of total federal revenues (Canadian Hospital Association, 1993).

Health-care costs for the 1990–1991 year ranged from 25 to 37 percent of total provincial expenditures (CMA, 1993). Governments have no flexibility left to alter expenses to meet new health needs of the population. The national and provincial economies are still recovering from a recession, so unemployment is high, income support programs are heavily used, and tax revenues are down. The federal government has had to reduce the growth rate of its transfer payments to provinces for health and education. Both levels of government are closely examining ways to make health care more economical and effective, as well as more appropriate for health needs.

Most of Canada's provinces and territories have completed major reviews of their health-care systems during the past few years. The problems with existing organizational structures for health care included a lack of accountability for health-care costs or results; a lack of continuity of care for the client who needed care from more than one organization; and territoriality between sectors such as community and long-term care, between organizations even in the same sector, and among professional groups. Some provinces had hundreds of independent layperson boards that governed the spending of taxpayer dollars, with each board attempting to expand a territory of control. The atmosphere did not lend itself to cooperation or to ensuring easy access or continuity of care for clients. Whenever a board was upset or wanted something, the chairperson and chief executive officer could go directly to the Minister of Health, bypassing the civil servants. With public support, politicians from all parties went on building sprees that coincided with the electoral timetable, neglecting to look at the longer-term issue of operating costs. A twelve-bed acute-care hospital in a rural area can cost $1 million per year to operate — all for an average daily census of two or three patients who may not even have acute-care needs. The federal government's sharing of construction costs on a 50–50 basis over three decades contributed to the overbuilding and the present Canadian emphasis on institutional care. This funding policy, combined with the cost-sharing of institutional operating costs, was to the detriment of community-health services, which were never cost-shared to the same extent.

Some of the provinces have responded to these economic pressures by attempting to reorganize the delivery of health services. (See the following section, Trends in Canadian Health Care.) Most provinces have taken measures to reduce the variety and amount of services insured, and private expenditures for health have increased nationally from 23.5 percent in 1975 to 25.6 percent in 1986 (Canadian Hospital Association, 1993). It is inevitable that the decreased coverage of health costs by the public purse would lead to an increase in the market for private insurance companies, with correspondingly higher premiums. The health-care system is increasingly looking toward QM as a means of "cost containment, downsizing, improving clinical outcomes, and improving health outcomes" (Health Canada, 1993, p. vi). Quality is redefined as the provision of effective health-care services for less cost.

Momentum has increased during the past five years. Federal and provincial government documents (from commissions, task forces, and working groups reviewing aspects of the health-care system) have produced recommendations remarkably similar to one another. Professional associations have produced major reports on the delivery of health services and the future role of their professions in a revised system. The Canadian Council on Health Facilities Accreditation (CCHFA) has been exploring new directions as it attempts to respond to the changing structure for the delivery of health-care services in the provinces. Provider associations such as the Canadian Hospital Association have released results of studies or major position statements on the future of the Canadian health-care system. The delivery structure is changing daily. And quality is a concept that underlies almost all of these reports, briefs, and position statements. Quality-of-care initiatives have become commonly touted as a means of attaining effective, economical, and appropriate health care.

TRENDS IN CANADIAN HEALTH CARE

In response to fiscal and provincial pressures, Health and Welfare Canada (1993b) organized a project team to study emerging trends in the organization and delivery of health-care services. This team identified and analyzed the trends for their strengths and weaknesses, and articulated an evaluation framework for the ongoing study of their impact on the health care of Canadians. A trend was described as "a response or proposed solution to an unstated problem" (Health and Welfare Canada, 1993b, p. 28), and the report included a survey of the range of health-care solutions being tried. The project team identified six major trends within Canadian health care: regionalization/decentralization, community-based health care, partnerships in health care, role redefinitions among health-care providers, consumer participation movement, and alternative medicine.

Regionalization/Decentralization

The complex trend of regionalization/decentralization involves the transfer of administrative authority, of political power, of managerial responsibility, or of service-delivery responsibility from a central government to a local body (Health and Welfare Canada, 1993b). That local or regional body may be a level of local government or a community board. Because each province has jurisdiction over the delivery of health services, there are several different methods of restructuring planned or in effect. There are common concepts among the various methods, however. Sometimes the four types of transfer are combined in a reorganization of health care, and sometimes they are applied separately. Power over allocation of money may or may not be transferred to the local body.

Most of the provincial commissions that studied health care recommended the establishment of health regions governed by lay health boards that would have responsibility for the delivery of all acute-care, long-term-care, ambulance, home-care, mental-health, substance-abuse, and community-health services offered in the region. The mandate of these new boards would include the rationalization of duplications in hospital care, reduction of bed usage in both acute and long-term care, promotion of community services, and the increase of illness-prevention activities. The intention was that a more integrated approach to health-care services would be more responsive to community and district needs. Several provinces and territories have begun to implement regionalization as a response to fiscal pressures. Each province is approaching regionalization somewhat differently, for health is within provincial jurisdiction. There are new developments daily, and the information following is current as of mid 1994.

APPLYING REGIONALIZATION/DECENTRALIZATION

This brief survey starts with northern Canada, and moves west to east across the country. Health-care planning in the two Canadian territories is complicated by their scarce populations over vast distances and unsettled aboriginal land claims. The Yukon has control over hospital services and is in the process of assuming direct control of other health-care services from the federal government. The Northwest Territories have already assumed complete control over their health-care delivery system. It has had regional health boards supported by local community councils for a few years, and these boards appear to be more successful than the former system of centralized planning and service delivery.

British Columbia has made a commitment to establish twenty-one Regional Health Boards by October 1994. These health boards will operate regional and tertiary-care facilities and allocate monies to Community Health Councils. These Councils are to be appointed in 1995 to manage major health services at the community level. Regional executive directors and planning committees have been in place for one year. A provincial agreement has been reached with health unions. The agreement, which guarantees no job losses for three years as a result of changes to the health-care system, has created real economic constraints. No cuts have been made to health budgets yet.

Alberta has announced a 25 percent cut to its health-care budget over the next three years, in lieu of a long-term plan. Layoffs of acute-care personnel have already occurred. Roundtable discussions have been held to ascertain the opinions of stakeholder groups regarding future directions. Members were appointed to seventeen new regional boards in 1994, although structures reporting to the boards have not yet been finalized. These boards were expected to prepare business plans for health services within the reduced budget allocations by October 1994.

In 1992, Saskatchewan was the very first province to reduce the health budget. The new Health Districts Act, passed in 1993, established thirty health district boards for this province of less than one million people. These boards will eventually be responsible for hospital, ambulance, long-term-care, home-care, community-health, mental-health, and drug- and alcohol-abuse services within self-defined district boundaries. All publicly owned institutions are directly governed by the new district boards. Private organizations, both nonprofit and proprietary, have the option of amalgamating to be directly governed, or signing an affiliation agreement wherein the new board will contract with them for the delivery of health services. As of 1994, funding for districts is global and determined according to a needs-based funding formula based on population rather than on utilization data. The new district boards will control all public taxpayer monies for both public and private health organizations, and will, therefore, have the power to redirect funds across the sectors of health care to meet community needs more effectively. The members are currently appointed, but, eventually, two-thirds will be elected by district citizens.

Manitoba has announced health-system reform, but the long-term plan is not readily apparent. There have been both cuts to acute-care funding and hospital mergers, but no firm indication of when the plans for health regions will become reality.

Central Canada contains two provinces: Ontario, which is primarily English-speaking, and Quebec, which is primarily French-speaking. In Ontario, District Health Councils have existed for many years as advisory planning bodies to the Minister of Health representing consumers, providers, and local governments (Joint Task Force, 1993). Over the past few years, these councils have been given increasingly more power, such as approval or veto of construction projects and allocation of selected monies to district hospitals. Although the assessment of community needs and the coordination of health services in long-term and community sectors is part of their mandate, the boards have given various degrees of priority to those responsibilities when balanced with their acute-care role. Hospital mergers and regional planning for individual programs such as cancer care have occurred independently. Attempts at regionalization in the long-term care sector were made in 1993, through the designation of fourteen funding regions. As a result, new structures called multiservice agencies will have power to allocate contracts for the provision of both community and facility services in an attempt to standardize assessment and care delivery for the elderly and disabled. The Ontario government has imposed a "social contract" on public sector unions. This contract, which requires a reduction in the hours of work for every employee in order to reduce labor costs, has created many difficulties for health institutions with fixed budgets. The Ontario Ministry of Health has traditionally been quite innovative and generous in its support of pilot projects and research into alternative methods of delivering health care.

Quebec has had twenty years of experience with decentralization, citizen participation, and outcome-centered management through the community network of health and social-service centers. With the passage of 1991 health-reform legislation, this province altered the health-care structure to further emphasize these three goals (Pineault et al., 1993). Elected membership on seventeen Regional Boards, which govern both institutional and community services, is according to a specified proportion of stakeholder groups. Unified Boards allocate funds for organizations serving the same population in the region, such as organizations serving new mothers. Funding will be according to program areas such as "mental health" and "social adaptation," which will have health-status indicators and specific goals for the region.

The maritime provinces in Eastern Canada are also moving toward regionalized health care and are working more closely with each other. Plans exist for establishing a common list of insured services, common prescribing guidelines and purchasing of drugs, cooperation on purchase of medical equipment, and targets for numbers of doctors and hospital beds. In 1992, New Brunswick established seven large hospital corporations encompassing thirty-one large and small hospitals that cover the whole province. Annual budgets have been reduced twice by 3 percent. Community and long-term-care services are not yet part of this regional structure. Nova Scotia has announced its intention to move to a regional health structure of governing boards with wide responsibilities, but there is no timetable established as of yet. A Provincial Health Advisory Committee has been established and internal health department changes have occurred. Prince Edward Island is very small and does not have some of the territorial problems that have divided other provinces. A 1993 act replaced all existing health boards with five regional health boards. The number of physicians and their fees are being limited. Newfoundland has taken several major steps toward a regionalized structure, the latest being in 1994. Hospital boards in this sparsely populated province have been reduced in number. A second regional board system has been established to direct the widespread reorganization in community, mental health, and long-term-care services.

Provincial efforts to increase the efficiency of the health-care system through reorganization of health-care structures are indicative of a definite trend in

Canadian health care. The attention given to the effectiveness part of the quality equation, however, has been much less. Some provinces and territories are earnestly attempting to involve citizens in health-care planning, to require needs assessments, to base funding on population needs, and to establish targets for improved health status. The unknown question for the future is whether a region with high needs will be given extra funds for those needs or be chastised with a budget reduction for not addressing those needs effectively. This question can only be asked in a country where the provincial government is the single payer for public health insurance.

Community-Based Health Care

Canada, largely due to historical funding policies, has an institution-centered health-care system. In 1990, Canada had 196.2 persons per acute-care bed compared to 267.6 in the United States (Canadian Hospital Association, 1993). Consumers of health care are demanding that, whenever possible, health services should be delivered in community settings rather than in hospitals and other residential institutions (Health and Welfare Canada, 1993b). Acute-care changes have contributed to this trend. Advances in medical technology have created a proliferation of increasingly specialized hospital units and a corresponding increase in the capital and operating costs incurred by hospitals. Governments have recognized that community-based care is less expensive than the equivalent care in an institution (although savings are only realized when institutional beds are closed). There is pressure to reduce lengths of stay, increase the use of day surgery programs, and keep only people with acute-care needs in hospital beds. In rural areas, the small hospitals have begun to close — particularly hospitals with fewer than fifteen beds. Everywhere the number of active acute-care beds is being reduced and whole wards (and, sometimes, whole hospitals) are being closed. British Columbia reduced the number of acute-treatment beds by 10 percent in 1982 alone (Sutherland & Fulton, 1988). Some rural areas had as many as 6 acute-care beds per 1000 people. Provinces have established targets ranging between 2.2 and 3.0 beds per 1000 people.

Long-term care changes have also stimulated the trend toward community-based care. As the population has aged and demand for long-term-care facility beds has increased, the acuity level of those admitted to long-term-care beds has risen. The largest increase in the long-term-care population has been seen in the cognitively impaired and young disabled groups that have heavy care needs. Governments, in an attempt to reduce expenditures on long-term care, are reducing or eliminating subsidies for light levels of institutional care, and announcing intentions to reduce the number of long-term-care beds. Saskatchewan's ratio will change from 164 to 140 beds per 1000 people. At the same time a corresponding need for enriched or assisted housing is emerging. Requests for the construction of new acute- or long-term-care facilities or the purchase of new capital equipment are subject to intense scrutiny and often are denied by provincial departments of health, which still control capital budgets.

These alterations in the use of acute-care and long-term-care services have changed the nature of community-based services. There is an increased demand for home-health care and home-support services, because the frail elderly are not being admitted as readily to long-term-care facilities. Families are expected to maintain caregiving responsibilities for a longer time, thus increasing daily stress on the relationships and health of the caregivers. There is an increased financial burden for families — both those who choose an institutional alternative with less subsidy and those who require help in the home from community agencies that have user charges. Home-care agencies are providing more acute-care services because of the shorter hospital stays. Hospitals are establishing outreach programs in an attempt to improve the continuity of care for clients as they move from institution to community. Community-health centers, health-service organizations (physician practice units or community-board controlled), health- and social-service centers, and comprehensive-health organizations have developed to offer coordination of **multidisciplinary** health services, health promotion, and alternatives to institutional care. The number of private providers, both profit and nonprofit, is also increasing, as existing and new gaps in the fragmented health-care delivery system become opportunities for new enterprises.

The rhetoric and activity regarding health promotion has escalated, but the transfer of money into community programs has been minimal thus far. Most of the dollars saved through acute-care budget cuts have been used to reduce provincial government expenditures and deficits, rather than to support health-promotion programs. Health education for the public and some specific population groups, such as prenatal clients, has mushroomed, however (Health and Welfare Canada, 1993b). Quality concerns related to this trend include the lack of monitoring of new organizations and programs (such as private long-term-care boarding homes), the absence of provincial regulations for some categories of workers, and the inequitable access to services that is part of the largely user-pay community-care system.

Partnerships in Health Care

Increasing economic pressures on operating budgets have encouraged institutions and organizations to consider partnership as a method of reducing costs and providing increased benefits to clients. Partnerships may attempt to blend a medical model and a social model of health care, or may solidify one approach. Partnerships range from mergers to the sharing of services. Shared services can include "hotel" services provided by one organization for another, such as purchasing or laundry; collaborative arrangements to offer particular services to clients of both organizations based on expertise; or fully shared services where the costs, risks, and accountability are shared equally (Health and Welfare Canada, 1993b). Hospital mergers, both with and without full merging of assets, have become common. Some hospitals have merged with long-term-care facilities, creating either an integrated facility with both acute- and long-term-care beds (as in small rural towns in Saskatchewan), or one organization on different sites (such as the Greater Victoria Hospital Society in British Columbia). Community-health organizations have also been forming partnerships, sometimes with institutions or housing developments. Consumer-group partnerships are becoming more common as national and provincial task forces and associations seek to obtain consumer input into health planning. National associations of professionals and providers have created partnerships such as the Health Action Lobby Group, or HEAL, which is lobbying the federal government to maintain the principles of Medicare in spite of fiscal pressures. Provincial governments are working with private providers, such as the pharmacists in Saskatchewan who are provided with on-line computer access to the prescription history and deductible level for each client when drugs are dispensed. The Healthy Communities Project, cosponsored by the Canadian Public Health Association and Health and Welfare Canada, has encouraged communities across the country to consider establishing partnerships to address problems with multiple aspects. Chances of success are much greater if education, health, and social services work together to combat issues such as child hunger. Many cooperative intersectoral planning bodies have been formed to examine health needs, devise broad solutions to health problems, and deliver services (Health and Welfare Canada, 1993b).

The impact of these broadly or narrowly based partnerships on the quality of care is assumed to be neutral or positive. There have been few studies to explore the impact on client services or health status, however.

Role Redefinition among Health-Care Providers

The trend that affects health-care providers directly is blurring of roles and settings for the delivery of health-care services. A wider scope of practice is being considered for many health professionals (Health and Welfare Canada, 1993b). Most professions in Canada have a national organization that disseminates information, lobbies on behalf of the profession, performs research, and develops **standards** or practice guidelines for the profession.

MEDICINE

Because they control access to hospital and medical services (and, in some provinces, to long-term-care services) physicians are gatekeepers to the system. Societal pressures for instant cures and high technology often drive physician choices; it is much more difficult to make lifestyle changes and give credence and dollars to health promotion. Public expectations of medicine will likely not become realistic or affordable until there is extensive public debate on these complex health issues. Physicians, however, are actively participating in the definition of health policy and priorities, and are sharing responsibility for the allocation of limited resources. They are also being expected to consult others, both professionals and clients, about decisions that are not solely clinical. Views regarding the role of physicians are changing. Physicians are no longer considered to be just private providers protecting their own and their patients' interests, but, instead, are increasingly viewed as providers with a responsibility to serve the collective goals of a publicly funded health-care system (Barer & Stoddart, 1991).

Medicine governs its own profession through provincial regulating bodies, which monitor quality of practice. Provincial medical associations, which exist in all provinces, serve as the political voice of physicians and are closely linked with the Canadian Medical Association (CMA). The number of physicians has been growing faster than the population of Canada; from 1974 to 1984 the number of physicians increased 34 percent compared to a general population increase of 12 percent (Institute for Health Care Facilities of the Future, 1988). In 1984 there were 49,916 physicians in practice (Institute for Health Care Facilities of the Future, 1988) and the growth rate has since leveled off. Physician billings have also increased exponentially. In most provinces monies available for physician reimbursement through Medicare have been reduced, and the provincial medical associations, which negotiate fee schedules with the governments, have accepted limits to the annual total. Several provinces are trying alternative methods of physician remuneration. Physicians in Quebec, for example, form two general groups — one group working on salary in the health- and social-service centers and the other group working in fee-for-service, independent practice.

A report on physician resource planning, entitled the Barer-Stoddart Report (1991), was commissioned by the provincial/territorial Deputy Ministers of Health. A twelve-point action plan on physician resource management was announced by the Ministers of Health in January 1992. The entry to practice in Canada for international medical graduates was restricted. The size of undergraduate medical classes was to be reduced by 10 percent. The size of postgraduate training was also to be reduced by 10 percent (Barer & Stoddart, 1991). The latter was implemented by the National Coordinating Committee on Postgraduate Medical Training, whose membership is from both government and national medical associations. Physician associations have been extensively consulted abut the implementation of these recommendations, and continue to advise government. Physician resource plans that restrict the number of practicing physicians have been implemented in New Brunswick, Prince Edward Island, and Quebec. Other provinces are working to develop a physician resource plan, in cooperation with local, provincial, and regional committees. These reductions are related to the 1988 ratio of persons per physician in Canada being 455 compared to 577 in 1976 (Canadian Hospital Association, 1993).

Through local utilization-management committees, provincial and national clinical-practice guidelines, and professional standards physicians have maintained a leadership role in the QM of their profession.

NURSING

Nursing is the largest health profession in Canada. In 1990 there were 256,145 registered nurses in Canada (Canadian Hospital Association, 1993). The Canadian Nurses Association (CNA) has endorsed the concepts of primary health care and the role of the nurse as an entry point into the health-care system (Canadian Nurses Association [CNA], 1993). Professional nursing associations have been innovative in establishing pilot projects in New Brunswick, British Columbia, and Newfoundland. These projects use nurses as the primary contact for the client needing health assistance (CNA, 1993). Nurses already have increased responsibilities in northern, isolated, and some community-health-center settings. Many occupational-health nurses routinely conduct physical examinations and histories. A few provinces have officially stated a wish to expand the nursing role as a means of reducing health-care costs. Unfortunately, the trend toward an increased role for nursing and an increased emphasis on community-based health promotion is not happening quickly enough to provide new jobs for the thousands of acute-care nurses who have been laid off because of the closure of hospital beds across the country (Paul, 1993).

There are a variety of avenues to attaining Registered Nurse designation. The most common educational program is a two- or three-year diploma in a community college setting, which has almost completely replaced three-year diploma programs based in hospitals. Four-year baccalaureate degree nursing programs have seen increased enrollments, including more men enrollees than ever before. The CNA has the support of all of the provincial nursing associations for its 1982 position that all new entrants into nursing should have a baccalaureate degree by the year 2000. Although that target will likely be missed, there is much activity evident in nursing education. University and diploma schools are designing and launching collaborative programs that may have a diploma exit after three years, but that will graduate most students after four years with a degree in nursing. The provinces and territories are at different stages. Prince Edward Island has only one nursing education program — a baccalaureate program. In the territories, the first diploma program has only just been established. Nurses with master's and doctoral degrees are primarily employed as administrators in health institutions and community settings, or as nursing educators, and are increasingly being employed as clinical experts or researchers in practice settings. Canadian doctoral programs in nursing did not exist until this decade.

The CNA is a federation of eleven member associations, representing the two territories and all provinces except Quebec. It speaks for Canadian nurses to other national and international organizations, provides national nursing leadership on health- and work-related issues, influences national health policy, and promotes high professional standards. The CNA Board has eight elected members, eleven provincial/territorial representatives, three consumers, and one representative from the CNA special-interest groups. Nursing, like medicine, is a self-regulating profession, conducting its own investigations of misconduct, and deciding its own disciplinary measures. Provincial nursing unions are very strong, particularly in acute care. The union positions are sometimes opposed to those of the professional associations, but there are increasing efforts from both groups to unify the goals and strategies used to promote nursing and nursing practice.

The close affiliation between the provincial/territorial nursing associations and the CNA has contributed to a coordinated national approach to the certification of nurses with a specialty practice. There is only one certification program, sponsored by the CNA since 1986. It has three phases (CNA, 1994). The designation of the specialty occurs in Phase One. It includes evidence of standards for practice, recurrent phenomena in practice, role definition, a specific body of literature and research, and a defined client population. A minimum of 1000 nurses from at least four provinces or territories must wish to establish specialty recognition, and there must be at least forty nurses with advanced preparation to assist with the development of the certification examination. The second phase is the development of an examination by the CNA Testing Service in consultation with members of that specialty group. Phase Three is the certification and recertification of nurses through examination, performance appraisal, work experience, and continuing education in the specialty. Four specialties now have full certification available: neuroscience, nephrology, emergency, an occupational health. In 1995, critical care, perioperative, and mental health/psychiatric nursing will be added to the list. There are presently twenty approved CNA interest groups and seven CNA affiliate groups; all twenty-seven represent a special aspect of nursing practice, administration, education, or research. A representative of the special-interest groups sits on the CNA board.

Quality management in health organizations has been largely designed and maintained by nurses. They have become experts in the use of **Quality-Assurance (QA)** tools and leaders in the movement toward implementation of **Total Quality Management (TQM)** in both hospital and community settings. National nursing-practice standards have been established by the CNA, the provincial/territorial associations, and by selected special-interest groups for particular client groups or settings.

ALLIED-HEALTH PROFESSIONS

There is increasing emphasis on multidisciplinary team work which includes the allied-health professions. All health professionals are struggling to solidify their roles in the midst of budget cuts to acute care. Many provinces have separate legislative acts relating to each profession. These acts give each profession the right to self-regulate and to specify the boundaries of practice (and, sometimes, to specify the relationship of the profession to other disciplines). Ontario passed the first Health Professions Act in Canada. It eliminated the separate legislative acts for each profession and established consistent guidelines for all professions. The professional associations interpret this act as a move to reduce their power to self-regulate; but acts such as this may "eliminate the existing confusion between the promotion of a profession's interests and the protection of the public, facilitate coordination among professional colleges, and address overlaps in existing scopes of practice among the health care professions" (Health and Welfare Canada, 1993b, p. 20).

Allied health educational opportunities are limited in Canada. For example, there are only two schools each for optometry, speech-language pathology, and podiatry. Opportunities to become an occupational therapist, chiropractor, public health inspector, and prosthetic technician are nonexistent in most provinces. Even physical therapy schools (of which there are more than for many other allied-health disciplines) have their enrollments restricted far below those of the medical schools — and this when the need for physical therapists is far greater than the need for physicians.

The quality initiatives of the allied-health professions are hampered by the low numbers of professionals combined with the vastness of the country. In spite of these limitations, most professions have established national standards for practice.

PARAPROFESSIONALS

Auxiliary-health-personnel (paraprofessional) categories number in the dozens. There are multiple health paraprofessional courses and certificates without transferability within one province, let alone between provinces. Similar paraprofessional designations, such as a Licensed Practical Nurse, may have different roles in different provinces; educational requirements and work settings may also vary from province to province. Educational programs may range from six weeks to two years, with a variety of titles, certificates, and diplomas being awarded on completion. Some programs are offered at community college, some at night school, and some on the job. Some workers are categorized according to the population they serve, such as youth workers, substance-abuse workers, and early-childhood-development workers. Others are categorized based on the clinical setting in which they practice, such as special-care-home (long-term-care facility) aides, home-care aides, community-health workers, and dental assistants. Some workers have a general focus, such as rehabilitation assistants, recreational therapists, and social-services workers. In some provinces pay scales have been established that give monetary recognition for the completion of a program; in other provinces, programs have been created to fill an employment need in the province. For example the dental assistant program was created in Saskatchewan when the Children's Dental Program was established as part of a political platform. When the government changed, however, the dental assistant positions were eliminated, and the training was not easily transferable to other existing positions in the health-care system.

Quality management in the paraprofessions is extremely diverse and uneven. There are very few national associations for these workers. Efforts to maintain quality are dependent on the policies of the employing agencies and the values of individual workers.

CONSUMER-PARTICIPATION MOVEMENT

Involving the user of a service in the planning, delivery, and evaluation of that service is acquiring increasing importance as organizations try to ensure that efforts and resources are not wasted on unwanted services. Consumers are also demanding more control over the services they receive. In health care, the consumer wants to be fully informed of options and consequences, as well as be treated as a partner when interacting with professionals. This trend manifests itself in several different ways. Self-help groups provide support to specific populations, usually organized around a particular health or social problem (such as Alcoholics Anonymous or caregivers of Alzheimer's victims). Self-help clearinghouses have become a distinct service by providing information and outreach to both affected populations and professional groups. Consumer-advocacy groups attempt to "bring about changes in either personal or institutional behavior (or) emphasize the rights and choices of the individuals receiving services" (Health and Welfare Canada, 1993b, p. 23). These groups can be organized around specific diseases like the Juvenile Diabetes Association, or be broadly based, like the women's health movement. National organizations cooperate with consumers through health promotion efforts that educate the public. Consumers are also being requested to participate in the governance of health-care organizations, sit on health-planning bodies, and offer opinions on the effectiveness and appropriateness of the services they receive. Several of the provinces now have advisory health councils of consumers to articulate the goals of health-care reform. People are also accepting more responsibility for the maintenance of their own health status, in large part thanks to Health and Welfare Canada initiatives such as Particip-action (to encourage exercise) and Break-Free Generation campaign (to reduce smoking). Although consumer participation does not usually equate to co-payment for services, the recent de-insuring of many health services has meant that the user must pay for all or part of the costs of nonessential procedures and prescription drugs.

The quality concerns related to consumer involvement are diverse, and often are driven by special-interest groups. Larger issues include the difficulty of defining "the public" or "the community," the scarcity of models for consumer involvement in health-care planning and delivery, and, particularly, the lack of evaluation of various approaches used with different client groups.

Alternative Medicine

The last major trend identified in Canadian health care is the growth and recognition of alternative therapies. In part, the consumer movement is fueling the growth of interest in alternative medicine. People want more choices and are looking for a more holistic approach to health than the traditional system provides. Alternative medicine includes diagnostic methods (such as iridology and hair analysis), therapeutic approaches (such as acupuncture, homeopathy, massage, and herbs), and traditional folk remedies (Health and Welfare Canada, 1993b). Resistance by the medical profession has limited official recognition and reimbursement for many of these practitioners; but that resistance is decreasing. Midwifery is an example. After decades of forbidding the practice of midwifery, Canadian provinces are changing policies. Ontario has recently made the practice of midwifery legal, and has established a three-year midwifery program; British Columbia's commission on health care recommended that midwifery be recognized in that province; and Alberta and Saskatchewan have established committees to study the matter. Some provinces reimburse chiropractors and podiatrists through their Medicare insurance. British Columbia has recently recognized the professions of acupuncture and naturopathy by establishing a provincial committee to study alternative therapies as a means of reducing health-care costs.

Quality management for this trend in health care is very difficult. The providers are a mixture of lay and professionally educated people who often practice in very small, private, for-profit enterprises. There are few national or provincial associations or standards, because of both the small number of practitioners in the country, and the differences in interpretation of practice.

QUALITY MANAGEMENT IN CANADIAN HEALTH CARE

The trends that have developed in Canadian health care have stimulated increased emphasis on the quality of care — both the effectiveness and the efficiency of health services. Several newly formed national organizations have quality care as their primary mandate; and the responsibility for quality care has increased for existing groups. The federal government has assumed an important role in the development of national policy and support systems for quality health care. Provincial governments have also undertaken a variety of initiatives to monitor the quality of care delivered in their jurisdictions. Most of the groups are in frequent contact with one another to minimize duplication of effort and ensure consistency of approach to similar issues.

National Associations for Quality

Interest in QM has coalesced into a number of national networks of health-care associations and organizations. Most of them seek to collect information on quality initiatives, disseminate the information, stimulate research, and lobby for a more coordinated approach to the management of quality in the process of health-care reform. Following is a list of the national collaborations including their primary purpose and membership (most information obtained from the *Inventory of Quality Initiatives in Canada* [Health and Welfare Canada, 1993a]).

- *Canadian Association for Quality in Health Care* — National, voluntary-membership organization devoted exclusively to quality in health care. Offers education, publication of journal, and the opportunity to collaborate with other national organizations regarding quality.

- *Canadian Center for Health Information* — Division within Statistics Canada. Maintains databases, conducts research, and takes priorities from National Health Information Council.

- *Canadian Coordinating Office for Health Technology Assessment (CCOHTA)* — Created by provincial Deputy Ministers of Health to collect, analyze, create, and disseminate information about the effectiveness and cost of technology and its impact on health. Recently added pharmaceutical assessment of effectiveness and economic impact to its mandate (Canadian Coordinating Office for Health Technology Assessment [CCOHTA], 1994).

- *Canadian Institute for Health Information* — Initiated by the National Health Information Council in 1993, including relevant sections of Health Canada and Statistics Canada, the Hospital Medical Records Institute, and the Management Information Systems group. Will provide and coordinate accurate and timely information for establishing health policy, managing the health system, and creating increased public awareness of factors influencing good health.

- *Canadian Network for Total Quality* — Facilitates the development of an integrated strategy to enhance the use of total quality concepts in Canada. Provides training services and assistance in implementation, and disseminates information. Four types of customers are businesses of all sizes; government departments; health and education bodies; and unions and community organizations.

- *Hospital Medical Records Institute* — Provides services to member hospitals by collecting and analyzing data regarding hospital care. Able to give national averages for particular procedures. Develops new reporting packages according to needs of customers. Working on outcome **indicators** and utilization management methods. Considering a change of name.

- *National Health Information Council* — Created by provincial Deputy Ministers of Health in 1988 to coordinate, produce, and disseminate health information.

- *National Partnership for Quality in Health* — Formed in 1992 by the national practice, regulatory, and educational physicians' associations in Canada. Focus is on the development and implementation of evidence-based practice guidelines for physicians.

- *National Quality Institute* — Independently incorporated, nonprofit organization to promote principles and practices of total quality and implementation of quality policies in Canadian workplaces. Board includes business, labor, health-care, government, and science and technology representatives. Has national awards program.

- *Quality Health Care Network* — Collaboration between health-care organizations and the Conference Board of Canada to assist senior executives in leading their organizations through major changes. Two types of networks exist, dependent on longevity of organization with implementation of **Continuous Quality Improvement (CQI)**. Activities include education, research, meetings, and quality tours.

Federal Government Quality Initiatives

The federal government in Canada has been very active in promoting quality within health care and within its own departments. Regular evaluation, using a framework devised by the Treasury Branch, is a required component of all national programs. Health and Welfare Canada, now Health Canada, has recently increased its production of studies and reports regarding QM. International leadership in health promotion came from the Canadian government with the release of the LaLaonde (1974) and Epp (1986) reports. Subsequent national grant programs have focused on the generation of health-promotion knowledge or the application of health-promotion concepts. Following is a list of selected national government initiatives (Health and Welfare Canada, 1993a).

- *Council of Federal/Provincial/Territorial Deputy Ministers of Health* — Has held several meetings (some with the deputy Ministers of Finance) to seek alternative approaches to the delivery of health care. Has hosted national invitational conferences and commissioned reports on national strategies for quality in health care, professional education, technology assessment, and medical human-resource planning. Currently planning a national health forum for 1994 or 1995.

- *Health Promotion Directorate* — Has funded small community programs and large national campaigns that address target populations for health-promotion activities. Publishes regular magazines and bulletins in the field, as well as documents to guide practice.

- *Health Protection Branch* — Responsible for testing and evaluating drugs, developing and monitoring national standards in relation to food safety, and regulating environmental health concerns.

- *Health Services Directorate* — Has produced guidelines for facilities in various program areas such as adult day programs, rehabilitation services, and palliative-care units. Collaborates with providers to improve the efficiency and effectiveness of health services and facilities.

- *National Health Research and Development Program* — Provides funding for scientific research on national health issues, training and career development of health researchers, and conferences on health research.

Provincial Government Quality Initiatives

Almost all provinces are sponsoring studies of particular aspects of health care, usually hospital usage, physician procedures, drugs, or alternative methods of reimbursement. Technology assessment committees exist in several provinces, with membership usually including physicians, government representatives, and representatives of provider organizations. These committees, most established since 1990, provide screening and cost-benefit analysis of new technologies, and coordinate capital purchases with provincial need. A sample of initiatives according to province follows.

BRITISH COLUMBIA
The Quality Assurance Branch in the Continuing Care Program of the Ministry of Health has the mandate of improving the quality of continuing-care services. It has developed standards in collaboration with providers for residential-care services, home-support (homemaker) services, and adult-day-care services. Monitoring capability was established in 1989 and full compliance monitoring was initiated in 1990. Standards are being developed for all continuing-care-contracted services, such as special-care units, group homes, family-care homes, and multilevel facilities. Standards for in-school services to special-needs children are underway, and a community-based workload-management system, which will measure client **outcomes**, is being planned. A Health Policy Research Unit has been established at the University of British Columbia within the Department of Health Care and Epidemiology. Researchers associated with the unit are renowned for their work on health-care utilization and economics.

MANITOBA
The Total Quality Management Coordinating Committee was established by the Deputy Minister of Health in 1991 to be a resource and catalyst for health-care facilities and agencies. Excellent health-care-utilization research has been conducted by the Manitoba Centre for Health Policy and Evaluation within the Department of Community Health Sciences of the Faculty of Medicine at the University of Manitoba in Winnipeg.

NEWFOUNDLAND
The Provincial Quality Assurance Committee of the Department of Health has been established to guide the development of quality indicators and research in the province. It is a collaborative committee of consumers, educators, professionals, and provider organizations.

ONTARIO
The Institute for Clinical Evaluation Sciences in Toronto is jointly sponsored by the Ontario Medical Association and the Ministry of Health. These researchers study physician practices in Ontario, including regional variations, urban-rural differences, and utilization rates of particular procedures. The Centre for Health Economics and Policy Analysis at McMaster University in Hamilton is part of the Department of Clinical Epidemiology and Biostatistics within the Faculty of Health Sciences. This unit has sponsored important conferences on health-care quality, and conducted significant health-care research. A large initiative on the cost-effectiveness of the Canadian Health Care System was jointly assumed by Queen's University in Kingston and the University of Ottawa when the federal government reduced its financial commitment to the project. The planned publication of fourteen extensive working papers on health-care costs and related issues is almost complete.

SASKATCHEWAN
In 1992 the provincial health research granting body had its terms of reference expanded to include utilization studies in all sectors of health care, and had its name changed to the Health Services Utilization and Review Commission. Reports on acute-care-hospital-bed usage by nonacute clients; usage of community and facility-

based long-term-care services; and thyroid testing have been well received. Studies on other diagnostic tests and services are underway in an attempt to provide evidence as a base for health-care planning.

CHALLENGES FOR GOVERNMENTS

During the past few years, there have been a multitude of reports, studies, surveys, and conference proceedings on issues surrounding the quality of health care in Canada. These documents have come from the federal government, from provincial and territorial governments, from professional associations, and from collaborative networks of providers and consumers. The consistency shown in the definition of major problems in the current health-care system and the unanimity of the recommendations for addressing these problems has been astounding. Many different sources of opinion have reached the same conclusions. These sources have challenged governments, health-care organizations, and professionals to put quality first in the redesign of the Canadian health-care system. Governments have been challenged to address five major issues: national health goals, financing, databases, research, and human-resource planning.

National Health Goals

Although the Canada Health Act of 1984 refers in broad terms to the responsibility of the government in promoting health, no national goals for health have been articulated. National principles such as the five principles of Medicare could be used as a foundation for national health goals. Establishing goals through discussion with all stakeholders would be preferable. National goals should clearly state the future direction of the health-care system, so that the provinces, which deliver health services, can articulate their own goals within that framework. Those goals could address the importance of quality in the delivery of health services, establishing a common definition of quality health care as a guide for organizations and associations. National health goals might also focus on priorities within health care. Is prevention of illness more important than treating someone who is acutely ill? What guidelines can be created to assist provincial governments and organizations as they face these decisions on a daily basis?

Equitable Financial Support for Health Care

The most important prerequisite to the stable funding of health care is a stable economy free of debt. The federal and provincial governments have the challenge of attempting to control deficits while reforming the health-care system. Until the recession is over, employment increases, and revenues stabilize, it will be a difficult struggle. Nevertheless, governments have a responsibility to support the health care needed by their citizens, and make arrangements to safeguard and stabilize health-care budgets. Perhaps alternative funding sources that do not conflict with national principles could be identified. Flexible and equitable funding mechanisms that would be responsive to regional needs and resources should be devised. Provinces with resources will not need transfer payments as much as will provinces with fewer resources. Equitable grants will ensure an equivalent level of health services for citizens across the country. Financial incentives for the provinces to deliver services needed by marginalized or less vocal groups are just as important as financial sanctions for undermining the principles of Medicare. Monitoring provincial compliance with expectations is important, as is the clear definition of rewards and sanctions.

Information Systems and Databases

A huge amount of data is collected by governments and other organizations about the delivery of health-care services. Most of this data is not useful because it has not been translated into information that is applicable to management of health care. Even when data is analyzed for the effectiveness or appropriateness of care, it may not be disseminated among the provider groups that need it in order to alter their patterns of care delivery. When information systems are incompatible, or when databases cannot produce new reports for new questions, statistics have no meaning. Technology assessment presents an ongoing challenge, because governments have traditionally been the primary source of funding for capital equipment in Canada. The establishment of provincial and national committees to collect and disseminate information is very helpful. The difficulty lies in the judgments that must be made. How can costs be measured against quality-of-life perceptions? How can decisions about new techniques be made in the absence of guidelines for client safety and outcomes?

Clinical practice guidelines and utilization management are based on accurate, specific data about client outcomes and professional practices. In the absence of common information systems and databases, no conclusions can be drawn from wide sample populations to indicate whether one treatment method is more effective than another. Governmental support to create and maintain national databases will shorten the length of time required for professions to reach conclusions about the best practice for a particular condition.

Health-Care Research

Research funding has decreased in real dollars over the past decade. It is recommended that the money devoted to research be gradually increased from the current 1 percent of health expenditures until it reaches 3 percent of the health-care budget for the country (Rachlis & Kushner, 1994). It is urgent that funding be made available because so little is known about what works, why it works, whether another approach would work as well, or whether watchful waiting would produce the same result. Health-status surveys of the Canadian population are needed on a regular basis to determine health needs, describe health status, and monitor the effects of health-care system changes on health status. Statistics Canada launched a six-part longitudinal national study in 1994, with measures to be taken every two years. There has been very little research into the determinants of health. How much influence do housing, shelter, and employment status have upon health status? What methods can be used by communities to address multifaceted issues such as poverty, unemployment, and racism? How can consumers be involved in health care? Which methods work best for which populations? Research into the various methods of QM is also scarce. Is TQM worth the investment in staff training? Would a results-oriented approach with minimal training create the same commitment to quality in staff? Which methods work best for implementing QM in an organization? Stakeholder satisfaction indices are needed. Many research questions, if answered, would be of immediate use. If funding is not provided for health-care research, there is a risk that resources will be wasted in approaches that either do not work or, even, do harm. Outcome studies need to be sponsored and coordinated, similar inputs and assessment tools need to be selected, and the information must be disseminated. The formation and maintenance of more research organizations to investigate broader policy, evaluation, and health issues should also be considered.

Human-Resource Planning

Canada is a vast country with a widely scattered population. It is difficult to provide accessible health care to everyone if the health professionals choose to locate only in urban areas. The national oversupply of physicians and of acute-care nurses could have been predicted. The undersupply of allied-health professionals has existed for decades. It is essential that a national health-care human-resource-planning strategy be articulated for two reasons: to avoid situations like the present one and to anticipate the needs of a restructured health-care system that emphasizes health-promotion services. Educational programs need time to change curricula, and organizations need guidance in the role descriptions for providers in a revised health-care system. Leadership from the federal government would encourage a consistent approach and similar definitions.

In order for governments to address some of these challenges, they must recognize and commit to the importance of a reformed, quality-driven health-care system in Canada. Until national, provincial, and territorial governments make that commitment, efforts of individual organizations will continue to be fragmented. Repetitive attempts will be made to develop guidelines, databases, and resources for health-care QM, with no central structure maintaining an inventory or taking responsibility for disseminating information. The call for quality, although very strong from many different sources, will not have sweeping national results without governmental support.

CHALLENGES FOR ACCREDITATION PROGRAMS

The largest accreditation program in Canadian health care is housed in the Canadian Council on Health Facilities Accreditation (CCHFA), which recogizes the quality of care delivered by health institutions. There are also some small programs that provide certification or other recognition for organizations which meet established standards. These programs tend to be restricted to a particular geographic region, or to a particular type of service delivery. The development of national standards leads to the question of whether accreditation is necessary to ensure quality services. One challenge for accrediting bodies is to keep relevant by altering standards or processes when there are changes in the health-care system. Another challenge has emerged with the trend toward consumer involvement in health care and the shift from QA to TQM.

Accreditation and Standards

The CCHFA is a nonprofit organization managed by a board of national health-care-association representatives who are committed to promoting "excellence in the provision of quality health care and the efficient use of resources in health organizations throughout Canada" (CCHFA, 1992a, p. i). The CCHFA is responsible for setting national performance standards for health-care organizations and monitoring compliance with those standards. The CCHFA is independent of government and is financially supported by the survey and annual fees received from members of the health-care community who voluntarily wish to be accredited. After many years of Canadian organizations contracting with American bodies for accreditation services, the Canadian Council was established in 1958. Its six goals include conducting research necessary for the development of standards; measuring the degree of compliance with standards; recognizing compliance with awards and noncompliance with recommendations for improvement; providing counseling for health-care facilities; monitoring trends in noncompliance; and providing educational programs on accreditation.

The Canadian Council has accreditation programs for acute-care hospitals, long-term-care institutions, mental-health institutions, and rehabilitation facilities. Current members include 1,316 facilities for a total of 220,399 beds (CCHFA, 1992b) — over half of the institutional beds in Canada. The Council has recently developed standards for small health facilities and for respiratory-home-care services. Standards development and testing is in progress for cancer-treatment services and community-health services. In keeping with its expanded mandate, the CCHFA Board has applied for a name change to the Canadian Council on Health Services Accreditation.

Participation in the Council accreditation program has been voluntary and generally reflects the size and stage of development of the participating organization. Larger and teaching hospitals are usually members. Small rural hospitals of fewer than fifty beds have found it difficult to comply with the large document relating to acute care; many smaller hospitals, therefore, are not members. The new document for small facilities may encourage more participation in the program among small hospitals, however. Long-term-care facilities also tend to belong if they are larger, and not belong if they are smaller. The decision to participate in an accreditation program often reflects the availability of staff to do the work in preparation for an accreditation visit, as well as the priority given to quality concerns by the board of directors and management.

Some standards have been developed for specific parts of the health-care system, with the support of the involved organizations. PriCare, an association of proprietary health companies in British Columbia, offers credentials when members meet the stated standards. The community-health units in Ontario have cooperated and accepted standards for practice, and units are accredited when the standards are met.

Challenges Related to Regionalization of Health-Care Services

Should the CCHFA continue to accredit individual organizations, or should the whole regional system be considered as one? Should the existing timetable of visits to individual sites be maintained during the transition? Some delays in accreditation visits have been accepted, but the decision to continue with the regular cycle of visits has been supported by both the Council and the organizations involved. A significant difficulty is that the Canadian Council does not yet have standards developed for the wide spectrum of services offered by the regional boards. Community-services standards are being developed, but no national accreditation standards currently exist for home-health-care, substance-abuse or community-mental-health agencies; for ambulance services; or for case-management or assisted-living arrangements for the elderly. It is accepted that the governing body standards must be the same for all organizations involved with the same board of directors.

The survey process itself presents logistical problems. Should all organizations under the jurisdiction of one board be surveyed at the same time or in rotation? Should the same surveyor be used? Is it going to be possible for some organizations governed by a board to be accredited and for others not to be recommended for accreditation? The Canadian Council is well aware of the issues implied by the restructuring trends and is already preparing for its first regional accreditation of hospitals in New Brunswick. Active discussions with Saskatchewan health districts are working toward district-wide accreditation within five years.

Challenges Related to Consumerism and Quality-Management Trends

The CCHFA is facing many challenges as it tries to anticipate and respond to changes within the health-care system. In preparation for major decisions on its future direction, the Council hosted a consensus conference on quality (CCHFA, 1993b), and conducted and published a survey of its membership on the implementation of QM (Heidemann, Coulton, Davidson, Baker, Murray, & Barnsley, 1993). The Board of Council subsequently approved "significant new directions, the incorporation of a continuous quality improvement philosophy and the introduction of a clearer focus on the patient care process, both within the standards and the survey process" (CCHFA, 1993a, p. 4). The four underlying principles for the revisions are: customer focus; leadership and commitment to quality; empowerment/team functioning; and **process** and outcome management. Implementation of these new directions will be seen first in the standards that are being developed for new accreditation programs: community-health services, cancer care, and small health facilities. Implementation of revised standards for the major programs in hospital, long-term-care, mental-health, and rehabilitation facilities will occur between 1995 and 1997 (CCHFA, 1993a).

In its exploration of outcome versus **structure** and process indicators, the Council commissioned research to explore the "development of innovative and cost-effective approaches to the monitoring of outcomes of care in health care facilities" (MacKenzie, Greenaway-Coates, & Djurfeldt, 1992, p. 1). The study focused on hospital services. Various indicators, or flags, were compared for sensitivity, predictive value for identifying quality problems, and significance; methods of chart review were compared for cost. The fourteen quality flags, particularly when used in combination with severity indexes, were significantly better at detecting quality problems than was random-chart selection, and significantly more efficient in their use of physician time for chart review (MacKenzie et al., 1992). The Council's challenge will be to convince organizations to develop information systems to track and use these indicators in their QM programs, and to develop comparable indicators for other sectors in the health-care system.

The draft standards for new accreditation programs make references to the importance of health programs being based on community need. Health professionals, particularly from acute-care settings, are not usually competent in assessing this area. Standards for needs assessment do not yet exist. There are many different versions of measurement indications, tools, and even definitions of service populations. The validity and reliability of needs-assessment instruments are uncertain, and research for evaluating the linkages between community needs and health-care services is very scarce. Implementing the principles of customer focus and team functioning will be a challenge for both the Canadian Council and health-care organizations in the future.

CHALLENGES FOR ORGANIZATIONS

Health-care organizations exist within a social, political, and economic context. As the values of Canadian society have changed, the pressure to evaluate organizational goals has increased. Political and economic shifts have created changes in financial status and sources of funding. Additional challenges for organizations delivering health care include information systems, research, and QM issues.

Goals

Health-care organizations are being forced to reexamine their goals in the context of the six trends in Canadian health care. Most organizations are client-centered on paper but not in reality. The consumer is demanding a more active role. Involvement of consumers in planning, implementing, and evaluating health-care programs may be threatening for professionals and health-care administrators. It will be a challenge to make consumer involvement meaningful and not just a token gesture. Very few organizations can claim that partnerships are part of their goal statements, or part of the strategies used to attain those goals. Territoriality has existed for decades, and it will be difficult for health-care professionals and organizations to think and act collaboratively. The other challenge related to goals lies in the responsibility to promote health, regardless of the primary purpose of the organization. When workers are oriented to treatment, it is difficult for them to expand their perspective to consider how to anticipate client needs, and, perhaps, prevent a future admission. Organizations are also challenged to establish principles by which to act. These principles will serve as a promise to both staff and public that administration and board will follow behaviors that are predictable — even when decisions are difficult.

Financing

Making decisions on the funding of programs is difficult for all organizations. When an organization has both acute-care and community-health-promotion activities, the decisions are even more difficult to make. There are few guidelines, vague criteria for priorities, and almost no information on the comparative impact of the acute-care or health-promotion alternatives on client outcomes. Challenges for organizations include, first, articulating decision-making frameworks, and, then, evaluating alternatives against their ability to fulfill the goals and mission of the organization.

Information Systems

There are many challenges to the delivery of quality health care in a regional governance structure. One is size. With one board being responsible for community, long-term, and acute-care services in a region, as many as two dozen organizations could be governed by one board of directors. The operational challenges of combining the organizations are staggering. The standards of care, priorities for practice, definitions of client groups, computer systems, and accounting and reporting practices may be different for each organization. In order to rationalize services, common information systems must be established to provide the data necessary for decision making. The rapid changes in information technology complicate matters, because decisions must be made regarding investments in items such as electronic transfer of X-ray images. Consolidation must occur where duplication exists, consistent approaches must be devised and accepted, and monies have to be reallocated to ensure that sound information is obtained for decision making. The greatest challenge in this process-reengineering is to maintain the quality of care in the midst of required organizational changes.

Research

An activity often omitted at the local level is study of the populations served by the organization. Until the client population can be described, no one knows whether the programs and services match the needs. Needs assessments of the client community become a foundation for both other research projects related to the principal functions of the organization and related outcome indicators.

Research in an organization often means program-evaluation activities but may not be undertaken without the help of consultants or academics. There is general support for the relationship between program evaluation and increased quality of services. The difficulty for many organizations is the first step of defining the programs. In acute-care and long-term-care facilities, services are offered under very vague categories, such as medicine, surgery, or pediatrics; or long-stay, chronic, or maintenance units. Without program definitions, it is difficult to identify measurable program goals against which outcomes can be compared. Clarification of goals is easier for smaller programs such as day surgery, pediatric outpatients, adult day care, or geriatric respite. Many programs, however, have goal statements that are too vague to guide the articulation of clinical indicators. By default, staff activities, rather than outcomes, are counted and described. A QA program based on structure and process issues may have little relationship to the effect of care on the clients or families. Challenges for organizations include defining the programs offered to clients, identifying client-centered outcomes, and building program-evaluation concepts into the ongoing monitoring of the activities for the unit.

The challenge for a multisite organization is to design a research or program-evaluation process that is feasible in terms of staff time and resources, that answers questions about appropriateness and effectiveness of care, and that is applicable across sites. Asking research questions is a skill that staff involved in the delivery of a service will be eager to learn. Finding the resources to investigate questions that are considered to be crucial to the principal functions of that department or program is a challenge. When some of the indicators can be built into the ongoing data collection processes for that program, it is easier for staff to identify quality improvement successes and failures.

The lack of availability of research funds at local, regional, and national levels in Canada has been a long-standing source of concern for practitioners, administrators, and academics in the health-care sector. Although some applied research in target areas has been funded, the vast majority of questions asked by health professionals as they attempt to work more effectively and efficiently have not been addressed.

Quality-Management Issues

The regionalization of governance in health care presents QM challenges for organizations. Because there are different sites involved, each has a different history of organizational culture, management styles, and expectations regarding performance. The developmental status of QM will be advanced in some sites and elementary or nonexistent in others. There will be different expectations for reporting and monitoring of ongoing processes, and different requirements of staff for ongoing quality measures. Additional resources will be required to create an inventory of existing quality practices, obtain opinions on future directions, and create and implement equivalent approaches across the multisite organization.

For the protection of the public and the maintenance of quality services within a profession or setting, standards have been developed as guides to practice. Canadian standards exist for some sectors of the health-care system through the Council's accreditation program. National standards have not yet been adopted for other sectors, such as home-health-care, community-mental-health, or substance-abuse services. Many organizations that deliver these services and are concerned about quality care have developed their own standards for practice. Because no central clearinghouse exists for practice guidelines or standards of care, several organizations or associations have developed very similar standards, resulting in unnecessary duplication of effort and resources. An example is the wide collection of standards for homemaking or home-health-aide services. A challenge for organizations is to form national coalitions to create inventories and resource libraries of approaches to QM.

CHALLENGES FOR PROFESSIONALS

As the system they work within changes, health professionals are forced to reexamine their roles and functions within that system. New professional goals may be required. The two largest health professions, medicine and nursing, could logically be expected to lead the way to a reformed, more effective and efficient health-care system. Unfortunately, these professions are comprised of many individuals and subgroups that often have differing opinions on the best future direction. Medicine and nursing face both internal and external challenges as they attempt to adjust to the changing workplace.

Goals

Professional goals usually relate to successful completion of a defined role. The new future in health care will require professionals and professional associations to become broader and more flexible in their interpretation of roles (Canadian Hospital Association, 1993). In the interests of continuity of care, client outcomes, and efficient use of health-care dollars, professionals must reconceptualize their roles. Partnerships with other disciplines and workers are necessary for quality care in all settings. Defining professional expertise according to tasks or geographical setting is a rigid approach that will not work in the future. Canada needs a multidisciplinary definition of the health-care professional, with a description of analytical and interactional skills held in common. Specific knowledge and technical skills that are usually, but not always, associated with a particular discipline could be appended. National and provincial professional associations sometimes cooperate in offering educational programs or conferences and may jointly sponsor position statements or research. There is an urgent need for cooperation on the development of new professional standards that are both based on research evidence and cognizant of the responsibility professions have to ensure that safe, appropriate care is provided by the most cost-effective worker. If individual professions are serious about putting client needs first and protection of their own territories second, then cooperation is mandatory.

It will be a challenge for most professions to place the needs of the client first and work with clients as partners in the delivery of care. Professionals have tended to think of themselves as experts and of clients as passive recipients of advice and care. The reality is that people only do what they believe will be helpful to them. Unless professionals start to listen to their clients more, much effort will be wasted in attempting to teach or rehabilitate people who are not ready to be taught or helped. The challenge is to alter the professional's definition of job satisfaction. It must change from, "He appreciated my help so much" to, "He did it by himself today."

A coordinated approach to the creation, training, and use of paraprofessionals is urgently required. Most issues regarding these health workers tend to be based in the political and economic context of health care, which provides very little rational basis for decision making. With little or no research available to demonstrate the comparable effectiveness of positions or training programs, it is a challenge for individual organizations to decide which workers should do what, where, and with whom.

Challenges for Medicine

Medical associations are taking the lead in monitoring and studying physician practice. The CMA convened a national conference in late 1992 to develop clinical practice guidelines for client groups (CMA, 1993). The effects of these guidelines are expected to include decreased use of invasive procedures, decreased physician billings, and savings to the health-care system, as well as more appropriate care for the client. Physician-resources planning was recognized as a national issue by the Deputy Ministers of Health, who commissioned a study known as the Barer-Stoddart Report. Medical associations are working in conjunction with governments to implement some of the recommendations of the report, such as a 10 percent reduction in medical school enrollment and residency placements. Alternatives to the fee-for-service payment system are being piloted in many areas of the country, with the support of physicians. The CMA continues to produce studies and reports related to the future of Canadian health care (CMA, 1993; Harrigan, 1992).

Challenges for Nursing

The CNA has been very active in producing position statements, briefs, and background papers for most groups that have reviewed the health-care system. The CNA has been proactive in selecting issues that require a higher profile and presenting association views on both the future contributions of the nurse and the risks of proposed actions for client care.

It will be a challenge for nursing to effectively deal with the large numbers of acute-care nurses without jobs, whose qualifications and training do not match the community need. The diploma nursing graduates do not have the background of family theory and practice — public-health and community nursing concepts learned by degree nursing graduates. Educational institutions and organizations must find creative ways of offering baccalaureate education to nurses in all geographic areas so that these nurses do not have to leave family to obtain their educations. There are several distance education programs in Canada now, and the demand is increasing. The risk for nursing is that short-term courses that provide nurses with increased technical skills may be touted as the solution. These courses will assist nurses in performing physical assessments of healthy individuals, but will not prepare them for the community-development and health-promotion roles that will be required in a reformed health-care system. Faculty will need to review their baccalaureate curricula to ensure that community diagnosis and development skills are part of the content, but that these skills do not detract from the necessary medical-surgical content and practice required to care for very ill hospital patients.

Human-resources planning and forecasting is required for nurses. The supply of nurses has traditionally followed a cycle of oversupply and shortages. Current trends in health care include the aging of the population, the increases in community-based services, technological advances, role redefinition, and the consumer participation movement (Haines, 1993). It is difficult to forecast the impact of these trends in health reform on the need for nursing positions. Professional associations need to work collaboratively with governments and other professions in this area.

Other challenges for nursing lie in the management and delivery of nursing services. Health-care organizations are adopting business approaches such as restructuring, cost containment, greater efficiency, and increasing quality. Concepts such as client-centered care, community case management and managed care, or critical paths for acute-care clients are being used in some organizations (Haines, 1993). Research on the impact of these changes on nurses or on clients is scarce. Various methods of nursing assignment have been tried in an attempt to increase nursing control over worklife and the quality of client care. Little is known about the impact of these systems on nursing morale or job satisfaction. Although nursing specialty groups and associations have articulated standards for nursing practice, research on practice guidelines for population groups has been minimal. When so much is unknown about the most effective methods of nursing care, it is difficult to design nursing systems for optimal impact on client care and outcomes. The relationship of nursing positions to those of paraprofessionals is also uncertain. It may cost an organization more money if paraprofessional positions are increased and there is a corresponding decrease in nursing positions; there may be longer lengths of stay, greater frequency of infections and other complications, and thus, more Registered Nurse time required for supervision. Collaborative approaches are needed between nursing service, education, and research to address some of the questions that are being raised by health reform.

CONCLUSION

The Canadian health-care system is on the cusp of change. The economic context for health care and the trends toward regionalization, consumer involvement, and community-based care will have an enormous impact on the quality of health care services. Although the concepts of QM are implicit and sometimes explicit in the multitude of reports and papers produced during the past few years, the implementation of those concepts during a time of upheaval will be very difficult. If quality care is to be attained and maintained, it will require the commitment and collaborative effort of all stakeholders in health care: governments; national associations and coalitions of organizational providers; health professionals; and consumers. The momentum has been created by pressures for efficient and effective health-care delivery. The future will tell whether an efficient and effective health-care system becomes a reality in Canada.

REFERENCES

Barer, M. L., & Stoddart, G. L. (1991). *Toward integrated medical resource policies for Canada* (report prepared for the Federal/Provincial/Territorial Conference of Deputy Ministers of Health). Vancouver, British Columbia: Manitoba Health.

Canada Health Act. (1984). c.6. Ottawa, Ontario: Government of Canada.

Canadian Coordinating Office for Health Technology Assessment. (1994). Changes at CCOHTA. *CCOHTA Update, 16*, Spring, 1.

Canadian Council on Health Facilities Accreditation. (1992a). *Accreditation in Canada.* Ottawa, Ontario: Author.

Canadian Council on Health Facilities Accreditation. (1992b). *Annual report 1992.* Ottawa, Ontario: Author.

Canadian Council on Health Facilities Accreditation. (1993a). New standards for 1995: Focus on care. *The Accreditation Standard, 1*(1), August, 4–5.

Canadian Council on Health Facilities Accreditation. (1993b). *Partnerships for the management of quality: Invitational consensus conference report.* Ottawa, Ontario: Author.

Canadian Hospital Association. (1993). *An open future: A shared vision.* Ottawa, Ontario: Author.

Canadian Medical Association (CMA). (1993). *Toward a new consensus on health care financing in Canada.* Ottawa, Ontario: Author.

Canadian Nurses Association (CNA). (1993). *Health for all Canadians: A call for health-care reform.* Ottawa, Ontario: Author.

Canadian Nurses Association (CNA). (1994). *Canadian Nurses Association certification program: An information booklet.* Ottawa, Ontario: Author.

Canadian Public Health Association. (1992). *Caring about health.* Ottawa, Ontario: Author.

Chernomes, R., & Sepehri, A. (1994). An economist's brief guide to the recent debate on the Canadian health care system. *International Journal of Health Services, 24*(2), 189–200.

Deber, R. B., Hastings, J. E. F., & Thompson, G. G. (1991). Health care in Canada: Current trends and issues. *Journal of Public Health Policy, 12*(1), 72–82.

Epp, J. (1986). *Achieving health for all: A framework for health promotion.* Ottawa, Ontario: Health and Welfare Canada.

Haines, J. (1993). *Leading in a time of change: The challenge for the nursing profession.* Ottawa, Ontario: Author.

Hall, E. M. (1980). *Canada's national-provincial health program for the 1980s.* Saskatoon, Saskatchewan: Health and Welfare Canada.

Harrigan, M. L. (1992). *Quality of care: Issues and challenges in the 90s.* Ottawa, Ontario: Canadian Medical Association.

Health and Welfare Canada. (1993a). *An inventory of quality initiatives in Canada: Toward a national strategy for quality and effectiveness in health care.* Ottawa, Ontario: Author.

Health and Welfare Canada. (1993b). *Planning for health: Toward informed decision-making.* Ottawa, Ontario: Author.

Health Canada. (1993). *Quest for quality in Canadian health care: Continuous Quality Improvement.* Ottawa, Ontario: Author.

Heidemann, E., Coulton, M., Davidson, C., Baker, G. R., Murray, M., & Barnsley, J. (1993). *Survey on Continuous Quality Improvement in health care: Key findings.* Ottawa, Ontario: Canadian Council on Health Facilities Accreditation.

Institute for Health Care Facilities of the Future. (1988). *Future health: A view of the horizon.* Ottawa, Ontario: Author.

Joint Task Force. (1993). *Moving forward: Strengthening health planning in Ontario.* Toronto, Ontario: Association of District Health Councils and Ministry of Health.

LaLonde, M. (1974). *A new perspective on the health of Canadians.* Ottawa, Ontario: Government of Canada.

MacKenzie, T. A., Greenaway-Coates, A., & Djurfeldt, M. (1992). *Outcomes monitoring project executive summary.* Ottawa, Ontario: Canadian Council on Health Facilities Accreditation.

Ministers of Health and Finance. (1992). *OECD health care reform project–National paper, Canada.* Ottawa, Ontario: Author.

Paul, A. (1993, April 20). Nurses vent rage at cost-cutting health consultant. *Winnipeg Free Press.*

Pineault, R., Lamarche, P. A., Champagne, F., Contandriopoulos, A. P., & Denis, J. L. (1993). The reform of the Quebec health care system: Potential for innovation? *Journal of Public Health Policy, 14*(2), 198–219.

Rachlis, M., & Kushner, C. (1989). *Second opinion: What's wrong with Canada's health care system and how to fix it.* Toronto, Ontario: Harper Collins Publishers Ltd.

Rachlis, M., & Kushner, C. (1994). *Strong medicine: How to save Canada's health care system.* Toronto, Ontario: Harper Collins Publishers Ltd.

Sutherland, R. W., & Fulton, M. J. (1988). *Health care in Canada: A description and analysis of Canadian health care services.* Ottawa, Ontario: The Health Group.

ADDITIONAL READING

Baker, G. R., Barnsley, J., & Murray, M. (1993). Continuous Quality Improvement in Canadian healthcare organizations. *Leadership in Health Services, 2*(5), 18–23.

Canadian Nurses Association (CNA). (1988). *The scope of nursing practice: A review of issues and trends.* Ottawa, Ontario: Author.

Canadian Nurses Association (CNA). (1990). *Select issues in health care delivery* (submission to Standing Committee of the House of Commons on Health and Welfare, Social Affairs, Seniors, and the Status of Women). Ottawa, Ontario: Author.

Fooks, C., Rachlis, M., & Kushner, C. (1990). Concepts of quality of care: National survey of five self-regulating health professions in Canada. *Quality Assurance in Health Care, 2*(1), 89–109.

Inglehart, J. K. (1990). Health policy report: Canada's health care system. *New England Journal of Medicine, 315*(12), 778–784.

Kerr, J. C. R. (1994). The Canadian healthcare system. In J. McCloskey & H. K. Grace (Eds.), *Current Issues in Nursing* (4th ed., pp. 467–472). St. Louis, MO: C. V. Mosby.

Larsen, J. (1991). *National nursing symposium report to the ministers of health of the provinces and territories.* Winnipeg, Manitoba: National Nursing Symposium Steering Committee.

Milio, N. (1986). *Promoting health through public policy.* Ottawa, Ontario: Canadian Public Health Association.

Ommanney, M. (1993, March 19). Steady decline in hospital beds promised. *The Star-Phoenix.*

Porter, B. (for Standing Committee on Health and Welfare, Social Affairs, Seniors, and the Status of Women). (1991). *The health care system in Canada and its funding: No easy solutions.* Ottawa, Ontario: House of Commons Canada.

Quality through health policy: The Canadian example. *International Nursing Review, 40*(16), (Issue 312), 167–170.

Siler-Wells, G. L. (1988). *Directing change and changing direction: A new health policy agenda for Canada.* Ottawa, Ontario: Canadian Public Health Association.

Thomson, A. (1991). *Federal support for health care: A background paper.* Ottawa, Ontario: The Health Action Lobby (HEAL).

PART IV

THE ORGANIZATIONAL CONTEXT FOR QUALITY

Mona R. Fields

CHAPTER *16*

Regulation of Health Care

INTRODUCTION

Regulation of health care in its broadest sense refers to that branch of **Quality Management (QM)** designed to ensure that an institution or caregiver meets some set of predetermined **standards** of performance and/or capacity to perform (American Hospital Association [AHA], 1977). Regulation is further defined as principles, rules, or laws imposed by an external authority for controlling or governing behavior. The term connotes the imposition of order, method, or uniformity. Regulation may be implemented by voluntary agreement or by government action. Within the context of regulation there are three specific processes that are discussed in this chapter: (1) **licensure**, (2) **certification**, and (3) **accreditation**. Each of these processes is defined and then discussed from a historical perspective. A practical application amplifies the certification process and includes discussions about licensure and accreditation as they pertain to the process of certification. The final part of this chapter presents a discussion of some of the social, economic, and political issues surrounding these three processes.

LICENSURE

Licensure occurs on two levels: personal and institutional. A *license* is defined as a formal permission authorized by law for someone or something to do some specified thing (Webster's, 1992). A license grants freedom or permission for an individual or institution to act in a certain manner, that is practice medicine or nursing or provide a service, such as hospital care or home-health care. Another word often used in connection with licensure is **registration**. Very often the word *registered* is attached to the title of the practitioner as part of the licensing process (for example, Registered Nurse or Registered Pharmacist). There is no formal process conducted by any of the regulatory agencies, however, that is termed *registration.* Use of this term in the context of governmental regulation is a misnomer.

Ironically, most caregivers and institutions seem to think of a license in a negative light. Using this negative perspective, the purpose of a nursing license is to prevent an unprepared person from practicing nursing. At the institutional level a license sometimes is viewed as a necessary evil related to constraining the organization's entrepreneurial activities. All licensure activities occur at the state level. Because licensure of health-care providers evolved before licensure of health-care institutions, professional licensure is discussed first, followed by a short discussion of institutional licensure.

Personal Licensure

Within the health-care professions the licensure of physicians occurred first. Texas led the way and in 1874 became the first state to require a person to seek a license in order to be called a doctor of medicine (AHA, 1977). Other states followed very quickly, and by the late 1800s all states required physicians to be licensed.

Nursing followed a similar path in some respects. In 1894 and 1896 two national organizations that eventually became known as the National League for Nursing (NLN) and the American Nurses Association (ANA) were formed. The primary objectives of both organizations were to establish some control over the profession and to stop the growth of substandard nursing schools (Roberts, 1961). Using the model set by the American Medical Association (AMA), the two organizations decided to seek licensure laws at the state level. The nurses in North Carolina were the first to succeed when a nurse registration act was passed in that state in 1903; three other registration acts were passed later that same year in New Jersey, New York, and Virginia (Robinson, 1933). By 1923 all states then in the Union had nurse licensure laws on their books (Roberts, 1961).

Every health-care specialty group has some type of licensure requirement for those persons in clinical decision-making roles. For some groups, competence is based on a test (for example, medicine and nursing), while for others it is based on having preparation in an area (for example, social work). In the example of social work, possessing a copy of a transcript or a degree establishes expertise in social work. The state then issues a license that permits one to represent oneself as a Licensed Social Worker. In some states instead of a license this document is called a *certificate;* and the social worker is a Certified Social Worker.

Many of the aforementioned groups include lesser-prepared individuals who assist the licensed personnel. Examples of assistants who are licensed by the state are Physician's Assistants and Licensed Physical Therapy Assistants. Individuals in these two groups must pass examinations in order to be licensed; but they practice under delegated protocols or plans of care prepared by their supervising practitioners. Other individuals may have completed short vocational-level training programs, such as those for Nursing Assistants; while others receive strictly on-the-job training, such as some Pharmacy Technicians. Most agencies establish some sort of institutional credentialing process for this level of personnel. These individuals must complete this internal credentialing process before the institution will allow them to function within the agency (a form of institutional licensure of personnel).

Institutional Licensure

Licensure of health-care agencies has been slower to develop. Some states still do not require a license for a hospital to operate. In its earliest regulatory activity, the government exercised its police power to protect the public. *Police power* refers to the authority of a governmental entity to limit the freedom of an individual or group for the good of all citizens. The states first invoked this power in an effort to limit the spread of contagious disease; they developed quarantine laws restricting infected individuals to their homes or a hospital and also restricting access of non-infected individuals to infected persons.

The authority of the federal government to regulate health care was first evoked in 1798 (Griffith & Johnston, 1990). Under its power to regulate interstate and foreign commerce, the federal government passed the United States Marine Act. This act called for the creation of an entity known as The United States Public Health Service. This organization was formed to promote research, demonstration projects, and interstate and international quarantines; provide advice on technical matters; and loan public health officers to state and local health departments and other federal agencies with particular health interests (Hanlon, 1969). The Public Health Service immediately began to operate and staff hospitals to treat illnesses of sailors and to prevent the spread of diseases contracted by sailors when in foreign countries. Thus, by 1798 both the federal government and various state governments were into the process of regulating the delivery of health care. The federal government did and does not, however, control through licensure but through laws and rules that must be met in order to qualify for federal programs and/or reimbursement through a federal program such as Medicare.

Although there were small changes in regulation by the federal government, nothing of substance occurred until the 1940s. After World War II, the regulation of health care, especially hospitals, underwent a major transformation. Hospitals had become the exclusive site for the performance of both sophisticated and routine medical procedures. The political climate had become more conducive to governmental involvement in all phases of commerce including health care. The growing effectiveness of medical treatments generated a huge demand for all types of medical services. And there was a tremendous increase in the number of third-party payers and the number of individuals covered by these payers. Thus, health care was on the verge of a tremendous expansion based on the demand for more facilities, more manpower, and a method to pay for these services.

In 1946 the federal government passed the Hill-Burton Hospital Survey and Construction act (AHA, 1977). Through this act the federal government became directly involved in financing health-care facilities, such as hospitals, for use by the general public. Although the specific intent of the Hill-Burton Act was to increase the number of hospitals, there were corresponding regulations that restricted conduct by those hospitals. This legislation established guidelines for surveying the community and determining levels of need for hospitals. In addition, the act sought to promote and elevate standards of design and construction. This, in turn, prompted the states to develop hospital licensing laws. An example of one such law states, "Hospitals are licensed in such manner that the Board of Health may promulgate and enforce rules that relate to '. . . (1) minimum requirements for staffing by physicians and nurses; (2) hospital services relating to patient care; and (3) fire prevention, safety, and sanitary provisions of hospitals'" (Griffith & Johnston, 1990, p. 24).

Most state licensure laws for health-care facilities have been developed since 1945. There is wide variation in which institutions are regulated by each state and in how that licensure process occurs. Some states accept accreditation by a private organization, such as the Joint Commission for Accreditation of Health Organizations (Joint Commission), as evidence that licensure standards have been met. Some accept certification for Medicare reimbursement as evidence of meeting licensure requirements. Still other states have separate licensing requirements and require inspections/audits/surveys by state employees apart from the accreditation and/or certification surveys in order for the facility to be granted a license. Even today some states do not require licensure of hospitals. Still other states have a dual system that both accepts accreditation by a private agency and also has a procedure for licensing a facility if the facility chooses not to be accredited by a private agency. Accreditation by a private agency is very expensive, and many smaller health-care facilities could not absorb such fees and continue to operate. Thus, the state provides a different method for agencies to meet licensing standards.

Most licenses are issued for one year. Even when the state accepts accreditation as a substitute for state validation of meeting licensing standards, the state retains police power. This means that if a consumer files a complaint against a health-care facility, the investigation of that complaint is a state obligation. This provides the state licensing entity an opportunity to validate that the health-care facility meets state licensing standards and that the accrediting agency is incorporating the state's standards into its accreditation process.

CERTIFICATION

Certification is a process that designates some entity or some group as worthy of some sort of recognition. This recognition may entitle a person to be recognized as an expert in a particular field, or it may allow an entity to participate in a particular activity or program. In the same manner as licensure, certification occurs on both an individual level and an institutional level.

Individual Certification

The first example of health professional certification involved physicians. By the early 1900s the practice of medicine had shifted from general practice to specialty practice. Some specialty physicians banded together and formed the American College of Surgeons. This group identified **criteria** for the practice of surgery and began credentialing physicians who held a license and met these additional criteria as surgeons. Thus, the Board Certification process was started for physicians.

Specialization in nursing did not occur to any recognized degree until the late 1940s and early 1950s. Two events appear to have influenced its development. The first event was the advent of the practice of medicine in a hospital setting rather than in just the office and home. The other was the rapid development of baccalaureate and master's programs, which occurred in the 1950s. The recognition of a nursing specialty was for many years dependent on the nurse holding a master's degree with a major in that particular specialty. In the 1970s specialist certification was developed by the ANA to recognize those who became specialists in particular practice arenas based on knowledge acquired during on-the-job experience, in-service education programs, continuing education programs, and self-directed study without the benefit of acquiring advanced degrees in the specialty areas. These persons are required to submit documentation of work experience and to pass a national examination. Another group to receive credentials beyond the original license as a Registered Nurse are termed Advanced Nurse Practitioners. Again, they are credentialed at the state level in order to practice; but the actual certification of competence derives from an educational program, or from the American Nurses' Credentialing Center, The American College of Nurse Midwives, or the National Certification Corporation (certifying body of the National Association of Women's Health, Obstetrics, and Neonatal Nurses). Certification by one of these groups is then presented to the state to indicate competence. The ANA now requires a master's degree to acquire this certification. Bulechek and Maas (1994) describe three models for nurse specialty practice certification: certification by professional organization, state, or institution.

Other disciplines also have certification. For speech therapists, the certification comes from the American Association of Speech Pathologists. The American Association of Dietetics provides certification for dietitians. There are a variety of certification programs for various types of professionals in counseling and psychotherapy. Some are offered through institutes designed to promote a particular approach, such as reality therapy. These certification programs usually involve an intense educational program followed by a short, guided internship wherein one practices with patients. Other certification programs require the earning of an advanced degree. In the interest of brevity these will not be explored in depth here. It is important to note, however, that many disciplines besides nursing and medicine have certification processes available for their practitioners. For all disciplines, certification represents the recognition of a high level of expertise in that particular discipline.

Institutional Certification

To understand the institutional certification process and its importance within the health-care system, the development of the Medicare/Medicaid programs must be examined. Medicare (Title XVIII) is a health-insurance program for people age sixty-five and older and for some disabled people under age sixty-five. It is a federal government program mandated by the 1964 Social Security Act and administered by the Health Care Financing Administration (HCFA) division of the Department of Health and Human Services (DHHS). Medicare has two parts: hospital insurance and medical insurance. Medicare hospital insurance (sometimes called Part A) helps pay for medically necessary inpatient hospital care, inpatient care in a skilled nursing facility following a hospital stay, home-health care, and hospice care. Certification and/or recertification of an institution means that the agency can bill Medicare and/or Medicaid for the health-care services provided if the patient is covered by Medicare and/or Medicaid (publicly funded insurance programs).

Medicare reimbursement does not always equal the full cost of certain services. In some states the Medicaid program (a matching federal and state program) reimburses those with very low incomes for authorized services not paid by Medicare. Some states also permit Medicaid for people with extremely low incomes who do not qualify for Medicare. Medicare/Medicaid claims and payments are handled by private insurance organizations under contract with the federal government. Those organizations handling claims from hospitals, skilled nursing facilities, hospices, and home-health agencies are called *intermediaries* or *fiscal intermediaries*.

The Secretary of DHHS designated HCFA to administer the standards and certification aspects of the Medicare and Medicaid programs. The HCFA's central office is located in Baltimore, Maryland, and is responsible for developing the certification policies and procedures; publishing and disseminating Medicare and Medicaid regulations; and responding to questions from regional offices, congressional members, and the general public. For administrative purposes HCFA divided the United States into ten regions. In each HCFA regional office the Division of Health Standards and Quality works with designated state agencies in administering the survey and certification program for Medicare/Medicaid. There is one designated agency in each state within the region. Agreements have been made between the Secretary of DHHS and the governors of the various states, territories, and the district of Columbia. These agreements stipulate that state agencies designated by the governors are responsible for the performance of the state functions created by Section 1864 of the 1964 Social Security Act (United States Congress, 1964). The agreement indicates that the state agency is responsible for conducting the safety surveys and quality surveys using the regulations written by HCFA. The state agency then makes a recommendation to the HCFA regional office as to whether or not the facility should be Medicare approved. Using the state's recommendation, the regional office determines whether the facility is in compliance and either certifies, recertifies, denies, or terminates the facility for Medicare participation.

The federal regulations become the standards that a health-care facility must meet if it wishes to participate in Medicare or Medicaid programs. The standards are titled "Conditions of Participation." Each type of facility has its own set of conditions of participation, and there are varying numbers of conditions. Each condition has a set of standards as subunits of the condition. The standards are designed to measure both the ability of a provider or supplier to furnish a service and the **quality** of that service. When a facility is certified to participate in Medicare, that facility can notify the state and participate in Medicaid. In the early days of the federal health-care programs, a great effort was made to certify as many facilities as possible for Medicare and Medicaid. The general approach to the quality issue was directed toward discrete measurement and enforcement. Today, a broader definition of quality prevails. Regulations require that quality assessment is to focus more on the needs of the individual patient/resident and less on the facility structure. Standards for long-term care hold that regulations are, to the extent possible, performance standards relying on the professional judgment of the surveyor. That official must determine whether the quality of service inherent in the standard has been achieved for the patient/resident. Neither Congress nor the federal agencies that administer health-care programs ever intended that quality be limited to minimum legal compliance with standards.

Federal standards for participation in Medicare and Medicaid programs determine what a facility is required to do in order to participate in the programs. These standards describe the structure, in terms of both the physical plant and organization, that a facility must possess in order to support its purpose in health care. Standards are created to control, to establish minimums or maximums, to guide action, and to improve procedures. Most importantly, they are intended to be realistic rather than merely legalistic. Surveyors of health-care facilities are concerned with three aspects of standards: capacity, performance, and product. *Capacity* concerns the physical plant — the professional and nonprofessional staff and the equipment. *Performance* refers to how the capacity of the facility is utilized. *Product* is based on the maintenance of the patient's well-being. Performance is a much more complex judgment for the surveyor to make than is a judgment of capacity.

Policy formulation, general management, and operational aspects of Medicare are delegated to the state by the Secretary of DHHS. The state survey agency (a division of the state health department), under agreement, conducts on-site visits to facilities to determine provider/supplier compliance with federal regulations; the state survey agency then completes the required survey report forms, and submits the forms to the appropriate office.

The State Operations Manual (SOM) and Regional Office Manual (ROM) detail the methods that are to be used in applying the Federal Survey and Certification Requirements (United States Department of Health and Human Services [DHHS], 1993). These manuals provide guidance to states in determining compliance with federal health and safety laws and regulations. The manuals also serve as a collection of pertinent data aimed at standardizing administrative judgments and detailing how programs are to be accomplished. Additionally, the manuals establish formats acceptable to the federal government prior to the submission of documents detailing costs to reimburse. The manuals are one attempt to standardize the application of federal regulations while maintaining freedom for each state to implement licensure regulations developed to meet the needs of its own citizens.

The two processes, licensure and certification, work together. A *statutory requirement* is a law that has been adopted or decreed by a federal, state, or municipal body and cannot be waived by a lessor authority. Because the federal regulations incorporate the requirements for state licensure, any additional requirement in state licensure must also be met for approval and eventual certification. Regulations, whether federal, state or local, seek to interpret the intent and meaning of law. Because they are legally based, regulations have the effect of law as soon as they are adopted and approved. Violation of regulations may be punishable offenses. The HCFA has begun implementing monetary penalties for institutions that fail to meet their conditions of participation. At present, however, the penalties are used very cautiously and only in the most blatant noncompliance cases.

Rules and regulations are developed by the agencies mandated to carry out the intent and meaning of the law, and are intended to assist in discharging these responsibilities. As previously discussed, certain federal rules and regulations (which are procedurally "laws of the land" when they pertain to the delivery of services by health-care providers) are known as Conditions of Participation. When applied to health-care suppliers, such as physicians and durable medical equipment companies, they are known as "Conditions of Coverage." By definition a condition of participation/coverage is described in federal regulations and sets forth requirements (that is, conditions) that must be met before the provider/supplier can be certified and reimbursed from federal funds specifically under Medicare and Medicaid programs. Certification for Medicare automatically makes an institution eligible for Medicaid reimbursement. Conditions of participation/coverage are subject to interpretation and, in many instances, to collective professional judgment. Regulatory bodies frequently publish formalized professional judgments. The philosophy here is one of uniformity. Under each condition of participation are lesser regulations that pertain to the topic of the condition. All providers and suppliers must meet statutory requirements. Providers/suppliers found by the survey/review process to have deficiencies at the standard level may be certified if they have an acceptable plan of correction.

THE SURVEY PROCESS FOR MEDICARE CERTIFICATION

There are three types of surveys for Medicare certification: (1) initial, (2) recertification, and (3) validation. As a general rule, surveys are unannounced; for hospitals, however, an exception to this rule often is made. Surveys may also be scheduled in advance for facilities that are mobile (for example, mobile X-ray units) or facilities that are not consistently staffed or open (for example, a rural health clinic open only two days per week). For an agency to have an initial survey, the institution must be open for business and have active clients. Resurvey/recertification occurs on a cyclic basis. The rules and regulations for home health-care agencies require yearly recertification surveys. The time period for all other institutions varies, usually based on the money available for certification activities. If a safety survey (Life Safety Code) is required, it is scheduled to coincide with the health survey of the institution. The safety survey should never precede the health survey because the safety survey would automatically announce the upcoming health survey.

It may be necessary to conduct a complete recertification survey at an earlier than planned date. Possible reasons for this would be a complaint about the standard of care, loss of Joint Commission hospital accreditation, an employee strike, substantial change in managerial personnel, or a significant change in the type of treatment provided. The decision to conduct a recertification survey at an earlier date than originally planned depends on whether there is a likelihood that the certification status could change. Change in size or location of an organization does not ordinarily require a special survey. The provider is expected to provide an adequate standard of care regardless of the physical location or the addition of new staff to serve more people. Only if the relocation raises significant questions as to the provider's ability to maintain standards is an early resurvey necessary. Thus, if an ambulatory survey center moved locations, a Life Safety Code survey would usually be considered necessary.

There are three types of validation surveys. The first is a survey conducted after a private organization, such as the Joint Commission, has conducted an accreditation survey in an effort to ascertain whether or not the accrediting organization's standards meet the federal conditions of participation. Another type of validation survey occurs when a survey team from a HCFA regional office resurveys an agency after a state survey has been conducted to determine whether or not the state surveyors are applying the conditions of participation appropriately. The final type of validation survey occurs when an agency challenges a survey based on claims of bias on the part of the state surveyor(s). This survey is conducted by other state surveyors with the original surveyor on site during the survey.

In preparation for a survey/resurvey the agency file is reviewed by the surveyors. Documents of interest include licensure records, fire safety reports, previous survey reports (including Life Safety Code), staffing reports, complaints, and other documents, as appropriate. The size and makeup of the survey team varies according to the type of institution, the size of the agency, and the purpose of the survey. For routine certification surveys, professional disciplines and experience represented by the survey team should reflect the condition of participation requirements for that provider/supplier group. In all instances members of the survey team must meet educational and training requirements.

Court decisions, both state and federal, have held that the acceptance of either the Medicare agreement or state licensure indicates implied consent by the institution to permit authorized officials to make unannounced visits. If access is refused, the team leader documents the identity (name and title) of the individual refusing admission and the reason for refusal. Refusal to allow a survey or complaint investigation to proceed is tantamount to surrender of the right to participate in the Medicare program.

During the actual survey, the surveyor or survey team looks at every condition of participation and the standards under that condition of participation; the surveyor or survey team then uses the interpretive guidelines to determine if the standards and, ultimately, the conditions are met. Interpretive guidelines provide guidance to both the agency and the surveyor as to the evidence that might indicate the standard has or has not been met; the guidelines also provide guidance regarding acceptable alternate methods for meeting a standard.

If the survey is of a hospital, the team considers all the appropriate conditions of participation. These conditions of participation, and their accompanying standards and guidelines, often are the basis for what is considered hospital routine in the delivery of health care. For example, federal regulations are the basis for such routine practices as stop orders on antibiotics and inclusion of key components for every clinical record. Conditions of participation also spell out well-known QM functions, such as infection control and **Quality Assurance (QA)**. When conditions of participation and their standards are developed, they are initially published in the Federal Register and then disseminated on a need-to-know basis.

During any survey the team first presents their credentials to the agency administrator. The facility representative provides a work space for the team and provides whatever assistance the team needs. The written policies of the agency are reviewed. Documentation of personnel credentials is ascertained. Patient/client records are reviewed. Normal operations of the facility, such as a home visit, or the passing of medications are observed. Both staff and patients are interviewed. If appropriate, physical facilities are inspected in order for the surveyors to gather the necessary data. After the data is gathered and analyzed by the surveyors, a decision is made as to whether or not a condition and its standards are met.

From a practical point of view, most agencies will receive deficiencies at the level of standards but are in compliance with the conditions of participation. If a deficiency is written, the facility has ten days to write an acceptable plan of correction and send it to the state health department. The facility has forty-five days to correct a standard-level deficiency. If a condition is out of compliance, the facility may have from three to ninety days to correct the situation, depending on whether a patient was harmed and the likelihood of continued harm to patients. Failure to correct a condition-level deficiency will result in the decertification of the facility for Medicare/Medicaid reimbursement and may also result in loss of the state license to conduct business.

ACCREDITATION

To *accredit* means to give credit, to authorize, or to give credentials or certification that a set standard has been met (Webster's, 1992). When used in a health-care context, the last part of this definition is the most appropriate meaning of the term. The HCFA refers to *accreditation* as verification that acceptable standards have been met (DHHS, 1992). In the context of regulation, accreditation is a voluntary process.

Accreditation of hospitals was established in 1916 by the American College of Surgeons (AHA, 1977). In 1952 the Joint Commission on Hospital Accreditation was formed by a joint effort of the American College of Surgeons, the American College of Physicians, the AMA, the AHA, and the Canadian Medical Association (CMA). The Canadian Commission on Hospital Accreditation was developed as a separate program in 1959 (AHA, 1977). The Joint Commission on Hospital Accreditation's name was more recently changed to the Joint Commission for Accreditation of Health Care Organizations to represent accreditation of other types of health facilities.

As stated earlier, accreditation is a voluntary process. Because of the prestige as well as the excellent marketing strategy of the Joint Commission, however, accreditation by that organization may be viewed as mandatory if a health-care organization wishes to survive in today's competitive health-care environment. For example, some insurance companies provide different levels of reimbursement or decline reimbursement entirely dependent on a facility's Joint Commission status — even when the organization has been granted a state license and Medicare certification. Possession of a certificate of accreditation by the Joint Commission is, in turn, used as a marketing tool by the holder of that certificate.

The initial Joint Commission "standards" were those that were used by the American College of Surgeons. The first revision of these standards was approved by the Joint Commission Board in 1956 and were published as the first set of standards in 1957. This publication consisted of twelve pages delineating minimal criteria for administration, medical staff, and nursing service within a hospital. In spite of the inclusion of nursing standards, the Joint Commission Board that approved these standards did not include a nurse. After more than twenty years of lobbying, the ANA finally won a seat for nursing on the Board of Commissioners of the Joint

Commission. In March 1992 Dennis O'Leary, President of the Joint Commission, created four additional seats on the twenty-four member board. Three new seats are for consumers and one is an at-large seat for nursing. In announcing these changes, O'Leary emphasized that the at-large seat was not for a representative of ANA. It seems likely that this unaffiliated nurse will receive scant notice on a board composed of seven physicians representing AMA, three physicians representing the American College of Physicians, three physicians representing the American College of Surgeons, seven representatives of the AHA, and one representative of the American Dental Association. "The decision to meet ANA half-way acknowledges the vital role of the nursing profession in addressing quality of care issues" according to O'Leary ("Joint Commission Makes Room," 1992, p. 100). It is ironic that one of the major reasons to admit patients to a hospital is that they need nursing care; yet, nursing is severely underrepresented in the body that accredits these institutions. This omission of persons qualified to speak to quality for the nursing profession has and continues to cause consternation within the profession.

When the 1965 Medicare legislation was passed, there was a provision that granted "deemed status" to any hospital accredited by the Joint Commission. *Deemed status* is a legal term meaning in accordance with federal law, agencies accredited by certain bodies are in automatic compliance with all the conditions of participation contained in the Federal Registry for that particular type of agency (United States Congress, 1964). The Joint Commission is the only organization with deemed status for the accreditation of hospitals. Despite the health-care industry's reluctance to be scrutinized by anyone outside the industry and the industry's stated opposition to regulation, the Joint Commission has continued to expand its criteria for accreditation. The complexity of accreditation requirements has prompted many facilities to hire consultants from the Joint Commission to help them prepare for accreditation visits. This involvement of Joint Commission consultants before the accreditation visit gives critics of the Joint Commission some grounds to question how objectively the accreditation visitation team members apply the standards when the team members are in effect reviewing their colleagues' work during the review of the agency. Because of this potential for loss of objectivity, HCFA conducts validation surveys on 10 percent of all Joint Commission-accredited hospitals each year.

The Joint Commission has continued to expand its voluntary accrediting role into specialized facilities; home-care programs; hospices; alcohol- and drug-abuse or psychiatric facilities; and freestanding ambulatory care centers. After a long delay, in 1993 HCFA granted the Joint Commission deemed status for home-health-care-agency accreditation. To comply with the federal regulation that home-health agencies be surveyed annually, the Joint Commission has developed two different survey processes for home-care agencies. Any home-care agency that does not wish to participate in the federal survey process conducted by state health departments can choose to have the Joint Commission come for accreditation on an annual basis. If the home-health agency is hospital based, however, it can be surveyed as a department of the hospital on the usual three-year cycle and continue to be surveyed by a state agency for Medicare certification.

Since 1992 the NLN-sponsored Community Health Accreditation Program (CHAP) has held deemed status for accreditation of home-health-care agencies. It is not anticipated that this will change. The Commission on Rehabilitation Facilities (CARF) holds deemed status for rehabilitation agencies. The American Psychiatric Association holds deemed status for the accreditation of psychiatric facilities. Depending on the prevailing political philosophy, the process of determining the quality of health-care facilities will probably continue to vacillate between use of private bodies, such as the Joint Commission, and use of federal, state, and local government employees, as is done in the certification process.

ISSUES

All organizations are developed to further a particular goal, to serve a specific client group, or to promote the good of a certain group. In effect, an organization stakes out a territory. And this is what happened with licensure of individual health-care providers. Now, of course, those provider organizations would argue that the purpose of licensure is to promote the public good — to protect consumers from unprepared persons. The same two-sided argument applies to accreditation. Is it to promote the public good or to make money for the organizations doing the accreditation?

Regulation of health care is controversial. People who believe in a totally unregulated free-enterprise system strongly believe that there is too much regulation of the health-care system. They further contend that the cost in both time and money is not justified in terms of the outcome. They contend health-care practitioners and facilities would function at just as high a level of care without regulation as they do with it. Those persons who believe the free-enterprise system has always flourished at the expense of the consumers of its services, however, tend to believe that the health-care system needs more, not less, regulatory oversight. Certainly anyone who followed the scandals in Florida and Texas (caused by facilities paying bounties for patients and, in some instances, kidnapping adolescents and forcing them into psychiatric facilities) might subscribe to this stance. Additionally, it is widely publicized that 95 percent of all hospital bills contain errors. Without regulations would these errors be for greater or lesser amounts? Obviously the current regulatory mechanisms have not prevented all the unnecessary patient deaths that occur today nor have quality standards eliminated decubiti or nosocomial infections. Regulatory standards have, however, forced facilities to develop QM programs wherein the intent is to investigate occurrences and develop methods to prevent untoward events from affecting other patients.

At this point no one can predict with any confidence what regulatory systems will exist after Congressional rejection of the Clinton administration's proposals for health-care reform. The money available for regulation at the federal level has decreased for the last several years. It seems safe to say, however, that regulation of the health-care industry will continue and will most likely increase rather than decrease in the future. Whether one believes this is beneficial or detrimental for health-care providers and consumers depends on where one's views align on the continuum from no regulation to total regulation.

CONCLUSION

Regulation of the health-care industry has to date served its constituency well. For the consumer of health care, regulation has provided caregivers who, at least at the time of licensure, demonstrate enough knowledge to meet minimum safety standards. Regulation has also promoted facilities that are, for the most part, clean and that operate with the intent to provide quality patient care. From a payer point of view (that is, the taxpayer who supplies the money to operate Medicare and Medicaid), regulations for reimbursement help to prevent fraud. While no system is perfect, the current regulations do strive to prevent the most blatant attempts to defraud the system. For the players in the health-care system, regulation provides a structure for quality care and can at times be used to prod to action those who are reluctant to make needed changes. There is no doubt that regulation costs money; but it can be a small price to pay for the benefits that accrue as a result of the regulatory process.

REFERENCES

American Hospital Association. (1977). *Hospital regulation: Report of the special committee on the regulatory process* (pp. 1–77). Chicago: Author.

Bulechek, G. M., & Maas, M. L. (1994). Nursing certification. In J. McClosky & H. K. Grace (Eds.), *Current issues in nursing* (4th ed., pp. 327–335). St. Louis, MO: C. V. Mosby.

Griffith, R. L., & Johnston, D. W. (1990). *Texas hospital law* (p. 24). Austin, TX: Butterworth Legal Publishers.

Hanlon, J. J. (1969). *Principles of public health administration* (5th ed., pp. 22–52). St. Louis, MO: C. V. Mosby.

Joint Commission makes room for nursing on its board. (1992). *American Journal of Nursing, 92*(5), 100.

Roberts, M. M. (1961). *American nursing: History and interpretation* (pp. 20–30). New York: Macmillan.

Robinson, V. (1933). *White caps: The story of nursing in Pennsylvania* (pp. 282–283, 306–307). Philadelphia: Pennsylvania State Nurses Association.

United States Congress. (1964). *The social security act* (Section 1864). Washington, DC: The Federal Registrar.

United States Department of Health & Human Services. (1992). *Basic health facility surveyor training course. HCFA/HSQB-Hospital Module* (p. 10). Baltimore: Author.

United States Department of Health and Human Services, Health Care Financing Administration. (1993). *State operations manual.* Baltimore: Author.

Webster's new world dictionary of the American language (pp. 10, 845). (1992). Cleveland, OH: The World.

ADDITIONAL READING

Anderson, G., Hyssel, R., & Dickler, R. (1993). Competition versus regulation: Its effect on hospitals. *Health Affairs, 12*(1), 70–80.

Larson, P., Osterweis, M., & Rubin, E. R. (Eds.) (1994). Licensure, accreditation, and institutional barriers to practice. In *Health workforce issues for the 21st century* (pp. 47–63). Washington, DC: Association of Academic Health Centers.

Mittelstadt, P. (Ed.) (1993). *The reimbursement manual: How to get paid for your advance practice nursing services.* Washington, DC: American Nurses Publishing.

Pickett, G. E., & Hanlon, J. J. (1969). *Principles of public health administration and practice* (9th ed., chaps. 1–3). St. Louis, MO: C. V. Mosby.

Webb, P. R. (1988). Adherence to the conditions of participation. In M. D. Harris (Ed.), *Home health administration* (pp. 61–79). Owings Mills, MD: National Health.

Carole H. Patterson

CHAPTER *17*

The Joint Commission and Organization Performance Improvement

INTRODUCTION

Nursing and health-care leaders individually and collectively use terms such as **Quality Management (QM)**, **Quality Assurance (QA)**, **Total Quality Management (TQM)**, and **Continuous Quality Improvement (CQI)** to describe efforts to control levels of quality in their organizations. They often ask the Joint Commission on Accreditation of Healthcare Organizations (Joint Commission) for detailed information on what is expected of health-care organizations in terms of complying with **accreditation** standards relative to CQI or TQM.

Because it is widely known that the Joint Commission continually researches and develops quality measurement theory, as Joint Commission **standards** evolve, questions become more focused on specific standards-compliance issues. Because the Joint Commission is now focusing on *organization* performance improvement, however, concerns relate to the new role of an *individual* nursing department or service in carrying out or participating with other departments or services in an **interdisciplinary** manner in an effort to measure, assess, and improve the organization's performance. As the Joint Commission continues to move incrementally from a focus on "pure" QA or CQI/TQM to a focus on "Improving Organization Performance" in 1995 and beyond, more questions naturally arise.

This chapter addresses those questions and includes:

- a brief overview of the Joint Commission — its mission, definitions, and applicable standards illustrative of a framework for improving organization performance

- a discussion of what all nurses and, indeed, all health-care providers need to know about the Joint Commission's general requirements for the ongoing measurement and improvement of patient-care quality

- a brief description of how to achieve compliance with specific standards from the "Improving Organization Performance" chapter in the 1995 edition of the *Accreditation Manual for Hospitals (AMH)*[1] (1994) — to provide the framework for a comprehensive quality measurement and assessment program

BACKGROUND AND HISTORICAL PERSPECTIVES

Consistent with the practices of all learning organizations, the Joint Commission has defined its mission, vision, and values. For example, the mission of the Joint Commission (Joint Commission Employee Handbook, 1994, p. 5) is

> ... to improve the quality of health care provided to the public. The Vision includes the creation of a performance-focused accreditation system for health care organizations while the Corporate Values include our employees' agreed upon definitions for:

- Quality
- Teamwork
- Respect
- Courtesy
- Integrity
- Empowerment
- Responsiveness
- Recognition
- Improvement

The Joint Commission is a private, not-for-profit organization dedicated to improving the quality of patient care provided in organized health-care settings. This is accomplished by developing standards through the use of expert panels and consensus building and testing processes to define and set the actual standards; evaluating the performance of health-care organizations against the standards through a combination of pre- and postsurvey document review and on-site survey activities; making accreditation decisions based on the findings of those activities; and providing educational and consultation services.

The Joint Commission accredits approximately 80 percent of the nation's hospitals (which account for 95 percent of all admissions) and other health-care organizations, such as those providing home care, hospice, ambulatory care, mental-health care, long-term care, laboratory services, managed care, and other organized delivery services.[2]

---

[1] The standards and scoring guidelines discussed in this chapter are from the Joint Commission's 1995 *Accreditation Manual for Hospitals (AMH)*, Volume I, Standards and Volume II, Scoring Guidelines, and are quoted with permission of the Joint Commission.

[2] Standards and scoring guidelines similar to the ones that will be discussed in this chapter are also found in the accreditation manuals for the other health-care organizations mentioned.

Health-care organizations voluntarily seek Joint Commission accreditation because it enhances community confidence; affects staff recruitment; expedites third-party payment; provides an educational tool to improve care, services, and programs; and may fulfill all or portions of state/federal licensure/certification requirements.

The Joint Commission's AMH has standards related to the organizationwide design of patient-care-focused quality measurement, assessment, and improvement. (Scoring Guidelines for all Joint Commission standards are found in a companion volume [Volume II] to each standards manual [designated as Volume I]. The scoring guidelines state the underlying principles and intent of the standards, and provide both examples of how to comply with the standards and scoring scales to be used in organizational self-assessment activities.)

Because all professionals working in health-care organizations share a responsibility to monitor and improve their performance, the standards in the *AMH* focus on patient-care quality. Patient quality of care is defined in the glossary of the *AMH* as:

> the degree to which patient care services increase the probability of desired patient outcomes and reduce the probability of undesired outcomes, given the current state of knowledge. (1994, p. 181)

Therefore, patient-care quality is viewed as the results of the actions of all care providers (the effect of multiple causes) and is composed of many **structures**, **processes**, and **outcomes** of the care provided by those individuals, both individually and collectively. Organizations can learn about their levels of performance by comparing their performance levels with

- themselves over time (historical patterns or trends)
- others (**benchmarking** with the best performers)
- standards (accreditation, national sets)
- best known practices (practice guidelines)

The remainder of this chapter discusses the Joint Commission's focus on performance measurement, assessment, and improvement as illustrated in the standards published in its accreditation manuals.

THEORETICAL/CONCEPTUAL ORIENTATION

The publication of the 1992 *AMH* (Joint Commission, 1991) marked the beginning of a carefully planned transition to standards that emphasize CQI. The standards in that edition de-emphasized some structural requirements that were not viewed as critical to the quality of patient care and services, and prepared the way for a shift in standards. Focus shifted from the performance of each department and service to the performance of those processes important to patient care that most often involve multiple departments and services.

Thus, a significant change in the 1992 *AMH* was the revision of the "Quality Assurance" chapter to make it more consistent with principles of CQI. The revisions to that chapter began with the change to its title: from "Quality Assurance" to "Quality Assessment and Improvement." This shift was in line with the Joint

Commission's plan to phase in over the years standards that reflect the approaches and methods of CQI. This process is to be substantially completed in all standards manuals published by the Joint Commission in 1995–1996. The Joint Commission wanted to ensure that the quality improvement standards included in future editions of AMH give health-care organizations as much flexibility as possible in the particular means they use to continuously measure, assess, and improve all levels of quality performance.

The Joint Commission's transition to CQI theory and standards draws from the insights of the originators and major developers of CQI, such as W. Edwards Deming, Joseph Juran, and Philip Crosby. Principles of CQI incorporate the strengths of QA as it was and is currently practiced, while broadening the scope, refining the approach to measuring and assessing care and service, and dispensing with the negative connotations sometimes associated with QA. In moving toward CQI, the Joint Commission wanted health-care organizations to build on the strengths of their existing QA mechanisms.

In 1994, performance-focused, functional standards that promoted appropriate cross-departmental attention to quality replaced most of those that previously referred only to departmental requirements: For example, rather than address patient-assessment requirements in multiple department- and service-specific chapters, a single chapter of "Patient Assessment" standards was published. Additional focus was given to interdepartmental review of care and service rather than continuing the tunnel-visioned view of individual professional or departmental quality reviews. An example of such a review might be the forming of a team representing nursing, operating room staff, and surgeons to assess and improve surgery scheduling.

The point is that quality is everybody's business. Focusing quality assessment exclusively on the activities of one department providing direct patient care often has led to an unwelcome and unnatural emphasis on finding problem practitioners rather than to people working together to improve whole systems of care delivery. In practice, improvement often hinges on redesigning and rethinking communication habits, the role of leaders and support staff, or the way departments work together, rather than on the performance of individual practitioners.

This new chapter of standards titled "Improving Organizational Performance" (IOP) was first published in the 1994 edition of the *AMH* (Joint Commission, 1993b). It represented a significant evolution in the understanding of quality improvement in health-care organizations and identified the connection between organizational performance and judgments about quality. The primary focus shifted from the performance of individuals to the performance of organizational systems and processes[3], while continuing to recognize the importance of the individual competence of all staff members. The chapter also provided flexibility to organizations in how they go about their design, measurement, assessment, and improvement activities. Thus, this chapter described the essential activities common to a wide variety of improvement approaches.

---

[3]Throughout the remainder of this chapter, *process* means a single process and/or a system of integrated processes.

Improving performance has been at the heart of the Joint Commission's activities since its inception. The focus of the 1994 manual was on the important patient-care functions performed by a health-care organization, and the IOP chapter described a framework for improving those functions. It should now be evident that the Joint Commission believes:

- Performance in health care is what is done (doing the right thing) and how well it is done (doing the right thing well)
- The level of performance in health care is:
  a. the degree to which what is done is *efficacious* and is appropriate for the individual patient
  b. the degree to which how it is done: makes it *available* in a *timely* manner to patients who need it; is *effective;* is *coordinated* with other care and care providers; is *safe;* is *efficient;* and is *caring and respectful* of the patient

The characteristics of *what is done* and *how it is done* are called the dimensions of performance, as shown in Table 17-1.

Table 17-1 • **DEFINITIONS OF JOINT COMMISSION DIMENSIONS OF PERFORMANCE**

I. DOING THE RIGHT THING

The *EFFICACY* of the procedure or treatment in relation to a patient's condition.

> The degree to which the care/intervention used for the patient has been shown to accomplish the desired/projected outcome(s).

The *APPROPRIATENESS* of a specific test, procedure, or service to meet a patient's needs.

> The degree to which the care/intervention provided is relevant to the patient's clinical needs, given the current state of the art.

II. DOING THE RIGHT THING WELL

The *AVAILABILITY* of a needed test, procedure, treatment, or service to a patient who needs it.

> The degree to which appropriate care/interventions are available to meet the needs of the patient served.

The *TIMELINESS* with which a needed test, procedure, treatment, or service is provided to a patient.

> The degree to which the care/intervention is provided to the patient at the time it is most beneficial or necessary.

The *EFFECTIVENESS* with which tests, procedures, treatments, and services are provided.

> The degree to which the care/intervention is provided in the correct manner, given the current state of the art, in order to achieve the desired/projected outcome for the patient.

Table 17-1 • DEFINITIONS OF JOINT COMMISSION DIMENSIONS OF PERFORMANCE (continued)

The *CONTINUITY* of the services provided to a patient with respect to other services, other practitioners, and other providers, and over time.
> The degree to which the care/intervention for the patient is coordinated among practitioners, between organizations, and across time.

The *SAFETY* to the patient (and others) with which the services are provided.
> The degree to which the risk of an intervention and risk in the care environment are reduced for the patient and health care provider.

The *EFFICIENCY* with which services are provided.
> The ratio of the outcomes (results of care) for a patient to the resources used to deliver the care.

The *RESPECT AND CARING* with which services are provided.
> The degree to which a patient, or designee, is involved in his/her own care decisions, and that those providing services do so with sensitivity and respect for the patient's needs, and expectations, and individual differences.

Source: Printed with permission from Joint Commission on Accreditation of Healthcare Organizations, "Improving Organizational Performance" (IOP), Accreditation Manual for Hospitals (AMH), Volume I, Standards (1993).

• The degree to which a health-care organization does the right things and does them well is influenced strongly by its design and the operation of a number of important functions. Many of these functions (for example, protecting the rights of patients, assessing patients' needs and expectations) are described in the accreditation manuals of the Joint Commission.

• Patients and others make judgments about the overall quality of the health care based on the patient-health outcomes (and, sometimes, on their perceptions of what was done and how it was done)."Patient health outcomes" include prevention, restoration, cure, maintenance, and comfort. See Table 17-2 for the Joint Commission's definitions of patient-health outcomes.

Table 17-2 • JOINT COMMISSION'S DEFINITIONS OF PATIENT HEALTH OUTCOMES

I.   PREVENTION .... Preventable illness or disability is prevented

II. RESTORATION... Restorable function is restored

III. CURE .... Curable disease is cured

IV. MAINTENANCE .. Maintainable function is maintained

V.   COMFORT....... Needed psychological and physical comfort is provided

Source: Reprinted with permission of the Joint Commission on Accreditation of Healthcare Organizations.

- Patients and others may also make judgments about the value of the health care by comparing their judgments of quality with the cost of the health care.

The 1994 IOP chapter was issued at a time when the health-care field was redesigning its performance-improvement mechanisms to incorporate concepts and methods developed by other fields (for example, TQM, which in our country had its foundations in industry; and systems-thinking, which was described by organizational theorists as being needed in learning organizations). Also, the health-service research community was making use of new data-driven and information-sharing mechanisms (for example, reference databases, clinical practice guidelines or parameters, functional-status and quality-of-life measures). The Joint Commission's new standards merged many of these useful concepts and methods with the best of current health-care QM activities.

For example, health-care organizations have begun to adopt some of the many approaches to CQI and TQM that have been successful in industry. Most of these approaches offer health-care organization leaders and staffs a powerful array of methods and tools that are useful additions to those already used in health care. Also, most of these approaches highlight the pivotal role of an organization's leaders and the importance of assessing the needs and expectations and listening to the feedback of patients. (See Chapter 5 for a detailed discussion of TQM in health care.)

Although the Joint Commission standards do not require organizations to specifically adopt CQI or TQM programs, the standards do reflect a selective incorporation of several core concepts of CQI and TQM, including:

- the key role that leaders (individually and collectively) play in enabling the systematic assessment and improvement of performance
- the fact that most problems and opportunities for improvement derive from process weaknesses, not from individual incompetence
- the need for careful coordination of work and collaboration across departments and professional groups
- the importance of seeking judgments about quality from patients and others and using such judgments to identify areas for improvement
- the importance of carefully setting priorities for improvement
- the need for both the systematic improvement of the performance of important functions and the maintenance of the stability of these functions

The standards in the IOP chapter did not, and do not, require adoption of any particular management style, subscription to any specified school of CQI or TQM, use of any specific quality-improvement tools (such as Hoshin planning), or adherence to any specific process for improvement (such as the Joint Commission's "10-Step Model"). (The reader is referred to *Using Quality Tools in a Healthcare Setting* [Joint Commission, 1992] for an overview of various approaches.)

The standards in the IOP chapter reflect the need for:

- monitoring to understand and maintain the stability of systems and processes (for example, statistical quality control)
- measuring outcomes to help determine priorities for improving systems and processes

- assessing of individual competence and performance (including by peer review) when appropriate

Finally, the scoring guidelines related to IOP chapter (Joint Commission, 1993a) were designed expressly to help organizations envision the long-term goals of the standards and to make incremental progress toward those goals. The activities described in the IOP chapter were seen as requiring varying amounts of time to fully implement, requiring varying types and levels of change, and requiring resource acquisition or reallocation. Thus, requirements for full compliance with many of these standards are being phased into the survey and scoring processes during the next several years at a pace consistent with the field's readiness.

APPLICATION OF THE NEW STANDARDS FOR ORGANIZATIONAL QUALITY PRACTICE

The new IOP standards address five specific processes: planning, designing, measuring, assessing, and improving. An overview of the specific focus of the five standards follows.[4]

1. Standard PI.1 requires the health-care organization to have a PLANNED, systematic, organizationwide approach to design, measurement, assessment, and improvement of its performance.

2. Standard PI.2, the DESIGN standard, states that whenever new processes are to be established, they are to be designed well.

3. Standard PI.3, the MEASURE standard, has an introductory section describing the specific intent of that standard.

Measurement (that is, the collection of data) is the basis for determining the level of performance of existing processes and the outcomes resulting from these processes. To provide useful data, measurement needs to be systematic, relate to relevant dimensions of performance, and be of appropriate breadth and frequency.

The standards in this section address issues such as the purposes of measurement, the selection criteria for functions, processes and outcomes to be measured, the important sources of data, and the continued role of measuring.

PI.3.1   The organization has in place a systematic process to collect data needed to:

- design and assess new processes;
- assess the dimensions of performance relevant to functions, processes, and outcomes;

---

[4]These standards were quoted and paraphrased from the Joint Commission's *Accreditation Manual for Hospitals (AMH)* Volume 1, Standards, 1995 edition (copyright 1994), and are presented with the permission of the Joint Commission. The companion document, *AMH* Volume II, Scoring Guidelines, provides additional information about these standards, the underlying principles and intent of the standards, examples of how to comply with the standards, and scoring scales to be used in organizational self-assessment activities.

- monitor the level of performance and stability of important existing processes;
- identify areas for possible improvement of existing processes;
- determine whether changes in the processes resulted in improvement.

PI.3.1   The data collected include measures of both processes and outcomes.

PI.3.2   Data are collected both for the priority issues chosen for improvement, and as part of monitoring.

PI.3.3   The organization collects data about:

PI.3.3.1   the needs and expectations of patients and others, and the degree to which these needs and expectations have been met.

PI.3.3.1.1   These data relate to the relevant dimensions of performance.

4. Standard PI.4, the ASSESS standard, also has an introductory section describing the specific intent of that standard.

Interpretation of the collected data provides information about the level of performance of the organization along many dimensions and over time. Assessment questions include, for example: the degree of conformance to process and outcome objectives, how stable is a process or how consistent is an outcome, where might a stable process be improved, was the variation in a process reduced or eliminated?

In addition to assessing performance over time, further information is gained from the comparison of data between and among organizations, when relevant reference databases exist.

The standards in the following section address the elements of a systematic assessment process, and emphasize the importance of asking the right assessment questions, and using the right processes and mechanism to answer these questions.

PI.4   The organization has a systematic process to assess the collected data in order to determine:

- whether design specifications for new processes were met;
- the level of performance and stability of important existing processes;
- priorities for possible improvement of existing processes;
- actions to improve the performance of processes; and
- whether changes in the processes resulted in improvement.

In Standard PI.4.1, following PI.4, the assessment process includes several additional items.

PI.4.1.1   using statistical quality control techniques as appropriate

PI.4.1.2   comparing data about

> PI.4.1.2.1   the organization's processes and outcomes over time;
>
> PI.4.1.2.2   the organization's processes to gather information from up-to-date sources about the design and performance of processes including practice guidelines or parameters of care;
>
> PI.4.1.2.3   the organization's performance of processes and their outcomes to that of other organizations (including participation in reference databases);

PI.4.1.3   intensive assessment when undesirable variation in performance may have occurred or is occurring.

> PI.4.1.3.1   Such assessments are initiated by important single events and by absolute levels and/or patterns/trends that are at significant undesired variance from those expected, based on appropriate statistical analyses;
>
> PI.4.1.3.2   when the organization's performance is known to be at significant undesirable variance from that of other organizations;
>
> PI.4.1.3.3   when the organization's performance is at significant undesirable variance from recognized standards.
>
> PI.4.1.3.4   when the organization wishes to improve already good performance;
>
> PI.4.1.3.5   in response to all major discrepancies, or patterns of discrepancies, between preoperative and postoperative (including pathologic) diagnoses including those identified during the pathological review of specimens removed during surgical or invasive procedures;
>
> PI.4.1.3.6   by all confirmed transfusion reactions;
>
> PI.4.1.3.7   by all significant adverse drug reactions.

When the findings of the assessment process are determined to be relevant to the performance of an individual:

• The medical staff is responsible for determining the use of the findings in peer review and/or as a component of the periodic evaluation of the competence of a licensed independent practitioner in accordance with the clinical privilege delineation process described in Medical Staff bylaws, rules, and regulations;

- The department or service director (for example, the Chief Nurse Executive, a nursing department leader) is responsible for the determination of the competence of individuals who are not independent practitioners in accordance with organization-performance-appraisal or competence-assessment activities.

5. Standard PI.5, the IMPROVE standard, also has an introductory section describing the specific intent of that standard.

The activities described in PI.3 and PI.4 will result in the identification of a variety of opportunities for improvement. These include improving already well performing processes, designing new processes, and/or reducing variation or eliminating undesirable variation in processes or outcomes.

The standards in this section address the elements of a systematic approach to improvement; planning the change, testing it, studying its effect, and implementing changes that are worthwhile improvements.

PI.5   The organization systematically improves its performance by improving existing processes.

PI.5.1   Existing processes are improved when an organization decides to act upon an opportunity for improvement or when the measurement of an existing process identifies that an undesirable change in performance may have occurred or is occurring.

The requirement to take action on identified opportunities to improve a system or activities continues in standard PI.5.4. The scoring guidelines for standard PI.5.4 state that "pilot testing" or phased implementation of modified ways to perform the activities or process being improved is a good way to demonstrate the organization's commitment to improving the process.

The five previously discussed standards for improving organizational performance clearly outline an *organizationwide* approach to planning a systematic, *interdepartmental*, and *interdisciplinary*, system of measurements related to specific prioritized issues of interest to that organization and its patients and other customers. The standards are provided in their entirety in Appendix 17-A.

THE FUTURE OF QUALITY ASSESSMENT AND IMPROVEMENT

A comprehensive quality-measurement-and-assessment plan will include evidence of the health-care organization's mission, vision, and values. Leaders will be knowledgeable in quality-improvement theory and methods and will show commitment to continuously and systematically designing (and redesigning, when necessary) all of its patient- and customer-focused processes and systems.

The organization's leaders will include, in addition to members of the governing body or authority, senior executive level people, such as the chief executive officer; the chief of medical staff; the nurse executive; and other department and service directors, including both administrative and medical staff directors. If the organization has group leaders, shift charge personnel, or other such middle managers, those people will have their degree of responsibility for the design and redesign of the organization's systems and processes spelled out in their performance expectations and/or job/position descriptions.

All of the health-care organization's leaders will be responsible for their organization's degree of success in improving both the frequency and rate of quality outcomes related to either the structures or the day-to-day activities and processes they manage. They will carry out various roles in coaching and facilitating the design, measurement, and assessment of all of those activities and important functions, both these functions directly related to patient care and those significant support functions. As stated earlier, quality is everybody's business; the leader becomes the facilitator and enabler for the professional and other staff members to do their daily work and their quality-measurement-and-assessment work.

As Joint Commission representatives started teaching and speaking on this new focus on organizational performance improvement, health-care professionals expressed high levels of acceptance and positive reactions. Health-care leaders, (including nurse executives and nurse managers, as well as staff nurses) have praised this new focus as both appropriate and timely and have expressed satisfaction that the new vision is becoming a reality. Indeed, representatives of all health-care professions have expressed satisfaction with the Joint Commission's new focus on the health-care organization or system as the change agent for quality.

Theorists outside of health care, including those in organizational dynamics theory and those predicting the future, state the belief that focusing on individuals as a means of improving anything is a *barrier* to improvement (Berwick, 1989; Peters, 1987; Hammer & Champy, 1993). If this is true in general industry and other organizations outside of health care, it seems obvious that it is also true for health care.

Nowhere in our society is it more imperative that people work as teams to carry out their activities on behalf of the customer or client than in health care. Third-party payers of health-care claims, in particular, have a vested interest in improving the efficiency of health care. The cost-quality equation has never been more visible on the American public policy agenda than since the introduction in 1993 of the Clinton Health Security Plan (and the subsequent various counterproposals). Thus, it becomes evident that the value that both patients and payers see in any one of the many measurable patient-care outcomes will vary with each individual's perceptions.

Health-care professionals have begun to recognize that no longer can one profession exist in a "Lone-Ranger" role and survive in the marketplace. The knowledge explosion and arrival of the information age have impacted every segment of our society; health-care provision is no exception.

Patient-focused organizational functions are the substance of the Joint Commission's initiatives to improve the health care provided to the public. This focus on improvement at the organizational level rather than solely at the individual level is believed to be a prerequisite to survival in the twenty-first century.

CONCLUSION

This chapter has described the Joint Commission's perspectives on health-care quality improvement. Focusing on the organization as change agent and contributor to constantly improving levels of quality performance is implicit in the new IOP standards directed toward improving organizational performance. When every individual professional sees himself or herself as an active, participating member of a **multidisciplinary**, multidepartmental team of players in the quality-improvement game, organizations will then be able to benefit from the expertise of all individuals and increase the power to improve organizational performance at an ever-growing rate. The tools exist. Health-care professionals must learn how to use those tools on behalf of each and every organization providing health care.

REFERENCES

Berwick, D. M. (1989). Continuous improvement as an ideal in health care. *New England Journal of Medicine, 320*(1), 53–56.

Hammer, M., & Champy, J. (1993). *Reengineering the corporation: A manifesto for business revolution.* New York: Harper Collins.

Joint Commission on Accreditation of Healthcare Organizations. (1991). *Accreditation manual for hospitals (AMH): Volume I, Standards.* Oakbrook Terrace, IL: Author.

Joint Commission on Accreditation of Healthcare Organizations. (1992). *Using quality improvement tools in a healthcare setting.* Oakbrook Terrace, IL: Author.

Joint Commission on Accreditation of Healthcare Organizations. (1993a). *Accreditation manual for hospitals (AMH): Volume II, Scoring Guidelines.* Oakbrook Terrace, IL: Author.

Joint Commission on Accreditation of Healthcare Organizations. (1993b). *Accreditation manual for hospitals (AMH): Volume I, Standards.* Oakbrook Terrace, IL: Author.

Joint Commission on Accreditation of Healthcare Organizations. (1994). *Accreditation manual for hospitals (AMH): Volume I, Standards.* Oakbrook Terrace, IL: Author.

Joint Commission on Accreditation of Healthcare Organizations. (1994). *Joint Commission employee handbook.* Oakbrook Terrace, IL: Author.

Peters, T. (1987). *Thriving on chaos: Handbook for a management revolution.* New York: Harper and Row.

ADDITIONAL READING

Joint Commission on Accreditation of Healthcare Organizations. (1990). *Primer on indicator development and application: Measuring quality in health care.* Oakbrook Terrace, IL: Author.

Joint Commission on Accreditation of Healthcare Organizations. (1992). *Striving for improvement: Six hospitals in search of quality.* Oakbrook Terrace, IL: Author.

Joint Commission on Accreditation of Healthcare Organizations. (1993). *Exploring quality improvement principles: A hospital leader's guide.* Oakbrook Terrace, IL: Author.

Joint Commission on Accreditation of Healthcare Organizations. (1993). *Implementing quality improvement: A hospital leader's guide.* Oakbrook Terrace, IL: Author.

Joint Commission on Accreditation of Healthcare Organizations. (1993). *The measurement mandate: On the road to performance improvement in health care.* Oakbrook Terrace, IL: Author.

Joint Commission on Accreditation of Healthcare Organizations. (1994). *Framework for improving performance: From principles to practice.* Oakbrook Terrace, IL: Author.

Joint Commission on Accreditation of Healthcare Organizations. (1994). *A guide to establishing programs for assessing outcomes in clinical settings.* Oakbrook Terrace, IL: Author.

Joint Commission on Accreditation of Healthcare Organizations. (1994). *A nursing guide to the framework for improving the performance of health care organizations.* Oakbrook Terrace, IL: Author.

APPENDIX 17-A

Joint Commission Standards

STANDARDS

Plan

If an organization is to initiate and maintain improvement, leadership and planning are essential. This is especially critical for coalescing existing and new improvement activities into a systematic, organizationwide approach. These standards point to the importance of a planned approach to improvement and to the need to have all units (for example, services) and all disciplines (for example, professional groups) collaborating to carry out that approach.

PI.1   The organization has a planned, systematic, organizationwide approach to designing, measuring, assessing, and improving its performance.

PI.1.1 The activities described in this chapter are carried out collaboratively and include the appropriate department(s) and discipline(s) involved.

Design

New processes can be designed well if done systematically and if at least four essential information sources (PI.2.1.1 through PI.2.1.4) are considered that can guide the design process. Each of these sources can identify design specifications and expectations against which success can be measured.

PI.2   New processes are designed well.

PI.2.1 The design is based on:

PI.2.1.1   the organization's mission, vision, and plans;

PI.2.1.2   the needs and expectations of patients, staff, and others;

PI.2.1.3   up-to-date sources of information about designing processes (including practice guidelines or parameters); and

PI.2.1.4   the performance of the processes and their outcomes in other organizations (such as information from reference databases).

Measure

Measurement (that is, the collection of data) is the basis for determining the level of performance of existing processes and the outcomes resulting from these processes. To provide useful data, measurement must be systematic, relate to relevant dimensions of performance, and be of appropriate breadth and frequency.

The standards in this section address issues such as the purposes of measurement, the selection criteria for functions, processes, and outcomes to be measured, the important sources of data, and the continued role of measuring.

PI.3   The organization has in place a systematic process to collect data needed to:

- design and assess new processes;

- assess the dimensions of performance relevant to functions, processes, and outcomes;

- measure the level of performance and stability[5] of important existing processes;

---

[5]A stable process can have very large common-cause variation. So it is possible to have a process that is stable, yet incapable of performing satisfactorily.

- identify areas for possible improvement of existing processes; and

- determine whether changes in the processes resulted in improvement.

PI.3.1 The collected data include measures of both processes and outcomes.

PI.3.2 Data are collected both for the priority issues chosen for improvement, and as part of continuing measurement.

PI.3.3 The organization collects data about:

PI.3.3.1   the needs and expectations of patients and others and the degree to which these needs and expectations have been met.

PI.3.3.1.1   These data relate to the relevant dimensions of performance.

PI.3.3.2   its staff's views regarding current performance and opportunities for improvement.

PI.3.4 The organization measures the performance of processes in all the patient care and organizational functions identified in this Manual.

PI.3.4.1   Processes measured on a continuing basis include those that:

PI.3.4.1.1   affect a large percentage of patients; and/or

PI.3.4.1.2   place patients at serious risk if not performed well, or performed when not indicated, or not performed when indicated; and/or

PI.3.4.1.3   have been or are likely to be problem-prone.

PI.3.4.2   Processes measured encompass at least

PI.3.4.2.1   those related to use of operative and other invasive procedures, including (1) selecting appropriate procedures, (2) preparing the patient for the procedure, (3) performing the procedure and monitoring of the patient, and (4) providing post-procedure care;

PI.3.4.2.2   those related to use of medications, including (1) prescribing/ordering medication, (2) preparation and dispensing, (3) administration, and (4) monitoring of the medications' effects on patients;

PI.3.4.2.3   those related to use of blood and blood components, including (1) ordering, (2) distributing, handling, and dispensing, (3) administration, and (4) monitoring the blood and blood components' effects on patients;

PI.3.4.2.4   those related to determining the appropriateness of admissions and continued hospitalization (that is, utilization review activities).

PI.3.5 The organization collects data about:

PI.3.5.1   autopsy results,

PI.3.5.2   risk management activities; and

PI.3.5.3   quality control activities, including in at least the following areas:

PI.3.5.3.1   clinical laboratory services;

PI.3.5.3.2   diagnostic radiology services;

PI.3.5.3.3   dietetic services;

PI.3.5.3.4   nuclear medicine services; and

PI.3.5.3.5   radiation oncology services.

Assess

Interpretation of the collected data provides information about the level of performance of the organization along many dimensions and over time. Assessment questions include, for example: the degree of conformance to process and outcome objectives, how stable is a process or how consistent is an outcome, where might a stable process be improved, was the variation in a process reduced or eliminated?

In addition to assessing performance over time, further information is gained from the comparison of data between and among organizations, when relevant reference databases exist.

The standards in this section address the elements of a systematic assessment process, and emphasize the importance of asking the right assessment questions, and using the right processes and mechanism to answer these questions.

PI.4   The organization has a systematic process to assess collected data in order to determine

- whether design specifications for new processes were met;

- the level of performance and stability of important existing processes;

- priorities for possible improvement of existing processes;

- actions to improve the performance of processes; and

- whether changes in the processes resulted in improvement.

PI.4.1 The assessment process includes:

PI.4.1.1   using statistical quality control techniques as appropriate;

PI.4.1.2   comparing data about

PI.4.1.2.1   the organization's processes and outcomes over time;

PI.4.1.2.2   the organization's processes to gather information from up-to-date sources about the design and performance of processes (including practice guidelines/parameters);

PI.4.1.2.3   the organization's performance of processes

and their outcomes to that of other organizations (including using reference databases);

PI.4.1.3   intensive assessment when undesirable variation in performance may have occurred or is occurring. Such assessments are initiated

PI.4.1.3.1   by important single events and by absolute levels and/or patterns/trends that are at significant undesired variance from those expected, based on appropriate statistical analysis.

PI.4.1.3.2   when the organization's performance is known to be at significant undesirable variance from that of other organizations.

PI.4.1.3.3   when the organization's performance is at significant undesirable variance from recognized standards.

PI.4.1.3.4   when the organization wishes to improve already good performance.

PI.4.1.3.5   in response to all major discrepancies, or patterns of discrepancies, between preoperative and postoperative (including pathologic) diagnoses, including those identified during the pathologic review of specimens removed during surgical or invasive procedures;

PI.4.1.3.6   by all confirmed transfusion reactions;

PI.4.1.3.7   by all significant adverse drug reactions.

PI.4.2 When the findings of the assessment process are relevant to an individual's performance,

PI.4.2.1   the medical staff is responsible for determining their use in peer review and/or the periodic evaluations of a licensed independent practitioner's competence, in accordance with the standards on renewing/revising clinical privileges delineated in the Medical Staff chapter; and/or

PI.4.2.2   the service director is responsible for determining the competence of individuals who are not independent practitioners, in accordance with LD.2.1.2.5.

Improve

The activities described in PI.3 and PI.4 will result in the identification of a variety of opportunities for improvement. These include improving already well performing processes, designing new processes, and/or reducing variation or eliminating undesirable variation in processes or outcomes.

The standards in this section address the elements of a systematic approach to improvement; planning the change, testing it, studying its effect, and implementing changes that are worthwhile improvements.

PI.5   The organization systematically improves its performance by improving existing processes.

PI.5.1   Existing processes are improved when an organization decides to act upon an opportunity for improvement or when the measurement of an existing process identifies that an undesirable change in performance may have occurred or is occurring.

PI.5.1.1   These decisions consider

PI.5.1.1.1   opportunities to improve processes within the important functions described in this Manual.

PI.5.1.1.2   the factors listed in PI.3.3 through PI.3.5.3.5

PI.5.1.1.3   the resources required to make the improvement, and

PI.5.1.1.4   the organization's mission and priorities.

PI.5.2   The design or improvement activities

PI.5.2.1   specifically consider the expected impact of the design or improvement on the relevant dimensions of performance;

PI.5.2.2   set performance expectations for the design or improvement of the processes;

PI.5.2.3   include adopting, adapting, or creating measures of the performance; and

PI.5.2.4   involve those individuals, professions, and departments closest to the design or improvement activity.

PI.5.3   The primary focus of design or improvement activities is on those processes that need to be improved and include:

PI.5.3.1   planning the action;

PI.5.3.1.1   When the plan includes testing on a trial basis, new actions are planned when tested actions are not effective.

PI.5.3.2   measuring and assessing the effect of the action; and

PI.5.3.3   implementing effective actions.

PI.5.4   Action is directed primarily at improving processes.

PI.5.4.1   Pursuant to PI.4.2, when improvement activities lead to a determination that an individual has performance problems that he or she is unable or unwilling to improve, his or her clinical privileges or job assignment are modified (in accordance with the standards on renewing and revising clinical privileges in the Medical Staff chapter and on determining competence in the Management of Human Resources chapter), as indicated, or some other appropriate action is taken.

Claire Gavin Meisenheimer

CHAPTER *18*

Organizational Issues that Impact the Pursuit of Quality

INTRODUCTION

The ability to demonstrate **quality** of care or service will determine whether an organization will effectively compete in the marketplace and survive into the twenty-first century — or die. Reich (1991) notes that the next century will bring fundamental change in global political, social, and economic systems. The past decade has already turned worlds upside down with increased competition, more sophisticated and demanding customers, a greater heterogeneous workforce, and decreased financial resources to provide the public with what they believe they need and deserve.

Federal health policies encouraging free enterprise; entrepreneurism; corporate acquisitions; and restructuring/reengineering of health-care facilities have all fostered the use of competitive markets, while regulations have simultaneously increased in an effort to control costs (Milakovich, 1991). In an attempt by the private and public sectors to address the three interrelated problems of access, cost, and quality, the health-care system is being transformed from a cost-driven, fee-for-service reimbursement system to a managed-competition system.

The mandate for change demanded by providers, payers, policy analysts, regulators, and legal constituencies is driving organizations to explore and develop integrated health-care systems, community networks, and accountable partnerships. Integrated delivery systems that draw primary, chronic, acute-care, home-care, and multiple-community services together under coordinated management are growing in number. These systems can demonstrate efficiency, effectiveness, and quality in a seamless delivery system. Outcomes can be measured as each episode occurs, as well as over time. Although patients may be discharged with a good outcome and within the prescribed lengths of stay, however, whatever happens physically, socially, and economically after that, is not measured.

The reality is that patients do not exit the health-care system. There is a difference between output of care and the final outcome of the total health-care process for the patient. Outcome variables that have more universal applicability and utility across varied and diverse settings will determine the health of the community and the quality of patient care. Shifting from episodic care, possible only through integrated systems, maximizes competitive strength and determines market survivors. As integrated systems increase in magnitude and complexity, however, significant challenges also increase for organizations attempting to demonstrate quality across the continuum of care.

The purpose of this chapter is to discuss the concept of customer-driven quality health care and the transformation that organizations must undergo as they find more cost-effective strategies to improve flawed processes. The pursuit of quality requires organizations to forge relationships with empowered clinicians and managers who share a common and well-articulated vision, and a commitment and cooperative approach to change, team work, and process analysis using rational, data-based information (McLaughlin & Kaluzny, 1994).

CHANGING THE QUALITY PARADIGM

Although individual practitioners in health-care organizations have always espoused the values of excellence and caring along with a commitment to improving, traditional **Quality-Assurance (QA)** efforts have focused primarily on the "bad apple." Clinical leaders, QA staff, and committees audit performance and monitor for deviations from preestablished **standards**. **Structure**, **process**, and **outcome** measurements, the three approaches to the assessment of quality proposed by Donabedian (1980), have rarely been interrelated sufficiently to make adequate judgments about quality. At one point in time, this fragmented approach did meet the requirements of external regulatory and **accrediting** associations, such as the Joint Commission on Accreditation of Healthcare Organizations (the Joint Commission). This approach, however, failed to stem health-care costs, increase access, or to continuously improve the quality of both clinical and managerial internal processes.

The renewed interest in quality has demanded that organizations (regardless of size, purpose, or affiliations) expand their quality programs. These programs would include the clinical orientation of QA and quality-assessment techniques leading to an integrated medical, managerial, and consumer model of quality improvement. McLaughlin and Kaluzny (1994) compared the traditional professional QA model and the **Total Quality Management (TQM)** model. They considered it as a paradigm shift to a new way of thinking about philosophy, research, and the practice of quality.

Total Quality Management and **Continuous Quality Improvement (CQI)** are similar in that they both must exist for organizations to succeed. But TQM and CQI are not interchangeable terms. Total Quality Management is a philosophy of leadership, grounded in statistical theory and driven by a shared set of values and beliefs. It is operationalized by top-down total employee commitment and participation in customer-focused CQI of all work processes throughout the organization or the continuum of organizations providing services. Continuous quality improvement refers to a set of process-improvement tools and practices used by empowered and satisfied employees and partners to systematically and statistically analyze opportunities for improvement.

A total-quality initiative requires transformation of an organization's management style and systems. There is a need to examine structure, processes, and outcomes, which encompass and treat costs and quality together. Because complex, multifaceted problems require a multidimensional problem-solving process, a systems approach that eliminates the conventional departmental and professional territories is required. Assuming multiple causation for organizationwide clinical and administrative processes places responsibility for ownership of each process in the hands of those directly involved. It is vital that management and administration provide support and oversight by optimizing a system of care focused on patients.

INITIATING A TOTAL-QUALITY FRAMEWORK

Although the health-care delivery system is comprised of diverse and complex entities that require individualized methods and applications, creating a corporate framework for quality does include several commonalities. Regardless of the specific model used, establishing a mature TQM environment requires recognition of **internal** and **external customers** and the identification of their needs and expectations. Customers — patients, providers, payers — are at the core of **Quality Management (QM)**; the assessment of their perceptions of quality, including satisfaction and performance measures based on data-based outcomes, must drive all markets, systems, and organizations (Laffel, 1993).

Quality management is customer-supplier focused, with the "customer" being defined as anyone who is the recipient of another's work. All work may be viewed as a process whereby a customer receives input from a supplier, adds value to that input, and then passes an output on to other customers. Because every individual's work in an organization is part of one or more processes, interdependencies become obvious; team work is critical to collaboratively identify and control variation in order to improve the process.

The path to health-care quality requires transformational leaders who are committed to dedicating significant and sufficient time and resources (economic and otherwise) to:

1. understanding the nature of organizations and of the whole system influencing outcomes

2. promoting strong participative leadership at the top of the organization, as well as complete employee participation, in managing the change

3. appreciating culture as a powerful force that can either drive or restrain innovation

4. functioning as collaborative teams with ongoing training resulting in learning all phases and processes of QM

Nature of Organizations

Three major theories have evolved in an attempt to understand the complexities of organizations. Classical theory focuses on the formal structure and functions of organizations and how these functions are divided, linked, delegated, reported, and controlled. Neoclassical theory centers on the existence of informal behavioral dimensions of workers and leaders. Both of these theories are important, but not sufficient. This is because quality issues, by virtue of their multidimensional nature, encompass various cultural, technical, administrative, and personal behavior systems both within and outside the context of the consumer-provider relationship (Ziegenfuss, 1993).

Systems, or modern organization theory describes organizations as open systems, integrating diverse interrelating elements and subsystems. This holistic orientation, which includes the external environment, requires that quality issues address the formal structure and functions, informal relations, and quality norms expected by competitors, purchasers, governmental agencies, accrediting bodies, and professional organizations. A "whole-systems" framework that integrates science and practice is needed to attack the complex **interdisciplinary**, cross-organizational problems that concern health-care consumers and practitioners alike. Improving a system's systems—human resource, information, diagnostic, finance, governance— requires honest examination of the culture, structure, clinical processes, and personnel management expectations.

As multistructures, organizations represent an amalgamation of individuals, work groups, and various coalitions of professionals and paraprofessionals (Kritchevsky & Simmons, 1991). Physicians, who enjoy considerable autonomy while significantly influencing organizations with their **gatekeeping** activities, have historically viewed themselves parallel to, and not necessarily part of, the formal organizational structure. Relationships among the various individuals and groups of an organization are crucial to both the social and technical aspects of the organization, because outcomes are achieved and quality is improved through clinical knowledge and application, as well as through attitudes and behaviors toward caregiving.

A systems model recognizes that organizations are a set of closely linked subsystems that must all be changed to achieve quality improvement. Quality is an organization-level problem, rather than a single-provider issue. Multiple strategies and actions are required to initiate and maintain quality. Improving clinical, administrative, and financial problems requires a whole team of clinical providers and administrative-support personnel using systems thinking.

Further, because they are open systems, organizations function within a larger environment and are influenced by external opinions and measures that require a locus of change within the organization if TQM is to succeed. For organizations to survive, planning quality into their design, functions, and behaviors must be contingent on the current situation or dictates of the environment at any given point in time. The total of all individuals and groups is greater than the sum of its parts; whole organizations, systems, and subsystems are interdependent in contributing to high or low quality.

Using the systems model to understand organizations blends with the principles of Crosby (1979), Deming (1986), and Juran (1988). As organizations continuously seek to attain the ideal, using data and the scientific method to solve problems — assessing the problem, planning responses, taking action, and evaluating with feedback — all elements of the system are involved. The behavior of each element has an effect on the whole; the whole cannot be divided into independent parts. The adoption of TQM principles and practices impacts everyone and every process, and thus requires total involvement. Leaders of an organization must appreciate work as a system and support collaborative work (Ferguson, Howell, & Batalden, 1993).

Participative Leadership

Total Quality Management provides a foundation upon which the governing body and chief executive officers establish a unique and distinctive vision and management philosophy exclusive to their organizations. Successful organizations are designed around a set of values and vision which must be demonstrated through a myriad of daily activities. As leaders of quality transformation, they commit themselves through the mission statement and strategic plan, to promote quality rather than exhibiting a bottom-line fixation.

Resources are required to train managers, physicians, and all employees about the philosophy of TQM and the tools of CQI; and the short-term results often are very limited (Jaeghers, 1991). Managing the tension resulting from differences between long- and short-term goals is a major struggle. It is very easy to start the process toward QM because many are looking for the "magic bullet" for survival. If an organization undertakes such a monumental endeavor simply because everyone else is doing it, a dysfunctional organization with distrustful employees may be created. Sustaining quality improvement efforts is a time-consuming, costly challenge that requires ongoing attention.

LEADERSHIP

The purpose of leadership is to influence individuals and events, and to cause significant happenings, by creating and sustaining an atmosphere wherein others can achieve their personal and professional best (Arnold, 1993). To effectively cope with an environment besieged with change, Schein (1985) states that one of the most decisive functions of leadership may well be the creation, management, and, if and when it becomes necessary, the destruction of culture. Top leaders must establish new vision, convince important stakeholders to believe in it, and engage in the process of designing strategies to achieve the vision. As part of everyone's belief system, the critical and central values reflected in the mission statement should direct all future efforts. Developing consensus about goals (including how to achieve them and how to measure the success of that achievement) requires systematic involvement of all people and use of multilevel change strategies.

Leaders who "walk the talk" have given considerable thought to why the organization is embarking on the quality path. Their self-esteem is strong; they are not afraid of taking risks and making mistakes as long as learning and improvement result. Successful leaders take the time to recognize the challenges and develop strategies essential to creating an effective and efficient organization. As suggested by Lewin (1947), effective organizational change requires acknowledgment of the current state, followed by an unfreezing of predominant attitudes and beliefs that inhibit acceptance of a new paradigm. Leaders must understand that removal of inhibitors and barriers is the only effective way to lower resistance and facilitate momentum toward change (Caldwell, 1993).

Organizations need visionary leaders who can build an organizational culture that is pervasively mission driven and directed toward the achievement of a clearly defined future state. This culture is characterized by the personification of values that reflect how the organization, and people who define it, live their daily work lives (Cesarone, 1993). An organization's culture reflects its leadership. Leaders influence the culture by how they behave on a daily basis, not necessarily by what they say or how they handle single events.

Organizational Culture

In spite of great hopes and expectations, early TQM efforts frequently failed because of the nature of organizational culture, commonly referred to as corporate culture. Further, the variety of subcultures was not understood. Creating a new culture takes several years; it does not happen overnight, nor does it occur because managers say it will. Workers learn to think like managers by analyzing constraints, resources, and receiving training in TQM principles and practices. Culture is not monolithic; it requires collective, networking relationships through which shared ownership results in shared rewards. Changing an organization's culture means that behaviors must change.

Schein (1985) describes organizational culture as the pattern of basic assumptions and shared meanings, or values, that a group develops to survive their common tasks and that works well enough to be taught to new members. Culture refers to the unspoken set of rules, beliefs, rituals, and customs that determine how an organization really works. It is a combination of symbols, language, thoughts, artifacts, and behavior patterns that overtly, and covertly, manifest an organization's norms and values. As social reality, culture is both a product and a process; it is the shaper of human interaction and of the outcomes generated by ongoing interactions.

Culture manifests itself explicitly in formal written arrangements, such as in mission statements or philosophies; policies and procedures; job descriptions; external reviews and reward systems; and organizational charts. These documents provide insight into the level of structure, accepted communication channels, and hierarchical and lateral relationships among services within an organization. The informal, unwritten rules and expectations relating to communication channels, dress and decorum, and other factors are implicit in the organization and permeate every aspect in which work is accomplished. These informal expectations may have great influence on the organization's culture. Explicit clues are more obvious and easier to change. Ignoring the key implicit indicators, however, will cause conflict and mistrust of management, thus prohibiting successful implementation of TQM.

Organizational culture differs from organizational climate; culture consists of common beliefs, values, and expected behaviors, whereas climate refers to feelings, perceptions, and thoughts about an organization (Thomas, Ward, Chorga, & Kumiega, 1990). Social-climate scales are useful for indicating problems that contribute to worker dissatisfaction and lack of productivity. Cultural assessment focuses on understanding how workers in an organization will behave in different situations (Flarey, 1991). Analysis of both work group ideologies and the extent of cultural homogeneity is necessary for organizational change to succeed.

Culture is a broad and powerful force based on values that manifest themselves in behavior. Deal and Kennedy (1982) describe culture as a broad, subtle, and powerful force consisting of patterns of behavior. Because most innovations impact the way individuals interact with each other, communication patterns and interpersonal interactions will undergo cultural changes. Culture is also a subtle force involving basic assumptions and shared meanings, which are usually hidden in the subconscious. Therefore, culture is not typically obvious to the casual participant, but is inferred or communicated informally to new members of a group by what seasoned members do and say. Group members will determine and strongly embrace solutions to shared problems. Stories, myths, rituals, and ceremonies that are symbolic of shared values and beliefs may distort reality and perpetuate conflict between organizational and personal goals. As different cultural behaviors combine to form a group's distinctive cultural pattern, leaders who are facilitating change must be aware of each group's uniqueness and how and why group behaviors may or may not change.

Because culture depends on an individual's ability to learn and transmit knowledge to subsequent generations, individuals and groups may differ significantly in their perceptions of an organization's culture. Preparing for a comprehensive cultural change requires an initial step of developing an overall, or superordinate, organizational goal, that includes spiritual, or significant, meanings and shared values compatible with the organization's members (Pascale & Athos, 1981). An extensive assessment of the organizational culture and climate must be conducted to identify the existing internal and external environment, including the competition, diverse customers, mix of services and personnel, technology, and fiscal resources. Managerial ideas for change are not likely to materialize if the work group culture is not carefully considered. Identifying values will determine congruency between personal and organizational beliefs and subsequent behavior patterns.

Creating and maintaining the strong and positive culture required in a quality organization is accomplished via various means. Distinguishing highly visible heroes who personify the values of the organization will assist in setting standards for performance. A cultural network of quality-conscious individuals, both clinical and administrative, is needed. These individuals will serve as role models, leaders, and teachers. Communication, social contacts, work, management, and recognition rituals characterizing important activities within the organization all serve to dramatize the values of the organizational culture. These data, transmitted by individuals via formal and informal channels of communication, will clearly define the existing culture and its congruence to the ideal culture needed by quality organizations.

A distinguishing quality of successful organizations is a visible belief system — a culture shared by staff and managers alike. A living, quality culture is created when thoughts, ideas, attitudes, and deliberate behaviors become automatic reactions to opportunities to solve problems for the purpose of continual improvement. Because workers are an intrinsic component of the service rendered in health care, it is essential that the cultural environment optimizes staff and organizational capability to accomplish the mission and vision. All managerial, structural, and operational innovations rely heavily on people processes. The power to effectively deliver high-quality services resides within individual providers who recognize the benefits of collaborative relationships.

Preparing for a comprehensive cultural change requires a redefinition of quality — from a strictly externally focused definition to an internally focused, value-based definition. Internal and external perceptions of quality provide the foundation for maximizing resources and effectively managing patient-care outcomes and consumer satisfaction. A customer focus permits members of the organization to define their respective customers, to define their collective meaning of quality, and to strive for continuous improvement. Accomplishing such a significant paradigm shift requires comprehensive and continuous education from the top down and the bottom up. Desirable educational emphasis includes TQM concepts such as communication, decision making, interdependence, collaboration, the ability to capitalize on the diversity of individuals, and work as a system. Continuous Quality Improvement requires a blending of cultures that mature and develop over time.

Collaborative Team Building

An inside-out process is needed to implement quality improvement. While top management may strongly support the initiative, making the paradigm shift to collaborative teams also requires the support of middle management, employees, physicians, and volunteers. Effective teamwork has been the central focus of team and organizational theorists for the past sixty years. Quality-improvement teams, however, are different from other task groups and committees in their purpose, leadership, membership, training, procedures, dynamics, and duration (Mosel & Shamp, 1993). Effective quality-improvement teams are able to:

1. share the same vision and goals

2. plan channels of communication

3. demonstrate mutual respect

4. exhibit successful problem-solving skills

5. manage conflict and disruption (Parsons & Murdaugh, 1994)

Skilled change agents (outside consultants *and* well-trained internal employees) must understand the differences between group process and team development. It is desirable that the change agent has expertise in creating tension for change so that individuals:

• believe process improvements are essential

• help identify improvements to the existing process

• develop the plan for change

• monitor process improvement efforts

The monitoring process will utilize evaluation data to ensure that the improvements become **benchmarks** for future review. Successful evolution through this transformation stage and the process of unfreezing of old and refreezing of new organizational values and culture, requires extensive education, support, and management.

Health-care organizations are highly differentiated, encompassing a variety of staff, educational backgrounds, special interests, **stakeholders**, and professional orientations and perspectives. These differences may create obstacles to interdisciplinary collaboration. Yet, in order for the processes of work effectiveness to be clearly defined and continuously improved, intra- and interfunctional collaboration and integration must occur. Total Quality Managment clearly focuses on external customers, such as patients, families, and payers. The ultimate quality of care or service, however, is determined by how well the internal supplier/customer relationships are developed. When employees begin to think of themselves as suppliers serving internal customers and **customers** of internal suppliers, relationships expand and mature. As barriers are broken and turf battles cease, trust and respect promote a collective spirit. Employees become colleagues and valued customers along a chain of processes that ultimately benefits both the internal and external customers.

Physicians are also both customer and supplier; therefore, they must be involved in the very early stages of the TQM process if continuous improvement in patient care is to occur (Berwick, Godfrey, & Roessner, 1990; McEachern, Schiff, & Cogan, 1992; O'Rourke, 1992). The physician's sense of responsibility is usually to the patient rather than to the institution. Physicians involved in TQM (whether through employment in an organization with semi-autonomous groups, involvement in private practices under self-governing medical models, or as clinical experts in medical centers) share a common thread with others; they want to provide quality care to their patients while benefiting their own work lives.

Physicians will participate in CQI as they come to recognize its value in promoting high-quality and more efficient and cost-effective care. Because the scientific approach is taught in medical school, physicians may readily accept the CQI process when dealing with endemic daily system problems that directly impinge on their ability to deliver quality care to their patients. Other more challenging issues are patient complexity, which creates significant medical uncertainty over the best diagnosis and treatment patterns for common medical conditions and procedures. A second issue relates to treatment for what is medically necessary or appropriate — one dimension of quality which is expected for third-party reimbursement.

The strong loyalty that physicians show their peers makes peer review difficult. Peer review among physicians is also difficult because there is limited agreement on a fixed standard of care that is easily discernible to all. Peer review based on integrated data collection is, therefore, of considerable benefit. Studying practice patterns on all activities by establishing both numerator and denominator data for all practitioners in a department or service (see Chapter 24) is much more useful than selecting only one critical process out of context. Using the former approach, clinically credible data-based information that is useful and accessible is made available. Total Quality Management tools such as care mapping, critical pathways, and guidelines, can be used for a system review of care. This review negates the former stance of assigning blame for deficient processes, thus leading to important positive organizational relationships. Although not a replacement for clinical judgment, practice guidelines (or practice parameters) based on outcome data have become a cornerstone of the CQI efforts of many health-care organizations (Kelly, 1993).

The deployment of an organizational change process driven from the top down, and requiring acceptance by successive layers of the organization, may not be accepted by many physicians. Physicians are educated and trained as independent professionals; they are taught to be critical thinkers. They may not be pleased with, or even familiar with, the organizational structures within which they practice. It is simply not possible, however, to mandate a new way of thinking and managing patient care without physician support. It is desirable for organizational leaders to choose physician TQM participants who are respected for their clinical skills and who are key to the organization's success. It is vital to consider physician needs regarding improvement of patient care and subsequently to incorporate their suggestions into the transformation process.

The ability to develop and maintain effective teams that include all practitioners (including physicians), administrative and support staff, and patients is a prerequisite for TQM success. Organizations traditionally have been designed around functional areas or disciplines, such as nursing, medicine, rehabilitation, and pharmacy. A hierarchical decision-making model has been employed, whereby issues are resolved by managers and their superiors. Ineffective decisions frequently have resulted because of indirect involvement in the issues, errors in translation, time constraints, inability to understand all processes involved, and focus on individual departments rather than on the flow of work across departments or disciplines.

Total Quality Management's emphasis on interdependence of the diverse activities involved in providing health-care services requires integrative thinking by cross-functional teams. Teams that cross traditional hierarchical lines are not limited to supervisors representing various functions or to subordinates who report to a common supervisor. Interdependencies promote team decision making which brings a greater sum total of knowledge and information to group deliberations.

With an appreciation of the system each member is responsible for improving, a skilled leader can help members develop a clear, shared vision for the organization and identify changes that will maximize the effects of resources applied toward improvement. The diversity of disciplinary and functional perspectives facilitates team-member understanding of expectations of other areas of service. This helps the team identify and plan simultaneous changes that optimize the entire system. In addition to recognizing their dependency on each other, team members must recognize their dependency on materials, equipment, environment, and methods to do their work. Adjusting to the notion of interdependence puts competition, with all of its attending tension and anxiety, in a different perspective; the power of cooperation and collaboration increases in value.

The success or failure of TQM rests heavily on people processes such as **multidisciplinary** teams, horizontal organizational design, point-of-service customer relations, and other managerial, structural, and operational innovations. While time must be spent determining broad managerial innovations and philosophies and new structural arrangements, equal effort must be dedicated to assist employees in appreciating the knowledge and skills needed to do collaborative work. Team success is promoted when individuals are able to manage themselves both as individuals and as members of a team. Team success is further enhanced when members understand how each others' attitudes and behaviors impact others (both positively and negatively). When individuals deal with conflict constructively, they become comfortable crossing traditional hierarchial lines of authority. It is important that all team members be treated as adult learners with knowledge, experience, and a need for self-esteem. Team members will be nurtured by a feeling of being needed.

TEAM DEVELOPMENT

Senge (1990) describes the team as a microcosm of the organization; a small system similar to the larger organization, which has unique communication patterns, cultural norms, and political agendas. Team learning is the process of aligning and developing the capacity of a team to create results that members truly desire. The team needs skills to think insightfully about complex issues and to take innovative, coordinated action. Because greater knowledge is gained by involving all employees, basic requirements for leaders include communication skills. These skills include listening, giving and receiving feedback, asking questions, and teaching. Meeting skills (such as the ability to formulate of ground rules for dialogue and discussion, and to facilitate group decision making) are also important.

Implementing CQI modalities is beneficial to an organization only if there exists a long-term commitment to the process. Unless physicians, senior administrators, and middle managers are willing to eliminate controlling practices related to group decisions, raising expectations of nontraditional team members may lead to distrust and deterioration of morale. Bice (1984); Laffel and Blumenthal (1989); Batalden and Buchanan (1989); and Ferguson, Howell, and Batalden (1993) have suggested ways to avoid the difficulties associated with cross-functional group decision-making efforts.

To ensure that nontraditional, cross-functional teams consistently make high-quality decisions, leaders must assist in choosing the teams, including selecting membership in appropriate workable numbers. Teams are most successful when they are comprised of members who need one another to do their work. Team size is determined primarily by the group's ability to gather the data needed to determine the cause(s) of a problem, identify solution(s), and monitor progress. It is desirable that individuals who have current firsthand knowledge of the process under consideration, regardless of their positions in the organizational hierarchy, be involved on the team. Heterogeneous groups with nontraditional members frequently can provide more creative solutions to quality problems than can homogeneous groups consisting of only senior-level managers.

Healthy levels of conflict allow more opportunities for improvement to surface. The collaborative leader welcomes diversity and, consequently, must be skilled in conflict management. Team members should have relationship-building skills that will allow for disagreement without denigration of team members. Effective leaders also recognize differences in behavioral and social styles of members. The ability to modify one's behavior to accommodate the styles of others optimizes the functioning of the system. Also, team members are likely to be intrinsically motivated when work assignments are compatible with their behavioral styles. When a behavior is disruptive to group work, focusing on the behavior, rather than the individual with the behavior, is the most constructive action.

Collaborative problem solving attends to the legitimate concerns and needs of all participants within given constraints. This type of problem solving searches for solutions that recognize the highest-priority concerns. Historically, power relationships have strongly influenced decision making in health care. Even today, physicians tend to hold the dominant position in multidisciplinary teams. Physicians generally focus on curing patients; administrators tend to focus on the bottom line; nurses emphasize caring for patients and their families; clerical staff are faced with scheduling problems; other staff members give attention to support activities that make the system work. Physicians have frequently been successful in implementing designs or programs that do not consider these other viewpoints. In contrast, the integrative approach explores the interests of all team members and attempts to seek solutions that incorporate high-priority values and enhance the quality of the group decision. (See Chapter 8 for a detailed discussion of interdisciplinary teamwork.)

In the past, intuition has often served as a basis for decision making; CQI, however, requires that all decisions be data driven. Pertinent and adequate data from multiple perspectives, whether the problem is operational or clinical, helps dissipate conflict and facilitate win-win solutions. Voluntary self-censorship may occur in groups with a strong sense of camaraderie. Another type of response called "group think" may occur when members limit their discussion and seek only information that supports the majority of group members. In both situations failure to consider the external environment and larger organization is likely to cause faulty decision making. While intragroup conflict is a means of integrating several differing, yet equally valid, opinions, managing excessive personal conflict between group members is important to future work. It is critical to separate the problem from the people in order to minimize long-term damage to relationships.

CONCLUSION

The health-care industry can learn from other industries. Reich (1991) implies that the rules by which we will operate in the twenty-first century are already emerging. The new emphasis on interdependency requires the skills of systems thinking. Evidence already exists of transition from the traditional high-volume, mass-production economy to an economy that embodies customized, high-value processes. The subsequent notion of enterprise webs, such as networks, partnerships, strategic alliances, and other various arrangements, promote an integrated health-care delivery system. Further, there is a need for individuals to "add value" to the services they provide. Health-care services are provided through the collaboration and cooperation of multiple, interdependent entities with a common purpose of providing appropriate, cost-effective and efficient care that meets the needs and expectations of the patient and family. Appreciation for this system of work is the foundation that underlies continuous improvement.

Quality-improvement and problem-solving experimentation by team members promotes the capacity to collaborate by engaging in teamwork and seeking out mutually beneficial solutions. Instead of placing blame when something is found to be dysfunctional, the problem becomes an opportunity to improve. In many organizations this is a totally new mind-set. Whether teams are established to address intra-organizational or clinical issues, or whether they span different organizations in order to address interorganizational problems, maintaining focus on a superordinate goal is critical for success. It is important to create structures that support both the vision and guiding principles that leaders profess. Evidence of these structures and principles are reflected in the organization's policies, procedures, reward systems, and emerging traditions.

An organization's fate rests in the hands of its leader (Locke, 1992). Effective leadership requires motives and traits, knowledge, skills, ability, and above all, the capacity to implement a vision. Transformational leadership occurs when individuals become engaged with one another in such a way that both leader and follower raise each other to higher levels of motivation and morality. They develop a singleness of purpose that is grounded in the vision of the organization.

Although organizations may provide different services and require employees with various skills and abilities, the overriding questions to be asked are, "What can actually be done to improve patient care?" and "What can be done to improve coordination and collaboration between disciplines/services/departments/organizations to improve patient care and work lives?" A shared appreciation of interdependencies promotes a new basis for communication, improved outcomes, and an improved approach to organizational change. A shared vision fosters change as an integral part of the strategic plan. This change will focus on the leader's vision for a health-care delivery system that will be a societal force for disease prevention and improved health for the community. By streamlining internal operational systems for admitting, caring for, and discharging or referring patients to other segments of the health-care delivery system, the interrelated issues of access, cost, and quality will be addressed.

The impetus for TQM often is the desire on the part of customers, payers, and employees to be associated with a quality institution. As the health-care industry becomes immersed in the principles and practices of TQM, as have other industries, a common language will emerge. The health-care enterprise will be driven by the fundamental soundness of quality. Providers working with customers in a TQM environment will stabilize cost levels, and health-care services will be purchased in a quality-based competitive market. Everyone is seeking value for their health-care dollars. Business will be conducted only with quality providers who demonstrate effective outcomes. Satisfaction will always influence the equation of *Value = Outcome and Cost!*

REFERENCES

Arnold, W. (1993). The leader's role in implementing quality improvement: Walking the talk. *Quality Review Bulletin, 19*(3), 79–82.

Batalden, P., & Buchanan, E. (1989). Industrial models of quality improvement. In N. Goldfield & D. Nash (Eds.), *Providing quality care* (pp. 133–159). Philadelphia: American College of Physicians.

Berwick, D., Godfrey, A., & Roessner, J. (1990). *Curing health care: New strategies for quality improvement: A report on the national demonstration project on Quality Improvement in health care (1st ed.).* San Francisco: Jossey-Bass.

Bice, M. (1984). Corporate culture and business strategy: A hospital management perspective. *Hospital and Health Services Administration, 29,* 64–78.

Caldwell, C. (1993). Accelerator and inhibitors to organizational change in a hospital. *Quality Review Bulletin, 19*(2), 42–46.

Cesarone, D. (1993). Vision, mission, and values: Putting it together. *Quality Review Bulletin, 19*(2), 47.

Crosby, P. (1979). *Quality is free: The art of making quality certain.* New York: McGraw-Hill.

Deal, T., & Kennedy, A. (1982). *Corporate cultures.* Menlo Park, CA: Addison-Wesley.

Deming, W. (1986). *Out of crisis.* Cambridge, MA: Massachusetts Institute of Technology.

Donabedian, A. (1980). *Exploration in quality assessment and monitoring: The definition of quality and approaches to its assessment* (Volume I). Ann Arbor, MI: Health Administration Press.

Ferguson, S., Howell, T., & Batalden, P. (1993). Knowledge and skills needed for collaborative work. *Quality Management in Health Care, 1*(2), 1–11.

Flarey, D. (1991). The social climate scale: A tool for organizational change and development. *Journal of Nursing Administration, 21*(4), 37–44.

Jaeghers, S. (1991). TQM: A CEO's perspective. *The Quality Letter, 3*(8).

Juran, J. (1988). *Juran on planning for quality.* New York: Free Press.

Kelly, J. (1993). Implementing practice parameters. *The Quality Letter, 5*(5), 28–29.

Kritchevsky, S., & Simmons, B. (1991). Continuous Quality Improvement: Concepts and applications for primary care. *Journal of the American Medical Association, 266*(13), 1817–1823.

Laffel, G. (1993). How professionals view their patients. *Quality Management in Healthcare, 1*(2), v–vii.

Laffel, G., & Blumenthal, D. (1989). The case for using industrial Quality Management science in health care organizations. *Journal of the American Medical Association, 262*(2), 2869–2873.

Lewin, K. (1947). Frontiers in group dynamics: Concept, method and reality in social science, social equilibria and social change. *Human Relations, 1*, 5–41.

Locke, E. (1992). *The essence of leadership: The four keys to leading successfully.* New York: Lexington Books.

McEachern, J., Schiff, L., & Cogan, O. (1992). How to start a direct patient care team. *Quality Review Bulletin, 18*(6), 191–200.

McLaughlin, C., & Kaluzny, A. (1994). *Continuous Quality Improvement in health care: Theory, implementation, and applications.* Gaithersburg, MD: Aspen.

Milakovich, M. (1991). Creating a total quality health care environment. *Health Care Management Review, 16*(2), 9–20.

Mosel, D., & Shamp, M. (1993). Enhancing quality improvement team effectiveness. *Quality Management in Health Care, 1*(2), 47–57.

O'Rourke, L. (1992). Involving physicians in Continuous Quality Improvement: Removing barriers and building successes. *The Quality Letter, 4*(4), 2–9.

Parsons, M., & Murdaugh, C. (1994). *Patient centered care: A model for restructuring.* Gaithersburg, MD: Aspen.

Pascale, R., & Athos, A. (1981). *The art of Japanese management.* New York: Alfred A. Knopf.

Reich, R. (1991). *The work of nations: Preparing ourselves for 21st century capitalism.* New York: Alfred A. Knopf.

Schein, E. (1985). *Organizational culture and leadership.* San Francisco: Jossey-Bass.

Senge, P. M. (1990). *The fifth discipline: The art and practice of the learning organization.* New York: Doubleday Currency.

Thomas, C., Ward, M., Chorga, C., & Kumiega, A. (1990). Measuring and interpreting organizational culture. *Journal of Nursing Administration, 20*(6), 17–29.

Ziegenfuss, J. (1993). *The organizational path to health care quality.* Ann Arbor, MI: Health Administration Press.

ADDITIONAL READING

American Nurses Association. (1991). *Report on case management by nurses* (Congress of Nursing Practice, pp. 1–63). Kansas City, MO: Author.

Bader, B. (1992). *Rediscovering quality.* Rockville, MD: Bader & Associates, Inc.

Burns, J. (1978). *Leadership.* New York: Harper and Row.

DeBack, V. (1991). The National Commission on Nursing Implementation Project. *Nursing Outlook, 39*(3), 124–127.

Joint Commission on Accreditation of Healthcare Organizations. (1990). *Agenda for change.* Chicago: Author.

Kramer, M., & Hafner, L. (1989). Shared values: Impact on staff nurse job satisfaction and perceived productivity. *Nursing Research, 38*(3), 172–177.

Melum, M. M., & Sinioris, M. E. (1993). Total Quality Management in health care: Taking stock. *Quality Management in Health Care, 1*(4), 59–63.

Perlman, D., & Takacs, G. (1990). The 10 stages of change. *Nursing Management, 21*(4), 34.

Peterson, M., & Allen, D. (1986). Shared governance: A strategy for transforming organizations. *Journal of Nursing Administration, 16*(1), 9–12.

Robinson, N. (1991). A patient-centered framework for restructuring care. *Journal of Nursing Administration, 34,* 29–34.

Michael R. Bleich

CHAPTER *19*

Implementing Continuous Quality Improvement

INTRODUCTION

Health-care-organization leaders who want to implement **Total Quality Management (TQM)** principles and **Continuous Quality Improvement (CQI)** methods will need to manage in new ways. Leaders must know that using TQM principles and CQI methods to improve work processes and achieve a quality-oriented culture requires dedication, involvement, and self-confidence. This transformation also calls for willingness to expand leadership boundaries beyond the traditional hierarchical approaches taken in most organizations. The transformation is from an industrial model, wherein workers understand only their singular part in how an organization's work is achieved, to a systems model, wherein workers understand how what they do contributes to the whole system.

In quality-driven organizations, leaders understand how all the major functions in the organization perform in order to meet or exceed customer expectations. They use their conceptual skills to design and re-engineer work to achieve the aims of these functions with the help of empowered employees who contribute input into the design process. Managers hire workers who understand and are committed to knowing that what they do impacts the outcome of the service being provided. All of this requires management commitment, passion, and courage to retool the organization internally to align with customer expectations and desired clinical outcomes. The external goal is to create improved relationships with suppliers of services, products, and information needed to fulfill services consistent with the organization's mission.

Leaders in the quality field contend that TQM is not just another program; yet there are those in health-care organizations who have been lured into quality initiatives by the charm of their programmatic elements. This chapter addresses the commitment required to transform an organization into a total-quality environment and introduces strategies to plan for this transformation.

BACKGROUND

Health-care executives traditionally have demonstrated business acumen but have had limited experience in the actual "product" of clinical care and service functions. Leadership activities have centered on gains in facilities, finances, and new services.

In the spirit of Frederick Taylor and other pioneers of the industrial age, hospitals and other health-care organizations were subdivided into "departments" according to body systems (respiratory care or cardiovascular services, for example) or technology (nuclear medicine or laboratory services, for example). The burgeoning growth of technology has required an increasing number of highly specialized practitioners who are able to perform specialized examinations and procedures, but who often are unable to comprehend how the patient as a whole person is affected by the outcome of their work; or who are unable to identify with the systems and other personnel who are involved in getting the patient to the technology. Rather than specialized services being brought to the patient's bedside, the patient frequently is required to go to the area of specialization to receive services.

Health care has been directly influenced by the dominance of American industry over other countries since World War II. At a time when mass production and a lack of global competition allowed the United States to maintain an unparalleled lead in the world economy, social policy was introduced to increase access to health-care services through Medicare and other entitlement programs. In fact, the industrial techno-revolution expanded and brought about the use of this technology into the health-care arena. The cost for employers to provide health care as a benefit for workers and their families was relatively inexpensive. The need and desire for, as well as the dependency on, health care expanded in this environment.

While mass-production and expansion orientation continued in America, the world economy began to shift. Other countries began to tap into the American dominance in the marketplace by focusing on quality. Although the genesis of creativity continued to be American, other countries demonstrated an ability to improve systems to generate superior products. As American industries began to compete from a less strategic position in the global marketplace, concern began to mount over the cost and quality of health care. As costs escalated, so did the degree of regulation; thus began the quest to limit access to care, assure clinical outcomes, limit the growth and utilization of high technology, and shift health-care services from hospitals to less expensive treatment centers.

This brief sketch presents a challenging scenario for health-care providers who want to provide care into the next century. The consumer demand for health-care services has grown to enormous proportions; the success of health-care technology has generated more treatment options; the dollar resources to invest in health care are increasingly restrained; consumers are willing to seek health care in alternative settings; and industry can no longer bear the expense of health care as a benefit. These factors coupled with unemployment and the predominance of entry-level workers in the workforce mean that a growing number of Americans do not receive even basic health care.

As the United States reconfigures its health-care system, it is becoming evident that cost factors must be balanced with quality services. The quality movement and the science of **Total Quality Management (TQM)** (described in Chapter 5, Total Quality Management in Health Care) furnish health-care providers with the methods to examine their mission, functions, processes, and outcomes, and begin to control costs by eliminating waste and rework. TQM also provides the tools to examine methods of work design, pursue enhanced relations with external suppliers, and focus on real versus perceived customer needs and wants. As reform progresses and integrated health networks form, services can be provided in the most appropriate low-cost settings; integrated health networks also will provide additional opportunities to streamline systems and processes that are essential to patient care.

Three types of quality must be balanced. *Clinical quality* is determined by health-care experts, physicians, nurses, pharmacists, therapists and others who make clinical decisions and determine the clinical methods and approaches to achieve desired health-related outcomes. *Patient-driven quality* focuses on the patient's experience with health-care systems and providers, and focuses on caring, communication, and concern. *Economic* or *finance-driven quality* is a measure of organization and practitioner-specific achievement in meeting clinical and patient-driven quality in the most cost-favorable manner (Cunningham, 1991). The use of TQM and CQI methods can achieve the necessary balance among these perspectives on quality.

THEORETICAL/CONCEPTUAL ORIENTATION

Committing to TQM and implementing CQI requires an orientation to, and applied experience with, several theories and their associated concepts. Leaders will be challenged to deepen their understanding of these and other emerging theories as quality initiatives are implemented within health-care organizations.

Key Concepts

There are several key concepts and theories that are foundational to the process of bringing about an organizational transformation that is focused on quality. The following section presents an overview of selected concepts and theories that are either explicitly or implicitly related to this organizational quality transformation.

QUALITY

There are a number of definitions of **quality**, including Crosby's "conformance to requirements" and "doing things right the first time" (1980), Deming's variance management through production of what the market expects (1986), and Juran's focus on "fitness for use" (Juran & Gryna, 1993). As mentioned previously, in health-care settings a definition of quality must encompass three dimensions: clinical, patient-driven, and finance-driven.

LEADERSHIP

Leadership is required to constantly assess and define the organization's mission, purpose, and goals. *Transactional leadership*, which requires a symbiotic relationship between leaders and their constituents, is required to improve existing processes; whereas *transformational leadership* is required to inspire *new* actions and events

(Burns, 1978). (See Chapter 20 for a detailed discussion of the qualities and tasks of leadership.)

If a quality-improvement initiative is to transform an organization, its leaders must: commit to current knowledge of their products, services, and functions; ensure the presence of working leadership to coordinate people, systems, and technology; establish clear job roles and performance expectations that include elements of clinical competency and teamwork; and remove procedural barriers when opportunities to improve systems and processes are evident.

Harrington (1987) notes essential behaviors for leaders to demonstrate in order to exert leadership in an environment where total quality is desired. Leaders must:

1. share power and responsibility
2. trust employees
3. receive training in problem solving and prevention
4. see work as a cooperative effort between themselves and their constituents
5. accept a system of decentralized decision making
6. believe that the contributions of each individual are necessary to derive best possible solutions
7. implement employees' suggestions when feasible
8. provide an environment that promotes loyalty
9. recognize group accomplishments
10. recognize all parties who contribute to a fully participative system
11. accept participation as a long-term management style that may not produce immediate results

CUSTOMERS

Customer definition and orientation is central to the continuous-improvement process. Melum and Sinioris (1992) define a **customer** as "anyone who receives and benefits from the product of an organization's labor" (p. 58). This includes recognition of both internal and external customers. **Internal customers** are those departments or individuals who are in the line of receiving information or services to carry out key functions; **external customers** include patients, referring physicians, payers, and regulators.

It is imperative that health-care providers interact with their customers in order to measure expected and perceived satisfaction with services. Frequent and consistent methods to measure customer satisfaction are essential to CQI. It is through measurement that comparison is possible and the organization can determine its course.

PROCESS

A **process** is a series of defined steps that, when executed in a planned, sequential manner, yields an **outcome** desirable to the customer. The key to CQI is for an organization to know its key functions and the processes that support each function. For example, in a hospital setting, patient education may be a key function that meets patients' expectations of being informed about procedures, disease entities, and the like. A hospital may have several processes that support this function. In one situation, formal one-to-one diabetes education is needed; the process will define how the request for education is received, how it is communicated to the provider, how the education is offered and documented, and how the outcome of the teaching will be measured. In another situation, patient education is provided over a closed-circuit television system; this "process" may intersect with the process used in the first example, but will have different components due to the use of electronic systems.

Berwick and Plsek (1992) identify a process as having six elements:

1. a sequence of actions
2. something passed along that sequence, changing as it moves
3. customers — those who depend on the process
4. outputs — what the process makes, with its salient characteristics to customers
5. suppliers — those who give the process what it needs
6. inputs — what comes from suppliers, with its salient characteristics

When **standards** are developed to describe customer expectations and define the steps in a process, it becomes possible to examine **variation** in the process. Controlling variation in processes designed to meet customer expectations induces quality.

Key Theories

There are several complementary theories that contribute to the successful implementation of CQI. These theories are complementary because each one in and of itself would not comprise a total-quality environment.

GENERAL SYSTEMS THEORY

According to Yura and Walsh (1983), general systems theory provides a framework for "dealing with complex societal, human, structural, and organizational problems and the changing relationships inherent within and among them" (p. 72). Each system has a purpose, defined functions that identify key services to meet customer expectations, and processes that reveal the interrelationships needed to secure the operations essential for the system to meet its objectives. As such, general systems theory provides the structure to examine the health-care organization as a whole entity, with each of its component parts. In this way the relationships among the component parts can be studied and managed.

According to the laws of general systems theory, several factors influence an organization — its purpose, development, and survival.

- Decisions are determined by interaction among various constituents who influence the organization
- Continuous interactions produce a dynamic state with infinite possibilities for the organization
- The evolution of an organization will move from a less to a more differentiated state
- Dynamic interaction between organizations and the environment will increase the complexity for both
- Systems will evolve to higher states of order, differentiation, and probability

- As open systems, organizations will self-differentiate, take in energy, information, or other resources, and return them to the environment

- Feedback on an organization's output will be used to adjust, correct, and accommodate interaction with the environment. (Duncan, 1978; Griffith & Christiansen, 1980)

General systems theory is useful in TQM for two reasons. First, it denotes the importance of using organizational performance information from external sources to adapt key functions, systems, and processes. This information influences the viability of the organization. Second, it promotes understanding organizations as a systems within and among other systems.

In order to think and act with a systems orientation, certain skills are required. Senge (1990) describes these necessary leadership skills:

- *Seeing interrelationships, not things; processes, not snap shots.* To continuously improve the organization, the emphasis must always be placed on the *context* in which events occur, and where the opportunity rests to improve an organizational system.

- *Moving beyond blame.* Most organizational issues result from systems problems rather than people problems. Leaders and constituents must address problems together.

- *Distinguishing detail complexity from dynamic complexity.* Leaders must stay focused on the nuances and subtleties of environmental changes so the organization maintains its responsiveness to customer needs (dynamic complexity) as opposed to getting mired down in operational detail (detail complexity).

- *Focusing on areas of high leverage.* Rather than trying to improve every aspect of every organizational function, the focus should be on those functions and processes that will yield the highest leverage for the organization. All functions and processes are not created equal.

- *Avoiding symptomatic solutions.* Examine the root cause of the problem, usually within the process itself, rather than focusing all energy on a short-term solution to the symptom.

There is a growing science of information available on systems thinking that has useful implications in the field of quality science. Tools that promote an understanding and application of systems theory include *brainstorming tools*, to promote qualitative and quantitative awareness of whole systems ("soft" versus "hard" data); *dynamic thinking tools*, to examine interrelationships and articulate systems issues within organizations over time (cause and effect analysis); *structural thinking tools*, to isolate and examine organizational variables for decision-making purposes; and *computer-based tools*, to allow for simulations, policy analysis, and the consequence of decision making (Kim, 1990).

VARIATION THEORY

Quality science is also closely tied to the pioneering work of Shewart and Deming — statistical theory of variation. Statistical control provides a mathematical description of a physical state, such as that associated with a function or process within an organization (Shewart, 1986). Through statistical forecasting, it can be determined whether an organization's processes are in control, that is, whether the processes are meeting the specifications of the customer in an efficient and effective manner. Deming (1986) was able to isolate **common cause variation** as the fluctuation generated by the design of a process. **Special cause variation** was isolated as a unique variable, generated by something or someone outside of the defined process. These isolating factors allow leaders to focus their energies on improving systems by examining the source of the variation.

As stated above, variation analysis is possible only as the result of measurement of a physical state. In health care, the physical state is measured in terms of clinical outcomes or by monitoring the processes that assure outcomes. Measurement of quality in health care requires careful consideration and the use of **indicators** that are reliable and valid. Patient-sensitive indicators may relate to untoward clinical results, functional status outcomes, patient satisfaction, success rates, or physiological parameters. Process-sensitive indicators may relate to timeliness of staff intervention, the sequence and performance of interventions, and the comprehensiveness of techniques and therapies used to provide care. (See Chapter 24 for a detailed discussion of indicators.)

CHANGE THEORY

Change theory allows for the ultimate application of general systems theory and variation theory. Change theory recognizes that when a system is in a state of disequilibrium, something needs to be done to restore it to a state of relative equilibrium. The essence of change theory is identifying symptoms, isolating the root cause of the problem within a process (or as a "special cause," when applicable), and acting on resolution of the problem.

Change theory represents the need for constant interaction between the change agent and the constituents who will be affected by the change process. In Lewin's (1947) classic work, the change process is described as unfreezing the current situation, moving to a new level, and refreezing the group at the new level. While this seems simplistic, given the current state of knowledge regarding human motivation, it represents basic principles that can be applied in the effort to continuously improve organizations:

- Without awareness of the need to improve, there will be no desire to change.

- When a state of awareness is reached where buy-in occurs among all constituents, a vision is needed to establish the standard for what will become. Quality improvement becomes possible when staff are compelled through vision to move from the current state to the new desired state. Standards will need to be agreed upon before successful change.

- When the process has been planned to achieve the new standard, the behavior of all constituents must support the new standard. Measurement of the improved processes must be ascertained on a regular basis to see if the standard has been achieved. If not achieved, an analysis must be performed to determine if the variation is a result of the process or other special causes.

APPLICATION TO PRACTICE

In order for the theoretical aspects of CQI to have meaning it is important to consider their application to practice. The section that follows emphasizes the practical considerations necessary for the successful quality transformation of any health-care organization.

Leadership Commitment and Practice

Without the commitment of the governing body, senior management, and all other organizational leaders to the principles of TQM and CQI, it is impossible to influence an organization's culture to accommodate the values of customer orientation, continuous improvement, cross-functional work teams, and decentralized decision making. The commitment to quality ideally is driven by the governing body itself via the support it provides for senior managers to enact methods to transform the existing organization. Support takes the form of establishing mission and vision for the organization; becoming educated in quality concepts and principles; seeking and promoting senior managers who have a participative-management style; and providing capital, material, and human resources for the strategic and operational improvements that will arise from the quality initiative.

Another function of the governing body is to receive and act on quality-related information regarding the organization's key functions and processes. Too often, governing bodies are still committed only to acting on the financial performance indicators of an organization's success. For balance, the governing body must actively seek information on the performance of organizational systems and processes as it relates to customer outcomes. Clinical and patient-satisfaction indicators will need to be added to the governing body's data set for their review and action.

Yet another function of the governing body is to oversee and approve the organization's quality-planning initiatives. The strategic plan of the organization should include specific elements related to the quality-transformation process. Quality improvement requires structures to support the coordination and measurement of quality, and job roles and responsibilities to carry out strategic directives to achieve quality improvement.

The commitment of senior managers and other organizational leaders to CQI should not be underemphasized. In addition to the expectations already mentioned, organizational leaders are challenged to: commit to acquire knowledge and skills in systems thinking; exert leadership to improve key functions and processes from a systems perspective, rather than from the traditional departmental viewpoint; and demonstrate skill and competency in problem-solving methods, basic and advanced statistics, and the use of other quality tools.

Quality Planning

To convert an organization to an environment of continuous improvement is a formidable task that requires initial and ongoing planning efforts. Too often the initial quality plan centers only on the programmatic element of staff development (which focuses on team functions and the use of quality tools). A more realistic plan centers on significant strategic objectives: assessing the organization's culture for change (see Chapter 18); examining its information-systems capacity; determining leadership competency in problem solving and leadership willingness to engage in participatory management; and evaluating the functions and processes that are stable enough to begin improvement activities.

VISIONING
The quality plan begins with a brief and compelling vision statement. This statement should set the tone for creating the desire to enhance the organization's ability to meet or exceed customer's expectations. In addition to the vision statement, the key values of the organization are often stated, defined, and operationalized through quality-improvement activities, and are included in the quality plan.

ASSESSING
Quality planning continues by initiating assessment activities centered on reviewing *techniques* to improve the processes of work; determining the context of work by examining the organization's *culture;* and understanding the needs of the people who depend on the organization by assessing the organization's *alignment* with external and internal customers (Berwick & Plsek, 1992).

A framework based on the principles of quality science is useful in achieving this assessment and ensuring a comprehensive and organized review. Two examples of frameworks commonly used to conduct initial readiness assessments are the Malcolm Baldrige National Quality Award Criteria and Deming's 14 Points. (See Chapter 5 for details.) For future planning and evaluation purposes, it is desirable that the assessment be written. When the assessment is complete, the organization will have identified its key product lines, functions, and patient populations; the type, location, and accessibility of clinical, patient-driven, and finance-driven information; the roles and responsibilities of staff who provide quality services; the type and effectiveness of committees that support quality functions; the clinical approaches for providing patient care; the development and use of clinical standards of care and practice; the ability of the organization to coordinate services and provide "seamless" care; and the relationship of the organization to suppliers, payers, regulators, and other health-care providers in a defined community.

MODEL SELECTION AND PROGRAM DESIGN
Planning for the implementation of the quality initiative requires establishing a direction that will ease staff acceptance of and adaptation to the quality transformation. The first step in establishing direction is selecting the most desirable problem-solving/continuous-improvement model. All models are similar in terms of the outcomes they attempt to achieve; semantics and processes, however, differ from model to model. Staff needs with regard to semantics and processes should, therefore, be considered when choosing a model. Examples of problem-solving models include Deming's PDCA cycle (plan-do-check-act), the Joint Commission's Framework for Improving Performance (design, measure, assess, improve redesign), and Organizational Dynamic's FADE process (focus-analyze-develop-execute) (Joint Commission, 1993). The second step in establishing direction is choosing a method for selecting processes for improvement. The method should include a balance between *functional-improvement opportunities* (related to functions such as

patient education, discharge planning, medication usage, clinical record keeping, and admissions that cross all boundaries of patient types) and *clinical-improvement opportunities* (related to significant care-management opportunities associated with specific patient populations, such as the care of congestive heart failure, caesarean-section, and terminally ill patients).

Improvement activities are targeted for processes that are stable, important to the organization, and able to yield visible and practical results. This means that prior to improving care, customer demands and outcomes, and the methods to facilitate care, should be known and practiced. When a process is targeted for improvement, a charter is written to describe the nature of the improvement opportunity and its impact on the organization's strategic positioning. Improving a process needs to involve those disciplines and departments responsible for its success.

The system for recording and reporting improvement results should be carefully designed. Tools most commonly used in CQI initiatives include **flow charts, cause and effect diagrams**, line graphs, **histograms**, and descriptive statistics. The quality plan should indicate the nature of the tools to be used during the quality-improvement process, and some standard manner for reporting information so as to facilitate communication and organizational interpretation.

The organizational structures for initiating improvement activities and reporting results should be known to everyone in the organization. Most organizations will establish a quality council to oversee and coordinate quality activities. The functions carried out by the quality council are stated as a part of the quality plan. Functions commonly assigned to the quality council include: clarifying mission, purpose, goals, and values of the quality initiative; defining *quality* and other operative terms associated with QM; planning and prioritizing opportunities for improvement; establishing the educational and leadership-development plans; providing methods for team recognition; and evaluating the outcomes of the quality initiative in the context of organizational resource management, clinical outcomes, and cultural transformation.

Other structural elements in the quality plan include defining how functional and clinical teams will be established and operate to accomplish their charters, and defining how risk management, infection control, utilization management, and other organizational functions that provide information about quality care will be integrated into the quality initiative.

Quality-Improvement Teams

Regardless of how the quality-improvement process is planned and designed in an organization, cross-functional teams will need to be established in order to activate the improvement process. Cross-functional teams are organized so that through the collective participation of each member, each element of a function or process can be flow charted. In this way, the "whole" and the "parts" of a process are known and a complete cause-and-effect analysis is possible. Assembling the right people — those who intimately "know" their part in a process — promotes participation and buy-in, enhances whole-systems knowledge among the participants, and generates ideas for process improvements, such as the elimination of waste and rework.

Teams require education in order to support the quality-improvement process. First, they need to know how they fit into the quality-planning process (described earlier). They also need education — promoted as "just-in-time" training — in the areas of standard setting, process definition and documentation, problem identification and analysis, documenting improvement, measuring results, and **control charting**/sampling techniques.

The challenge for a team is to know its charter; have an intimate knowledge of the process being analyzed; have members who are expert in decision making, quantitative measurement, data collection and analysis, process control, and problem solving; and to facilitate so that members know what is expected of them, take active roles in the team process, are willing to share with and respect other members, and are able to stay on target to get the charter accomplished. Harrington (1987) suggests that roadblocks to effective team functioning and problem solving center on insufficient staff time to carry out processes right the first time; lack of problem ownership; lack of problem recognition, such as when errors become the way of life; either ignorance regarding the importance of problems or a belief that problems are insolvable; self-interest and blame seeking, rather than focusing on collective improvement; and a lack of perspective about the importance of quality in relation to factors such as outputs, schedules, and cost.

Effective team efforts are at the heart of quality improvement. Roadblocks to team success must be minimized. Through the efforts of teams, improvement initiatives can be identified so that individual workers can develop the knowledge, competence, and skill to carry out specific processes in an environment of support, recognition, and efficiency. (See Chapters 8 and 18 for more detailed discussion of teams.)

Information Management

Quality initiatives require the constant use of data; this data must be reliable, valid, and suited for its purpose in the quality-improvement process. As previously mentioned, ongoing data collection is necessary for assessing internal and external customers. The database for this aspect of quality improvement is aimed at broad analysis of the environment. The data needed to sustain a quality initiative, however, reaches far beyond that associated with broad-based assessment; specific organizational and clinical data is needed to support CQI.

Juran and Gryna (1993) state that an information system that is focused on quality is an "organized method of collecting, storing, analyzing, and reporting information on quality to assist decision makers at all levels. Such a system should be designed to be compatible with a company management information system" (p. 562).

For each function or process, elements must be selected for ongoing monitoring to determine if the system or process is meeting expectations. This requires the use of indicators. In health care, these are classified as **structure**, process, and outcome indicators. *Structure indicators* measure whether the right staff, equipment, or other resources are in place at the right time to activate a needed intervention or process. *Process indicators* measure critical points in the process or sequence of care and, therefore, measure staff interactions and actions. *Outcome indicators* measure the impact of the intervention or process on the customer, most notably, the patient.

In that structure indicators measure the availability of resources at the time a process is initiated, structure indicators are never useful in analyzing process or outcome factors. On the other end of the spectrum, when outcome indicators indicate a variance from the desired objective, analysis of all structure and process elements is required to determine the cause of the variation.

An excellent reference on developing a quality-focused information system is *The Measurement Mandate: On the Road to Performance Improvement in Health Care* (Joint Commission, 1993c). In this text three steps in developing a performance-measurement system are described:

1. establishing units of measure

2. developing and validating instruments capable of reliably quantifying the units of measure

3. using the instruments to produce measurement data for subsequent analysis and use in the performance-improvement process

These steps describe the process that must be used for determining quality indicators for each function and patient population served within a health-care organization.

Quality improvement requires extensive use of data in order to improve key functions. When a process is targeted for improvement, the nature of the indicators that will measure quality should be decided and planned. If the target of the improvement effort is to improve the timeliness of care, for example, the measurement of time will be the indicator of how the system is functioning. If the appropriateness of care is the aim of the improvement activity, some measure of clinical judgment against preestablished practice guidelines will need to be performed. If improved patient satisfaction is the aim, indicators tailored to measure patients' perceptions of care are required. The Joint Commission (1993c) suggests that indicators of quality fall into any of nine dimensions: efficacy, appropriateness, availability, timeliness, effectiveness, continuity, safety, efficiency, respect, and caring (see Chapter 17).

The resulting data set for a comprehensive clinical and organizational quality program will be very extensive. Because of the complexity of health-care organizations, computer systems will be needed to support data collection and analysis, tracking, and reporting. These systems will need to be able to both support a single patient-centered database and interface with functions such as pharmacy, laboratory, medicine, and nursing. The ability to review, manipulate, and abstract data "on-line" is also required. Data accuracy will be enhanced with point-of-care data entry. Databases will need to interface will external agencies, such as payers and regulators, for the purpose of **benchmarking** an organization's clinical and cost performance (Mowry, 1992).

EVALUATION

Too often, evaluating of the impact of quality efforts is done without predetermined objectives or the use of quantitative data. There are several dimensions of evaluation that should be considered. One dimension of measurement should be the impact of quality-improvement strategies on the workforce — that is, the degree to which quality behaviors are becoming part of the organization's norm. For example, one concept key to a quality culture is the use of quality data to drive day-to-day decision making. If this objective has been set, program evaluation should include measurement of the improvements and barriers to information management.

Another dimension of evaluation is measuring the impact of teams assigned to an improvement process. The indicators for the nine dimensions of quality (mentioned previously in this chapter) should be aggregated for overall improvement monitoring and evaluation. For example, if an emergency department were making a concerted effort to improve laboratory turnaround times so as to enhance timely diagnosis of patients, then a summative evaluation of overall improvement would help the organization to measure the impact of quality efforts.

An aggregate evaluation of the organization's ability to identify and respond to customers' changing requirements requires another data set useful for determining quality planning and priority-setting objectives. The data used for this dimension of program evaluation is usually generated on an annual or bi-annual basis via focus groups or structured surveys.

Ultimately, program evaluation measures the impact of an organization's culture in adapting to change aimed at continuous improvement for all of its customers. Culture change is evidenced through role clarification, job enhancement, and improved work flow.

ISSUES AND TRENDS

The adoption of TQM and CQI requires a major personal and professional commitment on the part of organizational leaders. In an age of health-care reform and increased regulatory expectations, it would be easy for leaders to fall prey to creating the *image* of being a "quality" environment without making a *commitment* to managing using quality-improvement concepts. Leaders are faced with the pressure of not wanting to appear disinterested in quality or in team-based management in an era of participation.

These factors create an interesting dilemma for health-care leaders. While the Joint Commission does not require a specific TQM program, it *does* require organizations to show continuous improvement and use data to substantiate the improvement of organizational performance. The Joint Commission is creating an indicator set for monitoring key patient populations, and it is only a matter of time before organizations will be able to compare their clinical performance with the clinical performance of other organizations.

Payers, including the government, are also requesting information regarding quality. For an organization to secure a managed-care contract through large industries or through third-party payers, a "report card" of the organization's quality performance is becoming a requirement. This information allows the payer to give patients attractive alternatives in terms of cost and quality of care. Although current report cards lack sophistication and in-depth information regarding quality of performance, data that is reliable, valid, and able to be used for comparative benchmarking will soon be required of organizations and will be a matter of public record.

Minimally, hospital leaders can accept that their organizations must include a matrix of key organizational functions and processes aligned with departments of service. If hierarchical organizational structures do not change, opportunities need to be created to begin cross-functional dialogue regarding how systems and processes work. Quality professionals and information-systems experts must be given the opportunity to create a comprehensive assessment and ongoing indicator base that can and will be used by the organization in decision making.

Add to these factors the emergence of a new generation of workers. Whereas workers of the past valued money, financial security, and ladder climbing, the new-generation workers want also to know that their contributions to the workplace matter in a larger, social context — that is, they want meaning from their work. The challenge for leaders, thus, expands. Quality of life, both in and out of the work place, is a goal to be achieved (Deutschman, 1990).

Leaders who face these realities will assess their leadership styles in the context of these changes. Ongoing education in the principles and tools associated with learning organizations and quality improvement requires exploration. This spirit of exploration and working knowledge of the health-care functions and processes within one's own organization becomes an education in and of itself. Ensuring that managers are in tune with customers, staff, and systems and have opportunities for leadership development is imperative in order to transform organizations. When these elements are in place, a decision to begin a broader transformation to a total-quality environment can be made.

CONCLUSION

There is increasing pressure on organizations to conform to a TQM style and to implement CQI. The decision to do so has far-reaching implications for the organization. It is important that trustees and senior managers make well-informed decisions about the methods used to transform an organization: avoid the pitfalls of cloning a program without knowing the customer base, work force, key functions and processes, and culture; do not fail to tie quality efforts to the organization's vision; and select projects that are strategic, manageable, and stable so that improvement is possible (Rosati, 1992).

Total Quality Management has enormous positive implications for organizational success. It is customer-sensitive, data-driven, and employee-engaging. Organizations that enter the arena of continuous improvement with the right attitude, skills, and knowledge, and that focus on improving the right aspects of service, should enjoy ongoing success in a changing market.

REFERENCES

Berwick, D., & Plsek, P. (1992). *Managing medical quality* (video series). Chicago: Quality Visions.

Burns, J. M. (1978). *Leadership.* New York: Harper and Row.

Crosby, P. B. (1980). *Quality is free: The art of making quality certain.* New York: McGraw-Hill.

Cunningham, L. (1991). *The quality connection in health care.* San Francisco: Jossey-Bass.

Deming, W. E. (1986). *Out of the crisis.* Cambridge, MA: Massachusetts Institute of Technology.

Deutschman, A. (1990, August 27). What 25 year olds want. *Fortune, 122*(5), 42–44.

Duncan, W. J. (1978). *Essentials of management* (2nd ed.). Hinsdale, IL: The Dryden Press.

Griffith, J. W., & Christiansen, P. J. (1982). *Nursing process: Application of theories, frameworks, and models.* St. Louis, MO: C. V. Mosby.

Harrington, H. J. (1987). *The improvement process: How America's leading companies improve quality.* New York: McGraw-Hill.

Joint Commission on Accreditation of Healthcare Organizations. (1993c). *The measurement mandate: On the road to performance improvement in health care.* Oakbrook Terrace, IL: Author.

Juran, J. M., & Gryna, F. M. (1993). *Quality planning and analysis* (3rd ed.). New York: McGraw-Hill.

Kim, D. H. (1990). "A palette of systems thinking tools." *The systems thinker, 1*(3). Communications (Reprint number 01303-1).

Lewin, K. (1947). Frontiers in group dynamic. *Human Relations, 1,* 34.

Melum, M. M., & Sinioris, M. K. (1992). *Total Quality Management: The health care pioneers.* Chicago: American Hospital.

Mowry, M. M. (1992, March). Computerization and quality. In M. Johnson, *The delivery of quality health care (series on nursing administration, volume 3)*. St. Louis, MO: Mosby Year Book.

Rosati, R. (1992, Winter). Total Quality Management: Is the love affair over? *Managing for Quality, 6,* 1–2.

Senge, P. M. (1990, Fall). The leader's new work: Building learning organizations. *Sloan Management Review, 32*(1), 7–22.

Shewart, W. A. (1986). *Statistical method from the viewpoint of quality control* (unabridged replication of original work published by the Graduate School of the Department of Agriculture, Washington, DC, 1939). New York: Dover.

Yura, H., & Walsh, M. B. (1983). *The nursing process: Assessing, planning, implementing, evaluating* (4th ed.). Norwalk, CT: Appleton-Century-Crofts.

ADDITIONAL READING

Anderson, C. A., Cassidy, B., & Rivenbaugh, P. (1991). Implementing Continuous Quality Improvement (CQI) in hospitals: Lessons learned from the international quality study. *Quality Assurance in Health Care, 3*(3), 141–146.

Berwick, D. M. (1992). The clinical process and the quality process. *Quality Management in Health Care, 1*(1), 1–8.

Betalden, P. B. (1993). Organizationwide quality improvement in health care. In A. F. Al-Assaf & J. A. Schmele (Eds.), *The textbook of total quality in healthcare* (pp. 60–73). Delray Beach, FL: St. Lucie Press.

Counte, M. A., Glandon, G. L., Oleske, D. M., & Hill, J. P. (in press). Improving hospital performance: Major issues in assessing the impacts of Total Quality Management activities. *Hospital and Health Services Administration.*

Gaucher, E. J., & Coffey, R. J. (1993). Organization and leadership. In E. J. Gaucher & R. J. Coffey, *Total quality in health care* (pp. 99–147). San Francisco: Jossey-Bass.

Jackson, F. (1994). The Baldrige/JCAHO Crosswalk. *Quality Connection, 3* (4), 4–7.

Joint Commission on Accreditation of Healthcare Organizations (1993a, November/December). A framework for improving the performance of healthcare organizations. *Perspectives* (insert), pp. A1–A6.

Joint Commission on Accreditation of Healthcare Organizations (1993b). *Implementing quality improvement: A hospital leader's guide.* Oakbrook Terrace, IL: Author.

Kibbe, D. C., Kaluzny, A. D., & McLaughlin, C. P. (1994). Integrating guidelines with Continuous Quality Improvement: Doing the right thing the right way to achieve the right goals. *Joint Commission Journal on Quality Improvement, 20*(4), 181–191.

Kratochwill, E. W., & Sonda, L. P., III (1993). Physician involvement. In E. J. Gaucher & R. J. Coffey, *Total quality in health care* (pp. 181–216). San Francisco: Jossey-Bass.

Peters, D. A. (1992). A new look for quality in home care. *Journal of Nursing Administration, 22*(11), 21–26.

Michael R. Bleich

CHAPTER *20*

Leadership and Development of the Quality Professional

INTRODUCTION

The role of the quality professional is rapidly emerging as the science of **Continuous Quality Improvement (CQI)** takes hold within the health-care system. As health-care organizations embrace **Total Quality Management (TQM)** as a leadership style, quality-professional positions are being offered. And opportunities for professionals in the field of **Quality Management (QM)** expand, so do the expectations placed on these highly specialized workers.

Gone are the days when the duties of a **Quality Assurance (QA)** worker consisted strictly of writing **standards**, selecting **indicators**, performing audits, and preparing reports for other professional disciplines to analyze. Today, the quality professional must demonstrate attributes consistent with other organizational leaders. Implicit in the role of the quality professional is a body of knowledge encompassing topics such as clinical outcomes, patient satisfaction, measurement, informatics, systems design, strategic planning, conflict management, and statistical analysis.

Within an organization, the quality professional is required to function as a consultant, motivator, educator, and systems designer. The focus of the quality professional is to assist management and staff in defining and influencing all key organizational functions and processes through the power of system and job design, measurement, **benchmarking**, and organizational redesign — all in the spirit of continuous improvement. It is envisioned that within a given organization, this type of quality specialist role will be kept in place until such time as the organization becomes mature enough to have these functions securely embedded in its culture. This chapter discusses the leadership behaviors and skills needed to function as a quality professional in the current rapidly changing health-care environment.

BACKGROUND

In health care, the emergence of workers whose jobs entailed measuring and monitoring aspects of **quality** occurred in conjunction with the emergence of medicine, nursing, and allied-health disciplines. Regulatory agencies, particularly the Joint Commission on the Accreditation of Healthcare Organizations (Joint Commission) and the government (through its Medicare program), played a major part in creating roles for workers who specialized in helping health-care professionals represent quality to regulators, payers, and consumers.

The Audit

Quality Assurance roles emerged rapidly after 1975. At this time the Joint Commission required hospitals to both continually evaluate patient care through the use of explicit, measurable **criteria**, and focus on expected patient outcomes. A nurse typically assumed the role of working with the hospital medical and nursing staff to guide them in developing criteria used to audit care. The criteria themselves started the movement toward developing institutional standards of care, and the quality worker was central to this organizational initiative. The primary skills needed by the QA nurse (beyond those needed for writing criteria) centered on extracting and analyzing data from medical records. The retrospective audits that were performed had large sample sizes laden with multiple **structure**, **process**, and **outcome** criteria. Not infrequently, the methodology used was research-based and retrospective, making its application to daily clinical practice impractical. The QA nurse generally was not required to implement the findings from these audit activities.

The Problem-Focused Era

The QA standard issued by the Joint Commission in 1980 moved hospitals — and the QA worker — to coordinate a hospitalwide approach to clinical problem solving. The QA staff were required to shift their focus beyond data collection, to problem identification, assessment, and resolution. This transition required the quality worker — still most often a nurse — to begin networking with key organizational leaders to effect change. Armed with useful clinical and organizational data, the quality worker was expected to document how change occurred and the degree to which clinical improvements were made. Using this problem-solving approach, QA still focused on monitoring the practice of *individual* professionals and how they created "problems" within the organization. Accordingly, the data was tracked back to individuals within the medical, nursing, or allied-health staff. When a problem was identified, the individual or individuals causing the problem were notified; change was effected through education or awareness-raising to suggest that the practitioner was individually responsible for the breach in quality. Rarely were the *systems* that may have influenced or caused the problem identified and improved.

Continuous Monitoring of Clinical Aspects of Care

The limitations of problem monitoring became apparent. By 1985 the Joint Commission issued standards that required organizations to monitor all *important aspects* of their services, rather than just problem areas. Based on this more comprehensive approach, quality workers had to achieve balanced reviews of key organizational services. They thus began monitoring these services for components of quality. Quality programs developed more systematic structures for monitoring and evaluation; increased the use of information systems and tracking methods to assure that needed action and follow-up occurred to resolve issues; and furthered the involvement of leadership and clinical staff in examining their services for quality performance. The aim was to assure continuous improvement of each medical and clinical service.

To determine the quality and appropriateness of care, the quality worker was now required to coordinate and use information from other committee and support functions that had significant amounts of information about quality issues. Infection control, utilization review, and safety/risk management data were incorporated into the **Quality-Assessment-and-Improvement (QA & I)** activities of the organization (Joint Commission, 1990). This requirement continued to expand the quality worker's role as an information worker.

Continuous Monitoring of Organizational Functions

Today, hospitals and other health-care organizations are adapting the principles of CQI to enhance their patient-care systems. This is a paradigm shift away from monitoring and evaluating *individual* performance to identifying, analyzing, and improving the key organizational *systems* that contribute to effective and efficient performance. The Joint Commission now focuses on how the governance, clinical, and support processes contribute in total to the organization's ability to meet desired patient outcomes (1990). Each organization is encouraged to improve its own performance through the activities promoted by the concepts of CQI, and to use comparative data to benchmark optimal performance.

The paradigm shift from traditional QA to CQI can be summarized in five points (Joint Commission, 1990). These points equate directly to the emerging leadership opportunities for the quality professional.

1. Traditional QA tends to be driven by external forces; CQI focuses on self-assessment and improvement. Therefore, the quality professional must provide leadership in designing quality initiatives based on patient-care needs and *all* of the factors that influence patient-care outcomes.

2. Traditional QA focuses solely on problems that have been identified; CQI focuses on important functions and the improvement of these functions, even when an overt problem does not exist. Therefore, the quality professional must provide leadership aimed at establishing a vision of improved services to meet patient-care outcomes, rather than focusing strictly on problem solving.

3. Traditional QA examines the parts of an organization along the lines of service departments; CQI examines systems of care extending beyond departmental boundaries and from the patient's perspective. Therefore, the quality professional must provide leadership in delineating key organizational functions and providing methodologies that reflect the patient/family perspective.

4. Traditional QA examines the quality of care provided by individual clinicians; CQI focuses on providing quality services and involving all roles and departments

that provide or interface with providers to accomplish patient-care objectives. Therefore, the quality professional must provide leadership by fostering involvement and consensus among all of the relevant roles and functions that influence patient outcomes both directly and indirectly.

5. Traditional QA can be effective based on *departmental* leadership and commitment; CQI requires sustained *organizational* leadership aimed at cultural transformation. Therefore, the quality professional must provide leadership that fosters cultural change and motivates staff at all levels of the organization to understand and embrace quality concepts.

This brief background highlights the dramatic changes that have occurred within health-care organizations as the science of QM has emerged. The role of the quality worker as a standard writer, data collector, and regulatory interpreter has evolved into the role of a professional who has mastered a specific body of knowledge and possesses expertise in influencing total organizational design. Today's quality professional must be an architect of organizational systems who is anchored to the mission of the organization and able to establish and sustain action toward a vision of excellence in meeting patient needs and clinical outcomes. It is expected that the quality professional will be an effective leader within today's health-care organizations; the tasks of leadership must be willingly and effectively acted on by individuals who fill this role.

THEORETICAL/CONCEPTUAL ORIENTATION

The need for leadership in health-care organizations is paramount to meet the fast-paced, information-driven, consumer-oriented demands placed on an organization's care-delivery system. The nature of work in health-care settings is complex; routines are varied, with multiple steps and decision points, and cannot be programmed in the traditional "top-down" manner. Add to this a workforce that is increasingly independent, is searching for meaning in the work performed, and is able to identify more with their chosen profession than the organization for which they work, and it becomes readily apparent that there are many challenges facing health-care leaders today.

Although numerous theories on leadership and management have evolved over time, the concept of *transformational leadership* is consistent with the felt needs in health-care organizations today and is congruent with the demands placed on the quality professional. What is transformational leadership and why is the quality professional drawn into this leadership arena? In his classic work on transformational leadership, Burns (1978) describes the differences between *transactional leadership*, where, through constituent exchange with a leader, *existing* work processes are improved, and *transformational leadership*, where constituents are inspired by the leader to *new* actions and events. The transformational leader is able to engage followers to move beyond their own self-interests by using highly interpersonal communication and role-modeling skills. The involvement with constituents is a critical characteristic of the transformational leader. Sayles (1993) contends that *working leadership* is needed if organizations are to make the fast-paced trade-offs needed to coordinate people, systems, and technology in complex and competitive markets.

Bennis and Nanus (1985) describe four leadership strategies used by transformational leaders. Transformational leaders gain the attention of their constituents through vision, transfer meaning through communication, establish trust through positioning, and stay involved with those they represent. Bass (1981) suggests that transformational leadership brings about a transformed fellowship by inspiring, legitimizing, guiding, enlarging the action arena, and effectively managing conflicts.

Transformational and transactional leadership as described previously are among the distinguishing traits of quality professionals. The quality professional in health care has the personal characteristics and knowledge of systems and people to influence constituencies to improve existing systems and create new systems, when needed. Transactional and transformational leadership are traits that can promote cultural change, but only when the quality professional:

- is passionate about and is willing to speak to the mission, purpose, and goals of the organization
- can establish vision by knowing how the parts fit into the whole of the organization
- has a working knowledge of the functions and systems that influence key organizational and clinical outcomes
- has knowledge of the line and staff people who work in the organization's key functions and systems
- understands the customer's satisfaction and clinical-outcome needs in terms related at least to issues such as safety, quality of life, functional status, and outcomes from medical diagnoses and diagnostic treatments and procedures
- is able to comprehend the interrelationship of technology and the people who make the systems work

It is only when the quality professional — along with other health-care leaders — embraces these personal characteristics and has knowledge in these areas of organizational performance that transformational leadership emerges to move the organization to a state of true CQI.

APPLICATION TO PRACTICE

The quality professional has an opportunity to enact a central leadership role in a health-care organization. This is particularly true when the organization allows the quality professional to deliberate in establishing its vision, purpose, and objectives. Although quality professionals rarely have line responsibilities for departments, there are multiple opportunities for professionals to influence systems, customers, and multiple levels of staff. Quality professionals must be able to distinguish themselves as leaders. Gardner (1990) suggests that leaders do this in six ways:

1. They think long-term, beyond daily tasks, to project future states of being.

2. They think of departments and services by grasping relationships of these smaller entities to the larger realities of the organization as a whole and to the macrosystem to which the organization is connected.

3. They reach and influence constituents beyond their jurisdiction or boundary; they network.

4. They emphasize vision, values, and motivation and are sensitive to incorporate their intuition when listening to those with whom they interact.

5. They have political skills to cope with conflicting requirements of multiple constituencies.

6. They think in terms of renewal, adapting to and creating new processes and structures needed to maintain efficiency and effectiveness in a dynamic environment.

What Gardner describes is a blueprint for leadership self-assessment and development for the quality professional. In a health-care organization embracing principles of TQM, the quality professional should be able to enact each of these leadership attributes.

The Tasks of Leadership

In order to operationalize leadership, the quality professional must engage in tasks that solidify the role. These leadership tasks are easily understood in the work opportunities present in promoting continuous improvement in the health-care organization. Although not intended to be comprehensive, Gardner (1990) describes nine tasks as significant to the transformational leader: envisioning goals, affirming values, motivating, managing, achieving workable unity, explaining, serving as symbol, representing the group, and renewing. Following is a description of each of these tasks, along with some implications for the quality professional.

ENVISIONING GOALS

A leader recognizes that organizational goals emerge from many sources, interprets the input from these sources, and then puts personal emphasis and interpretation on the goals.

The quality professional has access to a multitude of individuals in many layers and departments within the organization. This multidimensional access to staff is atypical of many positions within an organization. Additionally, it is not uncommon for the quality professional to have direct access to customers (patients, physicians, and payers), hearing their wants and needs. Finally, the quality professional has access to all levels of managerial staff in clinical, support, and business functions within the health-care organization. Envisioning goals becomes possible for the quality professional when the input is gathered from these sources and activated by defining a vision for the organization and its systems. According to Block (1987), this vision should be a statement that:

- comes from the heart; it should stretch the boundaries of what currently exists

- is possible for the organization alone to make about itself; it should be personal and identifiable to those who know the organization

- is radical and compelling; it should dramatize the organization's wishes for its future state

There are many opportunities for the quality professional to establish organizational vision, from establishing the vision for how a quality organization will function to establishing vision statements related to each organizational function and system. To this end, establishing vision is an ongoing process; for when an organization narrows the gap between its current reality and its desired state, a future vision will keep the organization in a state of growth.

AFFIRMING VALUES

In every excellent organization there are shared assumptions, beliefs, customs, and ideas that give meaning and serve to motivate its members to professional behavior; these are the values that drive organizational success. Gardner (1990) observes that "values decay over time. Societies that keep their values alive do so not by escaping the processes of decay but by powerful processes of regeneration" (p. 13).

Health-care organizations are complex and pluralistic; that is, there are multiple individuals with values that may not be clearly apparent to staff who operate systems and processes. Even values that are clearly articulated may be in conflict, such as the values associated with cost and quality.

The quality professional can use the opportunities presented in improving systems and dealing with issues of quality — some of which reflect negative or catastrophic clinical outcomes — to identify, clarify, and reinforce the values that undergird systems and events. As systems are improved and work roles and processes modified, the values driving these changes can be presented to staff in a manner that is inspiring, or at least clarifying.

MOTIVATING

The challenge of creating an environment that leads to motivating staff to improve and change, which is the essence of continuous improvement, goes beyond just the rational facts associated with making a change. In addition to **flow charts**, graphs, and statistical analysis — all of which appeal to the rational sense within people — the quality professional must have knowledge of the nonrational, interactive issues associated with the motives and motivations of staff.

Knowing how to motivate comes from truly understanding the staff who will be influenced by change. Staff must be understood both as individuals and as the groups they form. The quality professional and other organizational leaders must realize that the broader the educational, experiential, cultural, and personal backgrounds of the staff who work within a system targeted for improvement, the more knowledge, skill, and expertise the quality professional must have to congeal the diverse group toward the aim of the system. To achieve a high-performing system, each individual must know the components of the system, what is at stake if the individual's role in the system falters, and what the outcomes are to the organization and the patient. This reality underscores the importance of motivation as a leadership task; many "perfect" systems have been designed but never optimized because the leader failed to motivate the staff through knowledge of staff needs for involvement, reward, and recognition.

MANAGING

While all managers may not be inspired leaders, few excellent leaders do not get involved in managing. Gardner (1990) identifies five aspects of managing that leaders frequently engage in; these aspects are possible for the quality professional to introduce in any work setting by virtue of the nature of the position.

Planning and Priority Setting   The quality professional must engage in planning activities, because an organization must examine its systems and processes in light of its resources and strategic plans. Organizations that engage in improving processes that are not significant to their strategic plans find themselves investing tremendous resources in marginal or strategically insignificant improvements. In fact, it is possible to detract from an organization's mission with quality-improvement activities that are not in the mainstream of the organization's purpose. The quality professional has a major role in planning and priority setting so that the organization spends its resources improving the right systems and processes.

Organizing and Institution Building   All too often, a program or service meets its demise when the person responsible for the program leaves the organization. Quality programs are intended to transform the culture of an organization. It is essential that CQI becomes a shared process that is imbedded in the organization's culture. Institution building relates specifically to the broad ownership needed to successfully provide quality services. The quality professional must lead, avoiding possessiveness, through shared ownership for TQM.

Keeping the System Functioning   Systems function through the activities of allocating resources, staffing, directing, coordinating, developing key procedures, providing feedback, and evaluating key organizational and clinical outcomes. The quality professional can sometimes have a direct influence in keeping systems running, but also can encourage other organizational leaders to ensure that obstacles to system functioning are removed.

Agenda Setting and Decision Making   Leaders set organizational vision and goals, but visions and goals are acted on by agenda setting and decision making. Agenda setting and decision making can be detrimental to the organization unless agendas consistently reflect the organization's mission. Likewise, when decisions are made, they must contribute not only to day-to-day survival, but also to the organization's long-term vision. The quality professional is challenged to set agendas from current reality and promote decision making based on the organization's commitment to its mission (Fritz, 1989).

Exercising Political Judgment   It is important for quality professionals to realize the extent to which their role involves making political judgments to keep conflicts from blocking needed improvements. Making political judgments requires a sense of timing, excellent communication skills, a true commitment to the desired outcome, an understanding of the interests for the parties involved, and, when necessary, an ability to be decisive when all parties have been heard. Fisher, Ury, and Patton (1991) have developed a four-step method for demonstrating political sensitivity in problem resolution:

1. separating the people from the problem
2. focusing on interest, not positions
3. inventing options for mutual gain
4. insisting on using objective criteria

ACHIEVING WORKABLE UNITY

Most health-care organizations have been established according to the needs of the disciplines that they employ. Hospital organizations typically organize medicine, nursing, laboratory, housekeeping, respiratory therapy, pharmacy, and other services each as discipline-specific entities. Quality improvement does not focus on disciplines; it is centered on effective and efficient organizational functions and processes needed to meet patient-care needs. Consequently, success or failure of each department no longer exists; success or failure is now a product of how well the function or process operates in the total organization and how the function or process meets customer demands.

Achieving workable unity in a health-care organization requires the quality professional to take a leadership role by assisting department managers and staff to reorient to "success measures" that are process- rather than department-based. By creating opportunities for removing departmental barriers, the quality professional can dramatically impact the rate of organizational transformation.

EXPLAINING

Leaders are willing to explain, again and again. They know that what they are trying to achieve is important and represents the values of the organization and its constituents. Reality is that individuals and groups within organizations — no matter how good the system or process change may be — require opportunities to acquire and transform change as a part of their own being. Explanations — repeated frequently — help with transition issues (Bridges, 1991).

Most quality professionals are accustomed to explaining quality concepts to all levels of staff. Explaining quality concepts and organizational systems and processes must become a way of life for the quality professional. As more organizations go through substantive transformation, explaining will be ever part of the successful quality organization.

SERVING AS SYMBOL

The quality professional is a symbol of quality in an organization. The person who fills this role will be observed by many different external and internal constituents; the quality professional will be listened to for cues as to the congruence of "what is said" and "what is meant" in terms of the practice standards that are adhered to in the clinical setting. It is vital that quality professionals be aware of their symbolic roles in organizations and use the symbolic nature of the position with care.

REPRESENTING THE GROUP

The quality professional has ever-increasing opportunities to represent the organization and its practitioners to external constituents. In the managed-care market, quality professionals find themselves representing the scope and comprehensiveness of services to external payers. When "report cards" are issued, the quality professional is called on to interpret quality-related data to the community. Recently, the Joint Commission announced that it would make its survey data available to the general public. This has major implications for quality professionals, especially with regard to interpretation skills.

In today's health-care environment, quality professionals must expand their scope of influence far beyond that of internal customers and departments. The challenge is to know the scope of the quality program, know the meaning behind quality data, and interpret this data in a manner that fully optimizes the position of the organization to a variety of external publics.

RENEWING

The nature of organizational survival is constant renewal. The concepts that drive CQI are essential to see the organization through its life cycle. It is imperative that leaders understand the purposes of renewal:

> To renew and reinterpret values that have been encrusted with hypocrisy, corroded by cynicism or simply abandoned; and to generate new values when needed.
>
> To liberate energies that have been imprisoned by outmoded procedures and habits of thought.
>
> To re-energize forgotten goals or to generate new goals appropriate to new circumstances.
>
> To achieve, through science and other modes of exploration, new understandings leading to new solutions.
>
> To foster the release of human possibilities, through education and lifelong growth. (Gardner, 1990, p. 122)

The quality professional can renew the organization by involving staff and customers in the improvement process and releasing the talent and energy that evolve from those who have a vested interest in meeting customer demands. The continuous improvement process ultimately leads to jobs where workers can more fully exercise their skills and talents. By staying close to customers, staff members can stay in touch with their own purpose and can renew the culture within the organization.

Enacting the tasks of leadership requires a combination of physical and positive emotional energy; intelligence; a willingness to put oneself "on-the-line"; an eagerness to accept responsibilities; accomplishment in human relations, decision making and priority setting; self-confidence; trustworthiness; and adaptability. Although not fully developed in all individuals, these traits are needed by those who will lead health-care organizations into the next century.

ISSUES AND TRENDS

The quality professionals in most health-care settings have received their education and experience through informal means and on-the-job training. There is an obvious need for more formal educational development if the quality practitioner is to achieve professional status.

Kibbee (1988) writes that the quality professional must be a clinical information specialist with managerial, interpersonal, technical, and consulting skills. These skills align with the tasks of leadership previously identified. Norman, Randall, and Hornsby (1990) identify twelve broad areas for curriculum development for the quality professional. These areas include management information systems, risk management, quantitative methods, principles of management and financial management, QA program design, application of principles and standards, organizational change, standards and regulations, utilization management, legal and ethical questions in health care, basic concepts of health and disease, and the health-care delivery system.

Given the comprehensive scope of knowledge and the experience needed to enact a leadership role within a health-care organization, the quality professional is well served to possess a graduate degree as a requisite to full collegial functioning with other health-care leaders. Unfortunately, there are few graduate programs that focus on the leadership and professional development issues of the quality professional (Schmele, 1992). Most quality professionals have had to acquire knowledge without the benefit of an organized curriculum. Practical skills in writing standards, developing indicators, data collection and analysis, statistical quality control, and other essential competencies have been acquired without formal development and mentoring from other health-care professionals. Professional organizations that support professional networking have played a critical role in the development of quality leaders, who often are without peers within an organization.

The need for experienced professionals in the quality field is growing in all health-care settings, especially in the payer sector where the rapid evolution of managed care is leading to expanded opportunities for quality professionals. (See Chapter 30 for a detailed discussion of quality-management role redefinition.)

CONCLUSION

The role of quality professionals and the demands placed on these individuals are changing rapidly. Leadership qualities and a savvy understanding of quality-improvement theory and practice are requirements for these positions in health-care organizations. The quality professional is at the center of organizational influence and change. Essential attributes of this position holder include a well-developed knowledge of the aims of health-care both from a practitioner and a patient-satisfaction perspective; sensitivity to the nature of the health-care business; and expertise in the interpretation and implementation of quality systems from both a regulator and a payer perspective. A combination of knowledge and leadership attributes is needed to transform traditional organizations into quality-driven institutions.

It is possible to envision a future organization where management and staff have systems thinking, measurement, and regulatory interpretation intrinsically developed within their work roles. The transition to an organization where the right job is done right at the right time will only be realized, however, with the concerted effort and expertise of organizational leaders whose work it is to shape an empowered environment. The quality professional is one such leader who will serve as a catalyst for quality-transformed organizations through the leadership and work roles described in this chapter.

REFERENCES

Bass, B. M. (1981). *Stogdills handbook of leadership.* New York: The Free Press.

Bennis, W., & Nanus, B. (1985). *Leaders.* New York: Harper and Row.

Block, P. (1987). *The empowered manager: Positive political skills at work.* San Francisco: Jossey-Bass.

Bridges, W. (1991). *Managing transitions.* Reading, MA: Addison-Wesley.

Burns, J. M. (1978). *Leadership.* New York: Harper and Row.

Fisher, R., Ury, W., & Patton, B. (1991). *Getting to yes.* New York: Penguin Books.

Fritz, R. (1989). *The path of least resistance.* New York: Fawcett Columbine.

Gardner, J. (1990). *On leadership.* New York: The Free Press.

Joint Commission on Accreditation of Healthcare Organizations. (1990). *Primer on indicator development and application: Measuring quality in health care* (pp. 91–192). Oakbrook Terrace, IL: Author.

Kibbee, P. (1988). An emerging professional: The Quality Assurance nurse. *Journal of Nursing Administration, 18*(4), 30–33.

Norman, D. K., Randall, R., & Hornsby, B. (1990). Critical features of a curriculum in health care quality and resource management. *Quality Review Bulletin, 16*(9), 317–336.

Sayles, L. R. (1993). *The working leader.* New York: The Free Press.

Schmele, J. A. (1992). Teaching Quality Management: The graduate experience. In C. G. Meisenheimer (Ed.), *Improving quality* (pp. 260–281). Gaithersburg, MD: Aspen.

ADDITIONAL READING

Acquaye, M., & Schroeder, P. (1991). The nursing Quality Assurance coordinator: An evolving role. In P. Schroeder, *The encyclopedia of nursing care quality volume 1* (pp. 163–177). Gaithersburg, MD: Aspen.

Bennis, W. (1989). *On becoming a leader.* New York: Addision-Wesley.

Block, P. (1991). *The empowered manager.* San Francisco: Jossey-Bass.

Fromberg, R. (1988). *The Joint Commission guide to Quality Assurance* (pp. 10–15). Chicago, IL: Joint Commission on Accreditation of Healthcare Organizations.

Helgesen, S. (1990). *The female advantage: Women's ways of leadership.* New York: Bantam Doubleday.

Joint Commission on Accreditation of Healthcare Organizations (1994). *A guide to establishing programs for assessing outcomes in clinical settings.* Oakbrook Terrace, IL: Author.

Marriner-Tomey, A. (1993). *Transformational leadership in nursing.* St. Louis, MO: Mosby Year Book.

Parisi, L., Johnson, T., & Keill, P. (1993). The nursing quality professional: A role in transition. *Journal of Nursing Care Quality, 7*(4), 1–5.

Wellins, R., Byham, W., & Wilson, J. (1991). *Empowered teams.* San Francisco: Jossey-Bass.

PART V

QUALITY IN PRACTICE

Frances K. Masters
Amy S. Lesniewski
June A. Schmele

CHAPTER *21*

The Integration of Traditional Quality Assurance and Total Quality Management

INTRODUCTION

During the past five years, many health-care organizations with traditional **Quality-Assurance (QA)** programs in place have moved toward the adoption of **Total Quality Management (TQM)** to assist in reducing costs and improving customer satisfaction and **quality**. The separateness of the two processes is implied by references such as "bridging the gap," "providing linkages," "running parallel systems," and many other cliches. The purpose of this chapter is to explore the integration of QA, an already established system of assessing, monitoring, and improving quality, with TQM, a proactive, customer-driven, top-down management philosophy that encompasses the use of teams to continually improve work processes throughout the organization. (See Chapter 5 for a detailed discussion of the history and background of TQM.)

COMPARISON OF QUALITY ASSURANCE AND TOTAL QUALITY MANAGEMENT

Quality Assurance is defined as the classic or traditional program that health-care organizations have used to improve selected aspects of quality. During the past several years, however, QA usually has taken the form of a provider-specific, reactive program. For example, when standards were not met, blame was often placed on a single provider or service. Quality Assurance programs generally have been directed toward meeting external requirements, usually in the form of **accreditation** (such as Joint Commission on Accreditation of Healthcare Organizations [Joint Commission]); or **certification** by state or federal agencies (generally in order to qualify for external funding). This organizational motivation frequently has meant that most processes were viewed retrospectively. Often, a crisis-management response was precipitated as new mandates were placed upon an organization. These mandates or standards usually were defined by the outside accrediting or certifying agencies. (See Chapter 16 for a detailed discussion of regulatory mechanisms.)

The majority of QA activities are directed toward clinical care. Inherent in most QA programs are **structure, process,** and **outcome standards,** most often focusing on identified problem areas. These problem areas usually are selected from high-risk, high-volume, and problem-prone client/patient situations. For example, in a problem-prone geriatric population, patient falls may be considered high volume as well as high risk. Disorientation or confusion in a geriatric population specifies a problem-prone situation, especially when there is an environmental change such as hospitalization. Another example of a high-risk situation is when a teenage pre-natal patient experiences fetal distress. In order to deal with the aforementioned situations, QA standards are written to reflect the care that is to be given. **Criteria** subsequently are developed to use as specific measurable levels of compliance with the standard. The goal of QA, then, is to meet the preestablished standard. Once the standard is met, there may have been no further impetus to improve; thus the standard of quality is seen as a static goal. However, in the early phases of TQM, the formerly static goal may be moved incrementally to higher levels (see Figure 21-1).

With TQM, on the other hand, the standard is the starting point. It is assumed that the standard is being met and that there is a continual need for analysis and improvement, requiring the standard to be dynamic in an upward fashion. Thus, the original standard is the starting point and the new standard is the dynamic goal signifying continuous improvement as shown in Figure 21-1.

When taking a more in-depth view of the concepts of QA and TQM, the similarities and differences can most easily be determined by comparing the descriptors of each program. These descriptors are very effectively and succinctly compared by Gaucher and Coffey (1993), as shown in Table 21-1.

This table illustrates the similarities and differences between the key characteristics of QA and TQM. It is important to note that one process does not replace the other; nor are the processes mutually exclusive. The ultimate goal of both processes is the improvement of patient care; thus it seems reasonable, desirable, and cost-effective to integrate the two processes. (See Chapter 6 for a detailed theoretical comparison of the health-care quality model and the industrial model for quality.)

INTEGRATION OF QUALITY ASSURANCE AND TOTAL QUALITY MANAGEMENT

Integration can be defined as the forming or blending of separate entities into a new whole. The concept of integration might be envisioned as a continuum, beginning at a minimal level and evolving to complete integration. During the past several years many health-care agencies have implemented TQM with varying levels of sophistication. The information in the literature is sparse relating to the specifics of how to actually integrate QA and TQM programs. Many authors do agree that QA should not be discarded, but instead should be integrated (Green 1991; Marker 1992).

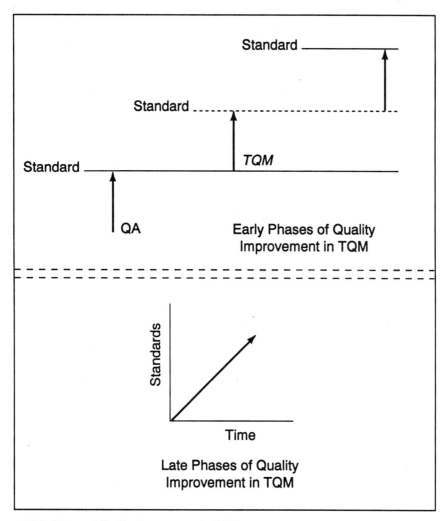

Figure 21-1 *Phases of Quality Improvement in TQM*

Table 21-1 • **COMPARISON OF TRADITIONAL QA AND TQM**

Characteristic	Traditional Quality Assurance	Total Quality Management
Purpose	Improve quality of patient care for patients	Improve quality of all services and products for patients and other customers
Scope	Clinical processes and outcomes	All systems and processes — clinical and nonclinical

Table 21-1 • **COMPARISON OF TRADITIONAL QA AND TQM** *(continued)*

Characteristic	Traditional Quality Assurance	Total Quality Management
Scope *(continued)*	Actions directed toward people studied	Actions directed toward process improvement
	Mandated by JCAHO and others	Optional, but in order to meet JCAHO performance measurement, some aspects of TQM needed
Leadership	Physician and clinical leaders; chief of clinical staff, QA committee	All clinical and nonclinical leaders
Aims	Problem solving	Continuous Improvement, even if no "problem" identified
	Identify individuals whose outcomes are outside specified thresholds — implies special causes	Addresses both special and common causes — most attention toward common causes
Focus	Peer review vertically focused by department or clinical process — each department does its own QA	Horizontally focused to improve all processes and people that affect outcomes
	Unacceptable few — education or elimination of those who do not meet standards	Improve performance of everyone, not just the unacceptable few
	Inspection	Prevention and design to improve the processes — then inspection to monitor process
	Outcome oriented	Process and outcome oriented
Customers and Requirements	Customers are professionals and review organizations — patient is focus	Customers are patients, professionals, review organizations, and others — everyone

Table 21-1 • **COMPARISON OF TRADITIONAL QA AND TQM** (*continued*)

Characteristic	Traditional Quality Assurance	Total Quality Management
Customers and Requirements (*continued*)	Measures and standards established by health-care professionals only	No long-term fixed standards — continuously improving standards established by customers and professionals
Methods	Chart audits Nominal group technique Hypothesis testing Indicator monitoring	Indicator monitoring and data use Brainstorming Nominal group technique Force field analysis Coaching/ mentoring Flowcharting Checklist Histogram/Pareto chart Cause and effect, fishbone diagram Run/control chart Stratification Quality function deployment Hoshin planning
People Involved	QA program and appointed committees Actions decided by committees appointed for specific periods Limited involvement	Everyone involved with process Actions decided by team of people familiar with process — no time period specified Total institutional involvement
Outcomes	Includes measurement and monitoring May improve performance of the few individuals addressed	Includes measurement and monitoring Improves performance of everyone involved in process

Table 21-1 • **COMPARISON OF TRADITIONAL QA AND TQM** *(continued)*

Characteristic	Traditional Quality Assurance	Total Quality Management
Outcomes *(continued)*	Creates defensive posturing	Focuses on process improvement — reduces threat to individuals, promotes team spirit, and can break down turf lines
		Includes QA efforts
Continuing Activities	Monitor for deviations from thresholds/standards	Monitor processes for deviations (QA) and to continually improve standards (QI)
	Follow up when there are special cause deviations	Follow up when there are special or common cause deviations

Source: From Total Quality in Heathcare: From Theory to Practice *(pp. 58–59), by E. J. Gaucher and R. J. Coffey, 1993, San Francisco: Jossey-Bass. Copyright 1993 by Jossey-Bass. Reprinted with permission.*

Experts suggest that it is desirable for preplanned integration and structural changes to occur early in the implementation phase of TQM so as to prevent duplication of work and reduce confusion (Anderson, 1990; Berwick, 1990). A study by Tindill (1992) substantiates the position of VA Chiefs of Staff to be supportive of early integration of QA and TQM programs. If the two processes are not integrated, it is likely that considerable overlap, rework, misunderstanding, and even power struggles will occur. Accrediting agencies such as the Joint Commission emphasize the value of building upon the strengths of existing QA mechanisms. (See Chapter 17 for a detailed discussion of the Joint Commission's perspectives.)

At the current time, some health-care organizations support totally parallel systems of QA and TQM with minimal or no integration, while others have developed completely integrated systems wherein traditional QA is subsumed into the broader concept of TQM. There are, of course, any number of varying degrees of integration between these two scenarios.

The continuum of integration most often is dynamic. Based on successes and failures, the degree of integration may or may not be sustained. It is sometimes necessary to go back to a previous level of integration to reassess and try a different strategy. Conversely, a success may cause a facility to surge ahead to the next level of integration.

The authors believe that the degree of integration will correlate positively with the degree of development or level of maturity of the TQM system in the organization. Further, the philosophy of the leaders may also facilitate or inhibit the growth or movement from one level of integration to the next. It seems self-evident that the most desirable position is one where the best aspects of both the QA and TQM processes are preserved as complementary to each other in an integrated system.

Because the ultimate goal of both processes is the improvement of health care, there is the expectation of a synergistic effect. For example, the gathering of data and the subsequent analysis of data are paramount to both processes. Freeland (1992) proposes that the integrated models should use data sources that are readily available, noting that only data that is relevant and meaningful should be collected. Similarly, staff who have been directly involved with the QA data gathering and other quality-management processes are likely candidates for a smooth transition to TQM.

The Use of Consultants

Instituting TQM in a health-care facility in an expert fashion may require an outside consultant. If this option is chosen it is desirable to use a consultant with previous health-care experience, because some industrial TQM experts may not be familiar with the health-care environment. Many of the principles previously discussed, however, can be applied universally, whether in industry or health care. In select health-care facilities, industrial engineers have functioned well in the role of consultant. It is noteworthy that many of the methods, tools, and techniques of TQM have long been known and used by industrial engineers.

The consultant's role in an organization is contingent on the specific agency's needs for guidance and direction. These needs are usually identified by agency leaders and mutually agreed upon by consultee and consultant. The timely use of a consultant can often prevent costly errors that can result from trial and error. The consultant can enhance and expedite the educational process. This includes training a designated individual or a select group of staff at the facility. This training ideally would consist of effective application of the TQM philosophy, tools, and techniques. The designated individual or group can assume the role of TQM expert(s) and continue guiding the facility to total integration after the consultant has gone.

Consultant roles are quite variable. For example, consultants may be called on to do organizational assessments; or during implementation of the TQM philosophy, consultants may be asked to help identify problems and problem solve with in-house TQM leaders. Consultants also may serve as objective sounding boards who see the big picture without becoming personally involved or invested in the outcome.

SELECT QUALITY ASSURANCE AND TOTAL QUALITY MANAGEMENT INTEGRATION MODELS

Although the literature discusses different models that integrate the concepts of QA and TQM, the goal of all the models is to improve quality. In addition, all of the quality-improvement models rely on the team concept to make them effective.

Each process-improvement project will have at least two assessment phases, each of which will include both data gathering and analysis. The first assessment phase includes the initial data collection for situational analysis, which may validate the need for subsequent improvement. After planning and implementing the improvement, the second phase of assessment (evaluation) requires additional data gathering to analyze and evaluate the improvement. Statistical methods of varying levels of sophistication are used in both phases to analyze the data and make it meaningful. The reader is referred to *Using Quality Improvement Tools in a Health Care Setting* (Joint Commission, 1992) for an overview of the various continuous-improvement models and methods. For purposes of this chapter three integration models are discussed in greater detail.

Joint Commission Ten-Step Process

Following the Agenda for Change (see Chapters 10 and 16), the Joint Commission suggested how the **Continuous-Quality-Improvement (CQI)** concept could be integrated into the frequently used Joint Commission Ten-Step Quality Assessment and Improvement Process (Joint Commission, 1992). Although the Joint Commission does not sanction this or any other specific model for CQI, many health-care organizations have found the Ten-Step Process to be a user-friendly approach. It therefore makes good sense to maintain and improve this familiar approach that emphasizes the ability to build on the strengths of traditional QA. Just as the first-generation model of the monitoring-and-evaluation process provided a useful tool for the implementation of QA, the second-generation Ten-Step Process provides staff with a familiar method to guide the transition from QA to continuous improvement. The integrated model uses the same ten steps of the original model but expands them. The following is a brief overview of the expanded process, emphasizing the changes.

> *STEP I — Assign Responsibility.* Not only is responsibility for QM identified, but emphasis is placed on the top-down commitment to continuous improvement. This top-down commitment ensures that the philosophy is given high priority. It follows that departmental or service lines will be crossed for purposes of team involvement when seeking opportunities for continuous improvement.
>
> *STEP II — Delineate Scope of Care.* The scope of care defines the customer population in relation to age, services provided, general customer expectations, and a general description of the group providing the services. Changes or additions include identifying **internal consumers** and **external consumers** in all departments. It is suggested that there be frontline involvement in determining the scope by using such tools as brainstorming, affinity diagrams, selection grids, and multivoting.
>
> *STEP III — Identify Important Aspects of Care.* Aspects of care are those areas deemed most important by the staff in relation to the customer population. They are usually service or group specific and are seen as opportunities for improvement that are high risk, high volume, or problem prone. The aforementioned tools can also be used by the frontline staff to determine the important aspects of care. When the aspects are identified, it is appropriate for the staff to prioritize them, based on the organizational mission.

STEP IV — Identify Indicators. Emphasis is placed on the interdepartmental formulation of objective and measurable criteria (**indicators**) that will show the degree to which the standards for each aspect of care have been met. It is desirable that there be frontline involvement in the development of these indicators, as well as feedback from patient and customer surveys. Patient-care indicators must reflect the current knowledge base and may be derived from such resources as standards of practice, standards of care, policies, and procedures.

It is noteworthy that the Joint Commission's Indicator Measurement System established in 1994 has identified three priority patient populations for the development of indicators: (1) patients having had a hospital stay after a surgical procedure under anesthesia, (2) delivered mothers, and (3) newborn babies. Ten rated-based indicators have been developed to serve as performance measures in the care of these specific populations (Joint Commission, 1993).

STEP V — Establish Threshold. The next step is the establishment of a **threshold** or trigger point beyond which the need for an in-depth evaluation of the area of deficiency is signaled. This step is facilitated by basic statistical tools that can be used to determine whether or not the threshold is met. For example, **run charts** and **control charts** are used as tools to identify the point at which the performance does not meet the desired threshold. **Sentinel events** or feedback from customers can also be used to trigger in-depth evaluations.

STEP VI — Collect and Organize Data. In addition to the usual collection and management of data, an integrated system entails the use of more formal data-management tools such as check sheets, run charts, control charts, **histograms**, **Pareto charts**, and **scatter diagrams**. Frontline employees frequently participate in collecting and managing data, which may add to their ownership in the quality-improvement process. (See Chapter 24 for a detailed discussion of data handling and TQM tools.)

STEP VII — Evaluate Care. All levels of staff, including various disciplines and departments (when appropriate), should be used to evaluate services. Data-management tools such as **fishbone diagrams**, brainstorming, and **flowcharting** can be used to involve staff in consensual problem identification, as well as in designation of areas for improvement. It is important that the focus for the improvement be on the work process or system, rather than on an individual or individuals.

STEP VIII — Take Action. Appropriate actions to improve care and service and/or to correct the root causes of problems should be directed by involved staff who have been empowered to take action to improve care and services. The action plan should be specific and identify the who, what, when, where, and how. This step is vital to establish the specific account-ability of the persons who are to carry out the plan.

STEP IX — Assess the Effectiveness of the Action. After follow-up intervention activities have been carried out as planned, appropriate staff begin the second assessment phase, using selected statistical tools to assess the result of the action that was performed to improve the service. This phase may also be called the evaluation phase. At this point a determination is made about the effectiveness of the action and the appropriateness of continuing the improvement cycle.

STEP X — Communicate Results. It is vital to establish and maintain regular reporting mechanisms for monitoring, evaluating, and reporting quality-improvement activities. It is desirable that these mechanisms include all appropriate staff throughout the organization. Therefore, quality-improvement information will be a necessary agenda item for staff meetings so that involved staff can benefit from receiving regular feedback.

In summary, the authors concur that the Ten-Step Process is a systematic and practical quality-improvement approach that is very amenable to the integration of QA and TQM. Further, some organizations may find it easier to adapt this model because the staff are already familiar with the process. Although the use of the Ten-Step Process has mainly been documented for acute-care facilities, it is useful in other types of health-care facilities as well.

University of Michigan Medical Center Model

The development of the University of Michigan Medical Center (UMMC) integrated model was spurred by the National Demonstration Project of Quality Improvement in Health Care. This model is discussed from the viewpoint of Gaucher and Coffey (1993). The UMMC model focuses on leadership, education, training, and incremental costs/benefits of TQM. The University of Michigan Medical Center anticipated several benefits that would result from integrating TQM with traditional QA. These benefits are enumerated by the following objectives:

- to define quality improvement of all care and services
- to expand quality to include both internal and external customers
- to redefine the scope of quality to include all work processes
- to place more emphasis on the use of data and statistical tools
- to change the goal of QA to become one of continuous improvement

The University of Michigan Medical Center leaders projected that TQM implementation would facilitate improvement of several areas. It was clear that some of these improvements would need to reflect changes in philosophy:

- Quality will not be defined only by QA indicators but also by indicators derived from customer surveys of patients, families, physicians, and suppliers;
- TQM will focus on the entire work process rather than just on the clinical performance of individual practitioners;
- Work processes will be analyzed using formal statistical tools and methods;
- There will be an emphasis on a positive approach to problem solving instead of the "bad apple" technique;

- The quality-improvement process will not be static, but will be constantly improved;
- The TQM approach will focus on improving work processes to build in quality rather than to inspect for the absence of quality.

According to Gaucher and Coffey (1993), the integration of QA and TQM began in 1988 and continues to the present. It has evolved through the following phases:

> *PHASE I.* Quality Assurance was independent of hospital structure and consisted of monitoring and evaluating high-volume, high-risk, and problem-prone areas. The QA process, led by clinical experts, was directed toward the review of outcomes of care.
>
> *PHASE II (Approximately two years).* The University of Michigan Medical Center began implementing TQM while maintaining QA as a separate program. The leaders were directly involved with both programs. The two programs, however, had different directors, monitored different aspects of care, and utilized separate surveillance mechanisms, techniques, and tools. The TQM program reviewed nonclinical situations, while QA monitored clinical aspects.
>
> The first steps of TQM implementation included the formulation of a definition of quality and the identification of both internal and external customers. The definition of quality was used to describe continuous improvement in terms that were meaningful to everyone in the organization. Many other philosophical changes were inherent in this new focus:
>
> - Everyone knew the mission and goals of the organization;
> - Goals addressed continuous improvement;
> - Frontline employees were members of the problem-solving team;
> - TQM education focused on teamwork and team-member involvement; thus, when processes were improved, the quality was built in.
>
> *PHASE III (Approximately two years).* The QA program began to use the TQM tools for data collection and management. The TQM experts started to use their skills in solving problems that were derived from the QA program. Quality Assurance liaisons were trained to become TQM facilitators and team leaders. To further provide for the integration, the leaders began by "combining the Plan-Do-Check-Act (P-D-C-A) process — a TQM technique — and the Standardize-Do-Check-Act (S-D-C-A) process — a QA technique" (Creps, Coffey, Warner, & McClatchey, 1992, p. 257). In S-D-C-A, a standard is established, implemented, and monitored. When compliance is not met and opportunities for improvement are identified, action for improvement is taken. If the process needs to be improved the P-D-C-A takes over. In P-D-C-A, the organization must have a "plan for improvement, implement the improvements, check and analyze the results and act on any changes the results indicate to fully implement the improvement" (Creps et al., 1992, p. 258).

PHASE IV. This phase involves the complete integration of QA and TQM. Problems that are identified through QA monitoring are used by quality-improvement teams as opportunities for improvement. The same leaders supervise and direct both programs. This model includes education and training, process identification, data collection and analysis, and actions to improve the processes.

Using the previously described approach, the UMMC has built on the strengths of its QA program and developed a strong management philosophy that continually improves patient care. The UMMC model, described in the writings of Marszalek-Gaucher and Coffey (1990) and Gaucher and Coffey (1993), is a major contribution to the field of TQM. The most recent book describing the implementation of this integrated approach to quality improvement, *Total Quality in Healthcare*, could very well become a classic in the quality-management field.

Hypothetical Model

The hypothetical model was developed from identification of the critical attributes of the previously described models, exploration of the literature, and the authors' own experiences. The critical attributes of this eclectic hypothetical model are as follows:

- customer driven
- proactive
- top-down management philosophy of quality improvement
- team approach
- continuous improvement of work processes
- use of existing QA data
- use of formal statistical tools for data management
- open communication

The hypothetical model to be described is based on the second-generation Ten-Step Joint Commission Process. This process, as previously discussed, has the potential for incorporation into most quality-improvement programs. The following discussion focuses on the various phases of implementation.

ORGANIZATIONAL ASSESSMENT

It is important to perform an organizational assessment to establish baseline data and pinpoint specific organizational needs through the identification of problems and opportunities for improvement. Various assessment tools are available. An organizational assessment, such as the one suggested by Gentling and Morrison (1993), can be used to examine the seven categories of the 1991 **Malcolm Baldrige National Quality Award**. These categories include leadership, information and analysis, strategic quality planning, human-resource utilization, QA of products and services, quality results, and customer satisfaction. Other agencies use tools such as the Quality Management Maturity Grid, which measures an organization's maturity in regard to quality matters (Schmele & Foss, 1989). A third assessment approach is the Innovation Quotient, which assesses five phases of managing organizational change. These phases are preparation, movement, team creativity, new reality, and integration (Manion, 1993).

The organizational assessment includes results of traditional QA as well as customer-satisfaction surveys. The results of the organizational assessment are vital to the development of an integrated program and are also helpful in selecting a consultant whose skills match the needs of the organization.

Implementation Plan

Many opportunities for improvement are identified through the organizational assessment. Based on organizational values, the opportunities can then be prioritized by a designated decision-making body or a TQM steering committee. Criteria for prioritizing might include opportunities that:

- impact a large proportion of the health-care organization's customers
- have the potential to be remedied
- could create a positive example of the TQM process
- have data readily available for problem analysis

In the hypothetical model, the hospital TQM steering committee is formed to guide the implementation process. The TQM steering committee functions as a formal decision-making body that guides the process of integrating QA and TQM. This six-to-twelve-member committee consists of the chief executive officer, medical director, chief operating officer, director of QA, and coordinator of TQM. Each service selects TQM steering committee members at large from their respective service steering committees. If there is a labor union, it is desirable for a union representative to be on the TQM steering committee.

During the development phase, early integration of QA processes into the TQM program is important. The TQM steering committee and other leaders of the organization will facilitate this integration by communicating how QA and TQM relate to each other and what the organizational configuration will be when integration of QA and TQM is accomplished. By discussing the similarities and differences of QA and TQM, the QA staff can begin to understand how the two processes fit together. In the early phases, it may be helpful if the QA and TQM staffs are cross-trained to become experts in both processes. The steering committee should also consider the availability of financial and human resources when planning for implementation. The combining of a traditional QA program with TQM offers more effective utilization of existing resources. When plans for implementation have been developed, the process can begin.

The TQM steering committee then surveys the employees to identify staff who are interested in serving on initial work-process teams, sometimes called *Quality-Improvement (QI)* teams. Team-member selection is based on previous or present involvement in QA, knowledge of the selected work process, availability of time, commitment level, and desire to be selected. Patient representation on the team is, of course, ideal. If this is not possible, however, teams can incorporate patient data from patient surveys or other sources.

Orientation and training of the QI team takes place before any general employee education. Following team training, problem identification is accomplished and the second-generation Joint Commission Ten-Step Process is then implemented. The team begins the process of gathering data that will be analyzed and used for problem solving and quality improvement. It is essential that the entire process of data-based decision making be evaluated for appropriate problem resolution and the actual improvement of quality.

APPLICATION OF THE HYPOTHETICAL MODEL

The following discussion describes the process that a medical center might use to integrate the TQM philosophy into an already existing traditional QA program. The proposed application is a hypothetical situation based on a combination of experience and suggested application from the literature.

Before any education or culture change can be attempted, an organizational assessment must be done. This will identify a number of problems and opportunities for improvement. Some of the most common areas identified by medical centers throughout the country are: patient education, employee reward and recognition, employee and visitor parking, patient waiting time in clinics, and clinical record retrieval.

For purposes of illustration, the opportunity for improvement discussed here is the process of patient education. Organizational rationale for selecting this particular process was that the process was viewed as easily improved, the QA data for at least twelve months already existed, and the patient-educational process was widespread throughout the agency. Within most organizations there are various levels of patient education. Examples of these are at the institutional level, where programs deal with every patient encounter; at the program level, where education focuses on diagnostic entities such as diabetes or hypertension; and at the unit level, where education is provided for specific patients such as those having had a total knee replacement.

After the decision is made to improve the process of patient education, the Patient Education Total Quality Improvement (PETQI) team will be formed. The hospital TQM steering committee will select the persons to fill the key PETQI team roles. These roles usually consist of a team leader, team facilitator, and a representative from the QM program.

The function of the team leader will be to provide content expertise in the area of patient education. The team leader will also have expertise in QM and can be a clinical nurse specialist, physician assistant, or some other specialist whose primary focus is patient education. The team leader will be responsible for providing direction and guidance to the team in matters of patient education. The team leader should be well organized and have a high tolerance for ambiguity, and must be capable of accepting and dealing with confrontation at the team level in order to accomplish team goals.

The team facilitator will provide process expertise and be someone who is not involved with the process being analyzed. This person will assist the team leader and other members to maximize the team process. The team facilitator also will monitor meetings to ensure that the rules of conduct are followed.

Although the membership of the team ideally will consist of no more than eight persons, it may be necessary to increase the membership to represent as many staff as possible who are directly involved in the work process of patient education. The members of the team will include various staff members who are involved in both inpatient and outpatient education and are interested and committed to improving the patient-education process. The representative from the TQM program will assist with the integration process and share QM expertise in problem solving and data management. Prior to the first team meeting, it is desirable that all members attend a team-building workshop.

At the first team meeting it is helpful to emphasize ground rules of conduct. These ground rules will eventually become the group norms and include such things as respecting each other, not interrupting while a member is speaking, responding to ideas rather than individuals, setting the time and place of meetings, setting the length of the meetings with adherence to stop and start times, and completing assignments on time.

After the group rules have been established, it is recommended that the group write a charter to define the quality-improvement goal and identify the customers and the patient-care requirements. The charter will also define the purpose, identify limitations, and specify how to assess the problem and how to measure the results. An example of a goal defined by the PETQI team might be as follows: "The goal of health education is to empower the patient, family and/or significant others to make informed decisions about and to take an interactive role in his/her health care" (Patient Education Committee, 1993).

Data-management tools will be helpful to facilitate purposive and orderly data gathering. For example, a flowchart outlining the current patient-education process will assist in identifying educational barriers or any other problems. The ideal desired patient-education process can then be outlined by a second flowchart incorporating the current knowledge base, available research, and the most effective patient-teaching protocols. The comparison of the two flowcharts and data from patient surveys will facilitate identification of problems such as limited or poorly organized patient-education programs, lack of material and human resources, and limited time availability to improve the process. The fishbone cause and effect diagram is an effective way to identify specific relationships that may have resulted in an ineffective patient-education program. The use of these and other tools will assist the team to isolate the cause of symptoms of dysfunction and help them identify specifically what needs to be changed.

At various time intervals, it is suggested that the team review the quality-improvement goals and accomplishments to be certain that they are doing what they set out to do. The development of a Gantt Chart or some other time-planning system is helpful in identifying goals and adhering to timelines. It is likely that there will be several months of weekly meetings and many lively discussions before the team is ready to make final recommendations.

The recommendations of the PETQI team may include such objectives as:

- accepting the definition and goal of patient education as defined by the team

- developing a medical-center policy assigning responsibility and accountability for patient-education functions

- budgeting for patient education

- completing staff education programs on patient-teaching skills

- prioritizing educational needs according to the most frequent DRG groupings

- developing patient-education resource guides

- increasing marketing of patient-education events/training to staff and patients

Recommendations need to be agreed on and prioritized in keeping with institutional values. These will then be presented to the hospitalwide steering committee for their concurrence. The hospital steering committee may also make additional recommendations. The selection of recommended activities for implementation will be based on the long- and short-term project objectives.

If the PETQI team is charged with carrying out their own recommendations, an updated quarterly progress report that tracks accomplishments will serve as a formative evaluation approach. This evaluation process may enhance project ownership.

Both patients and staff are expected to realize benefits from this QI project. Benefits may include improvement in structure, process, and outcome of patient education. Structure (resources) improvements may include such items as the addition of teaching materials, equipment, and facilities. Examples of process (activities) improvements would be additional or enhanced teaching activities and methods. Positive outcome (results) improvements may be demonstrated by evidence of increased patient knowledge and skills, which may be reflected in decreased readmissions.

Additional team-related successes may include the bonding of team members, team compatibility in further group work, improved group skills, effective communication patterns, and increased commitment of individual team members to quality improvement. After project completion, there are various options for the team members. They may continue as a patient-health-education committee, be dispersed to the hospitalwide steering committee, or serve on different subcommittees.

It is important to emphasize that the hypothetical model, or any other model of TQM/QA integration, needs to be adapted to the specific organization where it will be used. The hypothetical model was developed to identify and improve administrative and clinical processes, and, therefore, may not fit the specific needs of every organization.

CONCLUSION

While the hypothetical model may represent the ideal, it does not address all issues of controversy that arise when integrating QA and TQM. If certain underlying issues are not dealt with, integration may be slow or never achieved. While some interventions may not lead to a positive outcome, they should be viewed as a challenging, learning experience and an opportunity to improve the process. In all cases, QA and TQM should complement rather than replace each other.

It is noteworthy that a variety of TQM models have been developed to meet the needs of specific organizations. These models have been utilized successfully in various health-care institutions across the country to identify and improve administrative and clinical processes. There is no prescribed recipe for integration of the two processes, just as there are no easy answers to the questions that will arise. The process of integration, however, offers many benefits including improved work processes and customer satisfaction, reduction and elimination of rework and duplication, cost savings, and enhancement of the team concept with increased **multidisciplinary** problem solving. Perhaps the most desirable benefit of all, however, is that the whole will be greater than the sum of the parts.

REFERENCES

Anderson, C. (1990, November). *Introduction to statistical tools and techniques.* Presented at Joint Commission on Accreditation of Healthcare Organizations Third Annual Forum on Health Care Quality, Chicago, IL.

Berwick, D. M. (1990). Peer review and Quality Management: Are they compatible? *Quality Review Bulletin, 16*(7), 246–251.

Creps, L. B., Coffey, R. J., Warner, P. A., & McClatchey, K. D. (1992). Integrating Total Quality Management and Quality Assurance at the University of Michigan Medical Center. *Quality Review Bulletin, 18*(8), 250–258.

Freeland, B. (1992). Moving toward Continuous Quality Improvement. *Journal of Intravenous Nursing, 15*(5), 278–282.

Gaucher, E. J., & Coffey, R. J. (1993). *Total quality in healthcare: From theory to practice.* San Francisco: Jossey-Bass.

Gentling, S. J., & Morrison, J. P. (1993). Total quality within the VA healthcare system: A case study. In A. F. Al-Assaf & J. A. Schmele, *Total quality in healthcare* (pp. 288–290). Delray Beach, FL: St. Lucie Press.

Green, D. K. (1991). Quality improvement versus Quality Assurance? *Topics in Health Records Management, 11*(3), 58–70.

Joint Commission on Accreditation of Healthcare Organizations. (1992). *Using quality improvement tools in a healthcare setting.* Chicago: Author.

Joint Commission on Accreditation of Healthcare Organizations. (1993). I. M. system starts up with 10 indicators. *Perspectives, 13*(6), 1–3.

Manion, J. (1993). Chaos or transformation. *Journal of Nursing Administration, 23*(5), 41–48.

Marker, C. S. (1992). Total Quality Management and the Marker umbrella model for Quality Management, part II: An overview. *Aspens Advisory Nurse Executive, 7*(4), 5–8.

Marszalek-Gaucher, E. J., & Coffey, R. J. (1991). *Transforming healthcare organizations.* San Francisco: Jossey-Bass.

Patient Education Committee. (1993). *Patient education total quality improvement booklet.* Veterans' Affairs Medical Center, Oklahoma City, OK. (Available from Oklahoma City Veterans' Affairs Medical Center, Oklahoma City, OK 73104.)

Schmele, J. A., & Foss, S. (1989). The Quality Management maturity grid: A diagnostic method. *Journal of Nursing Administration, 19*(9), 29–36.

Tindill, B. (1992). *Evaluation of perceptions and attitudes regarding total quality improvement among Department of Veterans' Affairs Medical Center Directors and QA coordinators.* Unpublished master's thesis, University of Oklahoma, Oklahoma City, OK.

ADDITIONAL READING

Laughon, D., Ax, S., & Boyington, C. (1993). From unit-based Quality Assurance to multidisciplinary Continuous Quality Improvement in the coronary care unit. *Journal of Nursing Care Quality, 7*(3), 19–27.

Miller, S. T., & Flanagan, E. (1993). The transition from Quality Assurance to Continuous Quality Improvement in ambulatory care. *Quality Review Bulletin, 19*(2), 62–65.

Patton, S., & Stanley, J. (1993). Bridging Quality Assurance and Continuous Quality Improvement. *Journal of Nursing Care Quality, 7*(2), 15–23.

Ruden, J. C. (1994). The transition to Continuous Quality Improvement: A home care model. *Journal of Nursing Care Quality, 8*(2), 9–15.

Sherman, J. J., & Malkmus, M. A. (1994). Integration of Quality Assurance and Total Quality Management/quality improvement. *Journal of Nursing Administration, 24*(3), 37–41.

June A. Schmele
Avedis Donabedian

CHAPTER *22*

The Application of a Model to Measure the Quality of Nursing Care in Home Health

INTRODUCTION

The emergence of home-health care as a major alternative to hospitalization is evidenced by large-scale growth in home-health care, especially since the implementation of the Prospective Payment System (PPS) in 1983. This change has coincided with drastic shortening of hospital stays and a concomitant rise in the acuity of the homebound patient following hospitalization. The rapidly increasing elderly population has heightened the seriousness of the situation even more. In order to accommodate these changes, the demand for highly complex and skilled home care has burgeoned. A major responsibility for this care resides with the profession of nursing, because nurses are generally the major professional providers and managers of care in the home-health setting. In many instances, nurses are responsible for assisting the patient's family and/or significant others in providing highly complex care to the patient on a continual basis with only intermittent care from other health-care professionals and community resources.

These developments have heightened the concern of many about the **quality** of home-care services. Several years ago the classic *Black Box Report* by the American Bar Association (1986), presented to the Select Committee on Aging, emphasized the inadequacy of the present home-health-care system and the growing concern for the quality of care it provides. Key recommendations were to strengthen the content, increase the acceptability of **standards**, and increase consumer involvement. It was further recommended that there be increased **monitoring** and further research and data collection. Several years have passed since this report was presented, and the assurance of quality continues to be a major concern in the delivery of home-health care. Individual agencies frequently develop their own methods to measure and **evaluate** the quality of care, but it is well recognized that there is a lack of valid and reliable measuring tools that have generic applicability to various home-health-care settings.

The purpose of this chapter is to offer one such generic measure, describing the conceptual framework on which it rests (Donabedian, 1966, 1980), its antecedents (Schmele & Allen, 1990), and its step-wise development.

The chapter includes:

- the conceptual framework for defining and measuring quality[1]

- a discussion of the use of the nursing process as a framework for measurement, and the use of standards of care developed by the American Nurses Association (ANA) as a basis for measurement

- a review of select literature related to preexisting methods of quality in home-care nursing

- the step-wise development and testing of the *Schmele Instrument to Measure the Process of Nursing Practice in Home Health (SIMP-H)*

- a discussion of the operational quality-measurement approach

- a discussion of the use of the SIMP-H in research and service

CONCEPTUAL FRAMEWORK

The purpose of the following discussion is to define quality in health care, generally speaking; to describe the generic approaches to measuring quality; to describe the nursing process; and to show how each of these were used to develop assessment measures of the quality of nursing in home care.

The Meaning of Quality

It is useful to think of quality of health care as flowing from two sources: one is the science and technology of health care, the other is the application in everyday practice of that science and technology. The quality of health care that results from the confluence of these two sources can be conceived of as having a number of attributes that stand for, specify, and define the meaning of quality (Donabedian, 1990). These include:

1. *efficacy* — the ability of the science and art of health care to bring about improvement in health and well-being

2. *effectiveness* — the improvement in health that is achieved, or can be expected to be achieved, under the ordinary circumstances of everyday practice

3. *efficiency* — a measure of the cost at which any given improvement of health is achieved

4. *optimality* — the ability to obtain the most desirable balance of the costs of care against the consequences of that care

---

[1]See Chapter 4 for a detailed discussion of this topic.

5. *acceptability* — adaptation of care to the wishes, expectations, and values of patients and their families

6. *legitimacy* — conformity to social preferences as expressed in ethical principles, values, norms, mores, laws, and regulations

7. *equity* — the principle by which one determines what is just or fair in the distribution of care and its benefits among members of a population

The degree to which quality is or is not achieved with regard to its several attributes is judged by the extent of conformity to a set of expectations or standards derived from three sources:

1. the science and technology of health care, which determine what is achievable

2. individual values and expectations, which determine what is acceptable or desired

3. social values and expectations, which determine legitimacy

Which of the several attributes of quality deserve greater attention and how they are judged depends on what can be called the level and scope of concern. For example, when the focus of attention is the care provided to individual patients, it is the performance of health-care practitioners, in both its technical and interpersonal aspects, that is subject to the most detailed scrutiny. Technical performance depends on the knowledge and judgment used in arriving at the appropriate strategies of care, and on the skill with which these strategies are implemented. The caliber of technical performance is judged in comparison with the best in practice. The second element of practitioner performance is the management of the interpersonal relationship. The interpersonal exchange is the vehicle by which technical care is delivered. In many situations it is itself a therapeutic intervention and, by that token, a component of technical care. Through interpersonal exchange, practitioners and patients establish a relationship of trust and mutuality. The patient communicates both information necessary for arriving at a diagnosis and preferences concerning the risks, benefits, and costs of care; this information must guide the practitioner in selecting, in collaboration with the adequately informed patient, the most appropriate methods of care. It follows that at this level of analysis or assessment, conformance to technical standards and acceptability to individual patients become the determinants of quality.

The level and scope of concern are altered when attention shifts to assessing the quality of care received by a community as a whole. In this instance access to care and equity in its distribution become more salient elements in the assessment of quality. Moreover, what is effective, efficient, and optimal is judged from a perspective that takes into account not only what individuals desire to have, but also what is conceived to be the public good. (See Chapter 4 for a detailed discussion of how the social perspective on quality differs from the individual perspective.)

APPROACHES TO QUALITY ASSESSMENT

When quality has been defined, and the level and scope of assessment determined, it is time to consider an approach, or a combination of approaches, to assessment. Regardless of the attribute to be assessed, or whether the attribute is viewed from an individual or social perspective, there are three possible approaches. One may assess the characteristics of structure, process, or outcome (Donabedian, 1966).

- **Structure** comprises the relatively stable characteristics of the providers of care, the tools and resources they have at their disposal, and the physical and organizational settings where they work.
- **Process** comprises the set of activities, whether technical or interpersonal, that go on between practitioners and patients.
- **Outcome** is a change in a patient's current or future health status that can be attributed to antecedent health care.

These three approaches to quality assessment are possible only because good structure increases the likelihood of good process, and good process increases the likelihood of good outcome. Because of the multitude of uncontrolled variables in the care situation, it is difficult to establish firm causal relationships between structure, process, and outcome. It is necessary, however, to continue the search for cause and effect relationships, because when such relationships cannot be demonstrated or at least assumed, assessing quality becomes difficult, if not impossible.

SUBSEQUENT STEPS IN ASSESSMENT

To proceed to measurement, **criteria** have to be expressed in precise, quantifiable terms that specify what should exist or be achieved if quality is to be said to be present. Criteria are derived from prior knowledge of the relationships between structure, process, and outcome. Criteria reflect the science and technology of health care, as well as individual and social preferences. It is vital that criteria be measurable and lend themselves to quantification, at least at an ordinal level, but preferably higher.

The next step in quality assessment is to obtain accurate information about the criteria chosen as measures of quality. The patient record is the most usual and important source of information concerning the content of care. Additional information can be obtained from patients directly, by interview and questionnaires. Health-care practitioners and other workers can also provide valuable information. In certain instances, observation of the care episode has been used to assess care, especially with regard to aspects of care not likely to be found in the medical record. The outcome of care can often be directly verified as well.

Of course, each of these sources of information has weaknesses. The record says little about the interpersonal exchange and often is incomplete in other respects as well. Every method of obtaining information is subject to one or more of responder bias, observer bias, or error of measurement. Hence there is a need to pay strict attention to validity of the information being used in assessment of quality.

The preceding material provided a general framework for quality assessment. Following a discussion of the concept of the nursing process and the various ANA standards, the framework will be operationalized.

The Nursing Process

The nursing process, as a concept, was first described by Yura and Walsh in the 1960s to include the components of assessing, planning, implementing, and evaluating (1978). These functions occur within the context of a therapeutic relationship. In recent years some experts have added the component of nursing diagnosis, which previously had been subsumed in either the assessment or the planning component. Kenny (1990) defines the nursing process as "a deliberate activity whereby the practice of nursing is performed in a systematic manner" (p. 7). The nursing process is viewed as the core of practice. This position is legitimized by inclusion of the nursing process in both the licensing examination for Registered Nurses (RNs) and the ANA *Standards of Practice.* The ANA

> describes a competent level of nursing care as demonstrated by the nursing process, involving assessment, diagnosis, outcome identification, planning, implementation, and evaluation. The nursing process encompasses all significant actions taken by nurses in providing care to all clients, and forms the foundations of clinical decision making. (ANA, 1991, p. 3)

Kenny (1990) further suggests that "the deliberate use of the nursing process framework is especially valuable for the novice, while the expert begins to see the situation as gestalt" (p. 5).

The conceptual evolution related to the nursing process has been evident during the past few years. In 1978 Yura and Walsh described the nursing process as cyclic in nature, with constant movement between the elements. In contrast, Bleich (1991) likens the nursing process to a chain where the components of assessing, diagnosing, planning, implementing, and evaluating can be linked together for each clinical problem. This suggests a linear process where each step follows the previous step. McHugh (1991) also considers the nursing process as a linear process. She suggests that the concept fits into Donabedian's framework as the process component, which in the nursing situation represents behaviors and activities of the nurse.

More recently, the nursing process as a generic process has been integrated into various nursing conceptual models. Christensen and Kenny (1990) propose that the nursing models, such as those of Roy (1991), Neuman (1995), and others, provide a frame of reference for each component of the nursing process. Derdiarian's work (1991), using Johnson's Behavioral Systems model (Grubbs, 1980), supports the idea that the use of the nursing models enriches the data and quality of the nursing process.

In spite of the widespread evidence supporting the use of the nursing process as the basis for nursing, some authors suggest that this framework is less than facilitative to the development of the profession and practice of nursing. Kobert and Folan (1990) contend that the nursing process is a reductionistic approach based on the medical model and is only "associated with an immature level of professional development" (p. 309). They further suggest that this model is incompatible with a holistic approach. McHugh (1991) supports the belief that the nursing process is a restricting framework that may impede quality practice. Henderson (1987), in a critical analysis of the nursing process, believes that this scientific process is not unique to nursing but that it is common to all disciplines. She further observes that the jargon inherent in the nursing process has become an impediment to the delivery of care. She suggests that it would be timely for some other system that furthers collaboration to supersede the nursing process.

Previous well-recognized studies, such as Hegyvary (1979) and Slater-Stewart (1984), however, have documented the use of the nursing process as a valid construct. The ANA *Standards of Practice* (1973, 1991) support this construct in the generic standards of clinical practice. Further, various nursing specialty areas, such as community and home health, also base their practices on the nursing process and its well-defined standards.

In the context of this chapter, standards are considered broad goals of performance, while criteria are the essential, critical, measurable statements of care that, when met, signify the standard has been met. Neither practitioners nor the literature have offered valid and reliable instrumentation to measure the accomplishment of the ANA standards in home health. Thus, the purpose of this project was to develop a valid and reliable measure of quality of nursing care in home health as evidenced by the level of conformity to the ANA standards relating to the nursing process.

American Nurses Association Standards

Standards are defined as "broad statements that address the full scope of professional nursing practice" (ANA, 1991, V1). For at least the past twenty years the ANA has been involved in the development, testing, and promulgation of standards. According to the ANA

> Standards are authoritative statements by which the nursing
> profession describes the responsibilities for which its practitioners
> are accountable. Consequently, standards reflect the values and
> priorities of the profession. Standards provide direction for
> professional nursing practice and a framework for the evaluation
> of practice. Written in measurable terms, standards also define
> the nursing profession's accountability to the public and the
> client outcomes for which nurses are responsible. (1991, p. 1)

According to the ANA, there are two major classifications of standards. Standards of care describe "a competent level of nursing care as demonstrated by the nursing process . . ." (ANA, 1991, p. 2). Standards of professional performance describe a competent level of practice behaviors for professional nurses. It is noteworthy that the ANA *Standards of Home Health Nursing Practice* (1986b) are written using the framework of structure, process, and outcome for each component of the nursing process.

SELECT REVIEW OF THE LITERATURE RELATED TO QUALITY MEASUREMENT

Evidence in the literature regarding measuring the quality of the nursing process is scant. In London, Brookings (1988) developed a scale to measure the use of the nursing process in the acute setting. Her tool has three versions: the self-rating scale for ward nurses, nonparticipant-observers' ward-rating scale, and nurse-manager's ward-rating scale. She emphasizes that the scarcity of similar instruments is probably related to the methodological complexity of evaluating the multidimensional concept of the nursing process. She further notes that a valid and reliable method of measuring process is essential to the explanation of causal linkages of process to outcome:

". . . outcome measures alone without this sort of measure of process are of little value, as outcomes must be linked back to the process that brought them about" (p. 48).

Dolan, Pachis, and Skelton (1990) substantiate the value of the nursing-process framework for students in the home-care setting. She has developed an evaluation mechanism that utilizes the nursing process as an essential element in the episode of care. Several others have substantiated the use of the nursing process as a framework to evaluate the quality of care in the acute setting (Bleich, 1991; Brookings, 1988, Goldman, 1990; Hegyvary, 1979). This framework has also been used in home health to measure the quality of care (Ervin, Chen, & Upshaw, 1989; Reeder & Chen, 1990; Schmele & Allen, 1990).

Although not speaking specifically of home care, Lang and Marek (1990) emphasize the great need for valid and reliable tools to measure the quality of nursing care. "If nursing does not develop or identify indicators specific to nursing care the effectiveness of nursing care will remain invisible" (p. 163). According to Phillips, Morrison, and Chae (1990), the lack of clinical instrumentation is more pronounced in home care then in any other area.

Select Studies

A brief overview of select studies of the effectiveness of home-health care follows; it is recognized that this overview is far from exhaustive.

Ervin, Chen, and Upshaw (1989) conducted studies related to the use of the nursing process as a framework for quality measurement. They emphasize the necessity of using expert judgment to respond to criteria that fall in various places on the continuum ranging from explicit to implicit. *The Ervin Quality Assessment Measure (EQAM)* is a fourteen-item audit tool that is in the process of refinement and testing.

Over a span of several years, Schmele (1987) has developed, tested, and refined a measure of quality of the nursing process in home-health care based on Donabedian's conceptual framework (to be discussed in detail later in the chapter).

Building on the work of Schmele and others, Reeder and Chen (1990) have developed and tested in home care the *Client Satisfaction Scale (CSS)*, which is based on the nursing process and the concept of patient satisfaction. Each of the thirty-five items can be placed under one of the four components of the nursing process. By means of a mail survey, the client's perception of care is measured. Reeder suggests that following her preliminary study, further instrument testing is in order.

In a federally funded demonstration project, Oleske, Otte, and Heinze (1987) developed a mechanism to measure quality of nursing care for home-health oncology patients. This study emphasized the structure component and explored the effects of nurse-specialist availability and patient education on the quality of care. Oleske notes the need for refinement of this method of evaluating home care of oncology patients.

Several additional significant contributions have been made in home health. In a long-term project, Martin and Sheets (1992) have developed a patient-classification system for community-health nursing. This system includes a problem-rating scale for outcomes related to knowledge, behavior, or status. Rinke and her associates compiled resources relating to various physical, behavioral, psychosocial, knowledge, and function outcomes (Rinke, 1987; Rinke & Wilson, 1987). Saba (1992) has developed a method of classifying and assessing home-health Medicare patients in areas of service needs, resource utilization, and outcome measures. In her work at the Washington Home Care Association, Lalonde (1986) developed and tested the following outcome measures: taking medications, general symptom distress, discharge status, caregiver strain, functional status, physiological **indicators,** and knowledge of major diagnosis and health problems. Outcome measures of pain management, symptom control, physiological health status, ADL, sense of well-being, goal attainment, application of knowledge, satisfaction with service, family strain, and maintenance at home were contributions related to testing advanced by Sorgen (1986). Kramer, Shaughnessy, and Crisler's work documents the need for valid and practical measures of quality in home health, rather than the present emphasis on paper compliance. Shaughnessy and his associates conceptualize a focused-outcome approach directed toward homogeneous quality indicator groups (QUIG). They also acknowledge the need for structure and process measures (1990). Although not specific to home health, Lang and Marek (1990) have traced the historical development of outcome measures in nursing. Perhaps even more significant is their classification of outcome measures into the following categories: physiological; psychosocial; functional; behavioral; knowledge; symptom control; home maintenance; well-being; goal attainment; patient satisfaction; safe resolution of nursing diagnoses; frequency of service; cost; and rehospitalization.

In other instances, researchers have focused on the development of quality measures for specific types of problems or patients. For example, in response to documentation about elder abuse, the *Qualcare Scale* was developed by Phillips et al. (1990). This scale measures the degree to which the caregiver meets the client's needs in the domains of physical, medical management, psychosocial, environmental, human rights, and financial management. Edwardson and Nardone's *Dependency at Discharge Instrument* (1990), used to measure resource consumption in home care, has shown modest predictability of resource usage. Using a sample of 237 homebound elderly patients, Twarton and Gartner (1991) found that primary nursing did positively affect the patient's satisfaction with care. Although the study was directed toward the evaluation of primary nursing, the *Primary Nursing Evaluation Tool* may have potential for use in other nursing-care-delivery models.

One of the most significant ongoing projects of national scope is the *In Search of Excellence* project funded by the W. K. Kellogg Foundation and being carried out by the Community Health Accreditation Program (CHAP), a subsidiary of the National League for Nursing (NLN). Peters (1992) directs the long-term project, which is developing and testing a comprehensive approach to improve the quality of care in home health (Fahey, 1993). Project goals, based on the philosophy of **Continuous Quality Improvement (CQI),** are to:

1. define outcomes using consumer input

2. develop a system to use the outcomes

3. incorporate the process into the CHAP **accreditation** process

The development of measures combined with approaches to use them in a home-care-delivery system make this a valuable contribution to the improvement of quality in home care.

In summary, the literature generally shows there to be a lack of continuity in follow-up development, testing, and use of quality-measurement instruments. There is frequent documentation of relatively sophisticated instrument-development projects. There is a lack of evidence of subsequent follow-up testing and refinement experiences, however. It may well be that some of these tools are used in the service setting and there simply is no public record of the experience. The articles that do appear regarding quality evaluation in service agencies generally contain scant reference to instrumentation and deal mainly with the practice component. Conversely, research studies of instrument development may offer sophisticated psychometric discussions but lack in practical application. There is a definite need to integrate the research and practice goals directed toward the development and testing of instruments to measure the quality of care.

OPERATIONALIZING THE QUALITY FRAMEWORK

To assess the quality of nursing care in home health, an instrument was developed, guided by the conceptual framework previously described. In conformity with Donabedian's formulation, it was decided that the nurse-patient relationship would be the focus of attention, that both technical and interpersonal aspects of the relationship would be assessed, and that the attributes of quality to be assessed would be primarily effectiveness and acceptability as judged by practitioners and patients. Because acceptability to patients is a governing concern, special attention was given to detecting its presence and extent directly by surveying patients, and indirectly by looking for the modes of nurse-patient interaction that could be presumed to contribute to patient satisfaction.

The process of nursing care was the primary object of assessment, but attention was also given to outcome measures such as the accomplishment of mutually established goals. This melding of process and outcome as approaches to assessment was facilitated, and even improved, by the application of the second major component of the conceptual framework: that of the nursing process itself. In obedience to this formulation, the assessment instrument was divided into four major sections: assessing, planning, intervention, and evaluating. Whereas the first three segments of this four-part instrument focus entirely on the process of care, the last segment, on evaluation, is assessed in conjunction with process and outcome.

The standards and criteria by which the nursing care was judged were derived from the ANA *Standards of Nursing Practice* (1973, 1991), *Standards of Community Health Nursing Practice* (1974, 1986a), and *Standards of Home Health Nursing Practice* (1986b). These standards were chosen as the basis for specific instrument development because they consist of professional nursing standards related to the components of the nursing process. An example of an item from the *planning* component and dealing with a technical element is: "Was a short-term goal established?" An example exemplifying the *evaluation* component with an interpersonal element is, "Was the patient's progress toward nursing-care goals discussed with the patient?"

Three sources of information were used: direct observation, the clinical record, and a patient questionnaire. The selection of these data sources was dictated by objectives of the various phases of the instrument-development project, as well as the availability of existing resources. Variations in data sources, imposed by resource constraints, is discussed in greater detail in the sections that follow.

Multistage Instrument-Development Studies

The development, refinement, and testing of the Schmele Instrument to Measure the Process of Nursing Care in Home Health (SIMP-H) has been a multistage process over a period of several years. A brief overview of each of the studies related to the phases of development of the SIMP-H follows.

PHASE I

The major focus of the first study was to develop criterion measures to assess the quality of the nursing process based on the ANA *Standards for Community Health Nursing Practice* (1974). The rationale for selecting the process approach was based on the review of the literature and the experience of the investigator. The assumption was made that the nursing process was the core interpersonal and technical activity that was used in any nurse-patient caregiving situation in the community setting, and, therefore had generic applicability (Schmele, 1985).

An expert panel of eight nurses from various community settings reviewed and critiqued the criterion measures that had been developed by the researcher. The project included the development of three self-contained instruments known as the *Schmele Instrument to Measure Quality of Nursing Practice in the Community (SIMP)*. These instruments utilized three different data sources:

1. client record (audit tool)

2. nurse-patient interaction (observational tool)

3. patient (patient-satisfaction questionnaire)

Each instrument contained the four components of the nursing process: assessing, planning, implementing, and evaluating. The scoring value of each of the four subsections was 25, with each item receiving a value contingent on the number of items in that particular subsection. After pilot testing with fifteen sampling units, the study sample consisted of twenty-eight nurse-client interactions taking place in the following community programs: women, infants, and children (WIC); well baby; veneral disease; tuberculosis; and chronic disease.

Study findings showed that the client-satisfaction measure demonstrated the highest level of quality. This finding is in accord with the widely held perception that responder bias may have a strong influence on patient-reported satisfaction. The quality ratings for the components of the nursing process, from highest to lowest, were assessing, implementing, evaluating, and planning. Methodological challenges included the subjectivity of the observational measure; lack of reliability measures; the management problems inherent in the simultaneous testing of the three instruments with only a limited financial and human-resources budget; and the great number of variables in the home-health setting, for which there was no control. It is also noteworthy that in some of the programs the nurse-patient interaction was sparse, often consisting of the accomplishment of a program activity such as immunization or the issuance of WIC resources. In these situations there are those who would suggest that the only valid component to measure would be the "implementation" component. This "program versus practice" dilemma is governed by the philosophical underpinning of the agency. Thus, in order to continue the refinement of the SIMP, it was recommended that a more desirable program for testing the instrument would be one where it was more likely to be able to observe the nursing process in its entirety.

PHASE II

The purpose of this study was to test the SIMP specifically in the home-health setting, to strengthen validity, and to develop reliability measures (Schmele, 1987). Ten practicing home-health nurses validated the content of the items that made up the three self-contained instruments (observation, record, and patient), with each instrument containing the four parallel subsections (assessing, planning, implementing, and evaluating). The sampling unit was the nurse-patient interaction during home visits made by Visiting Nurse Association (VNA) nurses to patients of varying ages and diagnoses. Thirty-six observations were made by a nonparticipant nurse-observer. In addition to the SIMP, the *Slater Scale* (Hough & Schmele, 1987) was administered as a measure of construct validity. Cronbach's alpha was used as a measure of internal consistency. The alpha coefficients were 0.87, 0.75, and 0.25 for observation, record, and patient instruments, respectively. The very low inter-item correlation of the patient instrument pointed to the need for further refinement and testing. Findings were similar to the first study, which showed that scores for the assessment component were significantly higher (<.05) than those for planning, implementing, and evaluating. Although there were small differences between the total raw scores of the three data sources (record = 79, observation = 77, and patient = 76), these differences were statistically significant.

A correlation between the summated scores of the SIMP and the Slater yielded a lack of positive association. This lack of association could have meant that the two scales actually measured a different construct. The researchers concluded that there was a need for yet further refinement and testing of the three self-contained instruments in various home-health settings, using larger samples.

PHASE III

Because of the large number of uncontrolled variables present in previous studies, the complexity of administering three self-contained instruments, and a lack of resources, it was decided that Phase III would be directed toward the refinement and further testing of only one of the parts of the three-part instrument. Because of the low alphas and the observational bias inherent in the patient-satisfaction tool and the continued availability of the record for later audit, it was determined that this study would focus on strengthening the observational tool, which at the time seemed to have the greatest potential for refinement.

The study objective was to refine the somewhat complex scoring system, incorporate new ANA *Standards of Community Health Nursing Practice* (1986a) and *Standards of Home Health Nursing Practice* (1986b), and refine and strengthen validity for the home-health setting. Ten actively practicing VNA home-health nurses participated in several concentrated sessions directed toward refinement of criteria (Schmele & Foss, 1989). The group initially examined values about home-health nursing. The new ANA standards were then examined, as were the items from the

SIMP. Six additional content experts representing research, service, and education were also used to validate the items. The new sixty-item observational tool, which was then identified as the Schmele Instrument to Measure the Process of Nursing Practice in Home Health (SIMP-H) was developed specifically for home health.

The purpose of this study, then, was to evaluate the SIMP-H and compare it with three other observational instruments for use in home care (Schmele & Allen, 1990). All four instruments included the specific components of the nursing process. The *Stewart Evaluation of Nursing Scale (SENS)* (Slater-Stewart, 1984), based on the original *Slater Nursing Competencies Rating Scale* (Wandelt & Slater-Stewart, 1975), consisted of forty-seven items. The *Standards Rating Scale (SRS)* was simply an enumeration and Likert-type quantification of the forty-six items from the recently developed ANA *Standards of Home Health Nursing Practice* (ANA, 1986b). The final instrument was the observational portion of the original SIMP, now called the *SIMP-C* to differentiate it from the newly developed home-health instrument.

Because of resource constraints, the limited convenience sample for this preliminary study was made up of twenty-seven nurse-patient visits from eight metropolitan home-health agencies. The nonparticipant-observer gathered data using all four instruments during one episode of home-health care.

Psychometric findings revealed total instrument internal consistency (Cronbach's alpha) for each instrument as follows: SENS = 0.88, SIMP-H = 0.85, SIMP-C = 0.76 and SRS = 0.76. Correlation coefficients (Kendall's tau) done between each of the component subscales (assessing, planning, implementing, and evaluating) for all of the instruments showed a weak to moderate positive correlation among the four components. This positive correlation, although weak, may suggest the unitary nature of the nursing process. It is recognized in practice that although each component implies a different function, all the components are interdependent to some degree. Disappointingly, the SIMP-H yielded only a weak positive correlation with the other three instruments, perhaps illustrating that the nursing process is very elusive to measure and that there may be variation in the construct itself. The final part of this study was a comparative analysis of the four instruments using the Waltz and Bausell (1981) format for instrument evaluation. This included an evaluation of general information, design information, and practical concerns. Systematic evaluation of each of these areas was then quantified to yield a composite numeric score. Based on this score, the instruments were ranked as follows in order of highest desirability for use in the home-health setting: SENS, SIMP-H, SIMP-C, and SRS. As a result, instruments of choice for subsequent studies included the SENS and the SIMP-H.

PHASE IV

The major purpose of this study (Schmele, Henson, & Robinson, 1994) was the further testing of the SIMP-H in a sample of 100 VNA clients who were receiving nursing care from RNs. In an effort to minimize the number of uncontrolled variables, the convenience sample consisted of patients sixty-five years and older. Each patient was observed for one home visit during which the nonparticipant-observer completed the SIMP-H and the SENS, the latter being used as a concurrent measure of validity.

In contrast to an earlier study with a much smaller sample size, concurrent validity was supported in this study by a highly positive correlation (0.93, p = 0.08) between the SENS and the SIMP-H. Preliminary findings from a factor analysis identified fourteen factors in the instrument. A possible interpretation is that these factors are representative of specific nursing roles that occur *across* components of the nursing process. It is also recognized that the size of the sample (100) is less than ideal for a factor analysis.

The reliability measure of internal consistency was supported by Cronbach's alpha for both the total instrument and the subscales. Total instrument was 0.95, while the subscales were assessment 0.77, planning 0.94, intervention 0.83, and evaluation 0.71.

Inter-rater reliability was established between two raters on a sample of fifteen home visits. Inter-rater reliability for the total instrument was 0.95 (p = 0.000). Reliability for the subscales were assessment 0.71, planning 0.94, intervention 0.88, and evaluation 0.97, all with a significance level of 0.000.

Discussion

In the discussion that follows, attention is given to the operationalization of the conceptual framework and the evaluation of this study methodology. The major purpose of the discussion is to reflect on the strengths and limitations related to the application of the generic quality-assessment model to the specific measurement of quality of nursing care in home health.

CONCEPTUAL FRAMEWORK
The conceptual foundation for the studies will be discussed from the perspective of both quality and the nursing process which together serve as an integrated framework. Further discussion deals with methodological concerns.

Quality   Donabedian's formulation was useful as a general guide to devise the choice of attributes of quality to measure, the level and scope of assessment, and approaches to their assessment. In keeping with the level and scope of responsibilities in a home-health agency, quality assessment focused on the clinical encounters between nurse and patient. The perspective that structured the assessment was the welfare of individual patients as distinct from the public good.

It is recognized that a process approach to assessing quality may only receive its full value when it is related to beneficial outcomes of care. It should be understood, first, that the process of care is always judged by its presumed capacity to bring about the accomplishment of goals arrived at jointly by the nurse and the patient. In addition, the accomplishment of such goals, patient satisfaction among them, needs to be directly assessed. Because acceptability to patients is a governing concern, it is a key element in defining and assessing quality. This degree of attention to satisfaction is justifiable. It is a judgment by the patient on aspects of care that the patient perceives and values. Satisfaction is believed to contribute to success in current and future care by increasing the probability of patient cooperation. Because satisfaction is an outcome in its own right it is something to be aimed for and accomplished in the process of nursing care.

The approach to assessment was primarily, but not exclusively, oriented to process. The evaluation by the nurse-observer, and in the earlier phases by the patients themselves responding to the patient-satisfaction survey, does include elements of outcome. By contrast, assessment of structural elements is entirely absent from the instrument. But there is nothing to prevent including structural elements, assuming that it is known which structural elements are highly correlated with good nursing care. The combination of structure, process, and outcome is preferable to total reliance on process or outcome alone. It is recognized that there may be disparity in the assessments of quality using each of the three approaches. According to Donabedian (1992), some of the possible causes of disparity between judgments based on process and outcome include the following:

1. The probability of process contributing to outcome is so small that the relation has escaped notice: too few cases have been observed, measurements are too crude, etc.

2. The timing of outcome observations has been inappropriate, not matching the manifestation of outcomes.

3. Outcomes contain additional information not contained in the process measured, including:
   a. skill (or lack of it) in the execution of care
   b. contributions of many other caregivers
   c. contributions of patient and family to care;

4. Information about process or outcome is inaccurate or tampered with.

5. Case-mix adjustment is improper or insufficient.

6. Process and outcome are not matched as to mutual relevance.

7. Accepted (or assumed) knowledge about relation between process and outcome is erroneous (scientifically unverified).

The need to continue to search for cause and effect relationships and to assess quality by more than one approach is quite clear.

Nursing Process   Because of the unique relationship of the nursing process to the practice of nursing as well as the availability of widely accepted nursing process-based standards of practice, the nursing process is a strong conceptual base of study. As Donabedian (1992) has suggested, however, there are some problems inherent in assessing quality by the attribute of the patient-practitioner relationship.

- It may be a substitute for, rather than an adjunct to, the "goodness" of technical care.

- Information about the relationship may be difficult to obtain.

- Because there is considerable variation in patient preference, standards and criteria of process are difficult to formulate.

- Patient satisfaction (the relevant outcome) is not always a totally valid indicator because patients are reluctant to express their views or because their expectations may be too low as well as too high.

• The cost of the time needed to observe a patient-practitioner relationship is to be balanced against its immediate and remote benefits.

A key consideration is the extent to which what the patient says can supplement in a valid way what the nurse-observer sees during the sampled encounter.

The assessment of the presence and effectiveness of the elements of the nursing process is somewhat difficult because of the cognitive nature of assessing, planning, and evaluating. It is for this reason that a high level of professional and unbiased judgment on the part of the nurse-observer is required. The judgments of effectiveness are not quite as difficult when an observable mutual approach is used, for example, when the nurse actively engages the client in decision making regarding the plan of care. This, of course, is highly desirable. But if there is a lack of observable patient involvement, the nonparticipant-observer of the home visit may have only minimal, if any, evidence of the accomplishment of the given planning criteria. The very absence of observable mutual behaviors, however, may be a reflection of the lack of quality or an indication that there has been only minimal accomplishment of standards. The intervention component of the nursing process is much more easily observable. It is likely that problems arising because of difficulty in observing behaviors may be alleviated to some extent by also using the clinical record as a source of information.

Although the assumption is made that the nursing process is operational at any time there is a patient-care situation, the specific components of the process have varied applicability depending on the specific episode of care being observed. For example, one would anticipate that the assessment component would be most prevalent during the first visit, and the evaluation component during the discharge visit. Conceptually, however, all components should be present in varying degrees during each visit. Consideration could be given to using a composite measure, which could be attained by observing three visits (admission, midpoint, and termination) during an episode of care and calculating the mean as the measure of quality. Furthermore, in many agencies where the same home-health nurse does not provide care during all three visits, the quality of the nursing process would then be recognized as a "nursing service" quality measure, rather than a measure of the competence of a specific nurse. This approach seems to be quite reasonable if, indeed, this is the service-delivery method. One recognizes, of course, that this lack of continuity is less than desirable.

The nursing process is recognized in clinical practice as a unitary concept because of the cyclical and often overlapping nature of the components. It is possible and likely that several of the components occur together and that there is a kind of constant give and take, as in a conversation when two persons can shift and adjust as they hear each other speak. Another kind of "unitariness" might occur through the ability of the nurse (or patient) to engage in all components with equal skill (or, in the opposite case, disparate skills). There is also a kind of "cause continuity" something like the causality inherent in the structure-process-outcome chain. In other words, good assessment leads to a good plan and a good plan leads to good implementation; conversely, an unimplementable plan is not good. On the other hand, because the components are conceptually separable, license may be taken in the research situation to treat them as discrete measures in order to evaluate the quality of each component. In certain instances, from a pragmatic point of view, it may be desirable, then, for an agency to have the ability to evaluate the quality of the nursing process and offer remediation in particular areas of weakness.

Sample   It is acknowledged that in all phases of the project the samples were small and sometimes restricted to only one agency, which limited the generalizability of the findings. It is also noted that in three of the studies, the convenience sampling necessitated the observation of each nurse more than once. This could bias both performance and observation. A large random sample ideally would consist of distinctly different nurse-patient dyads from various home-health agencies. This type of sampling would support the generalizability of the findings as well as provide sufficient data for more highly sophisticated data analysis. As is frequently the case, sample size was, of necessity, contingent on the available resources.

Data Gathering   For each study a RN-observer, considered to be a highly competent practitioner, was selected and trained to be a nonparticipant-observer and recorder of the home visit. Because no effort was made to use more than one observer for each study, the observer acted as her own control. If more than one rater is used, it would be desirable to incorporate observer training for the use of the instrument. The *Training Guide for SIMP-H Data Collection* (Robinson, Henson, & Schmele, 1994) was developed for this purpose.

Instrument   Although every effort was made to objectify the criterion measures, it is recognized that each has a varying degree of subjectivity. This makes it desirable, if not essential, that the professional nurse-observer possess above-average nursing competence and the ability to make sound nursing judgments.

   Although the length of the sixty-item SIMP-H observational tool does not present problems in the research setting, this is not the case in the practice setting. In order to accommodate the instrument to practical use in the service agency, therefore, a shortened form may be desirable.

Application in Service and Research

In home-health agencies, where nursing is considered the major component of home-health care, the SIMP-H offers an observational approach to measuring quality. Because a current trend is for accrediting agencies and **certification** bodies to actually observe specific episodes of care, it may also be advantageous for internal evaluators to begin to use this approach to assess the quality of care. For agencies that philosophically value the nursing process as the core of practice, this ANA-standards-based instrument represents agreed-upon levels of practice. The instrument contains standards and assessment criteria for assessing, planning, implementing, and evaluating care. These criteria could be used as the framework to implement the ANA *Standards of Practice* in a comprehensive approach that includes setting professional-practice expectations. These expectations would be reflected in the performance expectations found in job descriptions, and, subsequently, in performance evaluations. (This process is described in an earlier work by Chu and Schmele [1990].) The SIMP-H itself could be used to assess nursing competencies as well as the process component of the quality of care. Although the instrument yields a unitary measure of quality, a determination could be made of the quality of each of the specific components of the nursing process. These results could be used as evaluation data on which to base programming emphasis for professional development.

In conjunction with the SIMP-H, or as a single measure, agencies may also wish to use the *Client Satisfaction Survey* (Reeder & Chen, 1990) as an outcome measure. As previously mentioned, this tool is also based on the components of the nursing process and could be considered a companion instrument to the SIMP-H.

There are numerous research implications of this project. In keeping with tradition, one might say that there is a need for additional studies using larger samples. A large sample would facilitate the establishment of further psychometric properties that would be of value, especially in further factor analyzing the nursing process. Because the nursing process is generic, there may be value in using the instrument with a heterogeneous sample. Additional studies might address such questions as:

- What is the relationship of the quality of the nursing process to structure and outcome variables?

- What is the relationship of the quality of the nursing process to patient satisfaction?

- What are the relationships among the data sources of record, observation, and patient?

- How might the SIMP-H be shortened to accommodate its use in practice and still maintain validity and reliability?

As with any research, there are always more questions generated than there are answers provided.

CONCLUSION

Although significant strides are being made toward ensuring quality of care in home health, the need for sound approaches and measures remains evident. The rapidly growing field of home health, the increasing acuity of patients, and the complexity of care demand the concerted efforts of both the academic and service settings to develop theoretically based systems of quality. It is then through the publication and subsequent promulgation of these systems that additional testing and retesting can be done. This chapter represents the integration of a theoretical view of quality with the paradigm of the nursing process.

Donabedian's generic framework for the assessment of quality, coupled with the model of the nursing process, provided a sound base on which to formulate this approach to assess the quality of care in home health. An instrument, the SIMP-H, was developed for the individual level of analysis, based on the attributes of effectiveness and acceptability (including the aspects of technical and interpersonal care, and the characteristic of process).

At the inception of the project, the development of a three-source instrument (observation, patient, and record) was envisioned as a valid and reliable device for measuring quality of care in home health. The logistics, as well as the limitation of resources, led to modification of these goals and subsequent refinement of only the observation portion of the instrument, called the SIMP-H. During Phase II, however, collaboration with Reeder led to adaptation and refinement of her patient-satisfaction measure, which is now viewed as a viable companion instrument to the SIMP-H. Reeder's tool is known as the *Client Satisfaction Survey* (Reeder & Chen, 1990). The third instrument, based on the record, is yet to be refined and tested. Ervin's audit measure known as EQAM, however, offers the possibility of triangulation in the study of nursing quality in home care.

In summary, the instrument development and testing studies resulted in the formulation of the SIMP-H, a sixty-item observational instrument with respectable validity and reliability, as well as a companion training guide. This instrument, based on the components of the nursing process and the ANA standards, is suitable for assessing the process component of the quality of care in home health.

It is recognized that the operationalization of a conceptual model to assess quality is a complex and long-term project when coupled with instrument development, testing, and refinement. Even then, this endeavor is recognized as only a beginning approach to apply a generic model of quality to the measurement of the quality of nursing care in home health.

REFERENCES

American Bar Association. (1986). *The "black box" of home care quality.* (Comm. Pub. No. 99-573). Washington, DC: U. S. Government Printing Office.

American Nurses Association. (1973). *Standards of nursing practice.* Kansas City, MO: Author.

American Nurses Association. (1974). *Standards of community health nursing practice.* Kansas City, MO: Author.

American Nurses Association. (1986a). *Standards of community health nursing practice.* Kansas City, MO: Author.

American Nurses Association. (1986b). *Standards of home health nursing practice.* Kansas City, MO: Author.

American Nurses Association. (1991). *Standards of clinical nursing practice.* Kansas City, MO: Author.

Bleich, M. R. (1991). Monitoring the nursing process. In P. Schroeder, *Monitoring and evaluation in nursing* (pp. 205–218). Gaithersburg, MD: Aspen.

Brookings, J. I. (1988). A scale to measure use of the nursing process. *Nursing Times, 85*(15), 44–49.

Christensen, P. J., & Kenney, J. (1990). *Nursing process.* St. Louis, MO: C. V. Mosby.

Chu, N., & Schmele, J. A. (1990). Using the ANA standards as a basis for performance evaluation in the home health care setting. *Journal of Nursing Quality Assurance, 4*(3), 25–33.

Derdiarian, A. K. (1991). Effects of using a nursing model-based assessment instrument on quality of nursing care. *Nursing Administration Quarterly, 15*(3), 1–16.

Dolan, M. G., Pachis, K. A., & Skelton, J. M. (1990). Evaluation of home visits using a nursing process approach. *Journal of Community Health Nursing, 7*(2), 69–75.

Donabedian, A. (1966). Evaluating the quality of medical care (part 1). *Milbank Memorial Fund Quarterly, 44*(1), 166–203.

Donabedian, A. (1980). *The definition of quality and approaches to its assessment.* Ann Arbor, MI: Health Administration Press.

Donabedian, A. (1990). The seven pillars of quality. *Archives of Pathology and Laboratory Medicine, 114*(11), 1115–1118.

Donabedian, A. (1992). *What is quality in health care?* Visual materials prepared for Ninth International Conference of the Israel Society for Quality Assurance, Jerusalem, Israel.

Edwardson, S. R., & Nardone, P. (1990). The dependency at discharge instrument as a measure of resource use in home care. *Public Health Nursing, 7*(3), 138–144.

Ervin, N. E., Chen, S. C., & Upshaw, H. (1989). Development of a public health nursing quality assessment measure. *Quality Review Bulletin, 15*(5), 138–143.

Fahy, E. T. (1993). In search of excellence: An interview with Donna Peters. *Nursing and Health Care, 14*(9), 466–471.

Goldman, R. C. (1990). Nursing process components as a framework for monitoring and (evaluating) activities. *Journal of Nursing Quality Assurance, 4*(4), 17–25.

Grubbs, J. (1980). The Johnson Behavioral System Model. In J. Riehl & C. Roy (Eds.), *Conceptual models for nursing practice* (2nd ed.) (pp. 217–254). New York: Appleton-Century-Crofts.

Hegyvary, S. T. (1979). Nursing process: The basis for evaluating the quality of nursing care. *International Nursing Review, 26*(4), 113–116.

Henderson, V. (1987). Nursing process — A critique. *Holistic Nursing Practice, 1*(3), 7–18.

Hough, B., & Schmele, J. A. (1987). The Slater scale: A viable method for monitoring nursing quality in home health. *Journal of Nursing Quality Assurance, 1*(3), 28–38.

Kenney, J. W. (1990). Relevance of theoretical approaches in nursing practice. In P. J. Christensen & J. W. Kenney (Eds.), *Nursing process.* St. Louis, MO: C. V. Mosby.

Kobert, L., & Folan, M. (1990). Coming of age in nursing. *Nursing and Health Care, 11*(6), 308–312.

Kramer, A. M., Shaughnessy, P. W., Bauman, M. K., & Crisler, K. S. (1990). Assessing and assuring the quality of home health care: A conceptual framework. *Milbank Memorial Fund Quarterly, 68*(3), 413–443.

Lalonde, B. (1986). *Quality Assurance manual of the Home Care Association of Washington.* Edmonds, WA: Home Care Association of Washington.

Lang, N. M., & Marek, K. D. (1990). The classification of patient outcomes. *Journal of Professional Nursing, 6*(3), 158–163.

Martin, K. S., & Sheets, N. J. (1992). *The Omaha System.* Philadelphia: W. B. Saunders.

McHugh, M. K. (1991). Does the nursing process reflect quality care? *Holistic Nursing Practice, 5*(3), 22–28.

Neuman, B. (1995). *The Neuman Systems Model* (3rd ed.). Norwalk, CT: Appleton & Lange.

Oleske, D. M., Otte, D. M., & Heinze, S. (1987). Development and evaluation of a system for monitoring the quality of oncology nursing care in the home setting. *Cancer Nursing, 10*(4), 190–198.

Peters, D. A. (1992). A new look for quality in home care. *Journal of Nursing Administration, 22*(11), 21–26.

Phillips, L. R., Morrison, E. F., & Chae, Y. M. (1990). The QUALCARE scale: Developing an instrument to measure quality of home care. *International Journal of Nursing Studies, 27*(1), 61–75.

Reeder, P. J., & Chen, S. C. (1990). A client satisfaction survey in home health care. *Journal of Nursing Quality Assurance, 5*(1), 16–24.

Rinke, L. T. (1987). *Outcome measures in home care* (Vol. I). New York: National League for Nursing.

Rinke, L. T., & Wilson, A. A. (Eds.). (1987). *Outcome measures in home care* (Vol. II). New York: National League for Nursing.

Robinson, W., Henson, R., & Schmele, J. A. (1994). *Training guide for SIMP-H data collection.* Unpublished document, University of Oklahoma, Oklahoma City, OK.

Roy, C., & Andrews, H. A. (1991). *The Roy Adaptation Model: The definitive statement.* Norwalk, CT: Appleton & Lange.

Saba, V. (1992). Diagnoses and interventions. *Caring Magazine, 11*(3), 50–57.

Schmele, J. A. (1985). A method for evaluating nursing practice in a community setting. *Quality Review Bulletin, 11*(4), 115–122.

Schmele, J. A. (1987). Measuring the quality of nursing care in home health (Abstract). *Proceedings of the 11th Annual Midwest Nursing Research Society Conference.* St. Louis, MO, 243.

Schmele, J. A., & Allen, M. E. (1990). A comparison of four process measures of quality in home health. *Journal of Nursing Quality Assurance, 4*(4), 26–35.

Schmele, J. A., & Foss, S. J. (1989). A process method for clinical practice evaluation in the home health setting. *Journal of Nursing Quality Assurance, 3*(3), 54–63.

Schmele, J. A., Henson, R., & Robinson, W. (1994). *The testing of a measurement of quality of nursing care in home health.* Unpublished report. University of Oklahoma, Oklahoma City, OK.

Slater-Stewart, D. M. (1984). *The Stewart evaluation of nursing scale.* Unpublished paper, Wayne State University, Detroit, MI.

Sorgen, L. M. (1986). The development of a home care quality assurance program in Alberta. *Home Health Care Services Quarterly, 7*(2), 13–28.

Twarton, C. C., & Gartner, M. B. (1991). Patient satisfaction with primary nursing in home health. *Journal of Nursing Administration, 21*(11), 39–43.

Waltz, C., & Bausell, R. B. (1981). *Nursing research: Design, statistics and computer analysis.* Philadelphia: F. A. Davis.

Wandelt, M. A., & Slater-Stewart, D. (1975). *Slater nursing competencies rating scale.* New York: Appleton-Century-Crofts.

Yura, H., & Walsh, M. (1978). *The nursing process* (3rd ed.). New York: Appleton-Century-Crofts.

ADDITIONAL READING

Buchanan, L. M. (1994). Therapeutic nursing intervention knowledge development and outcome measures for advanced practice. *Nursing and Allied Health, 15*(4), 190–195.

Colling, J. (1994). The status of Quality Assurance in home health care. In J. McClosky & H. K. Grace (Eds.), *Current issues in nursing* (pp. 310–315). St. Louis, MO: Mosby.

Christensen, P. J. (1995). Nursing process: Application of conceptual models (4th ed.). St. Louis, MO: Mosby.

Martin, K. (1994). How can the quality of nursing practice be measured? In J. McClosky & H. K. Grace (Eds.), *Current issues in nursing* (pp. 343–349). St. Louis, MO: Mosby.

Katherine R. Jones

CHAPTER *23*

Outcomes Analysis:
Methods and Issues

Patient outcomes research provides an opportunity to improve the quality
of patient care by modifying the structures and processes of care delivery.
Optimal application of outcomes analysis involves collaboration between
the health-care disciplines. The result of such an endeavor would be the
identification of health-care practices that lead to desired patient outcomes
in the most cost-effective manner.

INTRODUCTION

The overriding concern in today's health-care environment is preserving or
enhancing **quality** while delivering services in a more efficient and cost-effective manner. One response is through better management of the **outcomes** of care.
Outcomes management connects the issues of quality, costs, and productivity.
These issues have received increasing attention as a result of new payment systems
that restrict reimbursement, and the recurrent professional staffing shortages.
More specifically, prospective payment systems have provided nurses the incentive
to expand from a narrow, incremental task approach to care delivery to a broader
view wherein nursing care is primarily determined and evaluated by expected and
achieved outcomes (Servais, 1991).

Improvements in productivity in today's market-driven environment focus on
offering better quality services at lower prices. This requires measuring what happens to patients as a result of nursing interventions. In the past, nursing care plans
were developed for patients on an individualized, comprehensive basis. Many of the
interventions represented common practices in a particular setting, and were never
evaluated for their effectiveness or efficacy. Patient outcomes research presents the

Note: This chapter is reprinted with permission of Jannetti Publications, Inc., from *Nursing
Economic$, 11*(3), 145–152, May–June 1993.

opportunity to demonstrate how specific nursing practices contribute to patient outcomes, which in turn will add to the scientific base for nursing practice. Outmoded or inefficient processes will be discarded. The Institute of Medicine (IOM) has identified the following as advantages of outcomes analysis (Lohr, 1990): (a) it allows **monitoring** of the system while allowing providers to undertake their own quality-improvement efforts; (b) it collects systematic data that can be used to inform the field about how **process** components are related to outcomes; (c) it provides a means to look across time and to appreciate the temporal and service linkages within episodes of care; and (d) it emphasizes aspects of care that are most relevant to patients and society.

The Joint Commission on Accreditation of Healthcare Organizations (Joint Commission) issued a series of **standards** in 1992 that addressed the important role that hospital leadership plays in assessing and improving patient-care quality. The Joint Commission based its new 1993 standards on several principles: (a) a hospital can improve patient-care quality by assessing and improving those governance, managerial, clinical, and support processes that most affect patient outcomes; (b) some of these processes are carried out by medical, nursing, and other clinicians; others by governing body members, managers, and support personnel; some are carried out jointly by more than one of these groups; (c) whether carried out by one or more of these groups, the processes must be coordinated and integrated; this coordination and integration requires the attention of clinical and managerial leaders of the hospital; and (d) most governance, managerial, medical, nursing, other clinical, and support staff are both motivated and competent to carry out the processes well; therefore, the opportunities to improve processes and patient outcomes are more frequent than are mistakes and errors (Patterson, 1993). These principles reflect both the current interest in **Total Quality Management (TQM)** and the efforts to monitor and measure outcomes of care. In its *Accreditation Manual for Hospitals*, the Joint Commission defines patient-care quality as "the degree to which patient care services increase the probability of desired patient outcomes and reduce the probability of undesired outcomes, given the current state of knowledge" (Joint Commission, 1993). It follows that these desired patient outcomes for specific patient groups must be identified, and when desired outcomes are not achieved, it is necessary to determine the associated clinical, managerial, or support processes that must be improved.

The purpose of this chapter is to present the issues to be considered when developing an outcomes-based research program. The identification of appropriate outcomes, potential sources of data, measurement issues, and different methodologies are discussed. Several examples of outcome studies from the nursing and health-services literature are then provided. Finally, implications for nurse managers and executives are given.

IDENTIFICATION OF APPROPRIATE OUTCOME VARIABLES

Outcomes are the end-results of care, or measurable changes in the health status or behavior of patients (Harris, 1991). Traditional measures of outcome have been negative, and have included mortality, morbidity (iatrogenic complications), unscheduled readmission, unscheduled repeat surgery, and unnecessary hospital procedures (a reflection of inefficient use of resources). These are sometimes identified as short-term and intermediate outcomes of care. They are primarily focused on hospital-based care processes.

Alternative measures of outcome relate to quality of life, and may include the patient's health status, functional status, reduced pain, improved mobility, return to work or normal activities, and patient satisfaction with services received and providers delivering care. These measures are particularly relevant to nurses and their patient care plans. The trend in outcomes measurement and management is toward measuring outcomes across the continuum of care, or across defined episodes of care that transcend organizational boundaries (Hornbrook, Hurtado, & Johnson, 1985; Jennings, 1991; Keeler, Solomon, Beck, Mendenhall, & Kane, 1982). This is consistent with the introduction of case-management programs, which include critical pathways with prehospitalization, inpatient, outpatient, and home-care events. In addition, outcomes such as reduced pain and improved mobility are particularly appropriate for hospice and home-care services, which are growing segments of the health-care delivery system. The primary focus in these agencies is nursing services.

Lohr (1985) identified a comprehensive typology of outcomes. They represent the continuum of care, and include:

1. mortality in the hospital or shortly after discharge

2. adverse events and complications during hospitalization

3. inadequate recovery or complications requiring readmission

4. prolongation of a medical problem that was not adequately assessed because of treatment of an unrelated condition

5. decline in health status because of problems or situations that lead to delay or denial of admission

6. decline in quality of life, including poorer physical, emotional, or mental function

Hegyvary (1991) has proposed four categories of outcome assessment, which allow for the multiple perspectives of providers, consumers, and purchasers:

1. *Clinical* — patient response to medical and nursing interventions.

2. *Functional* — maintenance or improvement of physical functioning.

3. *Financial* — outcomes achieved with most efficient use of resources.

4. *Perceptual* — patient's satisfaction with outcomes, care received, and providers.

THE CONTEXT OF OUTCOMES ANALYSIS

Before discussing the data and measurement issues, it is important to understand the broader context of outcomes analysis and management. *Context* refers to who wants outcome information, what they want to know, and why. There are many differing, and possibly competing, perspectives. Purchasers (employers, insurers) want value for their health-care dollars (Geigle & Jones, 1990; Rettig, 1991). Thus, they may want to compare disease-specific outcomes and costs across different providers. Institutional providers, such as hospitals, want to ensure the highest professional performance from their clinical and managerial staff. Thus, the results of outcomes analysis may be used for credential renewal, or as one way to demonstrate a high level of performance. Individual providers, such as nurses and physicians, use outcomes to evaluate change in health status and other outcomes of a client or group of clients specific to a course of care and treatment. For example, do special mattresses make a difference in the prevention of decubitus ulcers? Patients also increasingly want information about outcomes — both those related to different treatment options and those that reflect the quality of different providers. Bowen (1987) believes there is a need to put more emphasis on what patients expect as the outcome of their treatment. Nurses have typically included the patient in the care planning process, but have not always asked what the patient expects as a result of their care; for example, how the patient evaluates success or defines a successful outcome. It is also important to remember that the importance of particular outcomes varies with the population being studied, and that the desirability of one outcome over another in any given clinical condition may differ markedly according to patients' values and preferences (Geigle & Jones, 1990; Lohr, 1988).

SOURCES OF DATA

Measurement of outcomes of care are based on three data sources at the macro level. These data sources are used to **evaluate** outcomes at the population level, and to compare outcomes across multiple facilities and settings. They include:

1. *Discharge abstracts.* Patient discharge abstracts consist of diagnostic and treatment codes and labels. These are easy to retrieve and allow generation of large samples for analysis; but they provide limited information per patient and are usually limited to one payer group. Examples include the UB82 form used for Medicare billing and claims against insurance companies.

2. *Medical records.* This requires abstracting information contained within individual patient medical records. This method allows for more detailed information, but it is a more expensive source of data given the time and personnel required for records abstraction. Generally, more detailed data are gathered for a smaller number of patients, as compared to the use of discharge abstracts.

3. *Large, public/private databases,* such as those from the Health Care Financing Administration (HCFA) and MedStat. These data sets provide extensive information on millions of hospital discharges and ambulatory-care visits for specific patient populations. The HCFA data set includes detailed information on patients receiving payment under Medicare or Medicaid, while MedStat contains records from privately insured individuals. Data elements are those that drive the reimbursement of patient bills. Limitations include few if any nursing-related variables; difficulty in determining the sequence of events within a single episode of care; and lack of depth in the clinical data. However, these databases do provide information on the utilization of services for specific patient diagnoses and procedures across payer groups and care settings.

These three sources of data allow for analysis of a limited range of variables (mortality, morbidity), which are not usually the desired focus of nursing-outcome studies. Therefore, micro-level data may be more appropriate. At the micro level, financial and administrative records may be used for cost and staffing data; surveys and focus groups may be used for staff and patient data. Specially constructed data-collection instruments that are employed concurrently or retrospectively in the study of processes and outcomes for specific patient populations may be developed. Sources of data may include direct observation, interviews, **flow charts**, financial reports, medical records, and critical-path variance reports. These sources of data allow identification and analysis of a wide range of process and outcome variables for specific patient groups.

MEASUREMENT ISSUES

There are several measurement issues that must be addressed when doing outcomes research. The first is timing, or the specification of the time period in which certain outcomes should be achieved (Hegyvary, 1991). Outcomes may be measured over the short term, such as when monitoring patient response to medication. Alternatively, they may be intermediate, such as length of stay, complications, or return to work after surgery; or long-term, such as success of an educational program one year post-instruction. Certain outcomes might need to be measured repeatedly. For example, patients in a rehabilitation program after suffering a cerebral hemorrhage might have certain outcomes measured every three to six months.

The second measurement issue relates to level of analysis, which is associated with the purpose of the study (Hegyvary, 1991). For example, the objective may be to study the results of the specific care and treatment of individuals, or it may be to study the effect of services delivered by a specific unit or institution. At the most macro level, the objective may be to determine the quality of care delivered by the entire health-care system. The different levels of analysis require different types of **indicators** and methodological approaches (Hegyvary, 1991; Verran, Mark, & Lamb, 1992).

Attribution is a third measurement issue (Hegyvary, 1991). The time delay between intervention and outcome may make attribution of cause and effect difficult to determine. Researchers must identify the multiple variables that may contribute to any particular outcome. For example, research done by Shortell, Rousseau, Gillies, Devers, and Simms (1991) and Knaus, Draper, Wagner, and Zimmerman (1986) examined mortality rates across multiple intensive-care sites, and included medical, nursing, managerial, patient-demographic, and environmental factors as potential contributing factors to **variation** in this outcome.

A final measurement issue concerns databases (Hegyvary, 1991). Currently, measures that reflect outcomes are not comparable across institutional systems, and there is basic incompatibility among databases and data systems. There are issues surrounding security and confidentiality of the data, as well as the validity and reliability of measures. Databases must be developed or modified so that they reflect nursing interventions as well as medical management. However, the nursing profession first must achieve consensus on these data elements. In addition, there is a need to organize data in a standard way and with a common data language

(Jennings, 1991). It is also time to develop **multidisciplinary** models of care. Inter-Study (Ellwood, 1988) is developing standardized data-collection instruments that can be used on a broad-scale, national basis. This effort has incorporated instruments from the Rand Medical Outcomes Study, which included scales for general health, and functional, social, and mental status (Stewart, Hays, & Ware, 1988). These are patient outcomes that are relevant to both nursing and medical practice, as well as that of other disciplines.

MEASURING VARIATIONS IN OUTCOMES

At the macro level, differences in outcomes across hospitals are compared in order to measure the level of hospital performance. Several other factors may also be influencing these outcomes, however. These include (Des Harnais, McMahon, Wroblewski, & Hogan, 1990):

1. variations in the types of patients treated, for example, the DRG mix

2. overall severity of patients' primary or principal diagnoses

3. the type and complexity of the patients' comorbidities

4. the social and financial conditions of patients

These possible contributing factors to outcome variation require the use of case-mix and severity-of-illness adjusters when analyzing and comparing outcomes of care. The first level of case-mix control usually uses one of the diagnostic classification systems, such as ICD-9-CM codes, the DRG distribution, DRG clusters (adjacent DRGs), Major Diagnostic Categories, or CCGs (clinically coherent groups.)

The next level of case-mix control is controlling for the severity and/or complexity of illness within each diagnostic grouping. Several commercial systems are available, including the Computerized Severity Index (CSI), Medis-Groups, APACHE III, and Disease Staging. Alternatively, one may use secondary diagnoses, weighted or unweighted, that reflect preexisting comorbid conditions. A third level of case-mix control is variation due to individual patient characteristics, including demographics and socioeconomic status (living arrangements, finances). The source of payment for the health-care bill can be a good proxy for socioeconomic status.

Additional contributing factors have been identified that can help explain variations in outcomes. These include: (a) the reason for admission — whether it is the terminal phase of an illness or the diagnostic phase; and (b) the patient's physiologic reserve — for example, the APACHE severity-of-illness measurement system for acutely ill patients in the intensive-care unit has a Chronic Health Evaluation component to determine the patient's preexisting health status (Wagner & Draper, 1984). When these patient-specific factors are identified and controlled for, the residual variation in outcomes is most likely due to provider performance factors, such as the adequacy of the staff or physical plant, quality of interpersonal relationships and technical performance, and unmeasured severity of illness.

Adequacy of staff refers to **certification**, educational, and skill-mix issues, among other things. Quality of interpersonal relations reflects the extent of customer focus, as well as caregiver-to-caregiver communication and cooperation. Technical performance refers to the interventions, treatments, actions, techniques, or practice patterns used in particular situations to elicit desired outcomes (Jennings, 1991). So far, nurses' specific contributions to improved outcomes have not been well-documented (Fagin, 1990). Testing of the influence of nursing interventions on outcomes should be done as a component of multidisciplinary studies, given that it would be difficult to isolate the effects of nursing interventions by themselves. It would also reflect the reality that no one professional group operates independently in the delivery of services to patients.

OUTCOMES ANALYSIS METHODOLOGY

There are several approaches to measuring variations in outcomes, each with certain advantages and limitations. At the macro level, these include:

- *Direct standardization* — involves isolating the effects of hospital care on patient outcomes. This should be the ideal measurement technique because it captures changes in the patient's health status following treatment. However, it is not possible to evaluate changing health status with existing databases. The alternate application is to measure variations in the rates of adverse consequences across hospitals. The assumption is that hospitals with lower rates of adverse events are producing better patient outcomes (Des Harnais et al., 1990). Thus, measures of adverse outcomes are used as proxies for positive measures of outcomes. This methodology usually focuses on specific procedures, disease categories, or hospital units. A limitation of this approach is that outcomes may vary because of underlying differences in the patient groups being compared, not because of different levels of provider performance.

- *Meta analysis* — involves the systematic evaluation and combination of results from separate studies of a particular subject (such as success associated with CABG procedures as compared to angioplasty). This is a useful methodology when individual studies disagree in their findings or if the sample sizes are too small to be conclusive.

- *Small area analysis* — population-based studies that focus primarily on utilization rates as reflections of quality, such as the performance of specific types of surgical procedures (T&A, hysterectomy, hernia repair, prostatectomy), hospital admissions, and physician visits. The difficulty with this methodology is in interpretation of the results: Is the one rate too high or the other too low? Are unnecessary procedures being performed on some patients, or are other patients not achieving access to potentially beneficial procedures? The health-care system currently lacks accepted standards of care, and there are no readily available **benchmarks** for comparison.

- *Indirect standardization* — the methodology most in use in the study of outcomes at the hospital or system level. Differences across hospitals in the types of patients treated (case mix) and their severity of illness are first accounted for statistically. Adjustments are then made for the differences in reason for admission, patient-demographic characteristics, and other variations across patients and providers.

Unless these adjustments are made, it is not possible to make valid comparisons — those treating more difficult cases will appear to have worse outcomes (Des Harnais et al., 1990; Schroeder, 1987).

At the micro level, various epidemiologic approaches may be used to study outcomes while employing necessary risk adjustments. These include case-control and cohort studies. Log-linear modeling has also been used to examine the influence of treatment variables on patient outcomes while controlling for the influence of case-mix factors such as gender and race. The results of retrospective and concurrent analysis of process-outcome relationships can suggest topics for further study using more sophisticated techniques, such as formal randomized, controlled clinical trials.

EXAMPLES OF OUTCOMES ANALYSIS

Outcome studies initially focused on mortality rates. Every major multihospital study on mortality demonstrated substantial variation in this measure across hospitals (Chassin, Park, Lohr, Kelsey, & Brook, 1989; Hartz et al., 1989; Scott, Forrest, & Brown, 1976; Shortell & Hughes, 1988). A consistent finding across these studies was that nursing care or nursing-care organization are among the factors that help explain variation in death rates across hospitals. For example, Scott et al. (1976) found that higher ratios of Registered Nurses (RNs) to Licensed Vocational Nurses (LVNs) and more highly qualified RNs were associated with lower death and morbidity rates. Better outcomes were also associated with decentralization of decisions to the unit level, standardization of nursing procedures, and higher ratios of clerks and unit secretaries. More recent, macro-level studies by Knaus et al. (1986) and Shortell et al. (1991) using indirect standardization techniques reported that differences in intensive-care-unit mortality appeared to be related to the integrative process of care, particularly the level of interaction and communication between physicians and nurses.

Behner, Fogg, Fournier, Frankenbach, and Robertson (1990) conducted a micro-level study on the relationship between cost and quality in nurse staffing decisions. They first determined staffing variances: hours of care actually delivered versus hours of care that should have been provided according to the Medicus patient-classification system. They examined patients within one DRG, hospitalized on one nursing unit, and calculated the staffing variance for each day of stay. They then analyzed the impact of staffing variances on patient complications and length of stay. The results indicated that staffing at 20 percent below the recommended level during the first 3 days of a patient's stay resulted in a 30 percent increase in the probability that the patient would experience a complication while in the hospital, which in turn would lead to an additional 3.5 days of hospital stay. They concluded that the additional costs associated with patients who experience complications is greater than the labor savings due to understaffing.

Weisman and Nathanson (1985) studied the relationship of organizational characteristics to professional-staff satisfaction in family-planning clinics, and the relationship of both organizational characteristics and staff satisfaction to client satisfaction and client compliance with contraceptive prescriptions. Staff satisfaction was the most important determinant for client satisfaction. Client satisfaction, in turn, predicted the rate of subsequent compliance, but compliance was more susceptible to variations in clinic structure than to variations in staff satisfaction levels.

These studies illustrate the important relationship between managerial and organizational processes and patient outcomes. How health-care organizations are structured and staffed, and how interdepartmental and **interdisciplinary** relationships are managed, makes a difference in the quality of services delivered. In addition, there may be important relationships between selected clinical processes for specific patient groups and resulting patient outcomes. For example, Wirtschafter, Jones, and Thomas (1992) analyzed the relationship between nutritional and respiratory-care treatment processes and outcomes experienced by very-low-birth-weight infants. They found that more conservative feeding and ventilation practices were associated with a higher risk of chronic lung disease and nosocomial infection, which in turn were related to significantly longer hospital stays.

IMPLICATIONS FOR RESEARCH

This discussion highlights several areas that need attention in order to move the field of outcomes analysis to a higher level. First, there is an urgent need to create large data sets and to conduct multisite studies of outcomes. The American Association of Critical Care Nurses has been pursuing this strategy with regard to several clinical research issues. Perhaps the American Organization of Nurse Executives (AONE) might follow a similar path with regard to structural and managerial issues in health-care settings. One a state level, the New York State Department of Health has developed a standardized data-collection process for specific cardiology procedures done in all hospitals across the state. State-level outcomes analysis is performed, plus hospitals have been shown how to calculate the expected probability of death for patients within their own settings so that cases requiring internal quality-of-care reviews can be identified (Hannan, Kilburn, O'Donnell, Lukacik, & Shields, 1990). These internal reviews might reveal deficiencies in medical, nursing, or ancillary care practices, or in care delivery processes. In California, the Office of Maternal and Child Health Services produces annual hospital-specific predicted and actual perinatal mortality rates for the state, again using indirect standardization techniques (Williams, 1979). Hospitals with higher than expected mortality rates must explore potential causative factors to explain the discrepancy.

IMPLICATIONS FOR NURSE MANAGERS AND EXECUTIVES

Research is critical to validating practice and developing theory. Nurse executives must support nursing research activities in their settings. The cost benefit of nursing research will be demonstrated by study results that show how specific nursing interventions directly improve patient outcomes, which in turn reduce cost and length of stay. The challenge in today's health-care environment is to continuously improve patient outcomes in shorter periods of time, at lower cost, while maintaining quality.

Nurse executives must become informed consumers of outcomes-analysis results. This implies the ability to review published reports and make informed judgments as to whether the findings should be disseminated within the institution and across the relevant peer groups. In addition, nurse executives must evaluate the results of outcome studies conducted within their own facilities to determine whether the findings are valid and reliable.

Changes in organizational structure, nursing-care delivery models, and caregiver roles must address cost, patient and staff satisfaction, length of stay, and quality issues. This focus on outcomes requires decision support systems built on a solid information base. Nurse executives need to build the internal capacity of their institutions to conduct outcomes analysis. This means building appropriate databases, hiring qualified personnel, and providing the requisite support structures. The organization's management team must link production-cost and revenue data with clinical and patient-based data on health outcomes. Computer systems must be designed that track nursing interventions, their costs, and patient outcomes that are attributable to these nursing actions. The costs associated with these activities should be recovered by the gains achieved by improving effectiveness and productivity.

At the unit level, nurse managers can conduct, support, or participate in studies on the impact of organizational/managerial changes on patient and organizational outcomes. These studies can be done with the assistance of the director of nursing research, in collaboration with faculty from area schools of nursing and public health, or as part of student theses or dissertation projects. Nurse managers should also work in collaboration with clinical nurse specialists to design and implement clinical outcome studies for specific patient groups on their units. The nurse executive and nurse manager should work actively to ensure that these research groups are multidisciplinary.

At the macro level, establishment of a minimum nursing-management data set, with uniform definitions and measurement techniques, would be particularly useful. This would be instrumental to conducting multisite studies of organizational outcomes, with improved validity and reliability of results. Nurse managers and nurse executives should also encourage dissemination of the results of outcomes studies, both internally and externally. The strategies may include nursing grand rounds, sponsoring local or regional conferences, presentations at professional meetings, manuscript production, staff development, and internal/external consulting.

CONCLUSION

Paying more attention to outcomes of care will lead to additional research questions for nursing, and growing interest in determining the most effective and efficient interventions for specific patient groups. This in turn will improve the overall quality of health care being delivered. Successful outcomes management depends on the ability of administration to control organizational costs while at the same time developing effective synergistic relationships with its clinicians and other health-care organizations to manage the health of the population over time (Conrad, 1991).

REFERENCES

Behner, K. G., Fogg, L. F., Fournier, L. C., Frankenbach, J. T., & Robertson, S. B. (1990). Nursing resource management: Analyzing the relationship between costs and quality in staffing decisions. *Health Care Management Review, 15*(4), 63–71.

Bowen, O. R. (1987). Shattuck Lecture — What is quality care? *New England Journal of Medicine, 316*(25), 1578–1580.

Chassin, M. R., Park, R. E., Lohr, K. N., Kelsey, J., & Brook, R. H. (1989). Differences among hospitals in Medicare patient mortality. *Health Services Research, 24*(1), 1–31.

Conrad, D. A. (1991). Editorial. *Frontiers in Health Services Management, 8*(2), 1–2.

Des Harnais, S. I., McMahon, L. F., Wroblewski, R. T., & Hogan, A. J. (1990). Measuring hospital performance: Development and validation of risk-adjusted indexes of mortality, readmissions, and complications. *Medical Care, 28*(12), 1127–1141.

Ellwood, P. (1988). Shattuck Lecture — Outcomes management: A technology of patient experience. *New England Journal of Medicine, 318*(23), 1549–1556.

Fagin, C. M. (1990). Nursing's value proves itself. *American Journal of Nursing, 90*(10), 17–30.

Geigle, R., & Jones, S. B. (1990). Outcomes measurement: A report from the front. *Inquiry, 27*(2), 7–13.

Hannan, R. L., Kilburn, H., O'Donnell, J. F., Lukacik, G., & Shields, E. P. (1990). Adult open heart surgery in New York State: An analysis of risk factors and hospital mortality rate. *Journal of the American Medical Association, 264*(21), 2768–2774.

Harris, M. D. (1991). Clinical and financial outcomes in patient care in a home health care agency. *Journal of Nursing Quality Assurance, 5*(2), 41–49.

Hartz, A. J., Krakauer, H., Kuhn, E. M., Young, M., Jacobsen, S. J., Gay, G., Muenz, L., Katzoff, M., Baily, R. C., & Rimm, A. A. (1989). Hospital characteristics and mortality rates. *New England Journal of Medicine, 321*(25), 1720–1725.

Hegyvary, S. T. (1991). Issues in outcomes research. *Journal of Nursing Quality Assurance, 5*(2), 1–6.

Hornbrook, M. C., Hurtado, A. V., & Johnson, R. E. (1985). Health care episodes: Definition, measurement, and uses. *Medical Care Review, 42*(2), 163–218.

Jennings, B. M. (1991). Patient outcomes research: Seizing the opportunity. *Advances in Nursing Science, 14*(2), 59–72.

Joint Commission on Accreditation of Healthcare Organizations. Standards. In *1993 Accreditation Manual for Hospitals*, (Vol. 1). Oakbrook Terrace, IL: Author.

Keeler, E. B., Solomon, D. H., Beck, J. C., Mendenhall, R. C., & Kane, R. L. (1982). Effect of patient age on duration of medical encounters with physicians. *Medical Care, 20*(11), 1101–1108.

Knaus, W. A., Draper, E. A., Wagner, D. P., & Zimmerman, J. E. (1986). An evaluation of outcomes from intensive care in major medical centers. *Annals of Internal Medicine, 104*(3), 410–418.

Lohr, K. N. (1985). *Impact of Medicare prospective payment on the quality of medical care: A research agenda.* Santa Monica, CA: The Rand Corporation.

Lohr, K. N. (1988). Outcome measurements: Concepts and questions. *Inquiry, 25*(1), 37–50.

Lohr, K. N. (1990). *Medicare: A strategy for Quality Assurance.* Washington, DC: National Academy Press.

Patterson, C. H. (1993). Joint Commission nursing care standards: The framework for a comprehensive program to assess and improve quality. *Journal of Nursing Care Quality, 7*(2), 1–14.

Rettig, R. (1991). History, development, and importance to nursing of outcomes research. *Journal of Nursing Quality Assurance, 5*(2), 13–17.

Schroeder, S. A. (1987). Outcome assessment 70 years later: Are we ready? *New England Journal of Medicine, 316*(3), 160–162.

Scott, W. L., Forrest, W. H., & Brown, B. W. (1976). Hospital structures and postoperative mortality and morbidity. In S. Shortell & Brown (Eds.), *Organizational research in hospitals.* Chicago: Blue Cross Association.

Servais, S. H. (1991). Nursing resource applications through outcome based nursing practice. *Nursing Economic$, 9*(3), 171–174.

Shortell, S., & Hughes, E. (1988). The effects of regulation, competition, and ownership on hospital rates among hospital inpatients. *New England Journal of Medicine, 318*(17), 1100–1107.

Shortell, S. M., Rousseau, D. M., Gillies, R. R., Devers, K. J., & Simms, T. L. (1991). Organizational assessment in intensive care units (ICUs): Construct development, reliability, and validity of the ICU nurse-physician questionnaire. *Medical Care, 29*(8), 709–726.

Stewart, A. L., Hays, R. D., & Ware, J. E. (1988). The MOS short-form general health survey: Reliability and validity in a patient population. *Medical Care, 26*(7), 724–735.

Verran, J. A., Mark, B. A., & Lamb, G. (1992). Psychometric examination of instruments using aggregated data. *Research in Nursing and Health, 15*(3), 237–240.

Wagner, D. P., & Draper, E. A. (1984). Acute physiology and chronic health evaluation (APACHE II) and Medicare reimbursement. *Health Care Financing Review (Ann. Supp.),* 91–105.

Weisman, C. S., & Nathanson, C. A. (1985). Professional satisfaction and client outcomes. *Medical Care, 23*(10), 1179–1192.

Williams, R. L. (1979). Measuring the effectiveness of perinatal medicine. *Medical Care, 17*(2), 95–110.

Wirtschafter, D. D., Jones, K. R., & Thomas, J. C. (1992). Using health outcomes to improve care in the NICU. Unpublished manuscript.

ADDITIONAL READING

Al-Assaf, A. F. (1993). Outcome management and TQ. In A. F. Al-Assaf & J. A. Schmele (Eds.), *Textbook of total quality in healthcare* (pp. 221–237). Del Ray Beach, FL: St. Lucie Press.

Betalden, P. B., Nelson, E. C., & Roberts, J. S. (1994). Linking outcomes measurement to continual improvement: The serial "V" way of thinking about improving clinical care. *Journal on Quality Improvement, 20*(4), 167–180.

Davies, A. R., Doyle, M. A. T., Lansky, D., Rutt, W., Stevic, M. O., & Doyle, J. B. (1994). Outcome assessment in clinical settings: A consensus statement on principles and best practices in project management. *Joint Commission Journal on Quality Improvement, 20*(1), 6–16.

Donabedian, A. (1992). The role of outcome in quality assessment and assurance. *Quality Review Bulletin, 18*(11), 356–360.

Gonnella, J. S., Louis, D. Z., & Gottlieb, J. E. (1994). Physicians' responsibilities and outcomes of medical care. *Journal on Quality Improvement, 20*(7), 402–410.

Lang, N. M., & Marck, K. D. (1990). The classification of patient outcomes. *Journal of Professional Nursing, 6*(3), 158–163.

Lang, N. M., & Marck, K. D. (1991). The policy and politics of patient outcomes. *Journal of Nursing Quality Assurance, 5*(2), 7–12.

U.S. Department of Health and Human Services. (1992). *Patient outcomes research: Examining the effectiveness of nursing practice* (NIH Publication No. 93-3411). Rockville, MD: Author.

P. Susan Wagner

CHAPTER 24

Guide to Identifying, Collecting, and Managing Data

INTRODUCTION

The focus of this chapter is sources of data for **Quality Management (QM)**, and methods of collecting that data. The chapter begins with a short discussion of changes in the health-care system and a brief overview of QM. Guidelines are then provided for making decisions regarding a QM program. The **indicators** selected for measurement determine the source of data and sometimes the data-collection method, as well. Alternate methods of indicator development are described. Specific dimensions of quality indicators guide the selection of priority areas for attention in the QM program. Discussion of factors influencing operational decisions about specific sources of data precedes a description of the different data sources and methods of data collection. Approaches used to present the data depend on the specificity of the data and the stage in the QM process. A brief discussion of data interpretation concludes the chapter.

CHANGES IN THE HEALTH-CARE SYSTEM

The health-care system has traditionally reflected the philosophical orientation of professionals and administrators within the system. During the middle of the twentieth century, this orientation was based on the adulation of the scientific discoveries of medicine, the expertise of the health-science professionals, and the subsequent dependence of the general public on professionals for health restoration and maintenance. The goal of the system was to improve health of patients through treatment of physical illnesses. The professional role was technical, and the organizational context was hierarchical and segmented by professional discipline. Concerns about the **quality** of care focused on medical procedures and structural requirements for implementing organizational routines, primarily in hospitals.

With recognition of the limits of scientific medicine, the increasing number of health disciplines, and the growth of the consumer movement, the concept of care and caring changed. The definition of health now includes mental, social, and environmental aspects in addition to the physical, with recognition that well-being is defined by the individual and community. The patient has become a client and **consumer** of health services, involved as a partner in decisions about the health care. The professional role is supportive, complementing the client's ability to accomplish self-care tasks with the provision of information or instrumental assistance. Management is expected to respect the opinions and contribution of employees and physicians in the organization, and work with them as partners. The focus is on a multitude of care providers, both institution and community based. These changes in philosophical approach are changing the nature of health-care organizations, and changing the expectations for QM. The effect of health care on client or community health status is considered the best evidence of quality performance by a health-care organization. Organizational **structure** and **processes** are viewed in terms of their contribution to the well-being of the client and the effectiveness of working relationships among departments, rather than as isolated entities (American Hospital Association, 1991; Van Maanen, 1984). Societal pressure for **accountability** within the health-care system is also influencing priorities as fiscal resources shrink. Health-care organizations are forced by regulatory bodies and fiscal realities to carefully examine their internal processes and end products. Quality-Management practices have become a tool for improving client health status and reducing unnecessary expenditures.

QUALITY MANAGEMENT

The purpose of a QM program is to improve the effectiveness and efficiency of client care by providing data for decision making. The client is central, so the most basic indicator of the quality of care is effectiveness or **outcome**, traditionally measured in terms of recovery, restoration, and survival (Holland, 1983). Outcome measures that are based in client experience and are related to well-being and quality of life are being developed by researchers. Efficiency is "the ratio of the product produced to the resources put in" (Holland, 1983, p. 20). The Canadian Medical Association (CMA) considers "efficacy, knowing what works; appropriateness, using what works; execution of care, doing well what works; and purpose of care, clarifying the values that determine what should be done" (Harrigan, 1992, p. 146) as the components of quality control. The Joint Commission on Accreditation of Healthcare Organizations (Joint Commission) lists twelve factors that contribute to the quality of health care: accessibility, timeliness, effectiveness, efficacy, appropriateness, efficiency, continuity, privacy, confidentiality, participation of the client, safety, and supportiveness of the care environment (Joint Commission on Accreditation of Healthcare Organizations [Joint Commission], 1989). (These elements of quality are discussed in Chapter 17.) It is evident that the client's perspective on care delivery and outcome has become central to the management of quality health care. The selection of indicators, data sources, and collection methods must include the experiences of people who are involved with the event (Sharp & Kilvington, 1993).

INDICATORS OF QUALITY CARE

The appropriate use of indicators requires an understanding of their development and dimensions. The section that follows deals with these topics.

Development of Indicators

Indicators are measurement tools used as guides to **monitoring** and **evaluating** the quality of important patient-care and support-service activities (Joint Commission, 1989). Indicators are not direct measures of quality, but, instead, focus attention on data about processes and outcomes related to the principal functions of the organization. They reflect events that occur to clients, staff, or the organization. The indicators selected reveal the assumptions and philosophical beliefs about clients, health, health care, and quality care (Krieger, 1992). A rate-based indicator is expressed as the number of events that occur compared to a specific universe of events. The resulting ratio can be monitored for its fit within predetermined parameters of functioning. A consistent approach to the development of quality indicators within an organization ensures application of common philosophical beliefs, use of common definitions, and a common format. When involvement of several disciplines in the selection of indicators is required and coordination of one department's indicators with those of other departments is expected, the potential for a comprehensive QM program is increased. After the organization establishes a broad statement of quality or **standard** for a given element of care, each discipline or department makes a unique contribution to the indicator(s) of that quality level. The results are specific guidelines for practice related to that indicator, followed by specific measurable **criteria** to evaluate performance by professionals or department staff. Wilson (1992) identifies four methods of developing indicators of quality care: by experience, by prescription, by audit process, and by activity mapping.

EXPERIENCE

The people who are involved with the event under consideration are the most direct source of quality indicators. The clients, professionals, or department workers have expectations regarding what the final outcome of the event should be, and what would indicate success or failure. Clinical practice guidelines developed by a health discipline are based on the experience of seasoned professionals and on research arising from that experience. These guidelines, developed around those population groups and events critical to that health discipline, are indicators of quality practice. The indicators suggested by the experience of workers focus on the outcome of care or the processes that contribute to that outcome. It is desirable to have a balance of practicing professionals and researchers on an indicator-selection committee (Kitson, Harvey, Hyndman, & Yerrell, 1994).

PRESCRIPTION

An indicator of quality is developed by prescription when an external body establishes expectations for quality processes or organizational performance. The external body could be an accrediting or regulatory body that defines the development process for indicators (Smith & Popowich, 1993). The process may include identification of the principle functions of the organization, the important components for those functions, the standards for quality related to the components, and, finally, the indicators that show the degree to which the standards have been met. Quality indicators may also be prescribed by a professional body and labeled clinical protocols, clinical practice guidelines, or a minimum data set (Anderson & Hannah, 1993). In Canada and the United States, funding bodies have rigid criteria for the reimbursement of particular services, and these indicators exist by prescription. The choice of indicators for reimbursement may also be based on extensive reviews of the literature, current research, or on the cost of certain procedures.

AUDIT PROCESS
Quality indicators may arise from the audit process, because results of care are often described in terms of the percentage of cases with a particular outcome. The indicator may be one of several indicators related to a particular standard, but is given special consideration because of an unusual pattern of practice, its importance, or the need for remedial action and future review.

ACTIVITY MAPPING
Identifying the steps in a particular process is described as activity mapping, criteria mapping, **flowcharting**, or creating a cause and effect or **fishbone diagram**. Naming the small steps that contribute to a result makes indicators of quality evident. An advantage of activity mapping is recognizing the myriad of factors and personnel that contribute to a successful outcome. (See the section on data presentation later in this chapter for further information.)

Selection of Priority Indicators

The priority indicators of quality need to be directly related to the principal functions of the organization. Principal functions are connected to the products or services that are outcomes of the organization's activities. Principle functions are results of staff activities and are most appropriately expressed in lay terms, using action verbs. Only six or eight principal functions account for 80 to 90 percent of an organization's or department's activities (Wilson, 1992). Keeping the list small ensures that the QM program is focused on work done rather than on recording of the work. Each written formulation needs to be requisite or essential for "either the department head in his or her management of the quality of the department's performance or senior management in the discharge of its duty to be accountable for quality to the [organization]'s board of trustees" (Wilson, 1992, p. 16). There is agreement that the most important indicators of quality include those activities that are high risk, high volume, problem prone, and high cost (Katz & Green, 1992). The American Hospital Association (1991) adds the criterion of high variability in practice patterns, particularly in relation to physician activities.

Wilson (1992) describes a process to guide decision making regarding which quality indicators are important. He classifies indicators as risk, key, descriptive, and dispensable. The first step is to categorize indicators by usefulness. Those unrelated to the principal functions of the organization or department are dispensable —

they are unnecessary because they are of questionable or no value. If indicators do not stand alone to communicate something important about functioning, they are dispensable. The second step is to classify indicators according to level of risk. Activities wherein the client or the organization is at high risk for negative consequences must have indicators of quality.

As mentioned earlier, key indicators refer to high-volume, problem-prone, or high-cost activities. High-volume activities are those that affect large numbers of clients or that occur frequently. If over 50 percent of clients receive a particular service, that service can be considered high volume (Katz & Green, 1992). Problem-prone activities are those that tend to produce complications or difficulties for clients, important others, staff, or the system. High-cost activities are key to the economic viability of the unit. These could be very expensive client, staff, or system activities, or high volumes of less costly activities. Descriptive indicators become important only if their values change significantly. They are not important enough and are too expensive to generate regularly. The Joint Commission (1993) has, for example, carefully selected rate-based indicators of quality based on client outcomes and the previously mentioned criteria of importance. These indicators are a result of several years of field testing. Examples of Joint Commission indicators are for medication use; infection control; anesthetics; and obstetrical, cardiovascular, oncology, and trauma care (Joint Commission, 1993). This indicator development program continues to be further developed and tested each year.

Dimensions of Clinical Indicators

Several different dimensions of quality guide the formulation of specific indicators. Five are discussed here: scope of care, aspect of care, appropriateness, seriousness of event, and type of event. Activities may or may not need an indicator for every dimension.

SCOPE OF CARE

The scope of care can be described by identifying activities or key functions. Katz and Green (1992) describe the domains within the scope of care as clinical, professional, or administrative. Indicators within the clinical domain refer to client, family, or community customers of service. Characteristics of the most common population groups cared for by that department or organization must be identified to ensure that activities match their needs. The severity of illness, existence of comorbid conditions, and other health data are important, as is demographic information such as age, gender, socioeconomic status, and literacy level. Indicators from the professional domain refer to the staff and professionals involved with events, as the customers of the activities. Identifying the characteristics and profile of staff assists in matching activities to staff needs. The functions of a staff-development department are primarily in this domain, and indicators may be related to orientation, continuing-education activities, and educational-leave policies. The administrative domain includes management, governance, or system activities. A profile of management personnel or board members may also assist in determining the appropriateness of activities undertaken in this domain. For example, if low attendance at board meetings occurs, the score for that quality indicator may be improved by a survey of the trustees regarding preferred meeting times. A system policy related to the measurement of client acuity may be supported when the forms required are designed or adapted by the managers who have to complete them.

ASPECT OF CARE
Donabedian (1988) described an approach to the complexity of health care that attempted to make the measurement of quality easier. He divided aspects of care into *structure, process,* and *outcome.* Structural aspects of care refer to the organization's ability to deliver quality care, the resources provided, and the characteristics of the settings where care is delivered. Attributes of the process of care reflect the way that care is delivered, or the efficiency of resource utilization management, for example, a system of retrospective, concurrent, and prospective measures that describe the use of resources. Outcomes of care are the results — the effects of care on the health of individuals or populations. Structural and process measures are indirect indicators of the quality of care, and outcome measures are a direct measure of the quality of care delivered (Bard, Jimenez, & Tornack, 1994).

APPROPRIATENESS OF CARE
The quality of care is often categorized by its appropriateness, for that client, at that time, in that setting, with that category of personnel, with that approach. The care should have efficacy, meaning that the care provided must be known to be effective for that condition. It should be delivered in an effective manner, so that it works as expected. The continuity and consistency of the care provided is also a measure of appropriateness. The timeliness of care can be viewed from the client's perspective, but also from the viewpoint of the organization. The care in question may be routinely offered, offered as need arises or as requested, or offered only in emergency situations.

SERIOUSNESS OF EVENTS
A **sentinel event** is a serious, undesirable outcome of care. Whenever a sentinel event occurs, there is an investigation into the cause and circumstances. These events can simply be recorded to establish a trend and measured in detail only when the rate of occurrence exceeds predetermined **thresholds**, or shows significant differences when comparisons are made to like organizations elsewhere. A rate-based indicator can be applied longitudinally, measuring events over time to establish trends of occurrence.

ADVERSE EVENT OR DESIRABLE EVENT
An event can be desirable if it indicates the maintenance of quality care, or undesirable if it reduces the quality of care. The relationships between these dimensions of clinical indicators can provide a format for organizing a QM program (Katz & Green, 1992). The scope of care can be categorized into clinical, professional, and organizational domains; events then can be listed for each domain in the categories of structure, process, or outcome. These indicators can then be subcategorized as routinely offered, offered as need arises or as requested, or offered only in emergency situations. They can be tagged as high risk, high volume, high cost, or problem prone to assist in making decisions about which indicators to begin measuring.

THRESHOLDS

A threshold is the border between compliance and noncompliance as determined by a written clinical indicator that is standards based. The setting of threshold parameters for clinical indicators is guided by past performance of the organization, experts in the field, or empirical findings reported in the literature. There are upper and lower limits for the occurrence of the event, and the desirability or undesirability of the event determines which limit indicates better quality performance. When the limit is passed, intensive evaluation of that aspect of care is required to determine whether there is an opportunity for improvement of organizational functioning. Thresholds are dynamic, and are expected to improve with time. They need to be realistic, for there are always unique circumstances that cannot be controlled by organizational effort. When clinical indicators are selected carefully, thresholds are objective signs of the quality of care.

SELECTION OF DATA SOURCES

The importance of selecting priority indicators cannot be overemphasized. It is possible to collect many different types of data; but if the data is not related to the principal functions of the organization, it has little meaning. When a QM program becomes known more for the amount of paperwork required than for the value of the findings, too much data is being collected — and there is a risk of reducing staff commitment to the QM program (Burdick, Stuart, & Lewis, 1994; Kitson et al., 1994; Ruden, 1994).

Katz and Green (1992) identify four reasons to collect data. Data validates that events are happening the way that they are intended to happen. Monitoring confirms or denies whether the processes of the organization are operating smoothly, and whether the principal functions are being met. The second reason for collecting data is to provide a basis for change or improvement of the care, practice, or governance of the organization. Without data, knowledge of current status and planning for future change cannot occur. The third value of data collection is to provide rationale for the maintenance or change of resource allocation in the organization. Decisions made on factual information lessen the number of inappropriate decisions. The last reason for collecting data is to assist with the development of thresholds to be used as guides in monitoring the current practices and future goals of the organization.

Considerations in the Selection of Data Sources

The Joint Commission (1989) describes four "necessary attributes" of clinical indicators: validity, face validity, sensitivity, and specificity. There are several other factors that also influence the selection of data sources. See Table 24-1 for a list of considerations in selecting data sources. The relative importance of each factor will be unique to each organization and should be carefully considered prior to the launching of a QM program.

VALIDITY

The degree to which the indicator accomplishes its purpose reflects the validity of that indicator. The data must measure accurately what it is supposed to reflect.

Table 24-1 • **CONSIDERATIONS IN SELECTING DATA SOURCES**

Validity	Accuracy
Face validity	Confidentiality
Sensitivity	Flexibility
Specificity	Nature of the data
Significance	Volume of data
Practicality	Availability of data
Reliability	Resources

Proof of validity is whether situations are identified wherein the quality of care and services should be improved. The number of client complaints, for example, is not a valid indicator of client satisfaction. It is only one dimension of the issue.

FACE VALIDITY
The opinions of informed users of the data or experts in the field are the basis for face validity. If the data is considered suitable for answering the information need, then there is face validity. If the information need is general, general information is required. If there is a particular problem, then the data obtained must be clearly related to that problem to be of use in defining alternatives for improvement. Data that is widely used within a profession or sphere of work is respected by users, more acceptable to staff, and enhances communication and comparison with other like organizations.

SENSITIVITY
The degree to which the indicator or data is capable of identifying all cases of care where actual quality of care problems exist indicates the sensitivity of the measure. If the data reveals the major problems, but not the minor ones, then more sensitive data is required. It is important that data also be sensitive to changes in quality of performance for that issue.

SPECIFICITY
If the indicator or the data is able to identify only those cases where a particular problem exists, and not identify cases where there are other problems, then there is specificity. When problems not related to the issue in question are identified by the indicator, the examination of solutions becomes difficult; and the data is not specific enough.

SIGNIFICANCE
To have real significance, the data must be closely related to the principal functions of the department or organization. A few key pieces of data have much more meaning to staff and management than does a diverse array of unimportant pieces that are reluctantly collected with a higher likelihood of inaccuracy. The data should focus on the critical aspects of the service and address every subsystem of the care process.

PRACTICALITY

The data source must be relatively easy to access. If data is not readily available, it is more likely that staff will postpone collecting it, or collect it incorrectly. When data is difficult to collect, it defeats the purpose of efficient monitoring of performance. If hard-to-collect data is considered very important, redesigning organizational systems or forms to make collection easier may be worthwhile. The data could also be collected on an annual or irregular basis, to reduce staff stress.

RELIABILITY

The data must have the same definition to all those who will be involved in collecting it or in using the information. If the data means different things to different people, then no fruitful comparisons can be made, and the data is unreliable.

ACCURACY

The data must be accurate to be meaningful. It must be valid and reliable to be accurate. Many data sources are based in the documentation of the practices of an organization. When that documentation is not complete, comprehensive, or legible, accurate data is not possible. Increasing the quality of the documentation is sometimes required prior to establishing a QM program. Alternate methods include redesigning forms in terms of the principal functions of the department or organization, establishing protocols regarding documentation, or clarifying the expectations of staff. If there are concerns about the quality of the documentation but the data must be used, triangulation (use of three or more sources of data) increases the validity and reliability, and, hence, the accuracy of the data obtained. Knowledge of care delivered, for example, can be obtained from the client record, an interview with the client, and observation of staff.

CONFIDENTIALITY

If data is to be shared across the industry, the format for data collection must protect the confidentiality of clients, practitioners, and even the organization (Milholland, 1994). The data source is always found in particular events involving specific persons. It is the circumstances surrounding the event and the event itself, however, that are of importance in identifying patterns of practice. The information obtained in QM should not be used for performance appraisal of staff, for then the program will be interpreted as punitive rather than supportive of staff efforts. Data may be used by individual practitioners for educational purposes.

FLEXIBILITY

The data that will indicate performance quality must be possible to collect across situations, in different structural settings, with differing amounts of resources. Even within one organization, each department may have slightly different practices regarding the same issue, and the data source should be flexible to fit those different practices. When the organization is composed of several different components or care-delivery settings, this criterion becomes particularly important.

NATURE OF THE DATA

Data can be classified as qualitative or quantitative. Both types of data are important measurements of the quality of care, service, or governance. Qualitative data is descriptive, unique to the individual at that time and in that context. The items or observed behaviors are assigned to mutually exclusive categories that are representative of the kinds of behavior exhibited. Qualitative data can be anecdotal when occasionally gathered, but becomes a powerful tool for monitoring quality performance when it is purposefully gathered on a regular basis. Qualitative data is often used in an exploratory way to identify themes of concern and dimensions of an event in question. It is then possible to identify sources of quantitative data that will be meaningful in monitoring the quality of performance related to the event. Quantitative measurement assigns items of data to categories according to the amount of a given characteristic. Nominal, ordinal, interval, or ratio scales are used in quantitative measurement. Nominal measures are labels or classes of objects or events. The categories are mutually exclusive, and the number of times the event occurs is counted. Examples include the number of people according to gender, or the number of people present or absent at an activity. Ordinal scales also categorize data, but on a sliding scale of "most" to "least" in regard to some characteristic. Client satisfaction data fits into this category. Interval scales rank order the data according to a characteristic. The intervals between the readings on a thermometer, for example, are known; but there is no absolute zero point. Ratio scales are extensively used in QM programs. They represent variables that have an absolute zero point on the scale. The numbers can be meaningfully multiplied or divided. The Joint Commission (1989) describes a clinical indicator as being a ratio of events within a universe of events. The number of clients who acquire an infection divided by the total number of clients on the surgical unit is an indicator of one measure of the quality of care provided.

VOLUME OF DATA

The volume of data is related to the availability of data, but also has importance by itself. With a large volume of data, it is possible to randomly select clients or events for study, thus increasing the scientific rigor of the investigation. In contrast, there may be only a few sentinel events during a year; but those few have importance when compared to numbers either from the previous year or from other organizations. If the statistical probability of a certain event occurring is being investigated, it may be necessary to collect data over a longer period of time or cooperate with other sites to obtain a sample large enough for meaningful results. Katz and Green (1992) recommend that one-quarter to one-third of the activities in a given operational unit be monitored. Those activities that combine the characteristic of high risk with the characteristics of high volume, high cost, and problem prone should be monitored at least three times per year. They also suggest proportions: 60 percent of the monitored activities relate to client care, 20 percent to staff or professional activities, and 20 percent to the administrative domain.

AVAILABILITY OF DATA

After the principal functions of a department or organization have been identified and the indicators selected, it is important to assess the availability of the data required. The data either exists, or has to be created. Existing data sources can be external or internal to the organization. External sources include the information previously collected from many organizations by funders, licensing or accrediting bodies, or the government. This data external to the functioning of the organization can provide important comparative information about utilization practices, clinical protocols based on research, staff mix ratios, and many other aspects of the organization and its outcomes. Existing sources of internal data include all the information supplied at regular intervals to funders, licensing or accrediting bodies, or the government. Very few organizations undertake a comprehensive review of the data routinely generated for various **stakeholders**; and fewer still use that data for QM purposes. Other sources of existing internal data include the documents and processes used in the daily functioning of the organization. Much more data is collected regularly than is used regularly. New, primary, or original data is more expensive and time consuming than existing data, and often requires the involvement of researchers or other experts to ensure validity, reliability, and a match with the information desired. Developing surveys and designing software programs to generate new reports are examples of creating new data to support a QM program.

RESOURCES

The cost of the source of data is a necessary consideration for all organizations. When data is readily available, or staff are used to record it, cost is minimal because collection is part of ongoing operations. If staff have to be trained in new procedures for documentation or data collection, or if new data must be generated, the costs of the QM program will be much greater. Sometimes accessing external data banks costs money; consequently, there is value in comparing this data to that data available from other organizations.

DATA SOURCES

Data sources can be generally grouped into four categories: client, staff, organization, and external. Each category can be the source of both qualitative and quantitative data. The data obtained may be more or less valid, reliable, specific, accurate, available, confidential, or costly. There exists some overlap between the sources of the data and collection methods; in a few instances they may be the same. (See the section on data-collection methods later in the chapter). Client and staff data related to demographics, structure, and processes of care is the easiest to obtain, given that much of it is recorded for other purposes. Because this data collection is part of daily organizational functioning, it is also the least expensive data source. Client and staff data based on perspectives and opinions is not often recorded, and is more difficult to collect. Systemwide data not based in client or staff activities is more difficult to obtain, given that it involves information related to organizational philosophy, beliefs, and practices. When data is collected across many departments in an organization, careful monitoring is required to ensure that the definitions and collection methods are consistent. Externally recognized data sources have the advantages of consistency and comparability across the industry. The disadvantages may include expensive charges for access to the data, difficulty in obtaining access, greater chances of the data not being shared in a timely manner, and data being irrelevant to the organization's current needs.

Client Data Sources

The client is the recipient of care. The recipient may be an individual consumer of services, a family, other significant people, the neighborhood, or the community. Data may be obtained directly from the client, or may be obtained about the client from other sources. Data that can be provided only by the client includes expectations, perceptions of care, satisfactions, complaints, and ratings of services (Hennessy & Friesen, 1994; Scardina, 1994). Demographic information and events that occur as part of the process of care delivery are usually recorded in the client record; thus that record is a major source of data. The effects of care on the client are recorded less frequently. Effects of care are difficult to verify as being the result of the care, and some outcomes are not apparent until after the client has been discharged from the organization. The ultimate criteria for judging quality of care are longitudinal outcomes — the measures of heath status over time.

Sentinel events regarding the recipient of care are investigated every time they occur, and are often specified by organizational policy. Examples of these events include death within twenty-four hours of admission to the hospital and readmission to home-health care within one week of discharge. Rate-based events that occur to clients during the delivery of hospital care include admissions, diagnostic examinations, surgeries performed, length of stays, and discharges. Some outcomes of care are also rate-based indicators, such as mortality, changes in severity of illness, infections, and length of stay. Trends in these rates can be tracked over time, and comparisons can be made with other organizations.

Staff Data Sources

The workers within the organization include the staff (both professional and non-professional), physicians, ancillary personnel, and volunteers. Data from these sources can be obtained directly or indirectly. Information that can be given only by the people involved includes expectations, perceptions of role, satisfactions, complaints, and ratings of services or management (Nauright & Simpson, 1994). Data obtained indirectly comes from sources such as employee statistics, professional-association role descriptions, and the implementation of union or organizational policies. Age, gender, qualifications, seniority, and job classification information is readily obtained. Examples of sentinel events related to staff include drug or alcohol abuse, theft, and abuse of a client. Rate-based indicators for staff include sick time, leaves, overtime, attendance at inservice education, and **certifications** awarded. Sources of data about physicians also include both sentinel and rate-based events. A sentinel event for a physician would be an operating-room death. Rate-based events would include orders of formulary and special-order drugs, number of procedures for particular populations, and billings for diagnostic tests.

Organizational Data Sources

Sources of data that reflect systemwide information are organizational, such as utilization-management and risk-management activity results. Data about administrative personnel and the systems used within the organization can be obtained directly and indirectly. Expectations, perceptions of role, satisfactions, complaints, and ratings of services or departments can be obtained only from the people involved. Demographic information on management staff can be obtained indirectly; organizational documents are a source of this data. Sentinel events, which always require investigation in this sphere, might include fraud or the handling of a strike or disaster. Trend statistics show budget changes; workload-versus-staffing ratios; staff-to-bed or staff-to-client ratios; or degree of implementation of a QM program.

External Data Sources

The opinions or behaviors of other community organizations or of the public constitute external data sources. Data may include expectations, perceptions of organization roles, satisfactions, complaints, and ratings of services, as well as the more common indicators such as numbers of referrals, coordination meetings, or donations to the organization. Other sources of data outside the organization include the information collected across the industry by funders, licensing or accrediting bodies, or the government. This data, based on consistent definitions and categories, can provide important comparative information about outcomes of care or internal aspects of health-care delivery.

SELECTION OF COLLECTION METHODS

There are significant parameters to consider when selecting data collection methods. The importance of selecting methods that are congruent with the goals of the QM program cannot be overestimated.

Goals of Data Collection

Data can be collected for budgetary purposes, regulatory or legal reasons, or to provide required information to external bodies. Katz and Green (1992) describe six major reasons for data collection, all related to QM. The first reason is to establish a system to ensure the accuracy of information required for decision making. One example is the search for a minimum data set that will accurately portray the complexity of nursing work as a base for decisions (Anderson & Hannah, 1993). A second reason is to examine data rather than people; in this way, rather than punishing those who report errors, processes can be improved. A third reason is to identify the domain that needs improvement: clinical, professional, or administrative. Fourthly, data collection identifies the circumstances that allowed a sentinel event to occur, and does so for all three domains. The fifth reason for data collection is to establish the level of improvement that has been attained after implementation of corrective actions following the initial findings of the QM program. The final reason for data collection is to demonstrate a sustained level of improvement in client, professional, and administrative domains. All collection methods should be examined to ensure that they fulfill these expectations. See Table 24-2 for a list of considerations in selecting data-collection methods.

Considerations in Selecting Data-Collection Methods

As with selecting sources of data, there are several factors that must be considered prior to deciding on methods of data collection. Each organization will rate the

Table 24-2 • **CONSIDERATIONS IN SELECTING DATA-COLLECTION METHODS**

Objectives of management	Volume of data
Reliability	Ease of collection
Validity	Personnel
Timeliness	Resources
Frequency	

importance of each factor differently, according to the expertise of their personnel, their current budget situation, and their expectations for QM.

OBJECTIVES OF MANAGEMENT
Data-collection methods are only part of a QM program. The trustees and administration of the organization must decide whether the goal of the QM program is to "ensure that within the [organization] itself there is attainment of a quality ... and/or, second, to comply with an external control either legal or issuing from the private insurance companies" (Jacquerye, 1984, p. 117). When the goal has been identified, various methods of approaching QM can be evaluated. Different methods and tools exist for the partial evaluation as opposed to the global evaluation of the quality of care (Bard, Jimenez, & Tornack, 1994). Some are readily applied to organizations of any size, and others are only applicable to large organizations.

RELIABILITY
Reliability is the extent to which the measure consistently provides the same results, regardless of who does the measurement and when or where it occurs. It attempts to eliminate the influence of random errors of measurement on the results. Holland (1983) describes four types of reliability that are important in the measurement of health care. *Inter-rater reliability* means that two observers assign the same value to the characteristic being measured. A level of 70 percent consistency is considered acceptable for most collection tools. *Intra-rater reliability* means that the same observer assigns the same rating to that characteristic at two or more different points in time. *Split-half reliability* means that items measuring similar characteristics on a questionnaire or survey have similar scores, or consistency. *Test re-test reliability* means that the same test given at different points in time yields the same result, providing that change has not occurred. For most organizations, inter-rater reliability is the most important type of reliability measure. It ensures that information is obtained in a similar manner, that data is recorded in a consistent way, and that coding into categories is guided by consistent criteria.

VALIDITY
Just as a data source must be valid for the purpose intended, the data-collection method must be valid for the information needs of the organization. If a data-collection instrument is reported in the literature as reliable and valid, there is strong temptation to use it before ensuring that it will provide the information

needed for decision making in a particular organization. If the tool cannot yield the required data, it is not valid for that purpose. The tool may be used to provide other data, but the desired data must be obtained by another method.

TIMELINESS

Timeliness has two aspects: one for the QM process itself, and one for indicators. The urgency felt by the organization affects the process chosen for the whole system. If results from quality monitoring are wanted within a short period of time, a QM program based on partial evaluation methods (wherein departments or indicators have been prioritized) will be adopted. If the organization has the luxury of a longer time period within which to establish the QM program, then a comprehensive approach may be considered (Ruden, 1994; Sherman & Malkmus, 1994). The approach may include the massive inservice education of trustees, administration, middle management, and staff to a **Total-Quality-Management (TQM)** approach to care; the restructuring of internal systems for reconceptualization or recording of data; or the purchase, installation, and orientation to a new computerized infrastructure throughout the organization. A second factor related to the larger process is the time required for the implementation of corrective action. If data reports from a national data bank are the primary source of quality information, and these reports are collated and reported on a quarterly basis, corrective action is significantly delayed. If internal methods of QM are the primary source of data, then corrective action can occur much more quickly, while staff are still motivated.

Data can be collected within three time frames: retrospectively, concurrently, and prospectively. The data-collection method should be planned so that the data can be collated, analyzed, and interpreted prior to decision making. For example, information that is carefully collected using valid and reliable methods and that is presented in an authoritative, finished report has no importance if decisions had to be made before the report was received.

Retrospective data is derived from past events. Much can be learned by studying previous patterns of practice in an organization. Past information assists in establishing thresholds for quality performance in the future. The most common type of study is a retrospective chart audit of the clinical records of discharged clients. Another retrospective method is listening to the care experiences of clients who no longer need the services of the organization. This method provides important information regarding areas for improvement in practice. A disadvantage of retrospective information is that it cannot be verified. Possible reasons for events or trends cannot be definitively identified and are only subject to speculation. People who try to recall past events and concerns may have difficulty in being specific enough to guide changes in future practice. The data from the client record has to be accepted at face value, even though more service may have been provided than was recorded. The quality of recording is affected by other factors such as staff-client ratio, acuity of clients on a particular day, and the availability of written aids to documentation (Schroeder & Maibusch, 1984). Another difficulty lies in the resources required. Because of the extensive time involved in obtaining information from records, it is difficult for individual units or departments to conduct retrospective studies with samples large enough to be significant.

Concurrent data is collected and analyzed while processes are occurring. For example, information about care provided to a resident of a long-term care facility is recorded daily and could be collated and interpreted weekly to give a picture of the current practice pattern. An advantage of concurrent analysis is that comparison to existing protocols can occur while the services are still being provided; thus improvements can be made immediately. Staff motivation for quality performance is increased when feedback on performance is immediate. Data from concurrent audits is considered by staff to be more useful than retrospective audits; but concurrent auditing does cost more because of the release time required for staff to collect the data. A disadvantage of concurrent auditing is the requirement that standards, thresholds, and collection methods be well established before the data-collection system is able to work efficiently. Another disadvantage is the potential for reviewer bias. Because the auditor knows the difficulties of the current working environment, there is a temptation to make allowances for performance outside the threshold, and, thus, not give the findings the importance required to change that working environment.

Prospective data collection occurs as the events happen, but the collation and analysis is postponed until there is a sufficient number of events to provide significant information, or until a specified length of time has passed. A major advantage of prospective data collection lies in the fact that it is unpredictable; thus information on client outcomes tends to be unbiased. Organizational patterns may show either deterioration or improvement. Disadvantages include a delay in obtaining feedback and the requirement that standards and thresholds be articulated clearly prior to beginning data collection.

FREQUENCY

The frequency of data collection depends on practice variations for the indicator and how many of the indicators are built into the daily functioning of the organization. The tendency is to collect data too frequently, in the unfulfilled hope that someone will eventually analyze it. Organizations that succumb to the temptation of inventing new forms for every quality problem without removing any of the old forms are ignoring the cumulative negative effect on staff. If compliance for a particular indicator is above expectations two or three months in a row, perhaps that indicator should only be measured annually. A new practice difficulty encountered by the department could be the source of a new indicator. One advantage of putting the collection plan on an annual calendar is limiting the addition of items to the **Quality Management (QM)** program and, therefore, reducing staff time devoted to QM activities. Other advantages include giving the department lead time, and ensuring better planning and delegation of work, and timely completion of audits. When a quality-monitoring plan is agreed on by both staff and management, there is more resistance to adding extra indicators that may be important for running the department, but that are not related to the principal functions of the unit, and, therefore, are not needed in the quality-monitoring program.

Wilson (1992) describes a method for creating a Quality Assurance (QA) calendar that distributes quality-monitoring activities over the whole year. The calendar is written in pencil so that it can be easily changed as the clients or organizational practices change. The principal functions of the department are numbered and listed at the bottom of the page. Months are on the vertical left side of the calendar. The next column is the "management" column, which designates and is the place to note when workload within the organization will interfere with QM activities. These high-workload times may include summer holidays, budget, or year end. The second column calls for a listing of regular outside inspections and the months when QA reports are expected, keeping in mind the requirement of preparation time. A third column is labeled "audits." Wilson (1992) recommends that four audits, either new or reaudits, be identified for a one-year period. These will likely be criterion-referenced or focused studies covering several indicators. The audits are numbered according to the principal functions of the department. The fourth column is labeled "P/I/X," for patients, indicators, and external bodies. Whenever the department plans to approach clients for their opinions, to review the data for a specific indicator, or expects to report on a scheduled inspection, the activity is noted in this last column. The QA calendar should demonstrate that in a one-year period the department intends to review all of its principal functions in four regular audits (with additional entries for those indicators considered important) and that clients will be asked for their views at least once. Generally, there is one quality-related activity per month. Management may choose to reserve one or two months for activities it specifies for all departments, such as reporting on readiness for **accreditation**.

VOLUME OF DATA (SAMPLE SIZE)

The sample size (that is, the number of charts to be reviewed or the number of clients or staff to be interviewed) is a difficult issue for many departments. Katz and Green (1992) identify sample sizes according to the importance of the type of audit. Audits are classified as routine reviews, query reviews, intensive reviews, or sentinel-event investigations. These audits will reflect the increasing concern about variations from the established threshold parameters and may reveal the increasing seriousness of untoward events. A routine review is done to ensure that quality standards are being met; thus, problems or variations are not expected. It is recommended that the volume of routine reviews be 5 percent of the total number of cases or twenty cases, whichever is greater. A query audit is done to explore a variance outside the threshold when the variance cannot be justified or explained; the volume of query reviews should be 10 percent of the total cases or forty cases, whichever is greater. An intensive review is conducted when unusual occurrences or trends have negative outcomes for clients, staff, or the organization. The sample size should be larger to obtain more data — 15 percent of the total cases or sixty cases, whichever is greater. Investigation of a sentinel event should occur 100 percent of the time, because each event has a negative outcome that requires cause and circumstances to be identified.

EASE OF COLLECTION

Ease of collection is very important to staff, who often view paperwork as interfering with their primary responsibilities. There are two aspects to the ease of data collection — the prior existence of an instrument or tool and the tool's ease of use. If the data-collection instrument already exists, either externally or within the organization, the only task required is to evaluate the tool for its validity — for whether the data obtained will match the data needed for a particular quality indicator. If the tool requires some adaptation, it will need to be pilot tested for validity, reliability, and specificity before it can be used. Some orientation to the instrument and its analysis will be necessary if the tool is unfamiliar to staff. Sometimes existing forms used by an organization on a daily or monthly basis can be used "as is" or adapted very slightly to obtain data about the indicators of principal functions. Forms used for management rounds, end-of-shift reports, or departmental statistics may contain data that is desired for monitoring quality performance. When the data-collection instrument needs to be created, however, the situation is more difficult, more time consuming, and more expensive, in terms of both staff and consultant time.

The second aspect to ease of collection is ease of use, which is related to the characteristics of data-collection tools. The tool used should be "simple to understand, contain necessary data when completed, and (be) flexible enough to be used throughout the organization" (Katz & Green, 1992, p. 127). It should use terminology understood throughout the organization and applicable to every department. The tool or instrument should be "user friendly" by collecting data in a sequence that is logical and fits with current practices; by having both lines wide enough for handwritten entries and blank spaces for comments; and by making collation of data simple to complete. The data-collection form should include features such as clear print, headings in bold face, white space between sections, double spacing, printed lines not exceeding two-thirds the width of the page, and clearly marked areas for completion by the user. A data-collection tool that is designed with such features in mind will be used more willingly and completed more accurately than will a tool that does not reflect the importance of graphic design. Ease of use affects the acceptability of the task.

PERSONNEL

It must be recognized that a QM program takes time. The extra work involved may not require additional personnel, but it will take staff away from their normal responsibilities. The question of who should collect the data is answered differently by different organizations. Some organizations require each department to collect its own QM data. Others require departments to audit one another. The data collection may be done by management, by an assigned staff person, or by the whole staff. Organizations may create one or more positions for managing the QM program and collecting all of the data. Another option is to hire an outside consultant to design the QM program and monitor the performance of the organization on an occasional basis. The disadvantage of assigning specific personnel to the QM program is that the volume of work required may be too much for the assigned people, and other staff may not understand the program, acknowledge the findings, or accept accountability for the quality of their work. An alternate approach used by some organizations is "quality councils" or "quality circles." The personnel on these councils, which operate at the department and the division levels, coordinate the QM program. Different decisions are made at each level of the organization, so the roles of each council in relation to QM are different as well. The management quality council identifies indicators for the principal functions. The division-level quality council identifies division-specific indicators to be monitored, and locates or develops the required data-collection forms. These forms are then distributed to the department quality councils for data collection. The collation and analysis of data can be done by that department or by the division. The department or division often identifies an action plan for addressing the quality concerns prior to sending the data to the management quality council for review and trend forecasting.

Peer review is one of the most common approaches to quality monitoring, and it is a practice used extensively in the profession of medicine. Because they are from the practice environment, evaluators are considered credible, and their comments are more acceptable than those of outside evaluators. The major disadvantage of peer review is the subjective bias or prejudice that can occur when one assesses the work of a person one knows. This is of particular concern in a small organizational unit. The potential for bias is sometimes counteracted by requesting that a member of the same discipline from another unit in the same organization do the peer review.

Another consideration is whether new or experienced staff members should collect quality data. The advantage of involving inexperienced staff is the potential for increasing their understanding of the importance of quality monitoring in daily activities. They may develop an appreciation for the many factors that can influence a variation in quality; and it is hoped that they will develop a sense of increased personal accountability. The advantage of involving experienced staff, on the other hand, is that they may be able to anticipate reasons for the variations and look for additional data to support the hypotheses even prior to the whole data set being analyzed. A collection team composed of both new and experienced staff is the best combination, with members of the team changing so that each staff member is involved with quality monitoring over a period of time.

RESOURCES

Administrative personnel decide on the most desirable type of QM program and then allocate resources to the program. It is obvious that the investment of staff time in QM activities can translate into time and, therefore, dollars lost to direct client care or services. An organization may need to employ additional personnel to cover ongoing service responsibilities while regular staff are involved in data collection or meetings related to QM. Staff training is a cost that tends to be underestimated when planning a QM program. In addition to the training of staff employed at the time of QM program implementation, normal staff turnover makes ongoing quality training necessary. Another resource-related consideration is the equipment and materials that may be required for a given data-collection method. If the data-collection method selected requires a new computer system, new software, or even many new forms and documents, additional costs will be incurred.

DATA-COLLECTION METHODS

The methods of data collection are many and varied. This section discusses the formal and informal methods as well as other factors to be considered when putting a specific method to use.

Predictability Using Different Data-Collection Methods

Each data-collection method and data source inherently contains a degree of predictability about the categories of information that result from the process. Predictability is determined by who controls the selected indicators, and how much control is given to the respondent and the party collecting the data.

INFORMAL METHODS

Generally, the more informal the method of data collection, the more control given to the respondent, and the more unpredictable the results. Qualitative data collection often fits in this category. For example, when observation of behavior is used as a method of collecting data, the events that occur and the responses to those events are unpredictable. Observations are usually recorded in qualitative terms. The advantage of using an unpredictable method of data collection is that perceptions and issues may arise that were thought to be either irrelevant to the event in question, or unimportant. After the concerns are identified, further exploration of their influence on events can occur, using both qualitative and quantitative methods. Difficulties encountered using data-collection methods with high unpredictability include the recording of the information, retention of the information for future use, and the increased time required for the analysis, interpretation, and follow-up of the findings.

FORMAL METHODS

More formal, predetermined methods of data collection produce very predictable categories of data strongly controlled by those who designed the collection system. Quantitative methods of data collection fit in this category. When a structured questionnaire is administered in an interview, the results fall into very predictable, predefined categories, and are often quantitatively analyzed. The advantages of using a predictable method of data collection include ease of collection, ease of analysis, and ease of interpretation. Disadvantages revolve around the possibility of missing important issues because the people involved in the event are not invited to share their perceptions. They are, instead, presented with a finished list of factors that staff believe ought to influence the quality of care.

Some data-collection methods fit into more than one category, depending on the amount of structure used to guide the selection of topic for data collection. Methods with variable degrees of structure include, but are not limited to, interviews, questionnaires, and research. For ease of presentation, methods of data collection are grouped into the most common category. Most methods can be applied to client, staff, organization, or external sources. A few methods are best described by identifying the data source. An overview of data-collection methods is shown in Table 24-3.

Informal Data-Collection Methods

There are various forms of informal data-collection methods. These methods offer a wealth of quality-related data that is sometimes passed over because of the appearance of insignificance.

Table 24-3 • OVERVIEW OF DATA-COLLECTION METHODS

Informal Data-Collection Methods

Direct communication

Complaints, bouquets, and hot lines

Suggestion boxes

Observation

Client diaries, logs, or journals

Client newspapers or newsletters

Residents' councils, self-help groups, and advocacy groups

Semi-Formal Data-Collection Methods

Satisfaction surveys

Client rounds

Family conferences

Interviews

Focus groups

Organizational documents, reports, and minutes

Formal Data-Collection Methods

Existing forms

Chart audit

  Peer review

  National data-based audit

  Criteria-based review

  Exception review

Clinical or laboratory examination (observation)

Questionnaire

Utilization-management programs, practice-pattern analysis

DIRECT COMMUNICATION

Direct communication as a method of collecting data about the quality of services is so obvious that it is often overlooked. A client, family member, worker from another department, or fellow staff member will have an opinion about events they have just experienced. They may be surprised and pleased if someone inquires about their opinion. When asked one or two simple, open-ended questions, they will likely describe the aspect of the event that was most important to them. The respondents retain control of what is said; therefore the information provides important clues for the organization in planning the improvement of services. Two simple questions are "What pleased you most about . . . ?" and "How do you think we could improve . . . ?" The difficulty with this collection method is designing a system for recording, collating, and reviewing the data.

COMPLAINTS, BOUQUETS, AND HOT LINES

Complaints, bouquets (positive feedback), and hotlines give the respondent complete control of the information discussed. Monitoring complaints is a common method of measuring quality of services; but the information is not useful unless it is recorded in a consistent manner. The same information must be gathered about each complaint, each event that has caused problems, and the actions, if any, that were taken to resolve the problem. If the organization's response to the complaint and the person's opinion of that response are also recorded, the method of handling complaints can be evaluated. Bouquets should be handled in the same manner, and feedback provided to staff with just as much regularity as are complaints. Hot lines are usually justified by the volume of calls. For information obtained from hotlines to be useful to an organization, the content of the calls and the actions suggested by staff should be recorded. Relating the number and content of calls to other events occurring in the community may provide valuable data for orienting personnel and staffing the hot lines. Data from all three sources may also provide assistance with the review of organizational goals and services.

SUGGESTION BOXES

Many organizations use suggestion boxes to solicit opinions about services. Clients and staff members have complete control over the content of notes placed in a suggestion box. Management controls the location, size, color, and visibility of the box; the collection and review of suggestions; and actions arising from the suggestions. The frequency with which a suggestion box is used depends on the perceptions of clients and staff about how open management is to new ideas. When ideas submitted are regularly reported; when persons who suggest good ideas are acknowledged or rewarded; and when some of the ideas are implemented, the boxes are used more often.

OBSERVATION

In nonparticipant observation, there is no interaction between the observer and the individual being observed. Respondents have control over their own behavior, and their actions may provide insight into the quality of the services provided, the relationships that have or have not been established, or the influence of environmental variables on their behavior. For example, when someone walks out of a sexually transmitted diseases clinic after waiting half an hour without seeing anyone, and this event recurs several times a week, staffing patterns may need to be reviewed. There are several advantages of this data-collection method. Because events are recorded at the time they occur, there are minimal problems with recall. Further, this method is adaptable to any setting, and the event may be audio- or video-taped for later review. Problems with this data-collection method arise from the event, the observer, and the tool used (Schroeder & Maibusch, 1984). Because there is no control, the observer must wait for the event to occur. If the events are infrequent, or the allotted observation time too short, the sample may be too small to produce accurate conclusions.

Observer consistency in defining and recording activities is also a problem. Everyone is influenced by emotions, attitudes, values, and past experiences. Observer bias or prejudice can interfere with the selection of events to record and the manner of recording them. Also, interobserver consistency is difficult to obtain. When the observational method is used in a more formal manner, as in a research study, there may be written classifications for behavior. Consistency is easier to obtain, but training of the observers is still required. If the study has a very detailed form for recording data, the observer may spend more time filling in the form than observing events. Office-practice peer review uses this method to evaluate physician practice (Harrigan, 1992). Some tools such as the Slater Scale have been developed to evaluate nurses as they provide care to clients (Hough & Schmele, 1987). Self-appraisal tools for community nurses are also available (Knox, 1985).

CLIENT DIARIES, LOGS, OR JOURNALS

The use of client diaries as a method of collecting quality-of-care data is uncommon. Client self-reporting can be very informal, with almost no guidelines for content, or structured, such as when a twenty-four-hour nutrition history is requested. The self-reporting that is required has both advantages and disadvantages. It is valuable to have the person's opinion of events; and although the recording of events is biased, the information is accepted as valid — as that person's perspective of the truth. Further, changes in an individual's opinion can be tracked over time, and the degree of impact of various events discovered. It is sometimes therapeutic for people to record notes on their thoughts, fears, and responses to an illness. Diaries are also useful as an adjunct to treatment when evaluating the effects of pain medication on symptoms, or of educational sessions on client behavior. A disadvantage of all written records is the requirement that the respondent be literate (although a tape-recorded journal could be used for people who are illiterate). And, finally, because diaries often contain a mixture of feelings, activities, and opinions, it is difficult to classify and collate the data obtained from client diaries.

CLIENT NEWSPAPERS OR NEWSLETTERS

In settings where individuals reside for several months or years, newsletters or newspapers produced by the residents can be an important source of data for the staff. The residents are free to report or discuss from their own perspective any issue they wish. The organization has no leverage, other than persuasion, over the content. Various factors such as the importance given to issues and the consistency with which some concerns are raised are indicators for managers that quality of care in those areas needs review.

RESIDENTS' COUNCILS, SELF-HELP GROUPS, AND ADVOCACY GROUPS

Residents' councils, self-help groups, and advocacy groups are rich sources of data because they are controlled by people who have had direct experience with events, who have opinions about the events, and who want others to be aware of their concerns. Representatives of an organization may be ex-officio or voting members of the group, invited as special guests for particular meetings, or informed of the results of meetings after they have occurred. The critical factor that determines the amount of information these groups share with an organization is the degree of trust that exists in the relationship. An organization earns trust by being receptive to concerns raised, requesting details regarding those concerns, identifying reasons for events, and providing regular feedback on findings. The major advantage of this data-collection method is the uniqueness of the perspectives shown and the number of people for whom it is a concern. The major disadvantage is the classification, recording, and collating of the data.

Semi-Formal Data-Collection Methods

In addition to informal methods of data collection, there are a variety of methods that are considered to be semi-formal. These methods include satisfaction surveys, client rounds, family conferences, interviews, focus groups, and organizational documents.

SATISFACTION SURVEYS

Patient and client-satisfaction surveys have become more important in the accreditation and **licensure** of organizations. Increased emphasis on the outcomes of care and on client-centered approaches demands increased use of these tools. The most promising instruments compare client expectations with the reality of their experiences (Greeneich, 1993; Hennessey & Friesen, 1994; Scardina, 1994). These surveys are either semi-structured or structured methods of data collection. Respondents share control over the survey content with professionals. Closed questions result in specific answers in categories expected by the organization; and open-ended questions have the potential to raise new information related to the quality of care. Validity of these instruments is problematic. Some client-satisfaction instruments are composed of topics identified by professionals. The validity of those based on client experiences is much higher, because the respondent groups have more control. Another difficulty encountered with client-satisfaction surveys is the tendency of respondents to supply socially acceptable answers, which are overwhelmingly positive and, thus, of little use in identifying areas for improvement. Retrospective surveys done after discharge are sometimes used to obviate the social-acceptability problem; but then there is a problem with accurate recollection of detail, so specific improvements needed are difficult to identify. Advantages of this method, in addition to obtaining user perspective, include the potential to monitor the improvement of a particular unit's performance on a dimension that had a poor score previously.

CLIENT ROUNDS

The use of client rounds as a data-collection method is most common in institutional-care settings. The physician and nurse may conduct rounds together or separately, with or without students in their respective disciplines. Sometimes the whole nursing staff within a unit make rounds of all clients early in the shift, for assessment and client-orientation purposes. When professionals wish to obtain specific data, client rounds are structured and may include information on the previous night's sleep; recent eating, drinking, and bowel patterns; or pain and other symptom control. The effectiveness of treatment may also be assessed through the inspection of skin and wounds, auscultation of chests and abdomens, or checking of intravenous infusions. This information is related to outcomes of care, and, therefore, to the quality of care. The involvement of the client in these rounds is highly variable and depends on the client's assertiveness and degree of comfort with the staff. Two productive, open-ended questions that can produce concurrent data on a different aspect of quality-of-care issues are, "Were you satisfied with the care you received yesterday?" and "What are your expectations for today?" The answers will guide staff in their selection of priorities for care that day, and may lead to action to improve the quality of services provided to that client. The difficulty with using rounds for data collection lies in the recording, collating, and reviewing of data for trends. Further, the qualitative information on symptom control, satisfaction, and expectations is challenging to monitor.

FAMILY CONFERENCES

Attendance at family conferences usually includes the client, one or more family members, and at least two professionals of different disciplines. The purpose of the family conference may be to provide an update for client and family on the health status of or the progress made by the client; to coordinate the activities of the professional group with the family and with each other; or to make arrangements for discharge and community follow-up. Using family conferences as a method for collecting quality-of-care data adds another perspective and purpose to the activity. The agenda is often structured around the concerns and opinions of the professionals. Data related to quality of care may arise, such as inconsistencies in staff approach; unclear expectations of client behavior; or poor relationships between the staff and the client or family, or among staff. If the client and family feel confident in voicing their opinions, important information can be obtained about their perceptions of the care delivered and their hopes for the future. Topics may be raised that were thought unimportant by the professionals, but that require careful consideration on the part of the family. If the client and family feel threatened and outnumbered by the professionals at the meeting, they may be reluctant to express opinions. In order to facilitate client-centered care, it may be helpful for a single staff member to talk with the family after the meeting to discover their perspectives. The benefit of family-conference information for quality of care is evident in all three time frames — retrospectively, concurrently, and prospectively — and for future care after discharge. The difficulty, as with most informal and semi-formal methods, resides in the design of a system for the categorization, collation, and analysis of the data so that it provides useful information for improving care.

INTERVIEWS

Information regarding the quality of services or care can be obtained through interviews with the client, a family member, staff member, or member of the public. The interview can be conducted face-to-face in the health facility or at home, or by telephone. The amount of control the respondent has over the topics discussed depends on the amount of structure imposed. If the interview consists of only open-ended questions, the respondent has much more control; but the interviewer has no guarantee of obtaining specific information. If a very detailed questionnaire format is used, the interviewer has control over the topics, and the data is easier to categorize, collate, and analyze; but the respondent may not have the opportunity to discuss some issues of concern. Many interviews include both open- and closed-ended questions; this is considered a semi-formal method of collecting quality-of-care data. Self-reported information is assumed to be valid data, because it reflects the opinions of the respondent. One advantage of the interview method is increased accuracy of data, because answers can be clarified by the interviewer before they are recorded. Interviews are well suited for the exploration of attitudes, opinions, satisfaction with service, and beliefs about health care (Schroeder & Maibusch, 1984).

Interviewing is a method that can be used with almost all people, literate or not. The interview process may be therapeutic for the respondent, if it relieves boredom, stimulates thinking, or assists in adaptation to a changed health status. The interview may be the only method for acquiring information about the history of an event or an illness, and, therefore, is valuable in establishing factors that should be investigated for their impact on the quality of care. There are several disadvantages to the interview method. The reliability is not high. The interviewer becomes part of a relationship with the respondent. Both the exploration of topics and the recording of data may be influenced by that relationship, particularly in combination with the interviewer's personal biases, beliefs, and opinions. Reliability can be improved, however, with careful training of the interviewers. A low number of interviews also threatens the reliability of the results. Also, information obtained may not be accurate if the respondent is anxious and attempts to say what will please the interviewer. Data collected in an interview may also be faulty due to memory lapses on the part of the respondent. Again, poor recollection of events is common in retrospective studies. The causality of an event is difficult to establish through the interview technique alone; it is important to consider other perspectives prior to reaching conclusions. Interviewing takes more time — for the interviewer, for the respondent, and for the person categorizing, collating, and analyzing the data — than do some other collection methods. This method is, therefore, more costly in both staff-replacement dollars and contract dollars. Although an interview can be audio- or video-taped for future reference or research purposes, the review of tapes and transcription of words, if required, take an inordinate amount of time. The time required can be reduced by using more closed questions and creating more structure for the interview; but this will result in sacrifice of data related to feelings and the complexity of the issue.

FOCUS GROUPS

When the opinion of a specific population group or group of staff is desired on the quality of a service, the focus group method may be preferred. Representatives of the desired group are selected, approached, invited to participate, and informed that there will be discussion of a particular topic. They meet with a facilitator and follow a semi-structured discussion format. The content of the conversation is recorded for future reference. Because an in-depth exploration of the topic is desired, a focus group discussion will last a minimum of an hour. The intent of a focus group is to "look at the adequacy, appropriateness, and sensitivity of the system" (Wilson, 1992) in relation to the needs of clients or workers. Control of the content is shared by the group members and the organization, making the focus group a semi-formal method of data collection. The organization selects the topic and articulates initial questions and probing comments related to the aspects of that event thought to be important. The respondents are free to express their opinions, based on personal experiences and their knowledge of the subject. Advantages of this method include the unpredictability of the participants' perception of important factors related to the topic, and the potential benefit information may have for the improvement of future care. This method takes less time than individual interviews but may make a similar contribution to the organization's knowledge about its practices. A difficulty associated with the focus group method is selecting participants who have the related experience, are knowledgeable about the topic, are representative of the target population, and are also comfortable expressing their opinions in a group setting. Another drawback is the need for a very skilled facilitator who elicits information from others but does not express any personal opinions. If more than one focus group is held, there also exists the challenge of ensuring consistent approaches among all facilitators. Finally, there is difficulty in categorizing, collating, and analyzing the data so that it becomes meaningful.

ORGANIZATIONAL DOCUMENTS, REPORTS, AND MINUTES

Although every organization has documents, these documents are often considered data sources, rather than a data-collection method. Although the difference is slight, these data sources cannot be used unless there is an information-collection method that is specifically matched to the type of data in the document. This method is considered a semi-formal approach to data collection, because the respondent, or the organization, has control over which documents are considered in the QM program. If the minutes of the board of directors and its committees are excluded from data collection in a review of the operations of the whole organization, the activities of the board are not evaluated. Tracing the ripple effect of a board decision on the practices of the organization may be enlightening, because the policy may not have been implemented the way in which it was intended. The review of organizational documents requires careful construction of data-collection tools to ensure validity, reliability, and accuracy. The goal of the data collection must be clear and the principal functions and indicators clearly defined for the results to be useful. Assigning one person to review one type of document is a way to ensure consistency in the categorization and recording of items.

Formal Data-Collection Methods

Formal data-collection methods provide the most direct approach to obtaining meaningful data. These formal methods generally have the potential for the user to established increasingly highs levels of objectivity, validity, and reliability.

EXISTING FORMS

The use of existing forms as a method of data collection is considered a formal method because the respondent, the worker in that department or unit, has no choice about the information gathered. This method is highly structured, being determined by external regulatory or accreditation requirements, by professional associations, or by financial and statistical reporting guidelines established by management. As with organizational documents, data-collection tools must be carefully constructed to ensure validity, reliability, and accuracy. Temptation may exist to use data recorded on existing forms; but this data must be carefully scrutinized to ensure that it answers the information need of the quality-of-service indicator. A slight adaptation of the existing form may be necessary, and the adopted form should be pilot tested to check its validity with the indicator. There are many instruments for collecting data from existing forms, but some of them will not fit the need. Some organizations have specific quality-of-care data-collection methods built into their ongoing practices. For example, a discharge form may require a client to comment about services. A psychiatric outpatient admission interview may include a valid and reliable tool for assessing mood and behavior. This assessment tool is again used on discharge to determine changes that have occurred. These can be integrated into the existing forms used by personnel and are excellent additions to a QM program.

CHART AUDIT

The most common method of formalized data collection for quality monitoring is chart audit. This method may be done retrospectively or concurrently. (See the Timeliness section under Considerations in Selecting Data-Collection Methods earlier in this chapter for the advantages and disadvantages of each.) Chart audits can be classified into four types: peer review, national data-based audit, criteria-based review, and exception review. One or more of these types may be used by an organization for different purposes; but all of these methods are based on the record of client care. The chart audit has recently been interpreted more broadly to include audit of operational records of the organization. Support-service departments participate in the QM program by measuring their departmental records of performance against industry averages, established criteria for that performance, or past patterns of practice within the organization. This expansion of the definition of chart audit is important; it recognizes the contribution of all parts of an organization to the delivery of appropriate client care.

Peer Review   Peer review is also called chart-based review. It was the first type of review to use the client record, and it has been done for decades within the medical profession. The review traditionally was completed by fellow professionals to determine whether the care provided by the professional being reviewed was of an acceptable standard. According to Harrigan (1992), "There usually were no criteria and the peer's judgment was subjective. The process itself was very time-consuming for the clinicians undertaking the reviewing. As well, this method made judgments on the basis of individual records, and could not produce patterns of care" (p. 13). Because of these difficulties, this type of anecdotal chart review is seldom used today as a quality-of-care activity. It has been replaced by the criteria-based review (described following). Other types of chart-based peer review include ward rounds, clinical lectures, and presentations where the physician's decisions and actions in the process of care delivery are analyzed by a group of peers or students. These activities are common today for their value in teaching and continuing education, but are seldom associated with QM programs.

National Data-Based Audit   National data-based audits are usually large collections of data abstracted on discharge from every client record from multiple organizations. The data collection is done according to regionally or nationally prescribed rules and definitions. The data is compiled by staff from the organization, and categorized as prescribed, using the required instruments for collection. It is then sent regularly to a regional or national center, collated, and analyzed en masse with statistics from all other participating organizations. Decisions about the tools used, the statistics requested, the methods of analysis, and the reports produced are determined by regional or national health priorities. Professional associations at the national level may have some role in the decision-making process, but participating organizations have little or no involvement. In Canada, this data bank is known as the Hospital Medical Records Institute (HMRI) clinical database. In the United States, a comparable system exists for Medicare and Medicaid reimbursement through the Health Care Financing Administration (HCFA). Reports from these databases are invaluable to practitioners and administrators, because the large catchment areas enable reliable comparisons to be made between local statistics and regional or national statistics. Similarities, discrepancies, and trends can be identified, particularly in relation to institutional care indicators such as diagnostic groupings, rates of day surgery, use of particular procedures, and length of stays. Adverse outcomes of care, such as infection rates, complications of surgery, and postpartem problems, are also tracked. Many organizations use these data banks as guideposts in establishing thresholds and goals for performance in their organizations. The disadvantage of these statistics is that, for most of them, no one has established whether the average rates are appropriate rates. There is the possibility that the scientific approach to medicine in North America has created an artificially high incidence of particular procedures, which becomes the accepted standard. An example of this is the generally high rate of Cesarean sections. Comparing the rates to those of other countries and continents is one method of checking the level of the accepted standard; but it still does not guarantee appropriateness of care.

Other types of data-based audits are completed for support-service departments. There are industry standards available for organizational functioning, which are based on research as well as current practice. Facility design and maintenance, equipment safety, dietary processes, and housekeeping practices are examples of the wide variety of areas having established criteria. Meeting accepted standards in a field ensures that structural and process aspects of the organization create an environment within which quality care can be provided.

Criteria-Based Review   The chart review most widely used in QM programs is the criteria-based or criterion-referenced audit. The purpose of this audit is to examine and validate current and recent-past practice. By definition, data is collected from clinical or operational records to determine whether or not the care or service provided falls within the thresholds previously selected. The findings are expressed in terms of percentage compliance with expectations, or the percentage of the examined cases out of the universe of total cases within or above the threshold levels. Use of this formal method of data collection requires preparatory work prior to implementation. The preparation includes decisions on "explicit criteria for good performance, objective measurements of performance, comparison of results over time and among peers, and identification of review procedure and results" (Harrigan, 1992, p. 13).

Criteria-based review of records is particularly suited to the examination of structural and process aspects of care and services. Client records demonstrate structural factors such as the qualifications of staff, the anesthetic compounds used, or the supplies used by a particular client. Operational aspects of structure, including the adequacy of equipment and safety of the working environment, are also easily measured. Process aspects of care can be easily obtained from either the client record or organizational documents, and include the administration of intravenous solutions, the continuity of caregiver, and the procedure for changing a sterile dressing. Some examples of operational process factors having performance thresholds include the number of units packaged per hour in pharmacy, the average return time from printing services, and the number of complaints received by the home-health-care office. Client charts and operational records can provide some information for outcome measurement; for example, data on client mortality or readmission within one week of discharge, the rate of equipment breakdown, or the number of staff disability claims. This information, however, is incomplete, and other data-collection methods must also be used to obtain a comprehensive picture of the circumstances influencing outcomes of care or services.

There are many advantages to criteria-based review. Because the criteria are so clearly defined, charts or records may be screened by nonprofessional staff, thus saving professional and managerial time. Discrepancies between performance and standards are clearly revealed and action can be taken to improve the care or service delivered as soon as reasons for the discrepancy are identified. The focus of attention is on variance from the established pattern, rather than on particular staff members. Employee expertise is respected by involving employees in the process of establishing both reasons for the variance and ways of improving practice. The most common disadvantage of criteria-based review is the tendency to become preoccupied with the minutia of the monitoring process rather than maintaining focus on the larger picture. This tendency is demonstrated by the continuation of monthly audits of practices that have had several months of 100 percent compliance, rather than analyzing current practice problems, reviewing literature to identify standards, and developing meaningful and measurable criteria for a new audit. Another disadvantage of criteria-based audits is the tendency to view the item in isolation of the outcome of the care or service, illustrated in the classic saying "the operation was successful, but the patient died." The third drawback to the criteria-based audit is related to the importance of the audit itself. Because all criteria-based audits are numerical, inquiry is reduced to those aspects of care or service that are easily measured; it does not mean that these are the most important aspects of the care. Wilson (1992) states, "the importance of aspects of life is inversely related to the ease of measuring them. The more fundamental and important the issue, the more difficult it is to assess with any degree of precision" (p. 78).

Exception Review When an event occurs that causes concern for the organization, a focused study or investigative audit may be completed. This type of audit is called an exception review because these events are not expected to occur; they are exceptions. The exception review is considered a formal data-collection method because most organizations have strict protocol for the data required, the people who must be informed, and the corrective actions taken to prevent the event occurring again. Sentinel events, which cause negative effects for clients, staff, or the organization, are investigated, as are trends or events that fall outside the thresholds established for safe practice. An exception review is occasionally conducted because staff consider the issue to be of enough importance and relevance to merit investigation. Following the review, a criteria-based audit may be created to ensure that the care or services delivered continue to be of high quality. The exception review is a flexible, inductive method of assessing quality. It is flexible because it includes several data sources, which can be carefully selected according the nature of the event. The outcome of an event for clients or recipients of departmental services is determined by many factors including context, staff, environment, materials, and expectations. A conclusion about the quality of care provided is inductively derived from all the data available. Because of the broad investigation of influencing factors, the exception review comes closer to assessing outcome than does any other data-collection method.

Data sources used for an exception review may include organizational documents, to check the policy; statistics, to check prior occurrences; and client charts or organizational records, to check the services provided. Client, family, or recipient observation (to check current status) or interviews (to identify expectations and perceptions of care) may be performed. Observation of the location where the incident occurred may be indicated. A criteria-based review related to the issue may provide background information, as may reviews of previous complaints from recipients of the service. Staff interviews may assist in defining the circumstances under which the event is more likely to occur. A literature review may even be performed to identify the rates of occurrence for similar events in other organizations. Because of the increased validity that comes with the use of several data sources, the size of the sample does not need to be large. (See the Volume of Data section under Considerations in Selecting Data-Collection Methods earlier in this chapter.) The flexibility and comprehensive nature of the exception review method have several implications for the organization. The staff members in charge of the review must be knowledgeable to ensure that data sources are selected carefully. The staff must be somewhat removed from the incident so as to minimize bias; and they should have enough time and energy available to complete the investigation. Because of the expenses incurred in staff time, organizations must be very selective when choosing to use this type of data-collection method.

CLINICAL OR LABORATORY EXAMINATION (OBSERVATION)

Clinical or laboratory examination is a common method of collecting quality-of-care information in health-care settings. Clinical examination is a formal method because the observations made and tests given are decided by professionals, not clients. The results are essential in determining the appropriateness of drug and other therapies. For example, it is important to establish a baseline physical and mental status examination in order to monitor progress of treatment. The data obtained from clinical or laboratory sources is directly related to client health status, and, so, is one of the few data-collection methods that measures treatment outcomes.

QUESTIONNAIRE

When a questionnaire is listed as a data-collection method, it usually means that there is no interaction between the respondent and the researcher, particularly with regard to the questionnaire items. The respondent independently provides written, self-reported data to answer the questions asked. The questions may be open-ended, allowing the respondent freedom to identify areas of concern. Many questionnaires used for quality monitoring are highly structured, which does not allow the respondent any control over the topics. This method is, therefore, considered a formal method of data collection. The type of data requested in a questionnaire is highly variable. Information solicited can include one or more of the following: demographic information; facts about events or conditions; beliefs related to facts; attitudes, opinions, and feelings; knowledge; intentions related to the future; or behaviors (Schroeder & Maibusch, 1984). Questionnaires may or may not have a direct impact on the respondent, depending on how soon the results are applied. If, prior to an individual teaching session, an individual with diabetes completes a pretest on knowledge of diabetes, the results can be used immediately to design a personal teaching program for that individual. Professionals can use the results of direct-impact questionnaires to provide new knowledge, "correct information, prevent unsafe behavior or undue emotional hardship, or stimulate changes in attitude or behavior" (Schroeder & Maibusch, 1984, p. 137). The respondent must be identified in direct-impact questionnaires, so anonymity is sacrificed. If lack of confidentiality will affect the accuracy of the responses, respondents can be questioned as a group, feedback provided to the group as a whole, and the results used directly to influence the information presented to the group.

When a questionnaire is already designed, the advantages include low costs; minimal time for the respondent to complete; straightforward collation of data; minimal interviewer bias; and accurate data, especially when anonymity is assured. The costs incurred relate to obtaining permission to use the questionnaire, duplicating, distribution or mailing, and analysis (if consultant or computer time is required). Questionnaires are also easily adapted to a large sample size, and respondents do not need to be restricted to the local geographic area.

There are disadvantages inherent in questionnaires, however. These disadvantages may or may not be overcome via careful structure and administration. The primary disadvantage is that a questionnaire requires a literate respondent. With estimates of functionally illiterate persons in North America ranging between 21 and 38 percent, depending on the definitions used, literacy is a real problem with this data-collection method. Another disadvantage is the so-called a "halo effect," where all answers are colored by the respondent's experience with one particular event. This produces low ratings for many items, or high ratings for most items. The factor of social acceptability may result in inaccurate positive ratings provided by the respondent in order to please a staff member or the sponsoring organization. Responses to questionnaires focusing on past events may be inaccurate because of respondent forgetfulness; and those questionnaires that attempt to measure current emotional state need to be timed so that data is accurate, but also so that respondent anxiety does not affect the results. A common drawback in the use of questionnaires is low response rate. This is particularly the case with mailed surveys, where the response rate is often below 25 percent. Techniques such as including a stamped envelope, giving reminders, and personally collecting the finished product may improve the response rate. The return rate ultimately depends on the interest and commitment of the respondent to the topic, and the construction of the questionnaire itself. Effective questionnaires have a clear purpose, are relatively short, and are fairly easy to complete. Questionnaire construction is very complex, very time consuming, very expensive, and is best accomplished by experts. The literature cites a multitude of existing tools that have been pretested for validity and reliability, and will likely measure the indicators desired in a QM program. One advantage of using an existing questionnaire is the availability of comparative data on similar populations. If small adaptations are required for an existing questionnaire, a carefully designed pretest will determine whether it still has reliability and validity. Even short-answer, open-ended questionnaires are very tricky to design with any assurance of accurate replies that will answer the information needs of the organization. Advice from experts may save a tremendous amount of staff time, effort, and money, and obtain a better result, as well.

UTILIZATION-MANAGEMENT PROGRAMS AND PRACTICE-PATTERN ANALYSIS

Utilization-management programs and practice-pattern analysis are usually applied to physician practice. They are formal collection methods because physicians have no individual control over the items and topics included. A group of practitioners in a particular organization may have some collective input regarding topics; but the organization is more likely to be guided by regulatory and accreditation requirements. These initiatives are essential components of QM. This is particularly true in institutions, because the client pathway and many health-care costs are dependent on physician treatment decisions. (See Chapter 27 on utilization management.)

SELECTION OF TECHNIQUES FOR DATA PRESENTATION

Raw data is of no value until it is translated into information. The translation must be planned carefully, considering the purpose of the data collection, its relationship to the QM program, the audience, and the uses to which the audience will put the information. Thus the selection of appropriate and meaningful data presentation techniques is imperative.

Purpose of Data Presentation

The most important reason for presenting data is to contribute to the QM program and improve the delivery of care or services. Accurate, valid, and reliable information interpreted in context should be the only basis for decisions about organizational change. System strengths and deficiencies must be clearly described by their relationship to knowledge, behavior, and performance. Statistics and anecdotal comments out of context have no meaning. They cannot be used to interpret past patterns of practice nor to guide future decisions, because the full picture is not presented. The primary audience for the presentation of data are those staff and workers who perform the activity that was studied. Ideally there was team involvement in establishing the framework and indicators for the quality monitoring in that unit, and those team members would likely have participated in the identification of data elements and the collection of data on the indicators applicable to the unit. Their interpretation of the data will transform it into information that can assist others outside that unit to understand the relationship between results and circumstances that influence practice. If workers want to do the best job possible under existing conditions, the natural inclination will be to apply the data, now translated into information, to maintain and improve their current practices.

The specific purpose of the presentation of data may be to make persons aware of the report, to educate and begin to build interest in the data, to gain authority to perform further data analysis, or to report back on the results of a previously authorized study or quality-improvement project (Bader & Bohr, 1991). The same clear presentation of data can serve all of these purposes, even though the audiences and resulting actions may differ.

Translating Data into Information

Several factors influence the process of transforming raw data into information that is useful for improving the quality of care. First a preliminary analysis needs to be performed to identify key findings. The data must be presented so that it is easily understood, can be compared to similar data to establish context, and, also, is protective of the confidentiality of practitioners. The process of presentation should include sending materials in advance, particularly to key people, articulating options, and clarifying the feedback process. See Table 24-4 for a summary of considerations in presentation of data.

Table 24-4 • **CONSIDERATIONS IN PRESENTATION OF DATA**

Preliminary analysis performed

Easily understood data

Comparative data presented

Format protective of confidentiality

Manageable volume

Materials sent in advance

Options for action identified

Feedback processes articulated and followed

PRELIMINARY ANALYSIS PERFORMED

Raw data is often presented in columns filled with figures or qualitative statements in no apparent order. It may have little meaning, even for people working within the area, unless a preliminary analysis is completed. A cover memo or executive summary can highlight the most obvious findings. Nonjudgmental language is necessary to define review categories. Words such as *substandard* or *inappropriate* are actually clinical judgments about the quality of practice, and are best made by peer-review panels.

Key questions arising from the findings and decisions implied by the data may or may not be articulated prior to discussion with the group whose practice was measured. Conclusions, such as recommendations for proposed actions, can be omitted. The data will be self-evident if presented clearly. According to the theory of change, individuals will change more readily if they contribute both to the identification of the need for change and to decisions regarding alternatives. Respect for the intelligence of others is essential in behavioral change.

EASILY UNDERSTOOD DATA

Graphic displays are more easily interpreted than tables. Too many columns or numbers on a page discourages people from carefully examining the data and understanding its significance. A chart displaying many variables may show complexity of the data; but the same chart may not teach anything about relationships among data, because the high number of variables inhibits understanding. Jargon should be avoided, particularly if there will be a lay audience of either workers or board members. *Nocosomial infections* means much less to a lay audience than does *hospital-acquired infections.* Too many abbreviations without a key can frustrate readers and discourage them from reading further. The use of statistical terms without explanation can also discourage readers. The report should be reread carefully to pick up any possible misinterpretations of the findings. Wording or tables should be corrected and clarified prior to presenting the information to ensure that all information is clear.

COMPARATIVE DATA PRESENTED

When information is presented out of context or in isolation, it has no meaning. Comparisons are necessary to understand whether the quality of care is better than expected or needs improvement. Internal data across reporting periods, months, quarters, or years may provide thresholds or benchmarks for knowing whether QM is improving, stable, or worsening. Comparisons to other organizations or to an established industry standard also transforms the data into valuable information. Variations in rates for specific variables between the average rates of organizations, or between the observed and the expected rates, all stimulate exploration. If valid comparisons are to be made, a common time frame and similar definitions must be used when choosing and comparing data sets (American Hospital Association, 1991).

FORMAT PROTECTIVE OF CONFIDENTIALITY

Presentation of data must protect the identity of individual practitioners and sometimes even units within the organization. It is the patterns of care, not individual practice, that are the focus of study. Individuals should be identified by number, letter, or code name in both reports and tables. Profession-specific reviews should be done by the same profession, and the results kept within that profession. The only other entities who may see those results would be the QM committee and administration, and they are bound by confidentiality.

MANAGEABLE VOLUME

If the presentation of data is too detailed, major concepts or findings are difficult to see or understand. Preliminary analysis with a concise statement of the major findings stimulates the participant to look for more detail when searching for explanations of **variance** in the data. Potentially important implications should also be highlighted by the preliminary analysis. This channels discussion toward objectives for future planning in that department or organization.

MATERIALS SENT IN ADVANCE

It is respectful to inform people in writing of major findings prior to a meeting. If negative findings of the quality review are likely to be a surprise, defensive behaviors are the normal result, and meetings become frustrating and uncomfortable. Key decision makers concerned with the problem area must be informed of the results prior to the meeting. It will give them time to react in private, plan questions, and perhaps even begin an investigation of possible reasons for the unexpected findings. Prior consideration of information also yields more questions and comments from people who are not directly involved, thus making the meeting more productive.

OPTIONS FOR ACTION IDENTIFIED

It is desirable that either the person who does the preliminary analysis, or the participants in the first meeting held to discuss the results of the quality review, identify options for corrective action, including approaches used by other organizations. (Committees are effective at giving "yes" or "no" answers, but may not be as effective at identifying options for improvement.) The facilitator of the first meeting is then prepared to stimulate discussion by citing improvement approaches used in other organizations. The situation must be framed as an opportunity for improvement. Options selected should be easy to accomplish, recognizing that the timing of the action will be dependent on the readiness of the people involved. Changes to systems and processes within the organization may need be installed prior to the action, in order to support the new behaviors. A follow-up meeting date should be set to maintain momentum for quality improvement. Another method for maintaining momentum is to identify the next audience for the communication of these results, and to assign tasks to be done by group members prior to that date. Peer review and comment must be supported and encouraged in order to disseminate the results and obtain staff commitment to improving the quality of performance.

FEEDBACK PROCESSES ARTICULATED AND FOLLOWED

The unit or department involved in measuring an indicator of quality performance must have regular, consistent feedback to maintain commitment of its staff to the QM program. A time frame needs to be set for another review of the indicator in question to assure staff that improvement has occurred as a result of their efforts. A push for quality just prior to an accreditation visit has little meaning if there is no regular follow-up to ensure that corrective action is taken. Feedback received reinforces efforts for continuous improvement in performance (Farley, 1994).

DATA-PRESENTATION TECHNIQUES

It is easier to discuss an issue when the content is illustrated via some kind of audio-visual aid. Most people understand and remember information graphically, rather than linguistically or numerically. Data-presentation techniques can be grouped according to their purpose: idea generation, beliefs portrayal, data display, or data analysis. These categories roughly parallel the process used in designing and implementing a QM program and are adapted from an organizing framework used by Wilson (1992). See Table 24-5 for a summary of the techniques used in data presentation.

Table 24-5 • DATA-PRESENTATION TECHNIQUES
Idea Generation
Brainstorming
Boarding
Multi-voting
Decision matrices
Portrayal of Beliefs
Flow diagrams
Fishbone diagrams
Display
Check sheets
Bar graphs (histograms)
Line graphs (run charts)
Analysis
Pareto charts
Control charts
Pie charts
Scatter diagrams
Stratification

Idea-Generation Techniques

After a principal function of the organization or department has been identified, the people who are involved in an aspect of that function need to meet and identify indicators of quality. The underlying purpose of any group idea-generation activity is to build team participation, team spirit, and team commitment to a mutual goal. All of these group purposes are desirable when establishing a QM program. Group-process theory has therefore been a source of methods for generating ideas in a group setting. Four methods to be discussed include brainstorming, boarding, multi-voting, and the use of decision matrices.

BRAINSTORMING

Brainstorming is one of the oldest and most effective methods of stimulating creative thought. The facilitator establishes certain ground rules, including no idea is too silly, no criticism, and no explanations or discussion. A recorder is appointed to write down everything that is said, with no editing of the terminology or phrasing used. The facilitator encourages group members to suggest as many ideas as possible, reminding them that piggybacking of ideas is desirable. People are asked to let their imaginations run wild, be funny, and be accepting of all suggestions. Because the participants' ideas all have equal value in the group, the exercise builds a sense of team credibility.

BOARDING

Boarding is often used in conjunction with brainstorming. Suggested ideas are placed on a board, flipchart, or other visual display for everyone to see. This visual display assists people to revisit earlier suggestions and come up with new ideas. It helps focus the discussion on the issues. It builds a sense of team, because it assures individuals that their ideas have been heard, recorded, and given equal status with those of other people. Boarding also provides assistance in the initial sorting process, which separates trivial issues from more important ones. The sorting is made easier by recording ideas on "Post-it" notes or pieces of paper that can be moved and placed close to other similar ideas. This can be done with a felt board, funtack, or easily removable masking tape.

MULTI-VOTING

When a group wishes to arrive at some conclusions for further work, a process of voting can be used to both sort and discard ideas. Multi-voting occurs after ideas have been generated and written for everyone to see, whether it be in a group setting or by written information that is circulated. The ideas can be ranked according to importance, sorted according to topic, combined, eliminated, or articulated in more detail during discussion. If there are differences of opinion, decisions are made by group consensus or voting. The ideas that obtain low ranking are eliminated from the list, and more voting determines the final ranking. The Delphi process and nominal group technique are two formalized methods of multi-voting. Both methods are designed to prevent domination of the group results by powerful people. If results are not tallied in writing over two or three ballots, the individual rankings of junior group members are recorded before those of the senior members of the group. This process facilitates team building, because the opinions of all members are respected, and the product is truly representative of the whole group.

DECISION MATRICES

A decision matrix is useful when a choice has to be made between alternate priorities, actions, or proposals. A grid is developed to assist in decision making. The left side of the grid lists each option (that is, priority, action, or proposal). The top of the grid has columns labeled according to the criteria selected as important considerations in the implementation of the options (see Figure 24-1). The most difficult part of the decision matrix is establishing the criteria (either characteristics or consequences) that will be used to judge the relative merits of the different options. A scoring system is established to rank each option according to the criteria, such as zero through four points. Low scores may be the best choices if negative consequences are the column labels; high scores may be the best choices if aspects of quality are the column labels. Each individual in the group of people making the decision completes the matrix independently, and the scores for each cell are added. The final score for each option is the total or the average of all cells. The group still retains control of the decision and does not have to decide in favor of the option with the best score. The value of the decision matrix is the exploration of criteria by which options will be evaluated, and the ensuing discussion regarding the relative merits of each option. This method of encouraging team participation helps to focus discussion and add some objectivity to the always-present subjective opinions of decision makers.

Beliefs Portrayal Techniques

Subjective opinions are based on personal beliefs and experiences. These beliefs must be articulated and examined to identify which aspects of a situation should be explored for improvement of performance. People in one department often are convinced that poor performance is related to the actions of another department. The process of recording beliefs shows respect for all staff; it shows that their opinions have legitimacy and are worthy of being explored in efforts to improve performance. Two methods for identifying multiple aspects of a situation are flow diagrams and fishbone diagrams. Both diagrams may be created by using team-building, idea-generating processes such as brainstorming and boarding. The diagrams could even be accepted by using a multi-voting process.

FLOW DIAGRAMS

Every organization has processes that are integral to its functioning. When people agree on a flow diagram of a process, they are expressing their belief about how that process works within the organization. Some flow diagrams have different shapes to indicate aspects of functioning. A circle can mean a starting or ending point, a rec-

Action	Consequences				Scores
	Morale	Cost	Time	Access to Resources	
A	+3	−1	−3	+2	+1
B	−2	+3	+1	−3	−1
C	+1	−3	+3	−1	0
D	−3	+2	+2	+1	+2
E	−1	−2	+2	−2	−3

Figure 24-1 *Decision Matrix*

tangle a step in the process, and a diamond a decision point (See Figure 24-2). These diagrams are also called flowcharts, process pathways, or process maps. People are astounded at how complex a simple process can be when the steps are recorded in sequential order, with exits to different points according to decisions

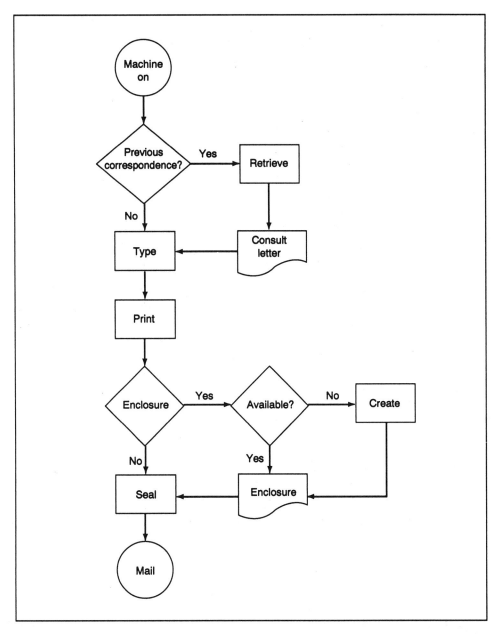

Figure 24-2 *Flow Diagram. (Reprinted with permission from C. R. M. Wilson [1992],* Strategies in Health Care Quality *[Exhibit 11.9, p. 324], copyright 1992 by W. B. Saunders Company Canada Limited.)*

made. Labeling each step and identifying responsibility for each decision point helps people to understand how many variables influence a single product. It is also surprising to see how many places something can go wrong. The draft flow diagram should be compared to actual practice, and changes made until it is an accurate reflection of the process. Indicators can then be developed, and monitoring of performance can begin. Recording the number of errors at particular points compared to the total number of services provided provides a basis for performance thresholds. Findings that do not match expectations may lead to exploration of other factors influencing the process. The people involved in the activity will then be able to base future quality-improvement efforts on local baseline data.

FISHBONE DIAGRAMS

The fishbone diagram of beliefs is a method of labeling and categorizing all variables that contribute to a particular problem. Wilson (1992) identifies five ribs to the fish skeleton. Each rib consists of variables that lead to the problem: people, places, provisions, procedures, and patrons. People variables may include apathy, frustration, or commitment to detail. Places are facilities that contribute to or hinder the desired performance, and the availability of suitable equipment. Provisions are financial resources and material supplies necessary for the process. The procedures rib includes the clarity, relevance, and use of policies, protocols, reporting systems, and the established pattern of accountability. Patrons are the funders who define the measurements that evaluate the problem; possible measurements of performance should be grouped along this rib of the diagram (see Figure 24-3). People who work in the area experiencing the problem are the experts; they are the best people to identify the factors for each rib of the skeleton. They will be aware of variables that must be in place before quality performance can occur, although they may not have listed them all before. Baseline data shows which aspects of the process are working well and which ones need improvement. If contributing

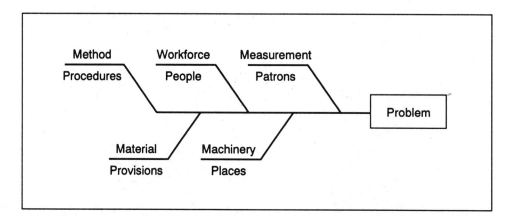

Figure 24-3 *Fishbone Diagram. (Reprinted with permission from C. R. M. Wilson [1992],* Strategies in Health Care Quality *[Exhibit 11.10, p. 326], copyright 1992 by W. B. Saunders Company Canada Limited.)*

factors are labeled according to category, and the process is monitored to discover where the breakdowns are occurring, then the specific cause of the problem can be addressed. Quality performance can be created by ensuring that each of those contributing factors is in place and working effectively.

Data Display Techniques

Data must be translated into information in order to be useful. Check sheets are a simple way of showing which characteristics are present in which items, and are easier for the receiver to process than a prose description. Tables of raw data acquire meaning when numbers are displayed graphically in bar graphs and line graphs.

CHECK SHEETS

When a group of items or processes is being examined according to the same criteria, a check sheet can illustrate which items have which characteristics. The items being compared are listed in rows on the left side of a graph. The characteristics or criteria that apply to each item create column labels across the top of the graph. A key to symbols will inform the reader at a glance: for instance, check marks might mean the presence of the characteristic; an "x" or "o" the absence; and a blank or "NA," not applicable (see Figure 24-4). Some consumer magazines rate products using an empty circle to indicate good performance, a black circle to indicate poor performance, and a split circle, half empty and half black, to indicate mediocre performance.

BAR GRAPHS

When the purpose of the display is to compare data sets, a bar graph or **histogram** is the preferred technique. A graph is created with the frequency of events or the

Product	Characteristics							
	1	2	3	4	5	6	7	8
A	x	x	x	o	x	o	/	/
B	x	x	o	o	x	o	/	/
C	x	o	o	x	x	/	/	x
D	o	o	x	x	/	x	o	/

Key to Symbols
x signifies the presence of the characteristic
o signifies the absence of the characteristic
/ signifies that the characteristic is nonapplicable

Figure 24-4 *Check Sheet*

volume of clients on the vertical axis. The horizontal axis is the base for two or more rectangular bars representing the categories of events or clients (see Figure 24-5). The graph is more accurate if it begins with zero at the bottom left corner for both axes. Data can be compared to that of similar organizations in a similar time period. The advantage of using bar graphs is the visual comparison between categories. Sometimes differences are dramatic, and the data becomes information that has impact.

LINE GRAPHS

When data has been collected over a period of time, and trends are of primary interest to the audience, a line chart or **run chart** is the method of choice. The graph has a vertical axis representing the quantity of events or clients, and the horizontal axis is marked according to times of measurement (see Figure 24-6). Trends in performance over time can be seen easily using this display method. The significance of improvement or deterioration in scores is readily understood when the line moves higher or lower on the graph, particularly if the incline is sharp.

Data Analysis Techniques

The separation of techniques for data display and analysis is somewhat artificial, because whenever data is displayed, analysis and comparisons are invited. For example, the bar chart is used for comparison of scores, and its interpretation requires analysis of influencing variables. A run chart can be used for trend analysis, if more than one event or time period is shown on the same chart and the inclines and directions of the lines are compared. These two methods can be further adapted specifically for data analysis. The bar graph can be transformed into a **Pareto chart**, and the run chart can become a **control chart**. Other tools used to analyze data include pie charts, scatter plots, and stratification of data into categories.

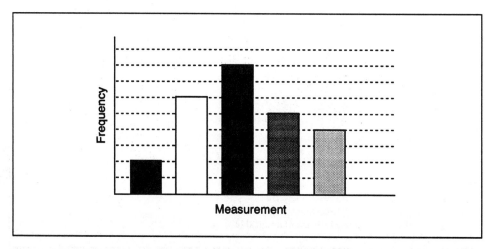

Figure 24-5 *Bar Graph or Histogram. (Reprinted with permission from C. R. M. Wilson [1992], Strategies in Health Care Quality [Exhibit 11.3, p. 318], copyright 1992 by W. B. Saunders Company Canada Limited.)*

PARETO CHARTS

These charts were named after an Italian who studied the distribution of wealth in nineteenth century Italy. Pareto charts are bar graphs of mutually exclusive types of events or clients totalling 100 percent of the population under consideration. The bars are displayed with the most frequent category on the far left, and the other categories in decreasing order of frequency. Sometimes a scale on the right side of the graph indicates the percentage of the total population, and a line is traced from one bar to the next, rising with the accumulated data until 100 percent is reached with the last bar (see Figure 24-7). A Pareto chart can be used to show how much particular factors contribute to variance in performance. It can also be used to show

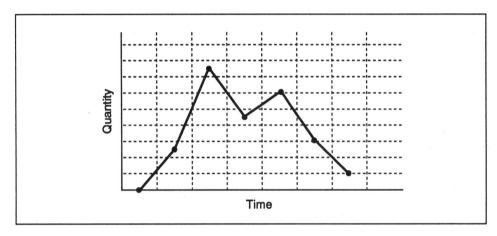

Figure 24-6 *Line Graph. (Reprinted with permission from C. R. M. Wilson [1992], Strategies in Health Care Quality [Exhibit 11.4, p. 318], copyright 1992 by W. B. Saunders Company Canada Limited.)*

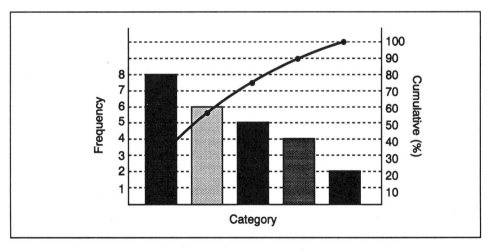

Figure 24-7 *Pareto Chart. (Reprinted with permission from C. R. M. Wilson [1992], Strategies in Health Care Quality [Exhibit 11.7, p. 321], copyright 1992 by W. B. Saunders Company Canada Limited.)*

the largest client groups within an organization's caseload. By illustrating analysis of data, identification of priorities is simplified.

CONTROL CHARTS

When line graphs have upper and lower control limits (UCL and LCL) shown on the graph, they become control charts. It is easy to see when the occurrence of events is above or below a given threshold, because the threshold is visible as a horizontal line drawn across the chart (see Figure 24-8). Analysis of data occurs at a glance. Variations between the upper and lower control limits are normal and expected as part of the process. When variations exceed the control limits, however, it is unexpected, and an investigation should be launched to identify the causes. Thresholds may be established when baseline data from monitoring the process are averaged, creating an average or mean score. One standard deviation on each side of the average score includes 68 percent of the random variation. Two standard deviations on each side of the mean includes 95 percent of the variation. Narrow control thresholds are used when consequences of the variation are severe for the client, staff, or organization.

PIE CHARTS

An alternative to the Pareto chart is the pie chart. Like the Pareto chart, the pie chart shows the sizes of mutually exclusive categories that, together, compose the whole population being considered. The size of the pie wedge represents the proportion of the whole belonging to that category (see Figure 24-9). Analysis is limited to relative proportions of the whole, however. No conclusions can be drawn about the relationship of that distribution to others at different times or from different organizations. Other comparisons would require more than one pie chart placed next to each other.

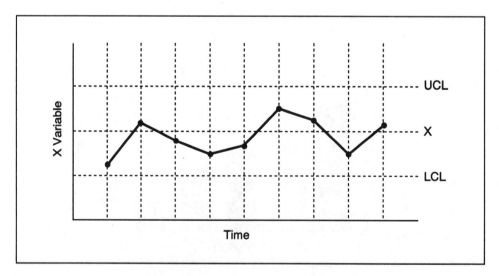

Figure 24-8 *Control Chart. (Reprinted with permission from C. R. M. Wilson [1992],* Strategies in Health Care Quality *[Exhibit 11.8, p. 322], copyright 1992 by W. B. Saunders Company Canada Limited.)*

SCATTER DIAGRAMS

When the group that is analyzing events wishes to explore the relationship between two variables, a **scatter diagram** can be used to discover whether there is a correlation — and in which direction. Each event is recorded as a dot on the graph, and the distribution of scores graphically illustrates the relationship between the horizontal and vertical variables (see Figure 24-10). For example, the number of hours of home-nursing services delivered compared to the age of clients served are

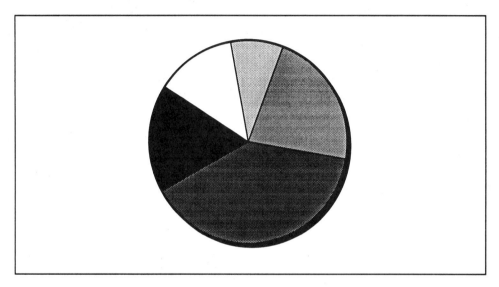

Figure 24-9 *Pie Chart. (Reprinted with permission from C. R. M. Wilson [1992],* Strategies in Health Care Quality *[Exhibit 11.5, p. 319], copyright 1992 by W. B. Saunders Company Canada Limited.)*

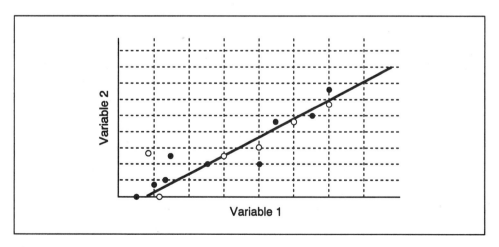

Figure 24-10 *Scatter Diagram. (Reprinted with permission from C. R. M. Wilson [1992],* Strategies in Health Care Quality *[Exhibit 11.6, p. 320], copyright 1992 by W. B. Saunders Company Canada Limited.)*

two variables that may be related. A positive correlation is shown if one variable increases as the other variable also increases. A negative correlation is shown if one variable decreases as the other increases. The most difficult aspect of using a scatter diagram is deciding which variables to compare. Visible results make correlations easy to understand.

STRATIFICATION

Stratification is used to examine data more closely and obtain more information about events. The average score may be within threshold limits for quality performance; but if complaints continue to be received, stratification will help identify the problem. The data is grouped by categories so that the average scores of each category can be seen separately. A bar graph can be used to visually display the numbers (see Figure 24-11). The average score, which was acceptable, now becomes information about which categories are outside the acceptable limits. A direction for quality-improvement efforts can then be easily identified.

The Transition from Data to Information and Action

Quality-improvement tools that generate ideas, portray beliefs, and display and analyze data are essential components of any effort to improve organizational functioning. When beliefs and data are translated into information, successes and failures can be labeled. Motivation to improve quality can then build naturally on the organization's and each individual's wish to do the best job possible.

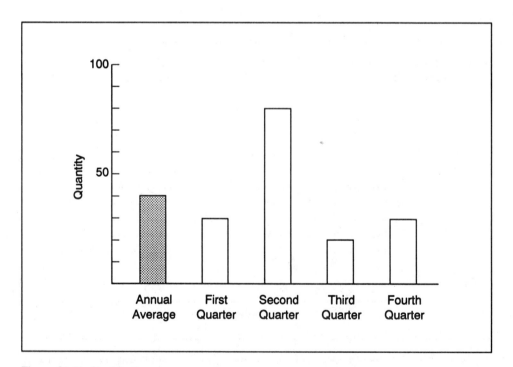

Figure 24-11 *Stratification*

DATA ANALYSIS

The sophistication of data analysis ranges according to the needs of the organization and the skill and knowledge of the individual performing the task. Much of the data collected for QM purposes is very straightforward and within the capabilities of front-line staff who understand ratios and percentages. Researchers who are interested in statistical significance of results may wish to use methods such as chi square, odds ratios, factor analysis, or computer-generated correlations. Controlling for certain variables that may confound results requires computer analysis of data. The method of analysis should be selected prior to data collection to ensure that the needed variables are gathered, and that the appropriate human and financial resources are in place to permit the planned analysis. There is no shame in using simple methods of data analysis such as arithmetic techniques; QM data can change practice only when staff understand the analysis.

DATA INTERPRETATION

The data collected in a QM program has no meaning until it is analyzed and translated into information through methods such as graphic display. That information has no value until it is interpreted by the people who will use it to analyze the quality of their own performance. Data analysis and interpretation then becomes an educational tool for assessing current status and determining future practice goals. When people have control over the use of information they are less threatened because data is not being used in a punitive manner. Their contribution to the quality of service is respected when they are trusted to make sound decisions regarding improvements in practice. If people have the freedom to identify the problem, provide alternate explanations for the results, or suggest methods of correcting it, they have some control over consequences. Variations in practice can be separated into **common cause variations** and **special cause variations**. Management of those variations can be discussed, explored, and attempted in the search for better-quality practice. The effectiveness of guidelines can be assessed and expectations changed by mutual consent. When there is a commitment to using the results of a QM program, a momentum toward increasing quality is created for the organization, its management, and its personnel.

Feedback is an essential component of any QM program. Results of data-collection efforts must be communicated to all stakeholders as soon as possible, including management, quality committees, and frontline staff. When the feedback comes quickly, the momentum of the staff toward quality is maintained, and energy can be used for the implementation of corrective action. Long delays in feedback mean that increased time and resources are required to reeducate staff about the purpose of the data collection, to review possible interpretations of the results, and to identify techniques for improving quality. Momentum must then be recreated for the implementation of corrective action.

CONCLUSION

This chapter provided an overview of the process of data acquisition and management in a health-care organization. Quality in practice requires the identification of principal functions of the organization as a basis for the articulation of quality indicators. The indicators that are most relevant to units of the organization often specify the best data sources to use and may even guide the selection of data-collection methods. When the data is gathered, it must be translated into information. Various techniques for the presentation of data, which portray beliefs and display data, were described. For complete understanding of all of the influencing variables, data interpretation, like other steps in the quality-improvement process, requires the participation of those who perform the activities.

Quality-of-care data is meaningless unless the organizational commitment to quality practice includes the allocation of resources to implement staff suggestions for improvement of daily practices. Administrative changes with monetary implications may be required in reporting or approval mechanisms, policies and procedures, or the QM process itself. Staff may need training in data management and release from regular duties for committee work. New staff positions devoted to quality concerns may need to be created. A revised system of information management may include the design of new forms, new computer software, new computer hardware, or the use of consultants in exploring options and their consequences. Almost every organizational change that contributes to the improvement of services has implications for the education of staff, which also costs money. Other barriers to quality-of-care initiatives were discussed as considerations that influence the selection of data sources, collection methods, or display techniques. These barriers can be grouped into three categories: human, statistical, and organizational. Decisions made will always be compromises balancing the commitment of the organization against the likely response of management and staff and the acceptable level of scientific rigor of the data. Organizations have differing strengths and limitations, and each organization works within a unique political and cultural context. The decisions made need to be the best ones possible at that time and under those circumstances. Every effort to improve the quality of health-care practices, however complete or incomplete, must be applauded. Through this approach, not only are things done right the first time, which saves money previously used for corrective actions; but staff morale and commitment to work are increased, with improved quality of service a natural by-product. The final result of quality practice is more acceptable, appropriate, and effective care for clients and families, who justify the existence of health-care services.

REFERENCES

American Hospital Association. (1991). *Practice pattern analysis: A tool for continuous improvement of patient care quality.* Chicago: Author.

Anderson, B., & Hannah, K. J. (1993). A Canadian nursing minimum data set: A major priority. *Canadian Journal of Nursing Administration, 6*(2), 7–13.

Bader, B. S., & Bohr, D. (1991). *Guide to the interpretation and use of quality-of-care data.* Chicago: Hospital Research and Educational Trust, American Hospital Association.

Bard, J., Jimenez, F., & Tornack, R. (1994). Outcome based management. *Canadian Journal of Nursing Administration, 7*(1), 42–61.

Burdick, M. B., Stuart, G. W., & Lewis, L. D. (1994). Measuring nursing outcomes in a psychiatric setting. *Issues in Mental Health Nursing, 15*(2), 137–148.

Donabedian, A. (1988). The quality of care: How can it be assessed? *Journal of the American Medical Association, 260*(12), 1743–1748.

Farley, E. (1994). How we survived a redesign. *American Journal of Nursing, 94*(3), 43–45.

Greeneich, D. (1993). The link between new and return business and quality of care: Patient satisfaction. *Advances in Nursing Science, 16*(1), 62–72.

Harrigan, M. L. (1992). *Quality of care: Issues and challenges in the 90s: A literature review.* Ottawa, Ontario: Canadian Medical Association.

Hennessy, L. L., & Friesen, M. A. (1994). Perceptions of quality of care in a minority population: A pilot study. *Journal of Nursing Care Quality, 8*(2), 32–37.

Holland, W. W. (Ed.). (1983). *Evaluation of health care.* Oxford, England: Oxford University Press.

Hough, B. L., & Schmele, J. A. (1987). The Slater scale: A viable method for monitoring nursing care quality in home health. *Journal of Nursing Quality Assurance, 1*(3), 28–38.

Jacquerye, A. (1984). Choosing an appropriate method of quality assurance. In L. D. Willis & M. E. Linwood (Eds.), *Measuring the quality of care* (pp. 107–120). Edinburgh, Scotland: Churchill Livingstone, Medical Division of Longman Group.

Joint Commission on the Accreditation of Healthcare Organizations (1989). Characteristics of clinical indicators. *Quality Review Bulletin, 15*(11), 330–339.

Joint Commission on the Accreditation of Healthcare Organizations (1993). IM system starts up with ten indicators. *Perspectives, 13*(6), 1–3.

Katz, J., & Green, E. (1992). *Managing quality: A guide to monitoring and evaluating nursing services.* St. Louis, MO: Mosby-Year Book.

Kitson, A., Harvey, G., Hyndman, S., & Yerrell, P. (1994). Criteria formulation and application: An evaluative framework. *International Journal of Nursing Studies, 31*(2), 5–167.

Knox, L. J. (1985). *The Knox guide to self-appraisal and goal-setting for community health nurses.* Ottawa, Ontario: The Canadian Public Health Association.

Koch, M. W., & Fairly, T. M. (1993). *Integrated Quality Management: The key to improving nursing care quality.* St. Louis, MO: Mosby Year Book.

Krieger, N. (1992). The making of public health data: Paradigms, politics, and policy. *Journal of Public Health Policy, 13*(4), 412–427.

Milholland, D. K. (1994). Privacy and confidentiality of patient information: Challenges for nursing. *Journal of Nursing Administration, 24*(2), 19–24.

Nauright, L. P., & Simpson, R. L. (1994). Benefits of hospital information systems as seen by front line nurses and general hospital staff. *Journal of Nursing Administration, 24*(4S), 26–32.

Ruden, J. C. (1994). A transition to quality improvement: A home care model. *Journal of Nursing Care Quality, 8*(2), 9–15.

Scardina, S. A. (1994). SERVQUAL: A tool for evaluating patient satisfaction with nursing care. *Journal of Nursing Care Quality, 8*(2), 38–46.

Schroeder, P. S., & Maibusch, R. M. (Eds.). (1984). *Nursing Quality Assurance: A unit-based approach.* Rockville, MD: Aspen Systems.

Sharp, T., & Kilvington. (1993). Towards integrative audit: A partnership for quality. *International Journal of Healthcare Quality Assurance, 6*(4), 12–15.

Sherman, J. J., & Malkmus, M. A. (1994). Integrating Quality Assurance and Total Quality Management/quality improvement. *Journal of Nursing Administration, 24*(3), 37–41.

Smith, T. C., & Popowich, J. M. (1993). Health care standards: The interstitial matter of quality programs. *Journal of Nursing Care Quality, 8*(1), 1–11.

Van Maanen, H. M. Th. (1984). Evaluation of nursing care: A multinational perspective. In L. D. Willis & M. E. Linwood (Eds.), *Measuring the quality of care* (pp. 3–42). Edinburgh, Scotland: Churchill Livingstone, Medical Division of Longman Group.

Wilson, C. R. M. (1992). *Strategies in health care quality.* Toronto, Ontario: W. B. Saunders Company Canada Limited.

ADDITIONAL READING

Connington, M. E., & Dupuis, P. (1990). *Unit-based nursing Quality Assurance: A patient-centered approach.* Rockville, MD: Aspen.

Fields, W. L., & Siroky, K. A. (1994). Converting data into information. *Journal of Nursing Care Quality, 8*(3), 1–11.

Green, E., Hobbs, L., & Mousseau, J. (1994). Introducing Quality Management in the community: The VON experience. *Canadian Journal of Nursing Administration, 7*(1), 62–75.

Joint Commission on the Accreditation of Healthcare Organizations (1991). *Primer on indicator development.* Oakbrook Terrace, IL: Author.

Plsek, P. E. (1994). Tutorial: Planning for data collection, part I: Asking the right questions. *Quality Management in Health Care, 2*(2), 76–81.

Schroeder, P. (Ed.). (1992). *The encyclopedia of nursing care quality: Vol. I. Issues and strategies for nursing care quality.* Rockville, MD: Aspen.

Schroeder, P. (Ed.). (1992). *The encyclopedia of nursing care quality: Vol. II. Approaches to nursing standards.* Rockville, MD: Aspen.

Schroeder, P. (Ed.). (1992). *The encyclopedia of nursing care quality: Vol. III. Monitoring and evaluation in nursing.* Rockville, MD: Aspen.

Simpson, R. L. (1994). Ensuring patient data privacy, confidentiality and security. *Nursing Management, 25*(7), 18–20.

Mary Jo Kreitzer
Judith Beck

CHAPTER *25*

Using Computers to Support Quality Management

INTRODUCTION

The delivery of health care has become inextricably entwined with the management of information. Timely, relevant, reliable, and accurate information is essential for clinical and managerial decision making. The increased demand for data is influenced by changes in the health-care environment and patient care. Health-care reform and the movement toward integrated service networks has accelerated the demand for information technology.

Under fee-for-service reimbursement, the goal was to capture charges. Computer systems were financially oriented and featured automated-billing, accounts-payable, and general-ledger processes. Health care was fragmented and inefficient, and there was no incentive to manage costs or coordinate care. In a managed-care environment, where health-care organizations are reimbursed a fixed dollar amount per capita, the dynamics are different. Purchasers of health care, whether they be individual **consumers**, businesses, or the government, are demanding information on services provided, the costs of care, the **quality** of care, and patient **outcomes** achieved. Information systems are required that help manage and coordinate the health care provided to an individual over a prolonged period of time, perhaps even a lifetime, as opposed to a discrete episode of care. There is a strong incentive to maximize quality and minimize costs on both an individual basis and for the entire patient population served.

Continuous-Quality-Improvement (CQI) tools facilitate the achievement of patient-care management, improved productivity, and improved quality of care. These processes are very data driven. Large data sets are required for **variance** analysis of key processes, outcomes assessment, and performance-based evaluations. It has become increasingly necessary to use computers to support these activities rather than rely on manual management of the data.

Benchmarking is an example of a CQI tool that continues to grow in popularity in the health-care industry. There is increasing recognition that the collection and use of objective information that describes delivery-system performance is critical. As described by Campbell (1994), benchmarking is firmly grounded in **process** orientation and is dependent on the collection and use of objective information. Simply stated, the steps of benchmarking include:

- definition of the process
- development of a database that describes process performance
- identification of extraordinary performers, as defined by data points
- identification of factors that drive system performance
- adoption of those factors by the benchmarking organization

Benchmarking requires resources to support data collection and analysis, as well as partnerships with other organizations to gain access to comparative performance data.

Patient data is the core or foundation of these data sets. Patient data acquired during the course of patient care can be used within the organization and across different organizational settings for multiple purposes. Patient data can be used to **monitor** or **evaluate** individual patient progress along a clinical pathway, or to support clinical decision making, research, quality-improvement monitoring, operations management, or financial analysis. Patient data that is captured and stored can be aggregated, analyzed, and summarized at a later date.

An information-technology infrastructure that links hospitals, clinics, and other health-care providers is a fundamental requirement for integrated-care management. Within health-care networks, clinical and financial data need to move seamlessly to achieve integrated care management. As a result, there are increased requirements for clinical information systems, such as those listed in Table 25-1.

Table 25-1 • **REQUIREMENTS FOR CLINICAL INFORMATION SYSTEMS**

- Timely, relevant, reliable, and accurate information essential for clinical and financial decision making
- Documentation, monitoring, and evaluation of interdisciplinary care processes and outcomes across the full continuum of care
- Systems that assure that care is delivered at the lowest level of resource utilization attainable
- Measurement of health status and other clinical outcomes on an individual and patient-population basis
- Integration of clinical and financial data to determine the impact of resource utilization on patient health status/outcomes
- Accessibility of clinical information to providers in various locations
- Access and utilization of public health databases

In the 1994 *Accreditation Manual for Hospitals*, the Joint Commission on Accreditation of Healthcare Organizations (Joint Commission) promulgates **standards** that apply to information management, whether automated or on paper. These standards include requirements such as combining data from many different systems, linking clinical and administrative data, and using external databases to monitor hospital performance. Functions such as these will be virtually impossible to achieve without computer support. The Joint Commission is also in the process of developing a new *Accreditation Manual for Health Care Networks*. As recently described by Corum (1994), this manual will include a set of information-management standards that emphasize the need for systems interfaces and integration.

This chapter focuses on the paradigm shift in computer technology that makes this vision of data integration possible. The processes and challenges inherent in capturing, transforming, and presenting **Quality-Management (QM)** data are described. Practical issues are also addressed: How can identified needs for information and tools be translated into system requirements and functionality? What are the advantages of designing versus purchasing an information-management system? What approaches can be used to evaluate information-management systems? What are the trends in technology and information science that will impact cost and functionality? The large, comprehensive databases created to support quality improvement and patient-care management also raise significant issues of information security and control, patient and provider confidentiality, and the legitimacy of public access to data.

PARADIGM SHIFT IN COMPUTER TECHNOLOGY

Changes in technology and the computer industry over the past few decades have occurred at a very rapid rate. The paradigm shift in information technology has impacted virtually every aspect of data management, including how data is entered, analyzed, retrieved, and stored. Table 25-2 summarizes the paradigm shift in information technology.

One of the most dramatic changes has been in the area of computer hardware. The industry has shifted from large, expensive mainframe computers to portable workstations and "networks" of computers. Workstations may be either personal computers (PCs), intelligent workstations, or portable devices. As hardware technology has evolved, there have been significant decreases in the price and size of computers, and corresponding increases in power, speed, and functionality.

Networks, called local area networks or LANs, provide physical connections that link computers together. Within a health-care organization, patient data that is stored in the computer system can be accessed from PCs or terminals that are on the network. This facilitates data access and allows software and data to be used simultaneously by more than one user. Whereas communication networks used to exist primarily within an institution, networks now cross institutions and are global in nature. An example of a global network is the *Internet*. The *Internet* provides a backbone that links smaller networks together around the globe. Academic, government, and industrial centers have the capability of exchanging data and electronic mail, engaging in interactive discussions, and accessing libraries.

Table 25-2 • PARADIGM SHIFTS IN INFORMATION TECHNOLOGY

Topic	Moving From	To
Computer hardware	Mainframe	Workstations and networks
Communication networks	Within institution	Multiple institutions Global
Mobility of computers	Stationary	Mobil, nomadic
Location of computers	Central areas	Point of care
Users	Clerical use Department defined	Professional staff use Multiple disciplines
Focus	Financial	Clinical
Programming tools	Labor intensive coding	4GL languages and beyond
Modifications	Custom programming	Tailored for each user and changed easily
Databases	Flat file, hierarchical	Relational, object oriented
Data storage	Disks and tapes	Optical disk

As changes in computer hardware have occurred, the accompanying shifts in the mobility and location of computers has increased access to new groups of users interested in applications that go beyond the financial domain. Computers are no longer stationary, located in central areas, and used primarily by clerical or technical staff. They are increasingly mobile, located at the point of care, and used by health-care professionals for clinical purposes. Technological advances such as high-resolution displays, graphics, menu-driven programs, structured notes, touch screens, pointing devices (such as track balls and mice), and voice input improve the ease and efficiency with which clinicians interact with computers.

The paradigm shift in information technology has created a new generation of software-development tools and applications. The old programming languages that required very labor intensive coding have been replaced with new computer languages that have shortened the development cycle for producing new applications and made it relatively easy to tailor software to meet individual customer needs.

The software application used most often in organizing quality-management data is the database program. Database programs provide a structure for organizing data. The first database programs developed were flat or hierarchical. Flat-file databases can be described as electronic card files, similar to a set of index cards or a catalog. These programs provide for useful sorting, organizing, and management of data. Although these databases are easy to use, they are limited with regard to sophistication of analysis. Relational and newer, object-oriented databases are also available. These databases can define an object along with associated descriptors or attributes. As a result, they can accommodate organization of data relationships and provide sophisticated data analysis. These characteristics are useful for clinical data where associated details are critically important. Medication documentation is an example. Relevant details include the generic name of the medication administered, the brand name, dose, dosage form, route, time, site, patient weight, dose calculation, and patient response.

The paradigm shift in computer technology has had a major impact on the focus of information systems, the users, the configuration and location of computer hardware, software technology, communication, and overall functionality. A vast array of tools are now available to support CQI efforts. These tools facilitate the capture of quality-improvement data, the analysis of data, and the subsequent communication and presentation of findings.

QUALITY-MANAGEMENT DATA

As the emphasis in QM has changed, so too has the demand for data. Increasingly, organizations are needing patient-related clinical data as well as administrative, financial, and operations data to support ongoing monitoring and evaluation functions. Capturing patient data poses several significant challenges related to how clinical information is described, recorded, and stored.

Data Acquisition

The clinical data of greatest interest at this time is patient-outcome data. Some patient-outcome data, such as mortality and length of stay, is relatively easy to obtain. Other data related to functional health status, nursing, or medical outcomes may either not be recorded or may not be recorded in such a manner that it can be easily retrieved, either manually or using a computer. The management of nursing data is a challenge because of the complexity of the care processes and the fact that nursing has historically had no common language. When nurses provide treatments such as airway management, bleeding reduction, or spiritual support, there is no standardized term to describe the care activity. While there is growing consensus that taxonomies are needed for nursing diagnoses, interventions, and outcomes, significant development work is still required in this area. Ozbolt (1992) notes that the

> absence of specific nursing data from national and regional
> databases is not the result of discrimination against nursing.
> Rather, it is the result of the profession's failure to agree upon
> and offer a set of clearly defined, valid, reliable and standardized
> data elements for inclusion. (p. 210)

The Nursing Minimum Data Set (NMDS) (Werley & Lang, 1988), the Nursing Interventions Classification (NIC) initiative (McCloskey & Bulechek, 1992), and the Omaha Classification System (Martin & Schect, 1992) used in community-health settings are examples of efforts to establish uniform standards for the collection of minimum, essential nursing data.

NURSING DATA ELEMENTS
The effort to develop the NMDS was initiated by Harriet Werley and Norma Lang in 1985. A national group of experts was convened and charged with identifying

the appropriate data elements and associated definitions. The work of the conference resulted in a list of sixteen elements in three categories. There are four nursing-care items, five patient- or client-demographic items, and seven service items (see Table 25-3).

Table 25-3 • **NURSING MINIMUM DATA SET**

Nursing-Care Elements

- Nursing diagnosis
- Nursing intervention
- Nursing outcome
- Intensity of nursing care

Patient or Client Demographic Elements

- Personal identification*
- Date of birth*
- Gender*
- Race and ethnicity*
- Residence*

Service Elements

- Unique facility or service agency number*
- Unique health record number of patient or client
- Unique number of principal Registered Nurse provider
- Episode admission or encounter date*
- Discharge or termination date*
- Disposition of patient or client*
- Expected payer for most of this bill*

---

* *Elements comparable to data elements in the Uniform Hospital Discharge Data Set.*

From H. Werley, P. Ryan, & A. Coenen. Brief Synopsis of the Nursing Minimum Data Set (NMDS) (June, 1994). University of Wisconsin-Milwaukee School of Nursing, Milwaukee, WI. With permission of H. Werley (noncopyrighted material).

More recently, McCloskey and Bulechek (1992) and a team of researchers developed the NIC, a taxonomy of nursing interventions. This taxonomy consolidates thousands of varied descriptions and often redundant terms for nursing treatments into 336 names and definitions. The National Library of Medicine now includes the 99 nursing diagnoses from NANDA and the 336 NIC nursing treatments in the *Unified Medical Language System Metathesaurus.* The metathesaurus is a computerized data locator that enables users to key in a word or term and find where that subject is covered in an extensive array of medical reference databases. With the exception of the nursing-care elements, most of the other data elements are already included in the Uniform Hospital Discharge Data Set (UHDDS). The UHDDS is one of several nationally recognized minimum data sets designed to meet the essential needs of multiple data users. Achieving consensus on data elements is critical, as is determining the most effective and efficient way to record data electronically or to transfer data into the computer.

Data Input

Data entry can be a very labor-intensive, expensive process. An increasingly feasible option is to have clinicians directly enter data into the computer as it is obtained at the point and time of care. This has the advantage of capturing data closest to the source, and integrates data collection into the care-documentation process. Dedicated workstations or bedside computer systems facilitate the integration of data entry into the work flow of the clinician. New technology can combine software that is designed for clinical use, high performance hardware and networks, and human interactive tools such as touch screens, pointing devices, or voice input. These combinations provide efficient and user-friendly ways for clinicians to interact with computers.

Patient data may already be available in an electronic format. Examples of this are some of the many instruments used in health care. Instruments in the laboratory read and report results without human transcription. Drug infusion pumps have computer chips that automatically display data. In the critical-care setting, integration of patient physiological monitors with clinical information systems offers the maximum efficiency and can achieve real time acquisition of data. Data from devices such as ventilators, pulse oximeters, and ECG arrhythmia monitoring systems can be transferred directly to the database in the computer. This data is periodically validated to ensure that the data entered accurately represents the physiological state of the patient.

Data Transformation

It is very possible to be data rich but information poor if tools are not available to transform data into meaningful information. Natural-language-processing (NLP) systems, databases, spreadsheets, and statistical and graphics software packages offer a wide variety of tools that format, trend, aggregate, summarize, and analyze data.

A significant amount of provider documentation exists in the form of text. From a quality-improvement perspective, it is a challenge to locate desired findings, conditions, and actions within text data. As Aronow and Coltin (1993) note, this task becomes more manageable when text is linked to coded data. Automated systems now have the capacity to extract meaning from text data via the use of NLP systems. Natural language processing can be used to index, codify, abstract, and interpret medical documentation and information resources.

Database management systems (DBMS) are able to store large amounts of data, which can be retrieved, manipulated, or transferred to another database system for subsequent analysis. Given the volume and complexity of clinical data, it will likely be necessary within a health-care setting to have multiple databases to store graphics, images, numerical data, sound, or even full-motion video. Databases generally are limited in the functions they can perform. Simple sorting or summarization of data may be possible, but more sophisticated data analysis requires the use of spreadsheets or statistical packages. Spreadsheets are ideal for the storage and manipulation of numbers. Simple calculations can be performed automatically as new data is entered. A spreadsheet can display, for example, the actual number of medication errors per patient-care unit, as well as the medication error rate (that is, the number of errors over the volume of medications administered).

Statistical packages vary considerably in ease of use and in the complexity of the functions performed. Basic descriptive statistics, including the mean, median, mode, quartile, standard deviation, and frequency distribution, are very useful in exploring numerical data. Assume, for example, that a patient-care unit has decided to collect information on the time it takes for a medication to be delivered to the unit after an order is written. A random-sampling process is used to collect data over a period of three weeks. Time in minutes is recorded for 520 medication orders. An analysis using descriptive statistics reveals that the delivery time for non-stat medications ranges from thirty minutes to three and one-half hours, with the mean delivery time being two hours. A frequency distribution of delays of over three hours confirms that 75 percent of all delays occur on weekends. This finding has significant implications for CQI. Further investigation may reveal, for example, that staffing patterns on weekends in the pharmacy need to change if service to the patient-care units is to be improved.

Statistical tests are used to evaluate relationships between two or more variables, or differences such as those between groups or over intervals of time. Data can be entered directly into the statistics software package or may be imported from a data file. In general, the larger the data set, the longer the analysis takes. More memory and disk storage are also needed.

Graphics software packages offer tremendous versatility in creating pictures, images, or graphs that bring QM data to life. The primary goal of a graph is to communicate a message or convey a story. Pie charts, bar graphs, **scatter diagrams**, **control charts**, and **histograms** are a few examples of commonly used presentation graphics that are useful in the quality-improvement process. Color, pattern, and different font sizes and styles add interest and clarity to graphs.

Tufte (1983) offers several excellence-in-graphics principles that provide direction in choosing a graphics software package and in designing graphs. Excellence in graphics, Tufte suggests, is the well-designed presentation of interesting data — a matter of substance, of statistics, and of design. Using graphs, complex ideas or information can be communicated with clarity, precision, and efficiency. A graph ideally should display the greatest amount of information in the shortest time, with the least ink, in the smallest space. Excellence in graphics is nearly always multivariate — that is, it shows the relationship between several variables. Tufte also notes that excellence in graphics requires telling the truth about the data!

Many graphics packages are limited in their ability to manipulate or analyze data. They frequently are used in conjunction with a spreadsheet or statistical package. Some newer products on the market combine word processing, spreadsheet, database, statistical, and graphics functions into a single software application. Although these integrated packages provide convenience and flexibility, they may not be as powerful or include all of the functions desired.

APPLICATION TO PRACTICE

An organization's objectives drive the selection and uses of information-system tools. In planning for an information-management system to support a QM program, an organization needs to consider the following questions:

> What do we want the information system to achieve (for example, concurrent variance analysis from critical pathways, patient outcomes, or ongoing performance data)?
>
> How can the computer tools help meet our objectives?
>
> What information-system infrastructure exists? What is the cycle time for our systems?
>
> Can we be on the forefront of technology?
>
> What will the cost of ownership be?
>
> What level of reliability do we need?
>
> What technical skills and staff are needed?

Selection Considerations

When an organization's objectives are clear and a strategic plan for information systems is developed, decisions need to be made regarding the information-systems infrastructure. The infrastructure includes: hardware and cabling; software tools and applications; database organization; networks and communication tools; and personnel.

It generally is helpful to identify the functions the system needs to perform. These functions can then be transferred into a requirements document or detailed system specifications. In evaluating information-systems alternatives, major factors to consider are the "buy-versus-build" question and the cost of ownership.

Designing and building a system offers the advantage of software designed to meet an organization's specific needs. Because this process requires staff attention during each phase of development (analysis, design, programming, testing, implementation, and post-implementation review), the cycle time to design and build needs to be considered. Other important questions for organizations to ask include:

> Do we have the staff skills to build and support a system?
>
> Are our time estimates realistic (that is, do they include *all* phases of the cycle)?
>
> Does our environment require that the software be changed frequently?
>
> How will the software be supported for troubleshooting and modification after it is built?

Buying software is advantageous because the software is tested, supported, and ready for use. Purchased software often can be tailored and configured to fit specific needs. Key factors to assess are the degree of configurability and fit of the software to the organization's needs.

Cost of ownership includes start-up and initial building costs, training costs, and licensee or annual service fees. One cost of ownership that requires careful analysis is the cost of system modification. This is especially important with rapidly changing clinical-data requirements, clinical-practice changes, and **accreditation** requirements. Questions to ask include:

How easily can modifications be made?

What is the cost?

How long does it take?

If on-site staff does the modification, what skill level does this require?

What are the training needs for both the technical staff and for the end users of the system?

Systems tailored for the specific work environments may be easier to use, and software that maximizes the "ease-of-use" features may fit better into the work flow and reduce the ongoing training costs.

Blending Systems for Patient Care and Quality Improvement

Patient care is a highly information-dependent process. Clinicians are increasingly relying on information systems for concurrent patient-care management (using data in the clinical information system to make decisions regarding patient care). Performing retrospective analysis of patient outcomes will influence approaches to future patient-care management. More sophisticated clinical information systems include "expert systems," built on mathematical models or decision trees. Fonteyn and Grobe (1994) describe expert systems as consisting of two components: the knowledge base (which stores facts about objects, actions, or processes and how they are interrelated) and the inference engine. The inference engine is designed to make decisions and judgments based on the data in the knowledge base. Based on external information about a problem, the inference engine uses the knowledge base to provide a potential solution to the problem. Expert systems may guide clinical decision making by recommending a course of action or a set of alternatives. A clinical information system with supporting communication systems can be used to obtain and record information about patients; consult with colleagues; access scientific literature; select appropriate laboratory tests and diagnostic procedures; access and interpret the results of tests; communicate plans or orders for patient care; and document patient progress and outcomes.

The following case study illustrates varying information-system tools and the infrastructures required to achieve different levels of quality-improvement activities. Also illustrated are differences in system requirements for data collection and data transformation, the timing and level of integration needed, and linkages between the clinical and quality-improvement systems.

CASE STUDY: *Three Hospitals, Three Information Systems*

Hospital A is a 250-bed community hospital that provides acute-care services to a primarily rural population. **Multidisciplinary** teams have identified important aspects of care and relevant **indicators**. Quality-improvement data is collected monthly. As illustrated in Table 25-4, the major objective from an information-management perspective is to have a system that provides data management including analysis, storage, and presentation of the data. A desktop personal computer and purchased software are sufficient to meet this objective. Hospital A was able to achieve a quick start-up with the purchased software and a minimum of staff time has been required for customization. The system has a high degree of reliability as long as regular backups are performed. A limitation of the system is that it requires manual data collection.

Table 25-4 • INFORMATION-SYSTEM REQUIREMENTS FOR HOSPITAL A	
System objectives	Data management, analysis, summary storage, and presentation.
Hardware and software tools	Desktop personal computer, purchased software for database, statistics, and presentation graphics; database customized easily.
Cost/support factors	Quick start-up with purchased software; staff time required for customization; widely used software selected for ready support.
Reliability	Regular backups completed.
Comments	Requires manual data collection. Data is organized and entered into one computer. Database design must accommodate trends in each indicator. Graphics or presentation packages used for summary presentation.

Hospital B is a 400-bed tertiary-care hospital located in a large metropolitan area. A highly sophisticated clinical information system supports ongoing management of patient data in the critical-care unit. The clinical system includes flowsheets, assessments, notes, and schedules. Data from bedside instruments and laboratory results is transferred directly to the database. Graphics tools are available to transform data. For research and quality-improvement activities, patient data is moved to a relational database for aggregation and analysis. Query and report-writer tools are used.

As illustrated in Table 25-5, high-performance workstations are located at each bedside to achieve the desired level of patient care and data management. A software bridge moves the data to a relational database. A system of this complexity requires a database manager and technical support. Collection of data occurs automatically, eliminating the need for manual data collection and data entry.

Table 25-5 • **INFORMATION-SYSTEM REQUIREMENTS FOR HOSPITAL B**

System objectives	Patient data management; summary and presentation of patient clinical status. Clinical system supports quality-improvement data collection as a by-product of service.
Hardware and software tools	High-performance workstations with graphics support are used at each bedside. Network configuration provides continuous access. Clinical system software is purchased and configured by the hospital to match clinical environment. Software bridge moves data to purchased relational database. High-performance workstations with graphics.
Cost/support factors	Primary expense is the clinical system. Research and quality-improvement database requires database manager and technical support to abstract data. Database organization must accommodate complex clinical data.
Reliability	Architecture of clinical system targets no single point of failure. All data has continuous mirror and is continuously accessible at all network locations. Data in research database has standard backup.
Comments	Automated data collection. Design supports one-time entry of data that is then available for multiple uses.

Hospital C is a 500-bed tertiary-care university hospital with a mission to support teaching, patient care, and research.

Table 25-6 • **INFORMATION-SYSTEM REQUIREMENTS FOR HOSPITAL C**

System objectives	Embedded knowledge-based tools assist clinicians in practice decisions. Incorporates expert opinion recommendations into practice setting.
Hardware and software tools	Hardware and software development tools selected to address knowledge-based feedback and graphics user interface. Client-server architecture.
Cost/support factors	Staff time for technical design and build process. Clinical time to develop and verify logic for expert knowledge tools. Development cycle time for all steps. Highly skilled technical support required during development cycle. Ongoing in-house support.
Reliability	Practice guidelines based on expert opinion are tested for reliability. All patient conditions are considered. Rigor in design and performance required. All elements must have backup.
Comments	Highly specialized system designed with specific care guidelines. Model uses real-time decision support. Development cycle expenses.

To achieve the goal of "effective and efficient" care, the hospital has automated parameters or guidelines that directly influence clinical decision making (see Table 25-6). For example, when a physician orders blood products or platelets, the expert information system automatically reviews all laboratory and clinical data and provides recommendations based on expert logic embedded in the system. If the order varies from the recommendation, a series of questions is posed to clarify the physician's rationale for choosing the alternative.

As noted in Table 25-6, a clinical information system that has embedded knowledge-based tools requires significant development time and costs. Highly skilled clinical and technical staff are required to develop and verify the logic for the expert knowledge tools. Systems of this nature generally are highly specialized. A major benefit of the system is that it has the potential of directly impacting patient care by focusing on concurrent decision support.

As the preceding case study illustrates, there are considerable costs associated with automation. Small institutions likely have different needs for data and may lack not only the resources to acquire sophisticated hardware and software and to support the training of personnel, but also the technical and professional staff required for ongoing operations of a large information system. Large institutions or institutions that are part of networks need a level of information-system support to integrate data across multiple units. In general, the type, volume, and complexity of data needed and the level of integration required will largely dictate the nature of information-systems support that is required.

DATA PRIVACY

The growing demands for patient information from peer-review bodies, third-party payers, government agencies, employers, and others who use health information for planning or research poses a threat to patient privacy. When patient privacy is disclosed, with or without patient consent, it is virtually impossible to control re-disclosure. One breach of a system's security can result in the unauthorized disclosure of extensive information about a large number of patients. Patient data that is computerized is perhaps more complete and accessible, and, therefore, more vulnerable than information contained in a paper record.

The legal and ethical duty to preserve confidentiality and prevent unauthorized access to patient records is the same with respect to both paper and computer-based records. Security mechanisms, policies, and procedures can provide some level of protection against unauthorized access to records contained in information systems. Even the most sophisticated security measures available today, however, will not provide fail-safe protection of patient records, especially in decentralized systems. At a minimum, an information system should include a security system that permits only authorized users to access only those portions of the records that are relevant to their particular functions. Some systems are capable of tracking and monitoring access, a feature that may be an additional deterrent to unauthorized review of records.

CONCLUSION

The demand for timely access to health-care data continues to mushroom. It is predicted that computer-based patient records will become a standard technology in health care within the decade. In fact, the Institute of Medicine, Committee on Improving the Patient Record (1991) has recommended that health-care professionals and organizations adopt the computer-based record as the standard for all records related to patient care. It is increasingly evident that information-management systems are necessary to support clinical decision making and quality-improvement processes critical to providing quality patient care.

The transformation to an integrated information-management system poses significant challenges and raises important legal and ethical issues. Hardware and software must be configured so that data is readily accessible to clinicians and is easily transferred and exchanged. Nomenclature and systems to adjust for patient severity need to be developed to the point where there is confidence that comparable patient data is aggregated and analyzed. The costs of investing in capital equipment and human resources to support the information-management infrastructure need to be weighed against the benefits accrued to patients, providers, and payers. One of the greatest challenges is the protection of patient privacy.

In reflecting on the future of computer applications in health care, Fagan and Perreault (1990) note that glimpses of the future can be both exciting and frightening. The future prospects are exciting as we see how emerging technologies can address frequently cited problems that confound current health-care practice. The future is also frightening as we realize how imperative it is that methodologies be applied wisely and sensitively if patients are to receive the humane and efficient health care that they have every right to expect. The question, Fagan and Perreault (1990) note, is

> not whether computer technologies will play a pervasive role in the
> health care environment of the future, but rather how we can
> ensure that future systems are designed and implemented effectively
> to optimize technology's role as a stimulus and support for the
> health care system and for individual practitioners. (p. 641)

A key for organizations is to first identify QM goals and then select information-systems tools that will support all phases of the quality-improvement process, from data collection to translating data into meaningful information.

REFERENCES

Aronow, D., & Coltin, K. L. (1993). Information technology applications in quality assurance and quality improvement, part II. *Journal on Quality Improvement, 19*(10), 465–478.

Campbell, A. B. (1994). Benchmarking: A performance intervention tool. *Journal on Quality Improvement, 20*(5), 225–228.

Corum, W. (1994). JCAHO standards and systems integration: Five years and counting down. *Healthcare Informatics, 1,* 22–28.

Fagan, L. M., & Perreault, L. E. (1990). The future of computer applications in health care. In E. Shortliffe & L. Perreault (Eds.), *Medical informatics: Computer applications in health care.* Reading, MA: Addison-Wesley.

Fonteyn, M., & Grobe, S. J. (1994). Expert system development in nursing: Implications for critical care nursing practice. *Heart & Lung, 23*(5), 80–87.

Institute of Medicine, Committee on Improving Patient Record. (1991). *The computer-based patient record.* Washington, DC: National Academy Press.

Joint Commission on Accreditation of Healthcare Organizations. (1993). *Accreditation manual for hospitals.* Oakbrook Terrace, IL: Author.

Martin, K. S., & Schect, N. J. (1992). *The Omaha system.* Philadelphia: W. B. Saunders.

McCloskey, J., & Bulechek, G. (1992). *Nursing interventions classification (NIC).* St. Louis, MO: Mosby.

Ozbolt, J. (1992). Strategies for building nursing databases for effectiveness research. In *Patient outcomes research: Examining the effectiveness of nursing practice.* Proceedings of a conference sponsored by the National Center for Nursing Research, pp. 210–218. Washington, DC: U.S. Department of Health and Human Services.

Tufte, E. (1983). *The visual display of quantitative information.* Cheshire, CT: Graphics Press.

Werley, H., & Lang, N. (1988). *Identification of the nursing minimum data set.* New York: Springer.

Werley, J., Ryan, P., & Coenen, A. (1994, June). *Brief synopsis of the nursing minimum data set (NMDS).* Milwaukee, WI: University of Wisconsin-Milwaukee School of Nursing.

ADDITIONAL READING

Ball, M. J., Hannah, K. J., Gerdin-Jelger, U., & Peterson, H. (Eds). (1989). *Nursing informatics: Where caring and technology meet.* New York: Springer-Verlag.

Darcy, L., & Boston, L. (1983). *Webster's new dictionary of computer terms.* New York: New World Dictionaries/Prentice Hall.

Harris, C., & Conner, C. (1994). Building a computer-supported quality improvement system in one year: The experience of a large state psychiatric hospital. *Journal on Quality Improvement, 20*(6), 330–342.

Kibbe, D. C. (1993). Computer software for health care CQI. *Quality Management in Health Care, 1*(4), 50–58.

Krol, E. (1992). *The whole internet: Users guide and catalog.* Sebastopol, CA: O'Reilly and Associates.

Shortliffe, E., & Perreault, L. (1990). *Medical informatics: Computer applications in health care.* Reading, MA: Addison-Wesley.

Ventura, M. R., Ackerman, M. H., Gugerty, B., Skomra, R., & Crosby, F. E. (1992). Selecting and using computer application software for Quality Assessment and Improvement. *Journal of Nursing Care Quality, 7*(1), 16–28.

Werley, H. H., Devine, E. C., Zorn, C. R., Ryan, P., & Westra, B. L. (1991). The nursing minimum data set: Abstraction tool for standardized, comparable, essential data. *American Journal of Public Health, 81*(4), 421–426.

Zielstorff, R., Hudgings, C., Grobe, S., & the National Commission on Nursing Implementation Project Taskforce on Nursing Information Systems. (1993). *Next generation nursing information systems: Essential characteristics for professional practice.* Washington, DC: American Nurses Association.

PART VI

RELATED PROCESSES

Betty R. Ferrell
Connie Leek

CHAPTER *26*

Linking Nursing Research and Quality Management

INTRODUCTION

This chapter provides an overview of the relationship of research and **Quality Management (QM)**. Understanding the current opportunities to merge QM and research activities begins with understanding the historical perspective of the research process and the **Quality-Assurance (QA)** process. Evaluation of the historical basis of QA reveals that it has emerged from the research tradition of nursing. The advances in nursing research and the evolution of QM have occurred simultaneously and now serve as complementary aspects of professional nursing practice (Frost, 1992; Masters & Schmele, 1991). This chapter also describes the significance of linking research and QM.

Both nursing researchers and other nursing professionals involved with QM can benefit from the marriage of the two forces. Research can serve as an important source of empowerment for nurses to make change. Quality Management links important patient outcomes as research variables. This chapter also illustrates the process of incorporating research within QM, using the clinical problem of pain management as a model example of applying the process of research to **Total Quality Management (TQM)**. This process is applied to clinical practice in a case study at the end of the chapter.

HISTORICAL BASIS OF QUALITY MANAGEMENT IN NURSING

The concept of combining QM and nursing research began with Florence Nightingale. Her professional commitment to **quality** led to the dramatic improvements seen in the Scutari hospitals during the Crimean War in the late 1800s. Conditions did not meet quality **standards**; disease was rampant and many soldiers were dying. Armed with foresight, influence with powerful friends, and the ability to organize and coordinate patient care, Nightingale and her nurses changed the conditions in the hospital wards at Scutari. Her carefully documented statistics became a powerful weapon, which she used in conjunction with persuasion and good management techniques. The results of her efforts became evident as the death rate plunged from 60 percent to 1 percent by the end of the war (Kelly, 1985). Throughout her life, Nightingale worked to improve the quality of nursing care provided to patients, much of which she accomplished through nursing education and research (Dolan, Fitzpatrick, & Hermann, 1983).

Although quality of care was emerging as a primary objective of the nursing and medical professions, little work had been done to explore the concept of quality. In the 1960s, Donabedian first wrote about his work with "quality of care" within the context of health care (Donabedian, 1980). Donabedian defined the quality of medical care as "the management that is expected to achieve the best balance of health benefits and risks. It is the responsibility of the practitioner to recommend and carry out such care" (Donabedian, 1980, p. 13). Most patient care has both risks and benefits. The aim of professional nursing is to enhance the quality of care given through careful **evaluation** and research. The quality-assessment process is one method by which the quality of **outcomes** is validated. This process is enhanced by use of research methods.

Quality was a major underpinning of the first constitution of the American Nurses Association (ANA). This focus on quality was reflected by the promotion of standards as goals of the first ANA constitution in 1897 (Schmidt, 1982). The nursing-education and nursing-practice standards developed by the ANA are further examples of activities designed to improve the quality of patient care (Schmidt, 1982).

In 1980, through the ANA Nursing Social Policy Statement, a social contract between nursing and society was recognized. Nursing, as a profession, was expected to "act responsibly, always mindful of the public trust. Self regulation to assure quality in performance is at the heart of this relationship" (ANA, 1980, p. 7). Such outcomes can only be evaluated through use of the research process. The nursing profession established authority over functions vital to itself; autonomy in conducting its own affairs was emphasized. The purpose of these regulations was to ensure quality in performance; Quality is implied throughout the Social Policy Statement. Nursing professionals are expected and obligated to provide quality care through this societal contract.

In 1980 the Joint Commission on the Accreditation of Hospitals (JCAH) formulated standards that addressed the organization of the nursing department to meet the nursing care needs of the patients and to maintain established standards of nursing practice (Patterson & Parsek, 1991). This quality care was to be achieved through the utilization of nursing standards. A *standard* is defined as "a quality or measure serving as basis or example or principle to which others should conform or by which others are judged; required or specified level of excellence" (Allen, 1984). Standards are only of benefit if they are evaluated through research. Standards of practice, then, are the measurements by which the quality of nursing practice can be judged (Dean-Barr, 1993). The research process provides consistent evaluation of outcomes. Standards reflect changes in **structure**, outcomes of care, and continuous improvement. (Joint Commission, 1994). (See Chapter 17 for a detailed discussion of current Joint Commission **accreditation** requirements.)

Nursing outcomes and quality are most effectively evaluated through nursing research. The steps of the **monitoring** and evaluation process encompass so much of the research process it would be a tremendous misuse of resources not to capitalize on the data and analysis gained from **Continuous-Quality-Improvement (CQI)** efforts (Cassidy & Friesen, 1990; Ferrell, 1993; Goode & Bulechek, 1992). Maintaining standards through the use of nursing research allows the testing and refinement of standards. Additionally, clinical evaluation of standards provides an opportunity for nursing staff to be included in the development and refinement of standards to which they will be held accountable (Western, 1994). Not only will nurses learn to apply the nursing process in ways other than patient care planning, they will also learn to utilize the process of nursing research and research utilization to implement the findings.

The evolution of nursing science, and of nursing as a profession, contributes to the opportunities for QM. Nursing as a profession is committed to quality care. Most health-care agencies choose to comply with Joint Commission requirements, and, therefore, quality assessment or CQI is an inherent part of professional practice. Nurses spend twenty-four hours a day with patients and families and are, thus, in an ideal position to identify both those interventions or systems that are working and those that could be improved or made more efficient. By linking the quality-assessment process with nursing research, the standards of nursing and health care can be accomplished at a higher level (Goode & Bulechek, 1992; Joiner, 1994). The QM process is incomplete without the critical component of research.

NURSING RESEARCH

The evolution of research in nursing has been documented in numerous texts. These texts generally emphasize the development of professional nursing since the 1950s and the development of nursing research. Burns and Grove (1992) report that research became a high priority during the 1950s and 1960s because of the development of several nursing-research journals and professional-association activities, such as the ANA Committee on Research and Studies (1956). In the early 1970s the ANA Commission on Nursing Research and the ANA Council of Nurse Researchers were formed. At the same time several notable research-utilization projects were inaugurated. Establishment of the National Center for Nursing Research (NCNR) in 1985 is also seen as a critical event in the development of nursing science. The NCNR was promoted to institute status in 1993 and now is recognized as the National Institute of Nursing Research (NINR).

The Research Process

There are several components to the research process. The process begins with identifying the problem area of research. A *problem statement* establishes what the researcher wants to know. It is a broad statement, but it serves to clarify the area to be addressed. An example of a problem statement might be, "What is the impact of case management on an orthopedic unit?"

The next step of the research process is to determine the *purpose* of the study. The purpose reveals why the investigator is interested in the research. An example of a purpose statement flowing from the previously mentioned problem area would be, "The purpose of this study is to explore select patient and institutional outcomes of case management as an aspect of the TQM process at Memorial Hospital."

The third step of the research process is establishing the *significance* of the study. The significance statement is also called the "so what?" statement; it establishes the importance of the particular area of research. A significance statement can be thought of as an attempt to sell the importance of the research to others. It is helpful to write a significance statement to define both the importance of attempting the research and the benefits that will be gained. An example of a significance statement would be:

> Orthopedic care is expected to become a predominant area of health care in the 1990s. Orthopedic patients are consuming a greater share of hospital and health-care resources because of increased technology in treatment. Case management has been documented as a helpful nursing process in other areas. This study will apply the case management process to the area of orthopedics and attempt to improve care of cancer patients as well as maximize the resources of the health-care system.

A *review of literature* is the next step in the research process. Literature review is useful in establishing what is already known in a particular area and helps refine what research needs to be done. Awareness of existing knowledge through other research is important so as to avoid reinventing the wheel. With the increase in nursing literature and, particularly, the increase in nursing research published over previous decades, there is an abundance of easily retrievable information that can be useful in the QM process. A careful review of literature also helps identify what methods or research instruments have previously been used. Furthermore, it often is possible to replicate the work of others.

Research is guided by careful selection of a *theoretical* or *conceptual framework for study*. The theoretical framework helps to refine the focus of the study, is useful in helping to select variables of interest, and provides a theoretical foundation for the inquiry. Many resources exist to guide the selection of a framework for study (Burns & Grove, 1992).

The next step in the research process is to determine the *study questions* or *hypothesis* that will be addressed in the research. Study questions are simply exploratory questions that do not predict an outcome. If the researchers can predict an outcome of the study, a hypothesis may be used. For example, simple study questions for the case-management research would be, "What is the impact of case management on overall patient satisfaction in orthopedics?" and "What is the length of stay of patients with a specific cancer diagnosis who receive case management?" If the investigators are predicting an outcome, hypothesis could be used in lieu of study questions. Hypotheses for the case-management research might be:

1. Patients receiving case management will have significantly shorter hospital stays compared to those patients who do not receive case management.

2. Patients receiving case management will have significantly higher satisfaction than those receiving traditional care.

Study questions or hypothesis are a very important part of the research process. They serve to determine what a particular study will address and help the researchers to prioritize those outcomes that are most important.

To further refine the research proposal, researchers select *independent* and *dependent variables*. Independent variables are those that the investigator manipulates or selects for study. In the case management example, the researchers may compare case management to traditional care, or case management to primary care. Investigators select how many groups will be compared. For example, two different forms of case management might be compared to a traditional care system, thus yielding three select groups or independent variables for comparison.

Dependent variables are identified to determine outcomes of interest. Dependent variables are those items or issues that are deemed important from the perspectives of the researcher and the manager. It is important to isolate select variables rather than attempt a "shotgun" approach to measure many, less-refined variables of interest. For example, in the evaluation of case management, one could select from several dependent variables including patient satisfaction, length of stay, staff satisfaction, physical complications, and patient anxiety, among others. Patient outcomes are often matched with institutional outcomes such as cost of care or staff evaluation.

It is also helpful in the research process to identify both *assumptions* and *limitations*. Assumptions are those facts accepted as true before initiating the study. For example, it might be assumed that decreased length of stay is a positive outcome and that patient satisfaction is an important **indicator** of effectiveness. Isolating assumptions often leads to recognition that things assumed to be true in a given situation are, in fact, not true. For example, it might be assumed that all staff on a particular unit have been trained in case management; and, yet, on closer examination it may become evident that case management has not even been fully implemented and, consequently, is not being conducted consistently. It is helpful, therefore, to pause to determine what assumptions are being held and whether those assumptions are, in fact, valid.

It is also helpful to recognize in advance the limitations of a particular study. A major area of limitation is the study's generalizability. Findings of a study are generalizable only to similar patients in similar situations. Thus, if the study on case management is to be conducted only on the orthopedic unit, the findings will be generalizable to similar patients on that unit; one cannot generalize findings from a postpartum unit to make decisions about the effectiveness of case management in an orthopedic unit. Recognizing the limitations of the study often leads to reevaluation of the design. There are many components of the research design that are critical to the quality of the research outcome.

Next, researchers select the *population* or group to whom they want findings to be generalizable and, therefore, the group that they will sample from. The *sample* then is derived from subjects within that group. Random selection of subjects is ideal, although not always practical, to enhance generalizability of the study. For example, if selection is limited to those patients who are extremely verbal and liked by the staff, outcomes might be quite different than if patients are chosen who receive case management but who are confused or for some other reason present management problems.

Another great challenge in the research process is to select those *instruments* or *measurements* that will be used to measure the dependent variables or outcomes of interest. In the case management example, it is important to take a global perspective in the selection of outcome measures. For example, it is wise to involve administrators, finance personnel, patient advocates, risk-management, utilization-review, and other departmental staff in determining the instruments or measurements to be employed. Because the TQM process is a global institutional effort, it is enriching for the study to include the perspective of others within the institution. It is desirable that selection of instruments includes strong consideration of the reliability and validity of the instrument, as well as the study procedures. Complete discussion of these issues is found in most standard research texts (Burns & Grove, 1992; Grant, Fleming, & Calvanico, 1990). The area of selecting research instruments also points toward the need for strong collaboration between researchers and managers. The findings of the study will only be useful to administrators or managers if the data are collected using strong research methods with reliable and valid tools.

A final note regarding the research process relates to use of the *pilot study*. Conducting a pilot study on a small sample, usually five to ten subjects, is invaluable in testing out the research methods. Conducting a pilot facilitates refinement of the procedures to be used, which enhances the final data obtained.

Another issue in QM research is related to involvement of staff. Involving nursing staff in QM research, such as using staff to conduct chart audits, participate in patient interviews, or perform other data collection, allows the staff to discover problems, as well as formulate solutions. Staff involvement in QM research can become a very positive process of discovery wherein staff learn and participate in the quality-improvement process.

LINKING NURSING RESEARCH AND QUALITY MANAGEMENT

Use of QM in conjunction with nursing research can be viewed as a source of empowerment for nurses in the process of making change. Rather than feeling like victims of the system, nurses, as professionals, can arm themselves with the power of data to improve the quality of care for patients. By using quality-assessment data to evaluate the impact of nursing care, areas of interest or deficiencies can be identified. With data as support, more credence is given to areas of concern relating to patient care. Table 26-1 identifies the link between nursing research and key terminology of QM.

The technological age presents a challenge and opportunity to combine nursing research and QM. The increased use of technology in health care is complex and expensive. Equipment is costly, training is expensive, and clinical errors occur despite efforts to avoid such problems. The direct cost of technology and the associated clinical errors contribute to the increasing cost of health care across all settings including the home, ambulatory clinics, and inpatient facilities (Ernst, 1994).

Table 26-1 • APPLICATION OF QUALITY-MANAGEMENT TERMINOLOGY TO NURSING RESEARCH

Quality-Management Terminology	Application To Research
QUALITY MANAGEMENT An umbrella term related to all systematic approaches to the assessment and improvement of quality.	The research process provides structure for systematic evaluation of outcomes.
QUALITY ASSURANCE The classic or traditional programs that organizations have used to assess, monitor, and improve quality.	Research methods provide a framework for identifying variables for assessment, reliable and valid monitoring measures, and outcomes on which to judge quality.
TOTAL QUALITY MANAGEMENT A leadership paradigm that subscribes to quality as a driving value for the organization. This value is operationalized by top-down total employee commitment and participation in consumer-focused continuous quality improvement of all work processes throughout the organization.	Nurse executives foster research throughout the organization as a means to quantify outcomes. Research is applicable across all nursing roles. Patient satisfaction is an outcome variable of interest.
CONTINUOUS QUALITY IMPROVEMENT A collaborative team process, usually interdisciplinary and statistically based, used to systematically respond to discrete opportunities for improvement.	Interdisciplinary research activities address the multidimensional needs of patients. Research results identify opportunities for continuous quality improvement.
STANDARD A broad statement of quality for a given element of care.	Standards determine variables of interest for research. Evaluation is based on standards of care.
CRITERIA A measurable statement addressing the intent of the standard.	Criteria facilitate selection of specific dependent variables for research.

While much attention is focused on the costs of providing care, much less attention is given to the costs of *failing* to provide care. Grant and Ferrell recently examined a hospital admission database for patients admitted over a period of twelve months. These records (N = 5,772) included 255 unscheduled admissions with a diagnosis of "uncontrolled pain," which represented the second most common reason for hospital admission. These unscheduled admissions were very costly to the individual facility as well as to the entire health-care system (Ferrell, 1993; Grant &

Ferrell, 1992). The cost of uncontrolled-pain admissions exceeded $5 million for one year alone for this institution. The data for this research project was collected through the quality-assessment process in conjunction with nursing research. When quality assessment data is linked with financial outcomes in this manner, it captures the attention of both staff and administration.

Quality-assessment reports can identify patterns that may impact the care provided to patients. New programs can be developed to correct deficiencies or enhance care in the areas of concern. Living rooms have become both hospital rooms and intensive-care units, as patients are either not hospitalized or are discharged after brief inpatient admissions. Increased use of techniques such as chronic spinal administration of opioids must be evaluated not only from the perspective of medical outcomes (for example, efficacy) but must also be evaluated from a nursing-research perspective. Research that includes outcomes such as patient anxiety, pain relief, burden, and the occurrence of infections, provides a more complete assessment of quality (Whedon & Ferrell, 1991).

The quality-assessment process can be compared to the nursing process, with which nurses are intimately familiar. Collection and analysis of data can be compared to the assessment phase of the nursing process. Nurses are so skilled at data collection that they often do not realize they are performing a unique research function. After conducting a thorough assessment of the situation, which may be either a problem or an area of interest that has the potential for improvement, a plan is established in conjunction with the patient or appropriate persons or systems involved. The quality-assessment plan or nursing-treatment plan is then implemented and evaluated to determine the impact of the change. Adjustments or revisions can be made, if necessary, and the process begins again.

In this context the nursing process takes the form of a process of continuous improvement. Nurses can use this familiar process to address any area of patient care. By using this process, positive nursing interventions can be implemented and evaluated. Not only can quality be improved, but dollars can be saved as well.

Utilizing quality assessment and the research process also serves to strengthen and ground professional nursing practice. The issue or problem area can be viewed in a professional manner, analysis can occur, a solution can be proposed, and implementation can take place based on advance planning. Evaluation is always included in the process.

Nursing as a profession can also benefit from the linking of QM and nursing research. The research process enables nurses to remain focused on areas of interest and importance to nursing. While many professions are involved in the process of CQI, nursing is the only profession focused on nursing-care outcomes. Thus, many patient-focused outcomes of care, such as symptom management or psychological responses to illness, may be neglected if not included in nursing research.

Linkage to the CQI efforts of other professions and disciplines is also important. Other health-care professionals may have unique perspectives of the patient or the system. The collaborative efforts of involved professionals frequently result in outcomes greater than those produced by any one particular discipline. Quality is improved through collaboration of various disciplines in assessing patient outcomes often in the form of research.

Nurses spend more time with patients across all settings — acute care, home care, clinics, and physician offices — than do any other health-care providers. Nurses are the first to evaluate changes resulting in the dramatic reforms in patient care. Nurses also evaluate system changes that may improve patient outcomes. Although nurses often see themselves as powerless to initiate change, this perception is far from true. By developing a well-grounded QM program, data can be collected, organized, and evaluated to affect patient outcomes. The process is very similar to the nursing process of assessment, planning, intervention, and evaluation. Nurses use the nursing process on a daily basis and are very familiar with the efficacy of this approach. This nursing process provides a strong power base upon which to make change.

The current emphasis on research utilization challenges nurses to incorporate research findings into practice (Goode & Bulecheck, 1992). Through the research process, data are collected, analyzed, and evaluated, and an impact is made on patient outcomes. Interventions are developed or devised to improve on the quality of care rendered to patients. Research is not an activity reserved only for doctorally prepared nurse scientists. Rather, research must be viewed as an integral activity and role component for all nurses whether they be staff nurses, advanced clinical specialists, managers, or administrators. Table 26-2 summarizes research activities across several nursing roles. The table emphasizes the distinct roles of nursing professionals in achieving quality patient care. The goals of TQM are best achieved through active participation in research by all nurses. Nurses acting in their unique roles, as well as collectively — as a profession — contribute to TQM.

Table 26-2 • JOB DESCRIPTION STATEMENTS FOR INCORPORATING RESEARCH INTO NURSING ROLES	
Clinical Nurse I	Demonstrates an awareness of the relevance of research in nursing.
	Assists in identifying problem areas in nursing.
	Facilitates research of others by cooperating with requests to complete instruments, collect data, or participate in studies.
Clinical Nurse II	Demonstrates competency in critiquing research for applicability to nursing practice.
	Shares research findings with staff.
	Assists in organizing a research interest group.
	Identifies practice issues for research.
	Facilitates research of others by assisting in the development of protocols for collecting data.
Clinical Nurse III	Identifies practice and nursing issues needing research and participates in the implementation of these studies.
	Facilitates the use of research findings by leading discussions at a research interest group or journal club.
	Promotes other's research by collaborating in the conduct of research and facilitation of data collection.

Table 26-2 • JOB DESCRIPTION STATEMENTS FOR INCORPORATING RESEARCH INTO NURSING ROLES *(continued)*

Clinical Instructor/ Educators	Actively participates in nursing research through collaboration. Assists others in applying research in nursing practice.
Clinical Specialist/ Nurse Practitioner	Facilitates the design and implementation of clinical research. Fosters collaborative health and nursing research. Facilitates collaboration between nursing staff and others involved in research. Uses research to monitor the quality of nursing practice and to make or recommend changes in practice. Initiates research interest groups.
Nurse Manager	Supports research activities of others by facilitating data collection. Promotes the use of research in evaluating and monitoring the quality of care provided. Evaluates trends and implements practice changes based on research findings.
Nurse Researcher	Fosters improvement in patient care by helping nurses develop systematic ways of studying and resolving problems. Assists in the acquisition of a database for administrative decisions and development of policies and procedures. Promotes research utilization for validating and importing clinical practice by assisting nurses in determining the applicability of findings to practice. Assists in developing techniques and tools for program evaluation. Facilitates research access to the clinical setting. Assists in disseminating study findings through presentations and publications.
Nurse Executive/ Vice President for Nursing	Creates an environment supportive of nursing research. Promotes a philosophy and standard of care that values research-based practice. Participates in Quality-Management research.

Adapted from L. Burnes-Bolton, Resources for Research. In M. A. Mateo & K. T. Kirchoff (Eds.) Conducting and Using Nursing Research in the Clinical Setting. Baltimore: Williams and Wilkins. Copyright, 1990.

APPLICATION TO PRACTICE

Quality assessment is the systematic evaluation of nursing care. Data generated from this type of evaluation determines changes that are necessary to improve nursing practice. Quality-improvement programs have developed within nursing organizations as a structure for evaluating the standards that have been established by regulatory or certifying bodies such as the Joint Commission.

Quality Management is coming of age in many ways. This is most likely because of the emphasis on cost effectiveness and the most appropriate use of resources in health care. This emphasis has also been fueled by **consumer** expectations of quality care and by professional organizations such as the ANA and the Oncology Nursing Society (Spross, McGuire, & Schmitt, 1991).

Pain Management as a Focus of Practice Improvement

Nursing is also concerned with patient advocacy. At present, there exists the opportunity for nursing to influence consumers of health care in a very positive and pragmatic manner. The concept of patient advocacy will become increasingly important in the future. Nursing organizations that excel in pain management, for example, are likely to make that service known to the public. Imagine a hospital that is so successful in relieving pain that this becomes a major component in its competition for surgical patients.

Pain, as the most frequently occurring symptom, is often targeted by accreditation and institutional review as an outcome for adults. For example, when the Joint Commission evaluates documentation of patient outcomes, complaints of pain and documentation of the measures taken by nurses to relieve that pain are often scrutinized. Effective pain relief is closely related to both patients' and families' overall satisfaction with care. Nurse administrators are increasingly concerned with patient satisfaction. As the health-care market becomes more competitive, consumer satisfaction is highly valued. Consumers are interested in health-care settings that provide comfort and expertise in management of pain (Ferrell, 1994; Ferrell, Wisdom, Rhiner, & Alletto, 1991).

A major limitation in previous years has been the lack of **accountability** for effective pain relief. Understanding the concept of pain and its treatment has now advanced to the point that professional organizations have begun to establish standards of care related to pain. The American Pain Society (APS) has provided leadership in developing guidelines for pain treatment. Several nursing specialty groups have included comfort or pain relief within their standards of practice. The Oncology Nursing Society recently completed a position paper on pain, which establishes standards of practice.

An additional standard from which to initiate quality improvement and research related to pain is the Agency for Health Care Policy and Research (AHCPR) Acute Pain Guideline (U.S. Department of Health and Human Services [US DHHS], 1992). In December, 1989, the AHCPR was established under Public Law 101-239 to enhance the quality, appropriateness, and effectiveness of health-care services and access to these services. These goals are accomplished through conducting and supporting research, developing clinical guidelines, and disseminating research findings and guidelines to persons involved in health care (US DHHS, 1992). The **interdisciplinary** approach to the development of the guidelines is a good example of the collaboration and communication that can occur with the combination of CQI and research. The AHCPR guidelines provide another example of utilizing research findings and the quality-assessment approach to define health policy.

The goals of the Acute Pain Guideline are to

> (1) reduce the incidence and severity of patients' acute postoperative or post traumatic pain; (2) educate patients about the need to communicate unrelieved pain so they can receive prompt evaluation and effective treatment; (3) enhance patient comfort and satisfaction; and (4) contribute to fewer postoperative complications, and in some cases, shorter stays after surgical procedures. (US DHHS, 1992, p. 1)

The three requirements identified in the pain guidelines are:

1. Pain intensity and relief must be assessed and reassessed at appropriate intervals.

2. Patient preferences must be respected when determining methods to be used for pain management.

3. Each institution must develop an organized program to evaluate the effectiveness of pain assessment and management.

Without such a program, staff efforts to treat pain may become sporadic and ineffectual. The third requirement listed, entitled "Requirements to Ensure Effective Management of Postoperative Pain," mandates that each institution develop a program to evaluate the effectiveness of pain assessment and management. The guideline emphasizes that a formal institutional process must be developed to ensure that different members of the health-care team cooperate to achieve optimal application of a variety of pain-control strategies.

The guideline builds on the recommendations made by the APS Committee on Quality Assurance Standards and states that "the institutional process of acute pain management begins with an affirmation that patients should have access to the best level of pain relief that may safely be provided" (US DHHS, 1992, p. 71). This affirmation requires more than just a simple philosophical statement on the part of an institution. The institution should develop an organized plan to evaluate the quality and effectiveness of acute-pain management.

The guideline acknowledges that the quality of pain control will be influenced by the type of pain-management program available, as well as by the level of training, experience, and expertise of the staff providing the care. Pain-management programs should be designed to meet the needs of a particular institution. In *every* institution, however, responsibility for pain management should be assigned to those professionals "most knowledgeable, experienced, interested, and available to deal with patients' needs in a timely fashion" (US DHHS, 1992, p. 71). One of the basic philosophical statements underlying the QA section of the guideline is that "only if institutions recognize the importance of effective pain control and assign responsibility to interested groups or individuals can the quality of care in this area [i.e., pain management] be at its best" (US DHHS, 1992, p. 72).

Professional guidelines such as the above become valuable only when put into practice through QM efforts and evaluated through research. An organized quality assessment and evaluation plan will both enable clinicians to systematically change practice and provide administrators with logical outcome measures to judge the efficacy of the changes in care.

CASE STUDY: *One Hospital's Approach to Pain Management*

One health-care facility determined, through the utilization of quality assessment and nursing research, that pain management was indeed a problem within the facility. The problem was prevalent throughout the medical and nursing departments and created a financial strain because of unscheduled patient readmissions for uncontrolled pain. An educational program was developed primarily for nurses, but for other disciplines as well. This educational program prepared staff nurses to assume the role of Pain Resource Nurses (PRNs) and to impact the quality of pain management on every unit in the institution (Ferrell, Grant, Ritchey, Ropchan, & Rivera, 1993). The forty-hour program covered all aspects of pain management, including pain assessment, pharmacologic and nondrug interventions, and use of the CQI process to improve the quality of pain relief.

When the nurses and pharmacists were educated, they began to educate the other nurses on their units, as well as the patients and physicians. This change process was a very slow and tedious one. In this particular institution, **multidisciplinary** educational meetings and seminars were planned for the continuing education of all disciplines. Most meetings were well attended. A multidisciplinary pain committee was developed. Representatives from all disciplines requested to become part of this committee. The committee met on a regular basis and accomplished several major goals to meet the stated objectives of improved pain management.

On the unit level, a multidisciplinary QA team was formed to meet the challenge of improved pain management for pediatric patients. Specific tasks were delegated to individuals, and results were reviewed at the regularly scheduled meetings. Documentation records were revised to include an objective assessment of pain on admission, as well as on the regular shift assessment form. Standards of care were revised to include more specific information about pain. Educational sessions were planned for the nursing staff, as were poster displays. The quality-assessment plan for the unit was revised to include pain management as an indicator. Chart audits were conducted by the nursing staff. Although the educational process is continuing, these efforts of the QA team have resulted in improved pain management for the pediatric patients. The problem of pain has been identified as an area for improved quality that involves medicine, nursing, pharmacy, and other related services. Table 26-3 summarizes an initial list of activities within the QA plan for enhancing pain management for children at the City of Hope Medical Center. Activities performed by the research person emphasize the inclusion of research within TQM.

Table 26-3 • **QUALITY-ASSURANCE PROGRAM FOR PEDIATRIC PAIN MANAGEMENT**

Goals	Target Date	Research Person
1. Improved assessment of pain by the staff and documentation of pain in the patient record.	4/15	Conduct staff knowledge-and-attitudes survey.
2. Review of current documentation procedures and assessment forms, and adopting necessary forms or alterations.	4/15	Conduct chart audit.
3. Education of the nursing staff regarding basics of pain assessment, drug management, and nondrug management of pain.	5/1	Repeat knowledge-and-attitudes survey.
4. Education of medical staff regarding the current knowledge of pain management in children.	5/15	Conduct physician knowledge-and-attitudes survey.
5. Development of structured protocols for drug management (for example, protocol for patient-controlled analgesia ([PCA]), continuous morphine infusions).	5/31	Use chart audit data to determine needs for protocols.
6. Education of patient and family, including written and verbal instruction.	6/1	Conduct parent knowledge-and-attitudes survey.
7. Establish means for continuity of pain management between inpatient, outpatient, and home care.	6/1	Chart audit of patients across settings.
8. Appropriate use of consultants (anesthesia, other medical consultants, physical therapy) as needed for pain.	5/15	Chart audit to determine use of consultants.
9. A forum (pain rounds, pain case conference) to discuss cases.	5/15	Compare case studies.
10. Integration of pain management into other areas in the medical center (care of adolescents on other units).	9/1	Chart audit on other units.
11. Appropriate use of adjuvant medications (neuroleptics, nonsteroidal anti-inflammatory drugs [NSAIDs], antidepressants).	6/1	Chart audit.
12. Assess and plan for improved management related to procedure pain.	6/1	Chart audit and parent interview.

CONCLUSION

This chapter addressed the relationship of nursing research and QM. A historical perspective of both nursing research and QM was presented, which specifically linked the two concepts. The utilization of quality-assessment data in conjunction with nursing research gives credibility and strength to the project being studied or reviewed. This process empowers nurses to make changes and achieve quality in patient outcomes and thereby enhance professional practice.

Several examples were provided to demonstrate combining the research process with QM. The application to practice was viewed from both a global and a unit-based perspective. Research also links QM with important health-policy considerations such as costs of care.

The overall focus was improved patient outcomes. These outcomes are based on objective data within a framework of quality. The benefits to society are obvious: more effective and efficient use of resources and a higher level of patient satisfaction. In the health-care climate of the 1990s, all health-care agencies must be as cost effective as possible. The combination of QM and nursing research can serve as a vehicle to help accomplish this arduous task. Research within clinical settings can be accomplished by nurses as well as other health-care professionals. Nurses can take pride in being in the forefront of this work, validating the effectiveness of nursing care, designing nursing interventions, and impacting patient outcomes.

REFERENCES

Allen, R. E. (Ed.). (1984). *The pocket Oxford dictionary of current English* (p. 733). Oxford, England: Clarendon Press.

American Nurses Association. (1980). *Nursing: A social policy statement.* Kansas City, MO: Author.

Burns, N., & Grove, S. K. (1992). *The practice of nursing research conduct, critique, & utilization* (2nd ed.). Philadelphia: W. B. Saunders.

Cassidy, D. A., & Friesen, M. (1990). QA: Applying JCAHO's generic model. *Nursing Management, 21*(6), 94–99.

Dean-Baar, S. L. (1993). Application of the new ANA framework for nursing practice standards and guidelines. *Journal of Nursing Care Quality, 8*(1), 33–42.

Dolan, J. A., Fitzpatrick, M. L., & Hermann, E. K. (1983). *Nursing in society: A historical perspective* (15th ed.). Philadelphia: W. B. Saunders.

Donabedian, A. (1980). *Explorations in quality assessment and monitoring: Vol. 1. The definition of quality and approaches to its assessment.* Ann Arbor, MI: Health Administration Press.

Ernst, D. F. (1994). Total Quality Management in the hospital setting. *Journal of Nursing Care Quality, 8*(1), 1–8.

Ferrell, B. R. (1993). Nursing and technology: The technology of pain. *Nursing Economics, 11*(1), 52–54.

Ferrell, B. R. (1994, April/May). An institutional commitment to pain management. *APS Bulletin,* 16–20.

Ferrell, B. R., Grant, M., Ritchey, K., Ropchan, R., & Rivera, L. M. (1993). The pain resource nurse training program: A unique approach to pain management. *Journal of Pain & Symptom Management, 8*(8), 549–556.

Ferrell, B. R., Wisdom, C., Rhiner, M., & Alletto, J. (1991). Pain management as a quality of care outcome. *Journal of Nursing Quality Assurance, 5*(2), 50–58.

Frost, M. H. (1992). Quality: A concept of importance to nursing. *Journal of Nursing Care Quality, 7*(1), 64–69.

Goode, C., & Bulechek, G. M. (1992). Research utilization: An organizational process that enhances quality of care. *Journal of Nursing Care Quality* (Special Report), 27–35.

Grant, M., & Ferrell, B. (1992). Is pain adequately controlled in patients with cancer? *Oncology Nursing Bulletin,* 9–11.

Grant, M., Fleming, I., & Calvanico, A. (1990). Research and Quality Assurance. In M. A. Mateo & K. T. Kirchoff (Eds.), *Conducting and using nursing research in the clinical setting* (pp. 8–21). Baltimore: Williams and Wilkins.

Joiner, G. A. (1994). Developing a proactive approach to medication error prevention. *Journal for Healthcare Quality 16*(2), 35–40.

Joint Commission on Accreditation for Healthcare Organizations (1994). *Accreditation Manual for Hospitals (AMH): Volume 1, Standards.* Oakbrook Terrace, IL: Author.

Kelly, L. Y. (1985). *Dimensions of professional nursing.* New York: Macmillan.

Masters, F., & Schmele, J. (1991). Total Quality Management: An idea whose time has come. *Journal of Nursing Quality Assurance, 5*(4), 7–16.

Patterson, C. H., & Parsek, J. D. (1991). Development of the nursing care standards. In Joint Commission on Accreditation of Healthcare Organizations, *An introduction to Joint Commission nursing care standards* (pp. 1–16). Oakbrook Terrace, IL: Author.

Schmidt, A. (1982). Quality Assurance. In Ann Marriner (Ed.). *Contemporary nursing management issues and practice* (pp. 348–366). St. Louis, MO: C.V. Mosby.

Spross, J. A., McGuire, D. B., & Schmitt, R. M. (1991). *Oncology nursing society position paper on cancer pain.* Pittsburgh, PA: Oncology Nursing Press.

U.S. Department of Health and Human Services. (1992). *Acute pain management: Operative or medical procedures and trauma clinical practice guidelines* (AHCPR Publication No. 92-0032). Rockville, MD: Author.

Western, P. (1994). QA/QI and nursing competence: A combined model. *Nursing management, 25*(3), 44–46.

Whedon, M., & Ferrell, B. R. (1991). Professional and ethical considerations in the use of high-tech pain management. *Oncology Nursing Forum, 18*(7), 1135–1143. (Also reprinted as a Professional Education Publication by the American Cancer Society, 1992.)˙

ADDITIONAL READING

Berwick, D. M. (1989). Health service research and the quality of care. *Medical Care, 27*(8), 763–771.

Bolton, L. B. (1991). Resources for research. In M. A. Mateo & K. T. Kirchhoff (Eds.), *Conducting and using nursing research in the clinical setting* (pp. 22–30). Baltimore: Williams and Witkins.

Brink, P. (1984). Are Quality Assurance studies really research? *Western Journal of Nursing Research, 6*(4), 365–366.

Crane, S. C., Hersh, A. S., & Shortell, S. M. (1992). Challenges for health services research in the 1990s. In S. M. Shortell & U. E. Reinhardt (Eds.), *Improving health policy and management* (pp. 369–384). Ann Arbor, MI: Health Administration Press.

Greenfield, S. (1993). A perspective on Quality Assurance research. In M. L. Goody, J. Bernstein, & S. Robinson (Eds.), *Putting research to work in quality improvement and Quality Assurance* (AHCPR Publication No. 93-0034, pp. 9–12). Washington, DC: U.S. Department of Health and Human Services.

Hegyvary, S. T. (1992). Outcomes research: Integrating nursing practice into the world view. In *Patient outcomes research: Examining the effectiveness of nursing practice* (NIH Publication No. 93-3411, pp. 17–24). Washington, DC: U.S. Department of Health and Human Services.

Kerfoot, K. M., & Watson, C. A. (1985). Research-based Quality Assurance: The key to excellence in nursing. In J. C. McClosky & H. K. Grace (Eds.), *Current issues in nursing* (2nd ed., pp. 538–547. Boston: Blackwell Scientific Publishing.

Lieske, A. M. (1992). Quality Management and research. In C. G. Meisenheimer (Ed.), *Improving quality* (pp. 183–196). Gaithersburg, MD: Aspen.

Nash, D. B., Carpenter, C. E., & Burnett, D. A. (1994). Clinical evaluation units: A research agenda. *Quality Management in Health Care, 2*(2), 27–37.

Patterson, C. H. (1988). Standards of patient care: The Joint Commission focus on nursing Quality Assurance. *Nursing Clinics of North America, 34*(3), 625–638.

Schmele, J. A. (1993). Research and total quality. In A. F. Al-Assaf & J. A. Schmele (Eds.), *The textbook of total quality in Healthcare* (pp. 239–257). Delray Beach, FL: St. Lucie Press.

U. S. Department of Health and Human Services (1993). *Putting research to work in quality improvement and Quality Assurance* (AHCPR Publication No. 93-0034). Washington, DC: Author.

A. F. Al-Assaf

CHAPTER **27**

Utilization Management and the Quality of Health Care

INTRODUCTION

Utilization management (UM) is a process of review and assessment of a patient medical record utilizing predetermined **criteria** based on expert opinion and/or care patterns. Originally referred to as utilization review (UR), this program has evolved into a broader scope, where principles of management and assessment are applied. The concept of UR was expanded to include management of the entire patient episode. Utilization management identifies the best possible medical-management procedures and protocols, combining the most efficient utilization of resources to render the best possible outcome for a given patient episode. Utilization management tends to provide optimum utilization of available health-care resources; it deters overutilization or underutilization of services of care, and at the same time, ensures **quality** of services based on designed criteria.

The purpose of this chapter is to introduce the processes of UM in health-care organizations. The objectives of UM, the methods, and the cost-containment implications are also discussed. The chapter concludes with a discussion of the relationship between UM and **Quality Management (QM)**.

OVERVIEW

The objectives of UM program are to *effectively* demonstrate the maintenance of high-quality patient care, to determine and ensure medical necessity of provided services, to practice and encourage cost-containment strategies to preserve resources, and to evaluate the effectiveness of these strategies. Utilization managers ensure guidelines are available to determine the appropriate allocation of resources. They also provide mechanisms for timely care planning and care delivery, as well as discharge planning. In addition, utilization managers may be involved in the evaluation and assessment of any variation between services rendered and services charged for, therefore, ensuring the preservation of resources.

The UM program should be designed to **evaluate** and ensure appropriate allocation of resources to deliver quality medical care in the most economical manner. Utilization management subscribes to the notion that more care is not necessarily better than less care, nor is less care necessarily better than more care. Utilization management ensures that patients receive the *appropriate* and *necessary* care needed for their medical conditions. A comprehensive UM program includes services at every stage of the patient encounter with the health-care field. A comprehensive UM program includes several distinct stages: preadmission review, concurrent review (during hospitalization or patient encounter with the provider), discharge planning, retrospective review, and follow-up evaluation. In certain cases UM may also involve case management and planning (to be discussed later). In each of these five stages, the issue under consideration at all times is whether there is an overutilization or underutilization of resources or whether there is efficient or inefficient use of provider services.

According to Roland and Roland (1991) four dimensions of utilization can be reviewed:

1. *What* care was provided and did it meet the patient's needs?

2. *When* was the service rendered? Was it appropriate? Was it rendered in a timely manner?

3. *How* much or how many services were rendered? Was the length of stay justified? Were ancillary services utilized optimally?

4. *Where* did the patient receive the care? Was a hospital stay necessary? Would outpatient surgery have been better?

These questions, and similar others, should be asked by the utilization manager. The answers to the questions should then be compared to predetermined criteria, based on national **standards** or **norms**. In other conditions where the prescribed medical service or procedure is new, judgment regarding appropriateness and necessity may be solicited from specific experts in the field, while the utilization manager acts as a liaison and coordinator to facilitate these services. It is desirable that the **customer** of the UM program be first the patient, secondly, the insurer, and thirdly, the provider. Patients' needs should never be compromised for cost, and the UM professional should evaluate and keep a balance between patients' needs and services provided. Utilization management focuses on the *efficiency* with which care is provided; thus its primary objective is decreasing cost while attempting to maintain the quality of care rendered to the patient. To do this, utilization managers take into consideration quality measures of **structure**, **process**, and **outcome**. Another element included in the UM plan is quality improvement. The objective to contain cost and *maintain* quality is not adequate; UM should identify ways to contain costs while *improving* quality. As much as possible, quality-improvement strategies should be incorporated into UM plans.

In summary, UM is based on cost-management and cost-containment strategies. The process is dynamic if applied comprehensively and objectively. The main objective of UM, which should also be the objective of the whole system, is to determine whether or not alternate methods of care are feasible and available. These methods of care, however, are expected to provide the same or better levels of quality, but at lower costs.

HISTORY OF UTILIZATION MANAGEMENT

It was not until 1960 that UR was included in the appraisal of medical care approved by the American Hospital Association (AHA) and the American Medical Association (AMA). The Joint Commission on Accreditation of Hospitals (JCAH) made reference to UR in its 1963 manual. In 1965, Title 18 and Title 19, better known as the legislation for the Medicare and Medicaid programs, were signed into law as part of the amendment of the Social Security Act of 1935. As part of efforts to ensure the provision of appropriate and necessary care, Medicare guidelines mandated a UR program for Medicare-participating organizations. This mandate was extended to the Medicaid program in 1967 (Kearns, 1984).

In another amendment of the Social Security Act, Professional Standards Review Organizations (PSROs) were established in 1972, as mandated by Public Law 92-603. The mandate of PSROs was to provide a peer review of the process of medical care rendered by providers to Medicare beneficiaries. The purpose was to ensure the most efficient delivery of care to Medicare beneficiaries. Professional Standards Review Organizations became heavily involved in the review of the practice of physician peers regarding Medicare recipients. This was an effort to adequately maintain the quality of care in the most economical manner (Kearns, 1984).

Utilization review received more attention in health care when the JCAH officially endorsed it in the standards for accrediting hospitals. In the *Accreditation Manual for Hospitals* (Supplement for 1976 and 1977), Standard II — Quality of Professional Services stated,

> The hospital shall demonstrate appropriate allocation of its
> resources through the conduct of an effective utilization review
> program. The results of the utilization review activity shall be
> contributory to the quality of patient care and shall be reflected
> in the other quality — protective functions of the hospital and
> the medical staff. (Joint Commission on Accreditation of
> Hospitals [JCAH], 1976, p. 28)

The UR standard evolved throughout the following years so that by 1989 UR was listed as a separate section of the manual. The UR standard stated, "The hospital provides for and demonstrates appropriate allocation of its resources through an effective utilization review program" (Joint Commission on Accreditation of Healthcare Organizations [Joint Commission], 1988, p. 281). The evolution continued in terms of the Joint Commission's emphasis on UR. Unlike previous manuals, the *Accreditation Manual for Hospitals* for 1994 lists UR program characteristics in a modified manner (Joint Commission, 1993). Although the content is somewhat similar, the method of scoring and, thereby, the emphasis on specifics, was changed. Utilization review standards are now spread over three main areas: leadership, information management, and planning.

COST CONTAINMENT AND UTILIZATION REVIEW

Over the past several years, the cost of health-care services has continued to increase. In an effort to control the rate of increase, both the AMA and the AHA joined with the Federation of American Hospitals to establish the Voluntary Cost Containment Program. The program objective was to efficiently distribute health-care services while maintaining high quality (Kearns, 1984).

According to Curtis and Al-Assaf (1990), *cost containment* became a buzz word in the late 1970s, especially when President Carter put major emphasis on this initiative. Health insurance companies took the lead in the movement and started to design and implement a variety of approaches in an effort to contain costs. These early approaches included a wide range of limitations on benefits, from limiting hospital stays and surgical schedules to limiting provider reimbursements and capping benefits. Reaction from different interest groups was rapid and prompted insurance companies to move to a phase of "benefit liberalization." Initially, major medical plans were added to existing basic hospitalization and surgical coverage. Subsequently, comprehensive medical plans replaced major medical plans.

In an attempt to further control the rising costs of health care, many indemnity plans and other comprehensive medical plans included a variety of approaches. These approaches included:

- exclusion of certain benefits considered to be medically unnecessary

- coordination-of-benefits provisions

- deductibles

- co-insurance

- benefit maximums specific to certain conditions, as well as to comprehensive care

- fraud control and establishment of both provider- and patient-claims investigation teams to audit questionable and outlier claims

- usual, customary, and reasonable fee profiles (UCR profiles)

These approaches were quickly put to the test and were incorporated in comprehensive medical plans. It soon became apparent that these approaches were effective at reducing benefits to beneficiaries, but they were not as effective at controlling health-care costs. Even with the addition of small deductibles and co-insurance, utilization of services, most often unnecessary services, still kept increasing. To control utilization of services and, ultimately, control costs, new measures therefore needed to be incorporated by insurers.

The first-generation cost-containment techniques were introduced in the early 1980s. The immediate approach used in first-generation cost containment was to increase the amounts paid by the insured for deductibles and co-insurance. In addition, this generation of cost containment added other features such as second surgical opinion, outpatient surgery, extended-care benefits, preadmission testing, and restrictions on weekend hospital admissions. These features did result in some stabilization of health-care claims; but rapid increases in utilization of hospital services continued as providers found alternate ways to maximize profits. The struggle for optimizing utilizations intensified as employers and insurers looked for ways to do so.

The overuse of resources lead to the development of second-generation cost containment — mainly hospital pre-certification and concurrent review programs. The intent of these programs was to encourage cost-effective utilization while providing disincentives for overutilization. These efforts to contain costs were encouraged by the JCAH. Emphasis on **accreditation** efforts relating to UR provided hospitals with specific criteria intended to discourage over- or underutilization of health-care services. Therefore, unlike the first-generation approaches of providing incentives for proper utilization, second-generation cost-containment measures relied on disincentives to discourage improper utilization.

During this same time period, the Federal government entered the field of cost containment by enacting the Prospective Payment System (PPS) in 1983, which also encompassed UR. The Prospective Payment System provided disincentives for lengthy hospitalization and shifted the burden for proper utilization of health-care services to hospitals. Peer Review Organizations (PROs) later replaced PSROs. Peer Review Organizations were charged with reviewing care rendered and ensuring effective utilization. But even with PPS and PROs, hospitals found ways to shift costs to the outpatient services, which at that time were not regulated. Again, through creative cost-shifting techniques and innovative resource-allocation approaches, the utilization of services was controlled in some patient-care areas but not in others. This discrepancy prompted insurers and employers to come up with the third-generation cost-containment measures, which emphasized negotiation with providers for fee reductions and utilization controls. Third-generation cost-containment measures ranged from negotiated fee schedules with hospitals, Health Maintenance Organizations (HMOs), Preferred Provider Organizations (PPOs), and Exclusive Provider Organizations (EPOs) to capitations and the use of **gatekeepers** (providers who regulate the use of services) (Curtis & Al-Assaf, 1990).

All of the previously mentioned approaches and measures were, and still are, attempts to effectively control utilization of health-care services. Utilization-review professionals are responsible for designing, implementing, and further evaluating those measures. Despite this, other approaches, such as managed competition, are being called for. President Clinton, in his efforts to reform health care in the United States, has emphasized the managed-competition approach. Managed competition is based on the concept that competition can produce excellence in quality, and if the utilization of services are managed effectively, both access to health care and cost containment may improve. At the time of this writing, the managed-competition approach is being tried in several locations, including Minnesota and California. Indications are that this approach might be the most effective so far in controlling utilization.

It must be noted that UM programs are used by both insurers and providers. This provides a check-and-balance type of system, where the ultimate winner is the patient. The UM programs sponsored by providers are mandated by a variety of accrediting agencies, in particular, the Joint Commission. The insurers' UM programs provide added checks on providers to ensure efficient resource utilization and maintenance of the quality of services.

STAGES OF A UTILIZATION-MANAGEMENT PROGRAM

As mentioned earlier, a comprehensive UM program in most health-care organizations includes five stages, or interventions, during the patient encounter with the health-care provider. A UM program should include preadmission, concurrent, and retrospective reviews, as well as discharge planning and follow-up. During each of these stages, the UM professional is charged with the review and identification of overutilization, underutilization, and inefficient use of provider services (Curtis & Al-Assaf, 1990).

Preadmission

Preadmission is the UR stage aimed at containing costs before hospitalization occurs. It requires that the insured person or the insured's provider discuss nonemergency admission requests with the insurer prior to admission. This process serves three main objectives. The first objective is to certify the medical necessity of the hospitalization. The insurer has the responsibility of suggesting alternate modes of care, such as outpatient or home care. Also, in a case where admission is deemed inappropriate or unnecessary, the insurer suggests an alternative. The second objective of the preadmission stage is to use national norms to establish predetermined length-of-stay criteria for the procedure or admission requested. This mechanism serves the insurer by determining overutilization, and at the same time serves the insured by preventing underutilization. The third objective of the preadmission stage is to identify potential need for individual case management early in the patient-management process. The preadmission progress helps to plan for the next UM phase — the admission and concurrent-review phase.

Admission and Concurrent Review

Concurrent review begins after admission of the patient to the hospital or during the receipt of health-care services. During this phase, the reviewer emphasizes deterence from improper utilization. Reviews of length of stay, appropriate procedures, and necessary care are all criteria for concurrent reviews. It is during this phase that requests for extended lengths of stay are handled and appropriate decisions are made. It must be noted that although one of the objectives of UR is ensuring quality of care, its main objective is cost containment.

Retrospective Review

Retrospective review is carried out after a patient is discharged or after services are rendered. Retrospective review attempts to identify whether the source of utilization problems is the hospital or the practitioner. During this phase, responsibilities of the UR professional include collecting and analyzing data to profile the resource-utilization patterns of physicians, hospitals, and patients. These profiles are helpful in determining local norms and identifying variations from the norms. Retrospective reviews are most effective when coupled with timely, provider-specific feedback. Retrospective reviews depend heavily on evaluation of patient care. Specifically, readmissions and adverse outcomes of care should be evaluated through a retrospective review to determine whether necessary services were rendered and whether inappropriate utilization was carried out. Other responsibilities of the retrospective reviewer are to identify unbundling of services (separating and billing for each ancillary service performed) and upcoding of DRGs (selecting the DRG with the highest reimbursement rate) and to evaluate the appropriateness of care.

Discharge Planning

Discharge planning is very important to ensure continuity of care beyond the acute-care received, thus maintaining the patient's health status. Discharge planning is, in essence, a team process wherein there is coordination of specific activities for each patient. This process of facilitating the discharge of the patient is another important aspect of UR. Discharge planning, according to the Joint Commission (1993), was developed to identify certain patients with conditions requiring discharge planning. Discharge-planning activities may include, but are not limited to, placement in long-term-care facilities, arrangement for referral to other needed health-care services, and coordination of transfer of care from an acute-care to a long-term setting. A UR professional maintains the responsibility of securing such activities for the sake of decreasing costs and improving patient health.

Follow-Up Care

The follow-up process is actually a continuum; it may start with a UR/UM professional, but it should be carried forward by other professionals such as patient representatives, administration, and marketing professionals.

Follow-up represents a process of continuous dialogue between the supplier (the provider) and the customer (patient). This process consists of review and continuous assessment of the patient's health status beyond the patient's contact with the provider. It ensures compliance with discharge planning, provides answers to questions regarding the continuity of care being received, and solicits the loyalty of the patient to the provider.

COMPONENTS OF UTILIZATION MANAGEMENT

While a distinct process in its own right, UM is also part of QM activities. Utilization-management professionals are included on several health-care facility committees, as prescribed by the Joint Commission; and the input of these professionals is important in facilitating committee tasks. In most major hospitals these committees include surgical case review, tissue review, blood utilization review, infection control, antibiotic utilization review, drug utilization review, pharmacy utilization, ancillary services utilization review, patient surveys review, profile analyses, and reimbursement agency utilization reports review. The extent of UM involvement in these activities varies among health-care organizations; but most organizations carry out these activities through UM. Following are brief explanations of each of these UM activities.

Surgical Case Review

Surgical case review is used to identify and provide solutions and feedback regarding surgical procedure problems, anesthesia time and practice, utilization of surgical suites, surgery schedules, problems in diagnosis (at admission and discharge), and deaths. Reviews are usually carried out monthly, and conclusions are provided to the facility's QM Committee for follow-up. Reviews of tissue use and handling are generally part of surgical case review. Procedure reviews and feedback are provided by the UM professional to ensure proper handling of tissues and associated activities by pathology services.

Blood Utilization Review

Blood utilization review is usually related to surgical case review. These reviews identify the over-use of whole blood versus the use of component blood elements; blood transfusions and any patient reactions following transfusions; amount of blood used or wasted; and whether blood was provided on an emergency or elective basis. Blood utilization reviews are usually carried out quarterly.

Infection Control

Infection control is another important activity requiring UM involvement. The UM professional is part of a team that identifies infections and carries out investigations of infection sources. This responsibility is important not only after an infection occurs, but also prior to an infection occurring. Infection-control teams facilitate an infection-free environment through establishment and maintenance of procedures and protocols such as initiating infection-control measures as promptly as possible. Infection-control reviews are usually carried out monthly.

Antibiotic Utilization Review

Antibiotic utilization review is usually carried out in conjunction with infection-control activities. These reviews identify proper and timely utilization of antibiotics both for prophylactic and infection-control use.

Drug Utilization Review

Drug utilization review includes quarterly reviews of therapeutic agent usage in terms of quality, frequency, availability, type, protocols, proper use, and repeated variations of recommended use. Utilization management professionals have the responsibility of identifying variations and providing usage patterns of therapeutic agents, especially frequently used agents. Drug-utilization categories may include special reviews for appropriate use of narcotics and heavy tranquilizers and will identify indicators of the necessity for using these drugs. This function is usually coordinated with pharmacy utilization review, in terms of patient-drug-use patterns as well as practitioner-prescription patterns. Frequent and heavy use of one or more drugs should be reviewed and justification for use provided. If justification is not provided, documentation of practice variations are provided to QM committees for follow-up.

Ancillary Services Utilization Review

Ancillary services utilization review is usually done as concurrent reviews to ensure proper utilization of services. For example, use of radiology or laboratory services is reviewed to determine whether or not STAT orders are overused or necessary. Utilization reviews of these services can be done retrospectively, thus identifying specific utilization patterns. Pattern variations from a specified norm are further isolated, and causes for such variations are identified by the UM professional for the purpose of developing a scheme for variation reduction. These reviews are usually carried out at least quarterly.

Patient Surveys Review

Patient surveys review is another important activity of UM. Patient surveys review has a major impact on care provided by the organization, as well as care provided by the practitioner. Patient surveys are important management tools that evaluate the outcome of care provided from the patient perspective. Therefore, care must be taken in the design, implementation, and analyses of these surveys. Information gathered from the surveys is often helpful in identifying challenges to the care process as well as opportunities for further improvement of this process. In some hospitals, UM professionals have the responsibility of surveying patients during the patients' encounters with health-care providers. In addition after discharge the UM professional may ask patients questions specific to the care received. In order to ensure collection of unbiased information, the methods of surveying, sample size, and patient characteristics are considered before patient surveys are conducted. Responder anonymity enhances the quality of feedback. Al-Assaf (1993) and Leebov and Ersoz (1992) discuss surveying techniques in more detail, and the reader is encouraged to pursue additional reading on this subject.

Profile Analyses

Profiles of practice and case patterns are usually designed and developed by UM professionals to compare with norms. Profile analyses may focus on physicians, patients, or hospitals. Physician profiles may consist of comparative analyses of staff physicians by specialty, by patient diagnosis in terms of admission frequencies, as well as in such areas as pharmacy utilization patterns, surgery, length of stay, and ancillary services. Patient profiles may include average length of stay by diagnostic related group (DRG), average cost by DRG, and type and frequency of procedures by DRG. Other qualifiers may include gender, age, or type of insurance. These profiles can be very helpful during process-improvement activities of both specific services and the organization as a whole. As variations in overutilization or improper utilization are identified, methods to reduce these variations can be developed and implemented.

Reimbursement Agency Utilization Reports Review and Other Roles of the Utilization Manager

Utilization managers may also be involved in reviewing reimbursement on an agency basis in order to identify patterns of error or denial, or to evaluate the comprehensiveness of reimbursement submission reports.

In addition to this activity, utilization managers may also be involved in budget reviews of specific departments or units in order to document allocation and utilization of monetary resources. The utilization manager's involvement in internal audit review should not be ignored, especially when the audit is in response to a specific UM report or data-gathering activity.

Finally, utilization managers often are involved in the credentialing process, continuing education, and training-improvement processes (Al-Assaf, 1992).

THE UTILIZATION-MANAGEMENT PLAN

A UM plan is an agreed-upon document that:

- establishes scope of care
- delineates program responsibilities
- sets forth objectives
- describes methods of implementation
- determines who evaluates and how effectiveness will be evaluated

As mentioned earlier, health-care organizations seeking accreditation must have a UR plan. For hospitals, the Joint Commission specifically asks for a detailed UR plan that describes both the method(s) for identifying problems related to utilization and whether the problems are results of inappropriateness, medical necessity, continued stays, or delays in or problems associated with the provision of supportive services. In the standards of the 1994 *Accreditation Manual for Hospitals,* the Joint Commission incorporated UR into several sections crucial to improvement of quality efforts relating to hospital care. Utilization review is included under a section on leadership: "The leaders allocate adequate resources for assessing and improving the organization's governance, managerial, clinical, and support processes..." (Joint Commission, 1993, p. 33). Utilization review is further emphasized in a section about information management, where the manual specifically refers to tasks at every stage of the patient encounter, including medical-record procedures (Joint Commission, 1993, p. 39). Utilization review is also referred to in the section entitled "Planning": "... processes measured encompass at least ... those related to determining the appropriateness of admissions and continued hospitalization (that is utilization review activities)" (Joint Commission, 1993, p. 55).

ADVANTAGES AND BENEFITS OF UTILIZATION MANAGEMENT

Roland and Roland (1991) list the following benefits of UM:

1. *Reducing costs* by reducing frequency of unnecessary procedures and length of hospital stays, as well as by reducing waste and putting an end to rework and duplication. All of these are potent cost-reduction measures.

2. *Improving the quality of care* through proper utilization of services, controlling of nosocomial (hospital-acquired) infections, and preventing iatrogenic (provider-induced) illness.

3. *Maintaining the quality of care* by preventing underutilization and promoting proper utilization of care services.

4. *Preserving access to care* by ensuring economical, physical, and availability access.

5. *Defining and articulating standards of care* by preventing potential malpractice and encouraging proper documentation and early identification of problems.

Depending on the rigor and type of UR method, as well as the training and performance of a reviewer, a UM program may elicit additional advantages. For example, *implicit reviews* (expert judgment, usually by a physician peer) enhance the reliability of the judgment rendered on a record. Also, implicit reviews may have the advantage of accessing professional judgment from a peer who is highly knowledgeable about the condition under review. The advantage of *explicit reviews* (objective reviews based on predetermined criteria and carried out by nonphysicians) is that judgments are objective and may not require additional assessment. It is merely a process of comparing the indicator under review to that of the norm and identifying the extent of and reason for variation or similarity. Also, when specificity and applicability of the review criteria are achieved, the review process becomes increasingly accurate and bias is reduced. Again, the effectiveness of the review with an experienced and adequately trained reviewer has a high level of objectivity with a small margin of error.

Biased reviewers and lack of objectivity are potential disadvantages of the UM process. In addition, if the criteria for review are not objective and effective, they may not be able to withstand criticism; in such cases the UM process will be ineffective. If the follow-up mechanism of the review process is not carried out equitably, and efforts to improve the system are not encouraged, UM will not be successful and will lose its credibility among providers.

UTILIZATION REVIEW AND QUALITY MANAGEMENT

When UM is appropriately applied and the original intention of *efficient* cost reduction is carried out, this process is a highly effective component of QM. It is the author's belief that (unmodified) UM principles are parallel with the QM goal of improving the quality of care provided to customers. According to Roland and Roland (1991), UR focuses on the *efficiency* of provided care — such as the cost of an inpatient day by DRG or the average cost of a procedure, and whether the care is provided in a cost-efficient manner. Quality Management, on the other hand, focuses on the *effectiveness* of provided services — that is, the benefits or impact of specific care on patient health status. Quality-Management activities usually place less emphasis on cost than do UM activities. The processes are, however, complementary and, thus, can enhance one another.

In the pursuit of QM, an essential component to achieving quality is resource optimization. The proper and appropriate utilization of resources is crucial to a QM effort. Quality Management calls for the decrease of waste, rework, and duplication. This is what utilization managers strive to achieve.

Both UM and QM are data driven, and most often the same data can be used for both processes. Kearns (1984) suggests that QM is the umbrella for several programs, including UR. Functions specific to UM may overlap somewhat with those of QM, and vice versa. Integration of UM and QM utilizes support staff more productively and can improve strategic planning and resource consumption (Miller, 1992).

Utilization-assessment data is usually comprehensive and specific — both of which are highly desirable characteristics of data for use in QM. Data for the process-improvement activities of QM can be derived from UM data, which is usually readily available, up to date, and accessible. When data are secured, analysis can be conducted for QM purposes. The utilization of standard QM tools is both feasible and cost effective. Rather than reinventing the wheel, UR data that is already available should be used. Tools such as trend charts, **control charts**, and **Pareto diagrams** can be used to manage large amounts of data (Al-Assaf, 1993; Leebov & Ersoz, 1992). Thus, the integration of UR with other QM processes is increasingly important to the quality improvement movement.

CONCLUSION

In this chapter, the concept of UM was presented, as was a discussion of UM roles, functions, stages, and impacts on health-care organizations. Utilization management is important in all health-care organizations. Its principles are as applicable to HMOs, other managed care arrangements, and nursing homes as they are to hospitals. The same goals and objectives apply, and the same focus and methodology are followed. In hospitals UM and UR are further mandated by external review agencies such as the Joint Commission and Health Care Financing Agency (HCFA). It is required that hospitals planning to participate in Medicare and Medicaid programs fulfill several conditions, one of which is UR. In order to participate in these programs it is necessary that the hospital have a UR plan in effect. This plan provides for the review of institutional and medical services rendered to patients entitled to benefits under the Medicare and Medicaid programs. The processes of UM and UR are essential for hospital participation in such resource-laden programs.

REFERENCES

Al-Assaf, A. F. (1992). Integrating Quality Assurance, risk management, and utilization review: The physician's perspective. In C. G. Meisenheimer (Ed.), *Improving quality* (pp. 166–182). Rockville, MD: Aspen.

Al-Assaf, A. F. (1993). Data management and total quality. In A. F. Al-Assaf & J. A. Schmele (Eds.), *The textbook on total quality in healthcare.* Del Ray, FL: St. Lucie Press.

Curtis, K., & Al-Assaf, A. F. (1990). *Report on the Oklahoma State Employee Insurance Board.* Oklahoma City, OK: Oklahoma University Health Sciences Center.

Joint Commission on Accreditation of Healthcare Organizations. (1992). *1993 Joint Commission Accreditation manual for hospitals.* Oakbrook Terrace, IL: Author.

Joint Commission on Accreditation of Healthcare Organizations. (1993). *1994 Joint Commission Accreditation manual for hospitals.* Oakbrook Terrace, IL: Author.

Joint Commission on Accreditation of Hospitals. (1976). *Joint Commission Accreditation manual for hospitals* (Supplement for 1976 and 1977). Chicago: Author.

Kearns, P. M. (1984). Quality Assurance and utilization review. In J. J. Pena, A. N. Haffner, B. Rosen, & D. W. Light (Eds.), *Hospital Quality Assurance* (pp. 237–252). Rockville, MD: Aspen.

Leebov, W., & Ersoz, C. J. (1992). *Manager's handbook on Continuous Quality Improvement.* Chicago: American Hospital Association.

Miller, D. K. (1992). Integrating Quality Assurance, risk management, and utilization review: The quality resource director's perspective. In C. G. Meisenheimer, (Ed.), *Improving quality* (pp. 151–165). Rockville, MD: Aspen.

Roland, H., & Roland, B. (1991). Utilization review. In *Hospital Quality Assurance manual* (pp. 10:1–10:18). Rockville, MD: Aspen.

ADDITIONAL READING

Allen, M. G., & Phillips, K. L. (1993). Utilization review of treatment for chemical dependence. *Hospital & Community Psychiatry, 44*(8), 752–756.

Baigelman, W., & Coldiron, J. (1993). The UR hot line: Purpose and process. American *Journal of Medical Quality, 8*(1) 6–12.

Cobb, A. B. (1993). The new PRO. *Journal of the Mississippi State Medical Association, 34*(11), 389–390.

Darby, P. W. (1992). Quick response teams: A new approach in utilization management. *Leadership in Health Services, 1*(5), 27–31.

Harrop, D. E. (1993). New methodology challenges PRO. *Pennsylvania Medicine, 96*(4), 42.

Hudson, T. (1991). PROs' new quality improvement focus: Will it work in practice? *Hospital, 65*(21), 48–50.

Joint Commission on Accreditation of Healthcare Organizations. (1992). *1993 Accreditation manual for hospitals* (pp. 171–210). Oakbrook Terrace, IL: Author.

Lenox, A. C. (1993). From theory to implementation: Integration strategies for utilization and quality review. *American Journal of Medical Quality, 8*(1), 12–20.

Payne, S. M. C., Campbell, D., Penzias, B. G., & Socholitzky, E. (1992). New methods for evaluating utilization management programs. *Quality Review Bulletin, 18*(10), 340–347.

Penchansky, R., & Macnee, C. L. (1993). Ensuring excellence: Reconceptualizing quality assurance, risk management, and utilization review. *Quality Review Bulletin, 19*(6), 182–189.

Shockney, T. (1992). The financial benefits of an effective hospital-wide Quality Assurance/utilization management program. *Quality Review Bulletin, 18*(8), 259–265.

Skipper, T. (1993). Utilization management: A rehabilitation approach to cost control. *Rehabilitation Nursing, 18*(4), 216–220, 230, 283–284.

Smith, D. G., & Perry, B. W. (1992). Toward effective hospital utilization management. Ten lessons from case studies. *American Journal of Medical Quality, 7*(4), 125–129.

Stone, C. L., & Krebs, K. (1990). The use of utilization review nurses to decrease reimbursement denials. *Home Healthcare Nurse, 8*(3), 13–17.

Work Group for Director of Research and Development of the Department of Health. (1993). What do we mean by appropriate care? *Quality in Health Care, 2*(2), 117–123.

Candace Friedman
Carol Chenoweth

CHAPTER *28*

Infection Control

INTRODUCTION

The tenets of infection-control (IC) practice have their roots in the epidemiologic work of Nightingale, Semmelweis, Lister, and Holmes. Hospital epidemiology, therefore, has as its main interest institutional infectious-disease control. The discipline of hospital epidemiology has changed dramatically over the past few decades — from an emphasis on data collection to one on intervention. Since the discussion regarding the use of **Continuous-Quality-Improvement (CQI)** techniques in health-care facilities began, it has become apparent that CQI techniques are similar to the epidemiologic method. Infection-control professionals (ICPs) use these techniques routinely in the control and prevention of nosocomial, or institution-associated, infections.

This chapter provides background on the historical changes in IC and hospital epidemiology, the maturing of IC programs, the role of health-care workers, and the relationship of IC practice to **Quality Management (QM)**.

HISTORY OF MODERN INFECTION CONTROL

Infection control is a relatively young and dynamic discipline that has undergone significant changes in a relatively short period of time. The modern concept of IC arose in the 1950s, in the midst of a global *Staphylococcus aureus* pandemic. During this time, *S. aureus*, which was previously uniformly susceptible to penicillin, developed the ability to produce penicillinase. Resistant strains of *S. aureus* spread from patient to patient via the hands of staff, causing nosocomial infections in susceptible patients, especially neonates and debilitated elderly adults. (Nosocomial infections include all infections that originate in a medical facility in patients in whom the infection was not present or incubating at the time of admission, or are the residuals of infections acquired during previous admissions.) The *S. aureus* epidemic spread worldwide, leading infection-control specialists to understand the mechanisms of spread, to determine causes of infection in certain patients, and to develop control measures (Decker & Schaffner, 1989).

Over the next decade, the staphylococcal epidemic resolved quickly, partially because of IC efforts and partially because of the widespread use of penicillinase-resistant antibiotics. The use of these antibiotics led to a shift in hospital microorganisms, and by the 1970s almost 70 percent of all nosocomial infections were caused by gram-negative bacilli. Unlike community-acquired strains, these nosocomial gram-negative strains were frequently resistant to multiple antimicrobials. These organisms infected patients who were in intensive-care units, and typically spread between patients via the hands of medical personnel.

During this period, hospital epidemiology established itself as a legitimate medical discipline. This was fostered by the requirements of the Joint Commission on Accreditation of Healthcare Organizations (Joint Commission) and reinforced by a large study reported by the Centers for Disease Control (CDC) — the Study on the Efficacy of Nosocomial Infection Control (SENIC). The American Hospital Association (AHA) was also recommending IC programs as a necessary function in hospitals. Based on these recommendations and regulatory requirements, most hospitals in the United States developed formal IC programs by the mid-1970s.

The practice of IC continued to change over the next decade. Several factors contributed to this change. The most dramatic was the AIDS (acquired-immune-deficiency syndrome) epidemic, which consumed much of ICPs time throughout most of the 1980s. At the same time, new resistant nosocomial pathogens began to surface. Most significantly, methicillin-resistant *Staphylococcus aureus* appeared, first in large training institutions then spreading to many smaller hospitals and long-term-care facilities. Other gram-positive cocci, such as coagulase-negative staphylococci and enterococci, also increased dramatically (Schaberg, Culver, & Gaynes, 1991). To further compound the situation, patients in most hospitals had become more susceptible to infections for various reasons. Generally, hospital patients were older and more immunocompromised, and more often required the use of invasive devices, such as intravascular lines, endotracheal tubes, and urinary catheters.

Along with internal changes, pressures from a number of external sources were also impacting the practice of IC. First was the development of the diagnosis related group (DRG) system of reimbursement, which placed an immediate emphasis on cost containment in the hospital setting. Hospitals previously were reimbursed for any additional costs if a patient developed a nosocomial infection. After DRGs were instituted, however, hospitals placed an emphasis on prevention of nosocomial infections because reimbursement was fixed. Secondly, the Occupational Safety and Health Administration (OSHA) had become increasingly interested in the medical industry to the point of promulgating the OSHA bloodborne pathogens rules in 1991 (Occupational Safety and Health Administration [OSHA], 1991). And finally, state and federal legislators developed many laws regulating the management of medical waste. All of these pressures contributed to stretching the limited resources of IC and also influenced the continuous change in the role of the ICP. The field of IC continues to evolve with changes in health care and as many programs expand

·their areas of expertise to include employee health, antibiotic utilization, and QM leadership roles.

INFECTION-CONTROL PROGRAMS

With the support of nationally based advocates, such as the AHA, the CDC, and the Joint Commission, health-care facilities began to develop comprehensive IC programs in the mid-1970s. The aim of these programs was to ensure **quality** of patient care through the surveillance, prevention, and control of nosocomial infections. Initially, surveillance or case finding of nosocomial infections was highly emphasized. Infection-control professionals spent the majority of their time collecting data on current infections. It soon became clear, however, that the collection of information on numbers and types of infections did not fully meet the objectives of prevention and control of nosocomial infections. It was determined that effective control programs required a balance between surveillance, education, and consultative activities.

Findings of the Study on the Efficacy of Nosocomial Infection Control

The need for surveillance, education, and consultation was recognized by practicing IC personnel and reinforced by a large study known as the Senic Project, reported by the CDC. This project was designed to determine effective components of an IC program. The essential components for an effective program as determined by SENIC included:

1. Conducting organized surveillance and control activities. These activities include **monitoring** segments of the patient population for the development of nosocomial infections and epidemiological investigation of clusters of infections.

2. An IC practitioner for every 250 beds.

3. A trained, effective IC physician, preferably trained in infectious diseases.

4. A system for reporting surgical wound infection rates to physicians.

The SENIC researchers concluded that IC programs with these four components decreased their infection rates by 32 percent. In contrast, the rate of nosocomial infections *increased* by 18 percent in hospitals with little or poor IC programs (Haley et al., 1985).

The Infection-Control Committee

The IC program is often directed by an authoritative committee, headed by a knowledgeable and interested person with training in microbiology, infectious diseases, or epidemiology. It is desirable that the committee include representatives from key areas, including administrative staff, nurses, physicians, microbiology laboratory staff, and ICPs. The key functions of an IC committee are to evaluate surveillance activities, to oversee investigations of infections, to review policies related to IC, and to disseminate information about IC activities. In most facilities, the IC committee is given the authority to review IC policies and to make changes when necessary.

The Infection-Control Professional

The ICP remains the cornerstone of an effective IC program. During the period of the SENIC project, 94 percent of these positions were filled by registered nurses, hence the title infection control nurse. Later, other professionals with clinical laboratory backgrounds began to take on the IC role. In 1972, the Association for Professionals in Infection Control and Epidemiology (APIC) deliberately chose a broader definition of the role, coining the term *infection control practitioner*. This term was subsequently expanded by APIC to *infection control professional (ICP)* in 1993. The prerequisite knowledge required for IC can be gained through degree or nondegree programs or experience as an ICP. In the United States, approximately 82 percent of APIC's members have nursing backgrounds — either diplomas, associate degrees, or bachelor degrees in nursing. Other ICPs include persons with bachelor degrees in medical technology or master degrees in public health. Individuals who meet certain requirements and successfully pass written examinations may become certified in IC. The daily activities of the ICP will vary in each health-care setting, depending on the patient population and type of surveillance performed. The surveillance method used must reflect the kinds and incidences of nosocomial infections found, the types of patients admitted, and the support services available. When the data is collected it is organized and analyzed before conclusions are drawn. Based on epidemiologic analysis of the data, specific control and prevention measures are instituted.

ROLES OF NURSES AND OTHER HEALTH-CARE PERSONNEL

Infection-control staff have overall responsibility for IC programs; *all* health-care personnel, however, have a role in making the program effective. Prevention of infection is crucial; therefore, health-care workers should assess each of their patients for the potential to develop an infection. Prevention techniques can then be emphasized for those patients deemed susceptible to infection. It is also important for all health-care workers to help develop and comply with the institution's policies on aseptic practice, handwashing, and other IC-related procedures. The success of an IC program depends largely on the degree to which its purposes are explained to the entire hospital staff. It is imperative that the hospital administration, IC committee, and medical and nursing staffs recognize that the ultimate goal of the IC program is to improve the quality of patient care.

INFECTION CONTROL AND TRADITIONAL QUALITY ASSURANCE

Quality Assurance (QA) is the traditional program used by organizations to assess, monitor, and improve quality. Quality Assurance is based on monitoring **indicators** that, at least theoretically, correlate with **outcomes**, such as duration of hospitalization, mortality, morbidity, and patient satisfaction. It is worth pointing out that IC programs have had experience related to QA issues. Infection-control personnel have long studied the impact of adverse nosocomial events on patient care; they have used epidemiologic tools to identify risk factors for nosocomial infections; and they have studied the efficacy of control measures in reducing rates of nosocomial infections. As such, they have vast experience with activities commonly referred to as *quality of care* (McGowan, 1990; Wenzel & Pfaller, 1991). Following is a discussion of these issues.

The impact of an adverse event is usually measured in morbidity, excess mortality, and increased costs. Several historical cohort studies have documented well the attributable mortality of nosocomial bloodstream infections and pneumonia (Green, Rubinstein, & Amit, 1982; Leu, Kaiser, Mori, Woolson, & Wenzel, 1989). Increased length of hospital stays has also been documented for these infections, as well as for urinary tract infections and postoperative wound infections. Measurement of the impact of infections may be used in a similar fashion to study any adverse nosocomial event. The study of the epidemiology of hospital-acquired infections has moved beyond the collection of numbers of infections and assessment of the economic impact of these infections. Several well-designed studies have identified important risk factors for nosocomial infections (Craven et al., 1986; Maki, 1989). Most of these studies used a case-control format and appropriate statistical methods to identify significant risk factors. Case-control studies evaluate two groups of subjects — one where subjects already have the outcome of interest and another where they do not — and compare the occurrence of the hypothesized exposure in the two groups (Moyer, 1994). The approaches used in these studies could be applied easily to any other adverse nosocomial event, such as falls. This type of controlled study provides a firm basis for the development of intervention strategies and policy making. After interventions are made, based on the known risk factors, it is imperative to determine if the interventions have worked. The design and conduct of carefully controlled trials to determine efficacy in reducing rates of nosocomial infections are of special concern to the hospital epidemiology team. A recent example of this type of study showed the efficacy of proper timing of administration of perioperative antibiotics (Classen et al., 1992).

Infection-control practice historically focused only on QA issues — that is, emphasis was placed on **evaluation** of surveillance data in order to identify *outliers*, or clusters of nosocomial infections that required epidemiological analysis. This analysis might result in identifying a health-care worker who did not follow proper procedures, finding a piece of equipment that was not cleaned or used properly, identifying a carrier of a microorganism, or finding a contaminated item that resulted in infections. Emphasis is now shifting toward CQI.

THE RELATIONSHIP OF INFECTION CONTROL, QUALITY ASSURANCE, AND CONTINUOUS QUALITY IMPROVEMENT

Continuous Quality Improvement is a natural outgrowth and extension of QA activities, as shown in Table 28-1. Data gathered from a QA indicator can provide the rationale or framework for a CQI project. The basic premise of CQI is that everything is a **process** — a systematic series of steps. In contrast, QA and IC focus on "outliers" rather than process. Whereas QA focuses on departmental problem

Table 28-1 • **COMPARISON OF QUALITY ASSURANCE AND CONTINUOUS QUALITY IMPROVEMENT**

Quality Assurance	Continuous Quality Improvement
Professional standards	Customer orientation
Subjective analysis	Statistical data
Case review	Trend analysis
Controls problems	Prevents problems
Departmental	Cross functional
Individual focus	System/process focus
Administrative control	Staff participation
Managing	Leading
Change as one-time event	Change as a constant process
Special cause	Common and special causes

Adapted from The Quality Letter, *by B. S. Bader, 1992, Rockville, MD: Bader & Associates. Copyright 1992 by Bader & Associates.*

solving, CQI uses cross-functional teams to solve problems; and whereas QA and IC staff "manage" the QA and IC activities, CQI techniques allow QA and IC staff to "lead" the activities of a team. Team involvement itself provides an incentive to improve outcomes.

Although CQI and outcome measurement (for nosocomial infections, for example) are sometimes classified as totally separate systems, they are, in fact, complementary. Continuous Quality Improvement incorporates outcome measurement to monitor efficacy, while outcome measurement identifies problems that may be amenable to the CQI approach (Goldmann et al., 1993).

As noted, IC staff use their expertise to assist other health-care workers in the development of rational IC practice, to provide surveillance for and epidemiological investigations of nosocomial infections, and to generally assist in problem solving by way of probing for root causes. The goal is to determine why nosocomial infections occur and develop strategies to reduce the probability of their occurrence. The epidemiological strategies used in successful IC programs are identical to those stressed in statistical-control and quality-improvement theories (Brewer & Gasser, 1993; Donabedian, 1993). When the epidemiological process is compared with the typical problem-solving format of CQI, the similarities are quite apparent (see Table 28-2).

Epidemiological/CQI activities involve the following steps:

- collect and stratify data to identify specific problems and establish a detailed statement reflecting the quality gap (develop hypotheses)

- identify and analyze contributing factors (root causes) to the effect (nosocomial infections)

Table 28-2 • **COMPARISON OF THE EPIDEMIOLOGICAL AND CONTINUOUS QUALITY IMPROVEMENT MODELS OF PROBLEM SOLVING**

Epidemiological Model	Continuous-Quality-Improvement Model*
Surveillance to confirm the problem	Recognize the process
Characterize the cases by person, place, and time	Organize the data
Identify and evaluate all potential risk factors; review charts	Analyze root causes
Formulate and test hypotheses, perform studies, institute control measures	Determine options
Evaluate efficacy of control measures with continued surveillance	Measure the change
Change policies and procedures, as necessary	Apply to work place
Routine surveillance	Plan for the future

Adapted from "Quality ROADMAP" (p. 21) in Total quality leadership program manual, University of Michigan Medical Center (1992). Ann Arbor, MI: University of Michigan Medical Center. Copyright 1992 by University of Michigan Medical Center.

- select options (control measures) that will decrease or eliminate the identified significant root causes
- measure results and success of the proposed option(s)
- standardize and maintain successful options to prevent recurrence of root causes
- generalize improvements to other areas
- investigate additional improvements

Surgical site infection (SSI) rates, for example, offer a means of identifying opportunities for improvement and for measuring the improvement. A study by Classen focused on the timing of antibiotic administration and the risk of SSI (Classen et al., 1992). Prophylactic antibiotics had been shown to be effective in preventing SSIs. This study prospectively monitored the timing of antibiotic prophylaxis (the process) and the occurrence of SSI (the outcome) in 2847 patients undergoing elective surgical procedures. The study determined that there was considerable variation in timing of prophylactic administration of antibiotics and that administration in the two hours before surgery reduced the risk of SSI (root cause).

Assessing the effectiveness of a particular clinical intervention requires a system of intense surveillance that is able to provide monitoring, analysis of variations, assessment of interventions, feedback, and education. Information can then be reported to staff, thus allowing them to alter their practice patterns and continually improve the quality of patient care (Classen et al., 1992).

Variation is inherent in hospital practices and outcomes. There are two types of variation in processes (Gabor, 1990). An unexpected, significant deviation outside predicted control limits is considered to represent a **special cause of variation**. These special causes tend to cluster by person, place, and time (that is, they are epidemiological). The cause of the problem is not part of the system — that is, it is external to the process. Therefore, the problem only occurs when the special cause is functioning. Special cause variation represents change that can be investigated and assigned to an identifiable source (Brewer & Gasser, 1993).

Common cause variation results from chance events that occur without a specific cause and from the inherent design of the system. As a result of common cause variation, rates of specific processes and outcomes fluctuate within statistically predictable bounds and over time. The success of a CQI initiative can be ascertained by determining whether it improves the rate of a process or outcome significantly when compared with the predicted rate based on previous experience. The goal is to improve mean performance incrementally through a continuous cycle of intervention and measurement (Goldmann et al., 1993).

Consider the example illustrated in Figure 28-1 (Decker, 1992), a **control chart** representing the monthly rate of ventilator-associated pneumonia.

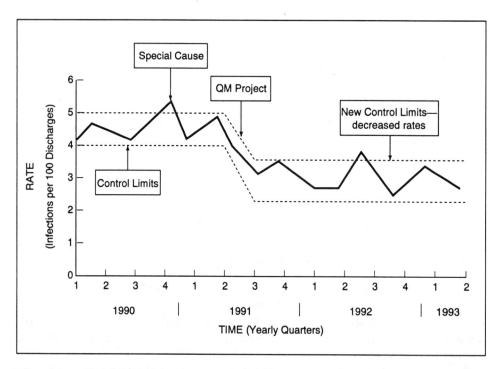

Figure 28-1 *Control Chart of Nosocomial Ventilator-Associated Pneumonia Rates. Adapted from* The Quality Letter *(p. 16), by B. S. Bader, 1992, Rockville, MD: Bader & Associates, Copyright 1992 by Bader & Associates, and from "Continuous Quality Improvement," by M. D. Decker, 1992,* Infection Control and Hospital Epidemiology, *13, pp. 165–169. Copyright 1992.*

Imagine that a persistent violation of the upper control limit is noted in the fall of 1990. A cause is sought, and it is discovered that Ambu bags are being shared among patients, allowing cross-contamination of airways. When the problem is corrected and this special cause eliminated, the rate declines. Apart from that deviation, the monthly rate fluctuates within the control limits. The month-to-month variations represent chance events, not correctable sources of variation. The processes underlying the development of ventilator-associated pneumonia may be investigated over the long-term to reduce the mean overall — and, thus, establish new control limits. Underlying determinants may be choice and use of equipment, duration of ventilator support, use or misuse of antibiotics, suctioning techniques, and head position, among others. Continuous-Quality-Improvement techniques assist in identifying these determinants, with a resultant overall improvement in nosocomial infection rates.

Integration of TQM concepts into IC practice has resulted in a shift in focus from special cause to common cause variation; a shift from reaction to prevention; and a shift from review of practitioners and equipment to review of processes. A new paradigm for IC, then, follows the CQI model. Instead of only using outcome data to focus on special causes of nosocomial infections, CQI techniques add the practice of redesigning processes in order to focus on reducing common causes. By changing the focus of how IC data are analyzed and evaluated, ICPs are moving toward meaningful process improvement activities (Ziacik, 1992). The addition of CQI techniques to IC practices will assist in bringing down the overall rates of endemic nosocomial infections; and it is the control of endemic disease that provides the greatest opportunity for improvement.

Continuous-Quality-Improvement skills have been used for many years in the field of IC and are now in demand in the study of quality in health care outside the realm of control and prevention of nosocomial infections. Those trained in epidemiology and experienced in the field of IC are being asked to apply their skills to broader concepts of quality care. With this, IC is becoming more integrated into the total-quality process (Wenzel & Pfaller, 1991).

One aspect of the **Total-Quality-Management (TQM)** process that is important to organizations and departments is the development of a mission statement and customer-satisfaction indicators. The University of Michigan Medical Center IC department developed the following mission statement:

> Infection Control Services' highest goal is to insure that the clinical
> community has the information to protect patients and personnel
> from adverse events. The department provides expertise in the
> epidemiological method through education, research, consultation,
> surveillance and investigation of disease clusters, environmental
> laboratory services, quality improvement and policy formation.
> These services exist to meet the needs of all persons associated with
> the University of Michigan Hospitals, particularly the patient, for
> the prevention of infectious complications. The department is a
> responsible and contributing member of its hospital community.
> (Friedman et al., 1993)

It can be seen from this mission statement that infection-control staff need to determine the quality of their work by assessing both the external and internal customer focus. Information is supplied in the form of surveillance data, which is then used by other staff members to impact IC practice. ICPs should determine customer satisfaction through surveys of customer groups, for example, nurses. They also should develop indicators of customer satisfaction to measure how well they are meeting their customers' needs and reasonable expectations. Infection-control departments also need to identify which data customers need in order to improve patient care.

CONTINUOUS QUALITY IMPROVEMENT IN INFECTION CONTROL

Kritchevsky and Simmons (1991) provide an effective example of TQM practice by focusing on standard aseptic techniques. These techniques form a system for preventing surgical infections. This system consists of rules and protocols outlining aseptic procedures, such as using prescribed soap products, scrubbing hands a specific length of time, preparing the incision site, and timing of antibiotic infusions. Even if these techniques are followed rigorously, some infections will still occur. This is because the number of causal pathways by which surgical infections occur is so large that no system of procedures can be designed to eliminate every one. Thus, the system of standard aseptic techniques permits a tolerably low level of infections to occur (common cause). This level is attributable to the system and cannot be reduced without changing processes.

In contrast, consider the patients of a surgeon who has a furuncle shedding *S. aureus.* These patients would be more likely to develop staphylococcal surgical site infections than would patients of other surgeons. In this example, there is a specific and identifiable cause of the patients' infections — a cause the standard aseptic techniques were not designed to control. By eliminating the surgeon's infection, many infections would be prevented. Left untreated, this surgeon would remain a special or extrasystemic cause of wound infections.

An IC/CQI examination of the processes that might lead to the development of surgical site infections could focus on the timing of prophylactic antibiotic administration. If all surgeons are using the same procedures, the rates of post-operative infections should be similar, on average. If there are outliers, it is important to determine why. A comprehensive group of CQI/epidemiological tools can be used to examine processes and answer the question, "Why is the antibiotic not given at the proper time?"

DIRECTIONS FOR THE FUTURE

Because of the changing demographics of individuals and new health-care technology, the potential for nosocomial infections in health-care institutions will continue to increase. Patients in hospitals will be sicker and there will be new antibiotic-resistant microorganisms; new instruments and procedures; and new infectious diseases.

To ensure that quality of care is not compromised, various organizations, such as the Joint Commission, are trying to understand and measure the effects of these changes. The Joint Commission incorporates an ongoing evaluation of the performance of health-care organizations in its survey process. The Joint Commission has developed various indicators to monitor outcomes in health care, including infections. These IC indicators monitor nosocomial infection outcomes.

There is an increasing demand for indicator data by various groups, including purchasers of heath care and governmental agencies (Scheckler, 1994). It is thought that this data can be used as a measure of quality. **Benchmarking** is an approach to establishing practices based on the best in the industry. An organization's performance can then be measured against that of others. The Joint Commission's indicator data is expected to be used for benchmarking purposes. Data from the CDC's National Nosocomial Infection Study is also useful for benchmarking.

Indicator data that measure outcomes, such as nosocomial infections, is strongly determined by patient characteristics and, thus, is largely out of the control of the medical system. Changes in outcome measures may represent changes in the system itself or changes in the inputs to the system. Sources of variation, such as underlying illnesses of patients that are not controllable by the system using adjustments for severity of illness and/or acuity, will need to be addressed (Kritchevsky & Simmons, 1991). Several severity of illness indices are available that allow for more accurate assessment of this outcome-measures data (Gross, 1989; Salemi, Morgan, Kelleghan, Hiebert-Crape, 1993).

CONCLUSION

Infection control has never really been the responsibility of only one department. All staff in a health-care setting are responsible for the prevention of infections in patients and clients. The emphasis on TQM in health care with its focus on **multidisciplinary** problem solving, has reemphasized this fact.

Infection-control professionals have espoused the fundamental principles of TQM for years; they are organized to maintain and improve. Hospital epidemiology represents a model for other QA and CQI activities; it is based in problem solving, with improving patient care its major goal.

REFERENCES

Bader, B. S. (1992). *The quality letter.* Rockville, MD: Bader & Associates.

Brewer, J. H., & Gasser, C. S. (1993). The affinity between Continuous Quality Improvement and epidemic surveillance. *Infection Control and Hospital Epidemiology, 14,* 95–98.

Classen, D. C., Evans, R. S., Pestotnik, S. L., Horn, S. D., Menlove, R. L., & Burke, J. P. (1992). The timing of prophylacwound administration of antibiotics and the risk of surgical-wound infection. *New England Journal of Medicine, 326*(5), 281–286.

Craven, D. E., Kunches, L. M., Kilinsky, V., Lichtenburg, D. A., Make, B. J., & McCabe, W. R. (1986). Risk factors for pneumonia and fatality in patients receiving continuous mechanical ventilation. *American Review of Respiratory Disease, 133*(5), 792–796.

Decker, M. D. (1992). Continuous Quality Improvement. *Infection Control and Hospital Epidemiology, 13*(3), 165–169.

Decker, M. D., & Schaffner, W. (1989). Changing trends in infection control and hospital epidemiology. *Infectious Disease Clinics of North America, 3,* 671–682.

Donabedian, A. (1993). Continuity and change in the quest for quality. *Clinical Performance and Quality Health Care, 1,* 9–16.

Friedman, C., Baker, C. A., Mowry-Hanley, J. L., Vander Hyde, K., Stites, M. S., & Hanson, R. J. (1993). Use of the total quality process in an infection control program: A surprising customer-needs assessment. *American Journal of Infection Control, 21*(3), 155–159.

Gabor, A. (1990). *The man who discovered quality.* New York: Times Books, Random House.

Goldmann, D. A., Saul, C. A., Parsons, S., Mansoor, C., Abbott, A., Damian, F., Young, G. J., Homer, C., & Caputo, G. L. (1993). Hospital-based Continuous Quality Improvement: A realistic appraisal. *Clinical Performance and Quality Health Care, 1,* 69–80.

Green, M. S., Rubinstein, E., & Amit, P. (1982). Estimating the effects of nosocomial infections on length of hospital stay. *Journal of Infectious Diseases, 145*(5), 667–672.

Gross, P. A. (1989). Expanding roles of hospital epidemiology: Severity of illness indicators. *Infection Control and Hospital Epidemiology, 10*(6), 257–260.

Haley, R. W., Culver, D. H., White, J. W., Morgan, W. M., Emori, T. G., Munn, V. P., & Hooton, T. M. (1985). The efficacy of infection surveillance and control programs in preventing nosocomial infections in US hospitals. *American Journal of Epidemiology, 121*(2), 182–205.

Kritchevsky, S. B., & Simmons, B. P. (1991). Continuous Quality Improvement. Concepts and applications for physician care. *Journal of the American Medical Association, 266*(13), 1817–1823.

Leu, H. S., Kaiser, D. L., Mori, M., Woolson, R. F., & Wenzel, R. P. (1989). Hospital acquired pneumonia: Attributable mortality and morbidity. *American Journal of Epidemiology, 129*(6), 1258-1267.

Maki, D. G. (1989). Risk factors for nosocomial infection in intensive care. "Devices vs. nature" and goals for the next decade. *Archives of Internal Medicine, 149*(1), 30–35.

McGowan, J. E. (1990). The infection control practitioner: An action plan for the 1990s. *American Journal of Infection Control, 18*(1), 29–39.

Moyer, V. A. (1994). Confusing conclusions and the clinician: An approach to evaluating case-control studies. *Journal of Pediatrics, 124*(5), 671–674.

Occupational Safety and Health Administration. (1991). Occupational exposure to blood-borne pathogens. *Federal Register, 56*(235), 64175–64182.

Salemi, C., Morgan, J. W., Kelleghan, S. I., & Hiebert-Crape, B. (1993). Severity of illness classification for infection control departments: A study in nosocomial pneumonia. *American Journal of Infection Control, 21,* 117–126.

Schaberg, D. R., Culver, D. H., & Gaynes, R. P. (1991). Major trends in the microbial etiology of nosocomial infections. *American Journal of Medicine, 91*(Suppl. 3B), 72S–75S.

Scheckler, W. E. (1994). Interim report of the quality indicator study group. *American Journal of Infection Control, 22,* 30A–36A.

Wenzel, R. P., & Pfaller, M. A. (1991). Infection control: the premier quality assessment program in the United States hospitals. *American Journal of Medicine, 91*(Suppl. 3B), 27S–31S.

Ziacik, E. (1992). An evolutionary process: Applying CQI techniques to Quality Assurance issues. *Journal for Healthcare Quality, 14*(4), 8–18.

ADDITIONAL READING

Bennett, J. V., & Brachman, P. S. (1992). *Hospital infections* (3rd ed.). Boston: Little, Brown and Co.

Haley, R. W., Quade, D., Freeman, H. E., Bennett, J. V. (1990). The SENIC Project: Study on the efficacy of nosocomial infection control: Summary of study design. *American Journal of Epidemiology, 111*(5).

Kelleghan, S. L. (1993). An effective Continuous Quality Improvement approach to the prevention of ventilator associated pneumonia. *American Journal of Infection Control, 21*(6), 322–330.

Nightingale, F (1898). *Notes on nursing: What it is, and what it is not.* New York: D. Appleton and Co.

Pollack, S. (1994). Applying TQM to infection surveillance. *Nursing Management, 25*(3), 74–75.

Wenzel, R. P. (1986). The evolving art and science of hospital epidemiology. *Journal of Infectious Diseases, 153*(3), 462–470.

Wenzel, R. P. (1993). *Prevention and control of nosocomial infections* (2nd ed.). Baltimore: Williams and Wilkins.

Jane M. Bryant
Mona R. Fields
Phillip Schaedler

CHAPTER *29*

Risk Management

•──•

INTRODUCTION

In 1976, in the *Medical Nemesis*, Ivan Illich proposed that the medical establishment had become a threat to health. In 1978 Columbia University's Jacques Barzum described the professsion as being "under seige," with the need of the public being weighed against the private practice of the physician (Barzum, 1978). During hearings on cost containment, Senator Edward Kennedy declared passionately to the leaders of the medical profession that they would surely bankrupt the country if their private practices were not constrained by legal means (Griffith & Johnston, 1992). With statements such as these being published in popular books and magazines and being stated openly in Senate hearings, it is little wonder that the public has sometimes adopted the belief that physicians cannot be trusted. Moreover, the lack of public trust has extended to the institutions where these professionals maintain their practices. These institutions, mainly hospitals, have done little to help increase public trust.

The provision of safe, cost-effective, and clinically effective care that meets the needs and expectations of both consumers and third-party payers will be the challenge that drives health-care management throughout the early part of the twenty-first century. Hospitals have institutionalized their response to this challenge and have given it a name: risk management (RM). Other health-care institutions practice RM in a less formalized manner. For example many physicians have adopted the practice of "defensive medicine" in an effort to decrease their risk.

What is RM? *Risk management* is defined as the science for identification, evaluation, and treatment of the risk of financial loss (Dankmyer & Groves, 1977). Sullivan and Decker (1988) define risk management as a planned program of loss prevention and liability control. Ashby, Stephens, and Pearson (1977) define it as the science of detecting, evaluating, financing, and reducing risk of financial loss.

Orlikoff, Fifer, and Greeley, however, offer the most comprehensive definition, which will be expanded on in this chapter. They note that hospital RM is the identification, analysis, evaluation and elimination and/or reduction of risks to employees, patients, and visitors. The RM program is a completely integrated program that involves quality assurance activities, safety and security activities, a patient feedback program, as well as a mechanism for dealing with incidents, claims, and insurance and litigation tasks.

As is evident from these definitions, formal RM activities are well suited for integration into nursing and other health-care areas, as guidelines to enhance the effective management of **quality**. Though sometimes considered only supportive of **Quality Assurance (QA)** activities, RM has long been a key source for data that relates to **outcomes** of care. Probably the best description of the relationship between RM and quality improvement is provided by J. Kelly Avery who states that "all risk management issues are not quality issues, but every quality issue is a risk management issue" (cited in Hudson, 1992, p. 30).

This chapter provides a short historical perspective of RM, a conceptual discussion of the components of an RM program, and an overview of some issues related to the practical aspects of an RM program.

HISTORICAL PERSPECTIVE

Risk management in health care is relatively new when compared to RM in other industries. Health-care organizations, particularly nonprofit organizations, were long protected from claims and competition by legislation prohibiting lawsuits against nonprofit and governmental institutions. For most of history, there were very few for-profit hospitals. In addition, third-party payment mechanisms did not promote competition among providers. More recently, the era of "risk" has slowly evolved.

Evolution of Internal Risk Management

Risk-management programs within health-care facilities were initiated in the 1970s. At this time the insurance industry began to raise premiums or cancel coverage for health-care providers because of the rapid increase in claim volume and award. Until this point, most RM activities had focused on purchasing low-cost insurance, maintaining a safe physical environment, and providing worker's compensation. In the late 1970s it became evident that health care was not invulnerable to the civil liability climate, where large sums of money were being demanded by patients and families to compensate for unanticipated outcomes. Up until this point, the relatively few medical malpractice claims had involved specific practitioners and not the organizations within which they practiced.

Evolution of Health-Care Competition

When organizations and their boards began to be named as defendants, the internal activities of clinical RM became a necessity in order to control costs. These initial RM programs had only a financial focus. During this time, increased competition in health care led to added emphasis on risk-prevention programs. Thus, the impetus for RM began to extend throughout the health-care organization as a part of QA initiatives.

Subsequent to this was the advent of diagnostic related groups (DRGs) and managed-care contracts, whereby set payments were made for each type of admission and service, regardless of the resources used in providing the care or service. Diagnostic related groups led health-care organizations to take a hard look at complication rates and outcomes, no matter what the perceived causes. Lengths of stay decreased, and use of ambulatory services and home care increased. Health-care services became less centralized, and organizations were more cognizant of their **accountability** for the services they provided and the outcomes associated with those services.

Evolution of Regulatory Agencies and Standards of Care

Regulatory and **licensing** mandates also broadened the scope of RM involvement in health-care operations. Governmental involvement in health-care **standards** and in reimbursement has extended into the clinical aspects of care. As a result, there are now quality standards that impact not only the claims area of RM but also an organization's operational activities at all levels. (See Chapter 16 for a more detailed discussion of regulation.) Added to this is the impact of requirements set by accrediting agencies such as the Joint Commission for Healthcare Organizations (Joint Commission). (See Chapter 17 for a detailed discussion of the Joint Commission.)

To the risk manager, all of these factors impact the organization by identifying standards and protocols that, if not met, can lead to fines and sanctions. These factors can also represent sources for bringing successful litigation against the organization, if during a **certification** or **accreditation** survey the organization is found not to be in compliance with the standards. Thus, RM today is a program that pervades every element of operation within a health-care organization.

RISK-MANAGEMENT CONCEPTS

Depending upon the organization there are various views of the specifics of risk management. However, the major objectives and other related concepts are common to most of these views.

Risk-Management Objectives

Obviously each health-care organization sets its own objectives for the RM program. It is generally agreed, however, that there are three major objectives of every program. The first is *loss prevention.* Loss prevention implies activity designed to prevent or reduce the frequency of preventable adverse occurrences that lead to malpractice liability. Areas of concern are hospital property, visitor and employee safety, and, most importantly, patient safety. The second objective is *loss control.* Loss control focuses on the development of systems to promptly identify, follow-up, and resolve patient, visitor, and employee safety problems. The intent is to minimize the financial, human, and intangible costs associated with these problems. The third objective is *risk financing.* Risk financing refers to an organization's search for the most economical method among alternatives in the insurance market or self-insurance programs for financing the institution's potential loss (American College of Surgeons, 1985).

The RM objectives can be carried out by the performance of six functions. The functions are:

1. protection of the financial assets of the facility or service

2. protection of human and intangible resources (that is, the reputation of the facility)

3. prevention of injury to patients, visitors, employees, and property

4. reduction of loss, focusing on individual loss or single incidents

5. prevention of loss by improving the quality of care through continuing and ongoing **monitoring**

6. review of each incident and the patterns of incidents through an RM system (Orlikoff & Lanham, 1981)

Comparison of Risk-Management and Quality-Assessment-and-Improvement Programs

Northrop and Kelly (1987) propose that RM and **Quality-Assessment-and-Improvement (QA&I)** programs are not identical, but rather are related programs. These programs differ in the following ways:

1. The motivation and focus of each function within the two processes is different.

2. Risk management is concerned with acceptable care at a minimal safe level (that is, the legal level), and QA&I focuses on the provision of optimal care.

3. Risk management is concerned with all facility exposures, while QA&I is concerned only with patient care.

4. Risk management is concerned with legal, insurance, and other distinct loss-prevention activities.

5. Quality assessment and improvement focuses on facilitating care through coordination of various activities — any activity with the potential for improving patient care; while RM is concerned only with the more-focused loss-prevention activities.

Risk management and QA&I also share many areas of concern. These include identification and prevention of adverse patient occurrences, emphasis on monitoring of trends to identify patterns of risk, correction of risks by education, changes in policies and procedures, and disciplinary actions. Both processes place strong emphasis on the importance of accurate and complete documentation. Implementing either or both processes, requires cooperation between the medical staff, nursing staff, and the administrative staff in all phases of the processes. Obviously, when change is needed, it can be accomplished only if these three groups support its implementation. Additionally, many of the data-collection activities used to identify risks are equally important to the quality-improvement program. Many organizations find that some sort of formal integrated relationship between the RM and QA&I departments maximizes the use of problem-identification data for both processes.

It is important to note that RM is a process to be embraced by all providers and is not the sole function of a designated area or department. Health-care facilities that have comprehensive RM programs in place have been able to focus on both reactive and proactive activities necessary to integrate prevention and risk control into quality improvement. Thus, as a result of findings generated by RM identification systems, quality within the entire organization improves.

Risk Management as a Process

To accomplish organizational goals, well-defined work processes are initiated and carried out by personnel. It is recognized that staff generally do not set out to disrupt the safe and effective delivery of care. Thus, when outcomes are different than anticipated, there is a need for a systematic process to evaluate the factors contributing to what has occurred. Organizations need to look at incidents, complaints, claims, and errors as symptoms of process problems and not as profiles of individual failings. If managers take the stance that mistakes and problems are the result of glitches in the process or in staff's understanding of the process, then the first step toward improving delivery of care is underway.

THE RISK-MANAGEMENT PROGRAM

Risk-Management Process

The RM process is a step-by-step approach used to identify, confront, and prevent risks and to accomplish the goals of an RM program. According to Sullivan and Decker (1988) the components of the RM process are:

1. Identifying potential risks for accident, injury, or financial loss.

2. Reviewing present institutionwide monitoring systems (incident reports, audits, committee minutes, oral complaints, patient questionnaires) and evaluating completeness of systems, to determine the need for additional systems to provide the factual data essential for RM control.

3. Analyzing the frequency, severity, and causes of general categories and specific types of incidents causing injury or adverse outcomes to patients. (It is necessary to plan risk-intervention strategies, estimating the possible loss associated with the various types of incidents.)

4. Reviewing and appraising safety and risk aspects of patient-care procedures and new programs.

5. Monitoring laws and codes related to patient safety, consent, and care.

6. Eliminating or reducing risks as much as possible.

7. Reviewing the work of other committees to determine potential liability and recommend prevention or corrective action.

8. Identifying educational needs of patient, family, and personnel and implementing appropriate educational programs.

9. **Evaluating** the results of the RM program.

10. Providing periodic reports to administration, medical staff, and the board of directors.

A discussion of the steps of the RM process follows.

RISK IDENTIFICATION AND INSTITUTIONAL MONITORING

As stated earlier, the first step of the RM process is risk identification. A variety of terms are used for those events with which risk management is concerned. An adverse patient outcome is defined by Craddick as "any untoward patient event which, under optimal conditions, is not a natural consequence of the patient's disease or procedure" (cited in Northrop & Kelly, 1987, p. 24). A potentially compensable event refers to any occurrence that could result in liability exposure. Other terms used frequently in risk identification include maloccurrence, mishap, patient safety problem, and incident. Regardless of what the event is called, there are a number of data sources that are used for risk identification.

The risk manager relies on data sources such as incident reports, verbal communication, surveys indicating client satisfaction or dissatisfaction, and committee reports. If the risk-identification process is functioning properly, all patient-liability and patient-safety problems are reported to the risk manager as soon as they occur or are detected. Some events are immediately recognizable. Examples of immediately recognizable events are things such as observing a patient fall, administering a medication to the wrong patient, or giving the wrong dosage or wrong medication. Not all events are immediately recognizable. One such event might be the occurrence of an unusually high rate of wound infections. This might not immediately be recognized if the infections are not localized in one hospital unit.

Incident reports have long been a standby as far as the risk manager is concerned. The term *incident*, according to Northrop and Kelly (1987), means "an accident, discovery of a hazardous condition, or any occurrence which is not consistent with routine operation of the institution or routine care of the patient" (p. 429). Attributes of an effective incident-report system are:

1. *Clear definition* of the term *incident*.

2. *Clear reporting forms* that are easy to complete and analyze. Reports using checklists and short, *objective* answers rather than formats that encourage open-ended, narrative responses, are imperative in helping to avoid documentation of conclusions or judgments about the appropriateness or inappropriateness of those individuals involved in the incident.

3. *Clear procedures.* All occurrences must be reported, even if no injury results, and all completed forms must be sent to the risk manager immediately.

4. *Prompt response.* Reports must reach the risk manager's office within twenty-four hours and an appropriate follow-up must begin immediately. Prompt investigation of reports shows providers that reports initiate follow-up action.

5. *Trending.* Incident-report data is recorded in a manner that allows for the identification of trends. This data is reviewed with the risk manager, QA&I committees, and the involved departments.

6. *Feedback.* Results of trending analysis, including both the desirable and the undesirable trends, are shared with staff.

7. *Education.* Inservice programs on incident reporting emphasize that the intended use of reports is to identify risk exposure, not to serve as a basis for disciplinary action against staff. Programs also include specific instructions for completing reports and a review of the laws affecting discoverability and admissibility of incident reports in the jurisdiction.

8. *Top level commitment* by administrators and medical and nursing staff leaders, who clearly and frequently express commitment to the incident reporting system. (Northrop & Kelly, 1987)

In addition to the incident-reporting system, some organizations have developed inspection surveys and questionnaires for health-care providers to use in identifing potential risk areas. These surveys may be nothing more than routine walking tours during which the assigned inspector looks for specific risks, such as equipment not returned to storage areas or dietary carts left in the hallway so as to form obstacle courses for patients ambulating in the hall.

Another source of risk-identification data is the patient-relations department. Some hospitals employ a person who acts as a patient advocate or ombudsman. Others use follow-up surveys to ascertain patients' perceptions of the quality of care delivered by the organization. Complaints about a particular practitioner, dissatisfaction with the care provided, refusal to pay the bill, or an angry letter alert the organization to potential risk situations. Any potential claims need to be reported to the risk manager immediately.

Another source of data for the RM program is peer review. Peer review data often are gathered as a part of the QA&I program, usually in the form of retrospective chart review. This type review cannot, however, identify liability situations unless they are captured in the patient record. Nor can it identify adverse outcomes that did not occur immediately (for example, if a patient falls and hurts her wrist, and is visually examined but not x-rayed at the time, and then, a week after dismissal, the wrist is still sore and an x-ray is taken revealing a broken bone). Retrospective chart review can, however, identify events that deviate from the standard that has been established for that particular type of patient or situation and is particularly effective in capturing medical occurrences such as misdiagnosis.

RISK ANALYSIS

When an event is identified, whether through those systems set up specifically for the RM program or through the institutionwide monitoring systems, the next step in the RM process is risk analysis. Someone or some group is required to decide whether the event was an isolated event or evidence of a trend. Whatever the answer, the next question becomes, "Is the loss potential, minimal, or serious?"

One approach to risk analysis is statistical or mathematical. According to Troyer and Salman, risk is assessed based on the following criteria: (1) probable frequency of the occurrence of the loss; (2) probable or possible severity of the loss; and (3) the effect the loss will have on the organization, both clinically and financially (cited in Northrop & Kelly, 1987). Quantification of this data allows the risk manager to assign priority and to tailor the needed interventions to the problem. In addition, statistical or mathematical rates help determine allocation of resources.

MONITORING PATIENT-CARE PROCEDURES AND PROGRAMS AND LAWS AND CODES

Reviewing and appraising safety and risk aspects of patient care procedures and new programs, and monitoring laws and codes are ongoing activities. Safety issues pervade all aspects of health-care organizations — from the parking lot to use of the most highly dangerous radioactive substances. The same observation is true for monitoring laws and codes. No one person in the organization can be responsible for these activities. Everyone in the organization must be responsible for prevention and early identification of events or information that might have risk implications for the organization.

Policies and procedures often are referred to as internal sources for standards of care. With the advent of integrated service units and the resultant expansion of the scope of duties to be performed, it will become even more critical to develop effective guidelines, policies, and procedures that address defined work processes. The reason policies and procedures exist is to support the staff in understanding the parameters under which quality outcomes may be achieved. Many policies and procedures have RM implications and support prevention activities. See Table 29-1 for a list of policies with RM implications.

Table 29-1 • **EXAMPLES OF POLICIES WITH RISK-MANAGEMENT IMPLICATIONS**

Release of information	Infant security
Report of unusual occurrences	Medical-staff/affiliated-staff privileging requirements
Consent policies — treatment, certain tests, information release	Handling of valuables
HIV testing	Laser safety requirements — training and protective equipment
Treatment refusal	
Drug screening	Exposure control plan for blood-borne pathogens
Use of restraints	Medical-device tracking
Patient categorization for treatment purposes (for example, do not resuscitate)	Medical-device failure reporting
	Biomedical inspection of equipment before use
Reuse of disposable products	Visitor control policy
Emergency consent	

There are several key points to remember about policy and procedure development and revision. First, it is vital to review the guidelines of speciality societies and boards, licensing agencies, and similar health-care organizations, and to explore the literature to ensure that practice is similar to that of comparative situations. Secondly, as policies and procedures are written, it is necessary to ensure that they remain consistent with all other policies and procedures already in effect in the organization. It is common for one unit of an organization to develop procedural or process guidelines that describe similar activities being performed in other areas of the organization. When there are discrepancies in policies within the organization, there is greater likelihood of system failure, which can result in quality failure. Thirdly, policies also need to be written in such a way as to meet realistic practice capabilities, and thus, become standards of practice. It is vital that these policies and procedures consistently reflect current practice based on available knowledge and research. Finally, it is important that both risk managers and staff participate in the development and the periodic review of policies and procedures. This encourages organizationwide compliance.

RISK REDUCTION

The correction, elimination, or reduction of the identified risk is probably the most important step in the RM process. In order to ensure effective remedial action, the organization must establish well-defined and well-understood lines of responsibility, authority, and accountability. If one person or group has responsibility for solving a problem, has the authority to do so, and is held accountable for the results, effective remedial action is usually taken.

Remedial action is a synonym for problem solving that involves decision making. Decision making is one of the primary components of the management process. Some situations require a certain course of action. Other situations may require decisions that use a combination of the possible courses of action. The key for the risk manager is deciding when to use each approach effectively.

Red tape and bureaucratic involvement can sometimes interfere with effective remedial action. Administrators who are alert to this possibility can take every step possible to eliminate this interference. It is important that the organization make every effort to encourage active management. One way to do this is to integrate active management into the organization's policies and procedures. This will facilitate effective remedial action — decision making that results in effective problem solving — and, ultimately, result in risk reduction.

Managers involved in remedial activities have four basic positive courses of action available, as well as one negative course. The four positive approaches are immediate action, nonaction, deferred action, and restricted action. The negative approach is default (Management Memos, 1965).

Immediate Action   *Immediate action* is the simplest type of decision. It is used when time is important or when the possible outcomes suggest that there is no other approach. Generally, the situation and the corrective action are very straightforward. An example might be a situation where someone notices that the carpet in a well-traveled hallway is torn, thus creating a danger of people tripping on the torn carpet. The manager might immediately dispatch someone to apply tape over the area until a more permanent repair can be accomplished.

Nonaction   If it is conscious and calculated, *nonaction* is an active decision. An example of nonaction is when an incident with possible risk occurs within a department and is brought to the attention of the responsible department head; and after thought and consideration, the department head decides to refrain from getting involved in the situation. For example, during the afternoon a patient gets out of bed and falls. The staff have the patient assessed. There are no injuries as a result of the fall. An incident report is filed. According to the incident report, the room was well lit, there were no obstacles, and the floor was not wet or slick; the patient stated, "I just got my feet tangled up"; and neither the patient nor family appeared upset by the incident. The manager therefore decides that the less done about the incident the better and, thus, chooses to take no action.

Deferred Action   The deliberate postponement of a corrective action is termed *deferred action*. Like nonaction, deferred action requires a deliberate thought process. The result of the thought process is to take an action sometime in the future. Deferred action often is used when there is not an immediate threat to the safety of patients, visitors, and staff and when the action is costly. The action may be deferred until the cost can be incorporated into the organization's budget.

Restricted Action   The alternative most often selected by the risk manager is *restricted action*; yet it is the least understood of all possible actions. This course of action involves delegation, an important key to productive and effective management. When restricted action is used, the manager restricts personal activity and places the responsibility for action on another person or group. The manager delegates. In delegating, the risk manager indicates what is to be done and offers assistance. The manager is careful, however, not to decide for the staff how to remedy the situation; rather the manager allows the subordinates to figure this out for themselves. This approach provides ownership of the problem, as well as a challenging growth process.

Default   The negative response of *default* is sometimes referred to as *passive management*. This type of management leads to organizational failure. Default means that a manager forfeits the opportunity to make a decision. Default often results from thoughtlessness or forgetfulness. It also may result from the unwillingness of the manager to make a decision. Some managers operate from the position that if they do not make a decision, they will never make a mistake. Initially, this approach may appear to work; but eventually the organization may cease to function effectively, or there may be mutiny on the part of the staff. At this point the manager is likely to be criticized for failing to produce results.

Because an organization is made up of humans, managers will be guilty of default from time to time. When this happens, the situation needs to be reevaluated and an action decision made. Sometimes the original action is still appropriate. Many times, however, the situation has escalated and is more difficult to resolve.

REVIEWING COMMITTEE WORK
Effectiveness of the RM process requires reviewing the minutes and actions of other committees and groups, with a view to integration of RM across the organization's activities. Risk-management-program **structures** vary depending on the size of the organization and the scope of services. Integration with organizational activities at all levels allows for efficient information exchange and proactive RM activities.

Many of the more traditional health-care activities include RM roles. Infection-control (IC) practitioners, patient representatives, utilization-review coordinators, case managers, safety officers, medical-information personnel, QA&I coordinators, patient-account representatives, administrators and managers, medical directors, staff developers, and nursing department managers all play key roles in the RM process, as do the various committees that exist in most organizations. Risk management programs today still address the key areas of risk identification, prevention, claims, and financing; with the integration of QM functions, however, RM becomes an organizational initiative rather than the activity of a single department. See Table 29-2 for a sample listing of RM activities.

Table 29-2 • EXAMPLES OF ORGANIZATIONAL RISK-MANAGEMENT ACTIVITIES BY DEPARTMENT

Administration
  Contracts
  Mergers
  Acquisitions

Patient Representation
  Complaint management

Dietary
  Nutritional management

Plant Engineering
  Building/exterior maintenance
  Water purity
  Temperature
  Construction
  Alarms

Environmental Services
  Waste management
  Needle disposal

Laboratory
  Release of pathological specimens
  Blood typing

Patient Accounts
  Billing
  Write-offs
  Complaint management

Social Services
  Discharge planning

Medical Information
  Release of records
  Attorney requests
  Coding

Medical Affairs Office
  Medical-staff applications
  Peer-review findings

Nursing
  Medication errors
  Patient falls

Personnel
  Applicant screening
  Disciplinary actions

Employee Health
  Drug screening
  Worker's compensation

Security
  Visitor control
  Intervention methods

Infection-Control Committee
  Policies
  Surveillance

Pharmacy-and-Therapeutics Committee
  Drug reactions

Institutional-Review Board
  Research activities
  Consents

Ethics Committee
  Treatment refusal
  Treatment conflicts

Bylaws Committee
  Medical-staff rules and regulations

Most clinical staff are involved on a continuing basis, in the review of RM and QM activities although not often defined as such. Traditional nursing problems and activities, such as medication errors, patient falls, and patient-staff relationships, are key identifiers of both risk and quality-improvement problems. These problems and activities become increasingly important as greater emphasis is placed on QM.

Traditional risk-identification systems such as incident reports, generic screens, outcome or event monitors, and reported complaints will become even more important as both data sources for identifying areas for improvement and as means to measure effectiveness of any changes implemented.

ASSESSING AND PROVIDING FOR RISK-MANAGEMENT EDUCATIONAL NEEDS

Identifying the educational needs of patients, families, and staff and then providing for those needs is a crucial step in risk reduction. For example, patient education is essential if a patient is to comply with orders of "nothing by mouth" before tests or surgery. In some instances, if the patient eats or drinks before surgery, there exists a danger of vomiting, aspiration, and, possibly, death. These are certainly complications an organization will insist in preventing. A second example is families needing education regarding both the use of the equipment in the patient's room and the procedure for summoning help for the patient. Failure to summon the nurse when needed can lead to untoward outcomes.

Staff education is also essential to the risk-prevention program. Staff education does not begin when the employee is hired; but, rather, it is a prerequisite to hiring. This means that it is essential that staff members be educationally prepared for the positions they hold. For example, it is desirable that a baccalaureate or master level nurse be selected for the position of discharge planner because this position requires a background in community-health nursing. The nursing preparation that includes this content is found at the baccalaureate and master nursing levels.

Some nursing leaders advocate that the nursing staff be as rigorously credentialed as the medical staff. Initial privileging, hiring, or contracting of professional staff should be thorough and include verification of all professional training and work experience. It is recommended that verification be confirmed in writing and supplemented with affirmation of applicants' abilities to perform the tasks of the positions for which they are applying. It is far simpler to prevent inappropriate privileging than it is to revoke staff privileges. While an unfilled position may appear to be a risk, it is a well-defined risk. Problems that could result from an unqualified practitioner constitute a much broader risk. It is important that essential competencies are predetermined and that personnel choices are made according to those competencies.

When personnel are hired, an effective orientation is essential to proactive risk reduction. New staff must be provided an extensive introduction to their job descriptions and how the organization supports their functioning within it. For example, Licensed Practical (Vocational) nurses need to be assured that they will not be expected to function as Registered Nurses. To avoid organizational risk in this example, the differences between the job descriptions of the registered and the practical nurse are explained. It is imperative that the organization orient the new staff to the environment, protocols, safety for self and those they serve, and the procedures they will be expected to perform. This process also allows the facility to observe the newly hired employee and confirm that the individual is prepared to take on the intended responsibilities.

As staff continue in positions, they are introduced to new techniques and technology, and they must relearn those functions that are utilized infrequently. Written standards dictate that there will be continuous evaluation of training methods and performance. Annual evaluations, based on objective data that incorporates patient safety and cost effectiveness, are required. It is no longer acceptable to base privileging or continued employment solely on initial training. And there will be an increasing need for competency-based evaluations that demonstrate ability to comply with accepted standards of practice.

RISK-MANAGEMENT EVALUATION

Like other programs and departments, it is important that the RM program be evaluated at least annually. There should be a comprehensive evaluation plan. Everyone involved in the program must be aware of which components will be evaluated, and the standard for each component must be clearly delineated.

REPORTS TO ADMINISTRATION

The final step in the RM process involves the production of reports. These reports are to be completed and forwarded to the appropriate committee or person. They may go to the medical staff, the various administrators, or the board of directors of the organization.

Risk-Management Committee

Most authors discussing the function of a RM committee agree that an **interdisciplinary** approach to RM, with representatives from medicine, nursing, medical records, legal counsel, education, and insurance claims, is preferential. The committee typically is composed of the risk manager; a nursing-service administrator; a nurse manager, a staff nurse, one to three medical staff representatives; chairs of the QA&I, utilization-review, IC, pharmacy, and operating-room committees; a patient-accounts representative; and legal counsel (ex officio). The education and training coordinator and insurance claims representative may be on the committee or may be invited to participate on an as-needed basis.

THE ROLE OF THE COMMITTEE

The committee's purpose is to develop and promote appropriate measures to minimize risk to patients and hospital personnel and to carry out the RM activities described earlier. The committee also establishes programs for increasing staff awareness, detection, education, and proper reporting of risk potential and incidents.

THE ROLE OF THE NURSE

In the hospital setting, nursing is the one department involved in patient care twenty-four hours a day. Nursing personnel are critical to the success of an RM program. It is imperative that the chief nurse administrator be committed to the program and convey this commitment to the nursing staff. If the staff is aware of the nurse administrator's support, this will influence their participation in the RM program. It is the nursing staff, with their daily patient contact, who actually contribute most to the implemention of a RM program. In many hospitals the risk manager is a nurse.

Claims statistics generated nationally by insurance companies have consistently shown that the five highest risk areas in acute care are: (1) medication errors, (2) complications from diagnostic or treatment procedures, (3) falls, (4) patient or family dissatisfaction with care, and (5) refusal of treatment or to sign consent for treatment. Nursing is involved in all five areas. Medical records and incident reports are used to document hospital, nurse, and physician accountability. If nurses are supportive of the RM program, their documentation can be expected to be more complete and acccurate. Also, they will be more likely to file incident reports, especially if they believe the report will be used in the RM program rather than in their personal evaluation.

Nurses are certainly the persons best positioned to develop an atmosphere where patients and their families feel respected as individuals and where the customers feel that care received has been adequate. Patients who express satisfaction with their care rarely sue, even when unanticipated outcomes occur. Key behaviors nurses can use to deal with adverse situations are (1) listening and being responsive to the patient and family, (2) documenting the facts and the patient's physical and psychological responses in the medical record, and (3) filing an incident report. The fact that an incident report was filed should *not* be documented in the record. The most important point from a RM perspective is that the nurse exhibit a caring attitude that reinforces the trustworthiness of the institution to the patient and family.

TRENDS AND ISSUES

There is no doubt that RM will continue to be a major concern within health-care organizations. Two pressing issues include the size of financial awards from litigated incidents and the adequacy of education and credentialing of professionals.

LIMITATION ON FINANCIAL LIABILITY

One solution to the ever-increasing number of claims and lawsuits, as well as to the amounts of these claims, is some form of legislation limiting these activities. Florida has led the way with this type of legislation, but other states have been slow to follow its lead. Whether health-care reform proposals will include this type of limitation is open to conjecture at this point.

Professional Credentialing

There does not appear to be any doubt that health-care organizations will provide improved credentialing of staff for purposes of reducing risk. The Association for State Boards of Nursing is discussing the possibility of requiring an internship for all new Registered Nurses, similar to that required for physicians. The body of knowledge that nurses must master has grown exponentially; it is no longer possible to provide enough clinical experience to allow new graduates to acquire both knowledge and highly developed technical skills. An internship is one solution being examined.

Another solution might be for organizations to extend the new employee orientation period. This is likely to become increasingly important as state boards implement computerized testing. This type of testing allows for earlier return of results; thus, new graduates will spend less time with temporary licenses. The advantage of the temporary license is the amount of supervision required. Under the new licensing format, the new graduate may start functioning independently much sooner than is presently the case. In addition, under the computerized-testing system, new graduates will be licensed at irregular intervals. This will necessitate new hiring and orientation procedures, or at least new vigilance in ascertaining that each new graduate becomes licensed.

CONCLUSION

As has been demonstrated, RM and QA&I are integrally related. But although the two processes are similar in form and function, there are significant differences. First, the motivation and focus differ. Risk management is concerned with protecting the health-care organization from liability and with diminishing the loss of corporate assets. Quality assessment and improvement focuses on protecting the patient. Risk management is concerned with delivery of a legally acceptable level of care, while QA&I strives to achieve an optimal level of care. Risk management must be concerned with all aspects of organizational operation and not just patient care.

Nevertheless, there are areas where these processes overlap. It has, therefore, been suggested that a system to prevent duplication between RM and QA&I would be beneficial. There are several advantages to such a proposal. Because health-care organizations have limited resources, integration of these two processes would help maximize the use of existing resources such as data and personnel. For example, being that data sources for the two processes are often the same, integration of the database would prevent duplication. Centralizing the database would allow risk trends to be identified, leading to timely elimination of the causes of risks and errors. Also, communication between risk managers and QA&I professionals would be enhanced. By way of the two programs working together, the loss-control and patient-injury-prevention systems would be augmented.

A successful QA&I program will significantly increase the likelihood that the objectives of the RM program will be met, and vice versa.

REFERENCES

American College of Surgeons. (1985). *Patient safety manual 101* (2nd ed.). Chicago: Author.

Ashby, J., Stephens, S., & Pearson, S. (1977). Elements in successful risk reduction programs. *Hospital Progress*, July, Vol. 58, No. 7, p. 60.

Barzum, J. (1978, October). The profession under seige. *Harper's*, 38–41.

Dankmyer, T., & Groves, J. (1977, May 16). Taking steps for safety's sake. *Hospitals, 51*(10), 60–62, 66.

Griffith, R. L., & Johnston, D. M. (1992). *Texas hospital law: Vol. 2 (2nd ed.).* Salem, NH: Butterworth Legal Publishers.

Hudson, T. (1992, October). Hospitals find ways to integrate risk management functions. *Hospitals, 66*(20), 32, 34–36.

Illich, I. (1976). *Medical nemesis.* New York: Pantheon.

Management Memos. (1965). West Orange, NJ: The Economic Press.

Northrop, C., & Kelly, M. (1987). *Legal issues in nursing.* St. Louis, MO: C.V. Mosby.

Orlickoff, J., Fifer, W., & Greeley, H. (1981, July). *Malpractice prevention and liability control for hospitals.* Chicago: American Hospital Association.

Orlickoff, J., & Lanham, D. (1981, September). Why risk management and Quality Assurance should be integrated. *Hospitals, 55*(11), 54–55.

Sullivan, J., & Decker, P. (1988). *Effective management in nursing* (2nd ed). Menlo Park, CA: Addison-Wesley.

ADDITIONAL READING

Al-Assaf, A. F. (1992). Integrating Quality Assurance, risk management, and utilization review: The physician's perspective. In C. G. Meisenheimer (Ed.), *Improving quality: A guide to effective programs* (pp. 166–182). Gaithersburg, MD: Aspen.

Albein, S. H. (1994). Quality as a risk management tool. *Rehabilitation Management, 7*(2), 105–6.

Brown, B. J. (1979). *Risk management for hospitals: A practical approach.* Germantown, MD: Aspen Systems.

Champion, F. X. (Ed.). (1990). *Grand rounds on medical malpractice.* Chicago: American Medical Association.

Fiesta, J. (1983). *The law and liability: A guide for nurses.* New York: John Wiley & Sons.

Freedman, T. J., & Gerring, G. (1993). Focus on risk management. *Leadership in Health Services, 2*(3), 29–33.

Harpster, L. M., & Veach, M. S. (1990). *Risk management handbook for health care facilities.* Chicago: American Hospital Association.

Harpster, L. M., & Veach, M. S. (1991). *Risk management self assessment manual.* Chicago: American Society for Healthcare Risk Management.

Rakich, J., Longest, B., & Darr, K. (1985). *Managing health services organizations.* Philadelphia: W.B. Saunders.

Youngberg, B. (1994). *The risk manager's desk reference.* Gaithersburg, MD: Aspen.

PART VII

TRENDS, ISSUES, AND OPPORTUNITIES

Margo MacRobert
June A. Schmele

CHAPTER *30*

Redefinition of Quality Management Roles in a Time of Shifting Paradigms

INTRODUCTION

The current state of health-care reform permeates the health-care environment. As has been noted in previous chapters, these evolutionary changes are far reaching and have strongly influenced the quality perspective of health-care delivery. Many believe that these rapidly paced changes have resulted in dramatic paradigm shifts, one of which is the move toward **Total Quality Management (TQM)**. In essence, TQM promotes the creation of a culture whereby consumers and health-care professionals are empowered to improve and sustain every facet of the health-care delivery process. As part of this paradigm shift, there has been a dramatic change in mind set from "quality at all costs" to the realization that **quality** and cost-effective care are compatible and achievable expectations.

Responding to these changed values and philosophies, leaders have both empowered and have encouraged health-care staff members to accept quality as part of their jobs. Therefore, quality has now moved from being the concern of a few isolated individuals to being everyone's concern. These changes have brought about the need to examine individual job functions. According to McLaughlin and Kaluzny (1990), specific actions must occur to make a successful transition to TQM. Of these actions, several are related to changes in job functions of health-care professionals. Specifically, these actions speak to the need to redefine roles and to empower the staff to solve the issues that impede the delivery of quality care.

The major purpose of this chapter is to reintroduce the concept of role and to examine the components of role theory that relate to the role-transition process occurring in health-care organizations. Additionally, this chapter examines individual roles related to **Quality Management (QM)** and delineates the redefinition of those roles as they evolve to reflect the QM philosophy.

THE CONCEPT OF ROLE

The concept of *role* is extremely complex and many faceted. The common usage of the term refers to the actual and expected behaviors of a position holder (Hardy & Hardy, 1988). Using the context of systems, Kuhn (1974) defines role as the "set of system states and actions of a subsystem, of an organization, including its interactions with other systems or nonsystem elements" (p. 298). This definition acknowledges that the behaviors and actions of a single person are affected by the behaviors and actions of other persons or organizational groups. Consequently, any change or adjustment in one organizational subsystem or associated system produces a corresponding need for change in another part of the system.

The operationalization of role, according to Kuhn's definition, follows. Executives of a health-care organization decide to adopt a formal framework of QM. This programmatic adjustment causes far-reaching changes throughout the organization. In order to respond, the organization needs to be aware that this change may have adverse effects on the staff. The organization needs to ensure that the staff are well informed about the change and that support structures are established to assist staff in making successful transitions to the QM environment. Individuals working in the organization need to receive education and training regarding their functions in this new environment.

Role Stress and Role Strain

Role stress is defined as a general condition "when a social structure creates very difficult, conflicting, or impossible demands for occupants of positions within it" (Hardy & Hardy, 1988, p. 150). Role stress is an organizational condition manifested by role obligations that are vague, conflicting, or impossible to meet. *Role strain*, on the other hand, is the subjective feeling of tension and frustration experienced by the individuals working in an organization undergoing role stress.

If the health-care organization does not provide adequate support, education, and training to its employees, the employees will experience some confusion regarding their responsibilities in the QM program. This situation is descriptive of the concept of role stress. In light of the rapid changes surrounding health care, varying degrees of role stress will always be present in health-care organizations. It is important for the organization to identify role stress and to employ interventions to minimize its effects on the work environment.

Concepts Related to Role Stress

In order to more clearly illlustrate the phenomenon of role stress, it is necessary to briefly review the concepts of conflict, ambiguity, incongruity, and overload. *Role conflict* occurs when the expectations of a certain position are incompatible. For example, conflict occurs when an incumbent is asked to carry out many roles at the same time or when conflicts exist between persons regarding the responsibilities inherent in a given role (Hurley-Wilson, 1988). Role conflict may occur, for example, in a situation where a staff nurse is reluctant to participate in the review of **Quality-Assessment-and-Improvement (QA&I)** activities. Although the staff nurse's job description clearly identifies **accountability** for review of QA&I activities, the staff nurse may choose to leave that function for the manager to perform. There are many and varied reasons why this might occur: the nurse might be honoring past custom, may not own the accountability, or may not understand the importance of participation.

According to Hardy and Hardy (1988), *role ambiguity* is present when unclear role expectations exist. Unclear role expectations may result from disagreement between individuals regarding the expectations, lack of information about the job, or job demands that are vague to the role incumbent. Role ambiguity is common in the health-care arena. Whereas technical job descriptions contain descriptive detail, professional job descriptions are usually written in vague and general terms. It is important that organizational leaders and managers make every effort to clearly describe job expectations. It is recognized, however, that within the current health-care environment, there is likely to be increasing role ambiguity and a concomitant need for flexibility of response in order to lessen role problems.

Role incongruity exists when the skills and abilities of a role incumbent are incompatible with the role obligations. It may also occur when a role incumbent's attitudes and values are incompatible with the expected role behaviors (Hardy & Hardy, 1988). For example, a nurse may be working in an administrative position because of a need for additional monetary compensation; but the nurse actually prefers more direct patient contact. This creates a situation of role strain because the nurse places more value on direct patient care and may not feel totally committed to the demands of the administrative job.

Role overload occurs when "a role occupant experiences difficulty in fulfilling role obligations which are excessive relative to the limited time available" (Hardy & Hardy, 1988, p. 224). Role overload can occur when the individual occupies one role but is given too heavy a workload, or when an individual is expected to cover several roles that seem excessive to the individual. According to Hardy, a situation is not considered role overload unless it occurs for a prolonged period of time. The current work environment contains numerous examples of role overload.

Role Transition

The preceding discussion demonstrates that role strain can be a serious problem detrimental to health-care organizations. As health-care-reform efforts spur rapid and abundant change, the already chaotic health-care organization will produce more role stress in its attempts to change and reform itself to maintain viability.

As the health-care delivery system continues to change, health-care professionals will, of necessity, experience major role transition. Some established roles will be redefined, and new roles will emerge. As professionals move into new or redefined roles, role transition occurs, and role strain is highly probable (Hardy & Hardy, 1988).

Role redefinition is likely to be very apparent in the area of leadership and health-care QM. As organizations adopt the TQM philosophy, quality professionals will experience role changes that reflect the evolutionary changes in health care. Deliberate approaches may be helpful to assist with role development and the subsequent progression to the redefined role.

Little has been written regarding role development of quality professionals. Kibbee (1988) describes steps outlining the development of the **Quality-Assurance (QA)** professional. These steps consist of skill building, establishing a close working relationship with a supervisor, obtaining **certification**, using a mentor, and networking with other quality professionals.

Benner's (1985) framework of role development is well known for describing the progression of skill acquisition and role development of clinical nurses. Benner identifies five stages that describe the process of development. Masters, Acquaye, MacRobert, and Schmele (1990) use this framework to describe their experiences progressing through various stages in the development of the nursing QA coordinator position. They identify experiences in each of the five stages of novice, advanced beginner, competent, proficient, and expert.

In summary, an understanding of role theory, especially the components related to role stress and role transition, will benefit individuals and organizations as they experience the effects of a rapidly changing health-care system. Additionally, the ability to redefine roles in response to the changes will enable organizations to facilitate transition. The position holder's ability to recognize and accept a certain degree of ambiguity and flexibility will be an asset to role redefinition.

QUALITY-MANAGEMENT ROLES

Following is a discussion of the various potential roles for health-care professionals involved in QM. Expectations of the specific role in the traditional QA environment are compared to expectations of the role in the TQM environment of today. In addition, preparation needed to successfully fulfill each of these roles is discussed. Table 30-1 lists these roles along corresponding role statements related to QM.

Table 30-1 • SELECT ROLES AND CORRESPONDING ROLE STATEMENTS RELATED TO QUALITY MANAGEMENT	
Chief Executive Officer	• Promotes the QM philosophy • Creates an environment supportive of QM activities • Demonstrates complete commitment to the QM program • Participates in the provision of QM education to staff • Provides necessary resources to ensure QM success • Serves as consultant to work groups concerning the QM process
Physician	• Provides expert clinical perspective for QM endeavors • Creates an environment supportive of QM activities • Promotes a "team player" attitude and creates an interdisciplinary environment • Serves as a consultant to other physicians and work groups • Demonstrates knowledge of QM processes • Assists with the development and implementation of practice guidelines
Chief Nurse Executive	• Same as for Chief Executive Officer, plus • Accountable for QM activities for the nursing department • Accountable for the development and implementation of practice standards

---

Table 30-1 • **SELECT ROLES AND CORRESPONDING ROLE STATEMENTS RELATED TO QUALITY MANAGEMENT** (*continued*)

Quality Manager	• Facilitates implementation of the QM plan • Disseminates information regarding QM activities • Evaluates QM findings and guides in problem-solving efforts to improve care • Serves as QM continuous-improvement leader/facilitator • Serves as consultant regarding QM continuous-improvement process • Provides education regarding QM continuous-improvement process • Demonstrates computer competency • Mentors unit-based QM coordinators • Maintains current knowledge of and interprets accreditation standards
Risk Manager	• Serves as consultant regarding safety and liability issues • Evaluates situations that are hazardous and takes corrective action to prevent • Provides education to staff regarding safety • Maintains current knowledge of safety codes and interprets same to the organization • Participates in continuous-improvement teams; may be team leader
Utilization Manager	• Monitors patient care to evaluate services and ensure maximum reimbursement • Maintains current knowledge and/or interprets reimbursement criteria • Facilitates organizationwide problem solving to maximize reimbursement • Participates in quality-improvement teams; may be team leader
Staff Nurse	• Provides expert nursing care perspective to QM endeavors • Maintains current knowledge of practice standards • Participates in the development of QM plan • Assists with data collection in QM studies • Assists with the formulation of action plans • Identifies opportunities to improve care • Represents nursing on QM committee and continuous-improvement work groups
Nurse Manager	• Accountable for QM activities on specific nursing units • Identifies opportunities to improve care • Models QM philosophy to staff • Participates in provision of QM education

Executive Level

The success or failure of any QM effort rests squarely on the shoulders of the organization's chief executive officer (CEO). The primary function of the CEO is to enhance the vision and mission by leading the organizational transformation from a provider to a customer focus. Subsequently, the CEO must emphasize and model the changed philosophy. Through the CEO's actions, it will become obvious to others in the organization that the priority is the customer. As Arnold (1993) states, "unless the leader is totally committed to the program both personally and professionally, the organization is better off not starting it at all. When leaders send mixed messages . . . this causes great dysfunction in the organization with disastrous results" (p. 79).

The role of the CEO extends to ensuring that partnerships with other organizational and medical-staff executives are sound and that they echo the commitment to the TQM process. Most importantly, the CEO must alter leadership style away from one of power and control to one that exudes and encourages trust, respect, and determination (Jaeghers, 1991). This role transition is often referred to as a shift from management and administration to leadership, which is a vastly different role.

This role transition or paradigm shift generally is brought about through knowledge acquisition that leads to attitude change. Most CEOs and other members of the executive level already have advanced degrees in health administration. The importance of formal or informal advanced executive-level education and training in QM concepts is made clear by TQM experts, who insist that TQM education and training begin at the executive level.

The Physician

The role of the physician in QM has undergone a major evolution. Previously, the physician might have participated in QA activities by chairing a QA committee or reviewing QA data. The physician is now required to maintain a level of accountability, to promote the TQM philosophy, and to work as a team player on an **interdisciplinary** level. This is quite a transition from the physician role of the past — where the physician focused on provision of medical care and had minimal involvement in organizational programs or concerns.

The physician has immense knowledge and understanding of clinical perspectives in the health-care environment. This input is very important as alternatives are explored and recommendations are made to change the health-care delivery **structures, processes**, and **outcomes**. One of the ways that improvements are being promulgated is through the use of clinical practice guidelines, especially those created by the Agency for Health Care Policy and Research (AHCPR, 1994). These interdisciplinary, **consumer**-based guidelines have been derived from the research and evaluation of scientific health and medical-care practice. (See Chapter 9 for discussion of AHCPR guidelines.) It is through the team development and implementation of practice guidelines such as these that physicians and members of other disciplines identify the components of quality health and medical care, and actively pursue mechanisms to demonstrate accountability for improvements in quality.

Physicians are assuming a more active role in QM activities. In order to participate in these activities, physicians are challenged to acquire knowledge and maintain skills in quality-improvement processes such as data management and group process, among others. For example, physicians may serve as consultants to other physicians or actively participate in work groups. In addition, physicians increasingly are gaining management and business skills through formal and informal educational avenues. This additional preparation is an asset and a necessity for those physicians actively engaging in the leadership of health-care organizations. Batalden, Berwick, Donabedian, and Laffel are among those physicians who are exerting strong leadership roles in the improvement of health care.

Chief Nurse Executive

The chief nurse executive (CNE) holds a key role in the TQM process as well as in all of the related QM functions. The CNE often is the "care expert" in the senior- or executive-level management group. In this capacity the CNE provides important information relative to clinical care and issues affecting consumer satisfaction, and does so from a nursing as well as a health-care perspective. In addition, the CNE, much like the CEO, models the TQM philosophy, especially to the nursing staff, but to the total organization as well.

The CNE may be accountable for those persons holding specialized staff positions in QM, such as the QA&I manager, the QM coordinator, and others. The CNE, therefore, has a direct role in **monitoring** and **evaluating** important aspects of service, and ensuring that these services are improved on a continuing basis. Ideally, the CNE has advanced formal educational preparation in nursing, as well as in administration. This preparation provides the CNE with an extensive knowledge base concerning nursing and management theories, delivery-of-care models, and clinical aspects of care. Ideally, this preparation will also provide formal training in the science of QM.

The Quality-Management Professional

Little has been written regarding the role of the QM professional until recently. The entire July 1993 issue of the *Journal of Nursing Care Quality* was devoted to the role of the nursing quality professional. Clearly this is a position that has experienced tremendous change in the past five to seven years.

Organizations differ greatly in the titles that they assign to this role. Titles such as QA coordinator, quality-improvement coordinator, QA&I coordinator, and quality manager are just a few of those in prominent use. The majority of incumbents in these positions are Registered Nurses, although members of other disciplines are assuming key QM roles as the field evolves.

With the evolution to TQM, this role has dramatically changed and greatly expanded. The QA position holders of times past were largely perceived as "police" — that is, these individuals were frequently data gatherers and monitors of indicators to determine compliance. They did not generally focus on the total practice environment, but only a segmented portion of the health-care organization. Kibbee (1988) states that the function of the QA nurse was "to assess and evaluate indicators of nursing care in actual practice. They conduct problem-focused studies, and more importantly, provide continuous, systematic monitoring of nursing processes and outcomes" (p. 30).

The advent of TQM and new forms of QM led to expanded roles as evidenced by both job enlargement and job enrichment. Today, quality managers are not so much involved in specific monitoring and evaluation activities as they are in acting as quality process experts in such capacities as coach, facilitator, and consultant. In many organizations these individuals are the knowledge experts in group process, continuous-improvement measurement, and statistical testing, among other areas. In essence, the role of quality professional has two major components. The first component is operational in nature and consists of facilitating the development and implementation of the QM plan, disseminating information regarding activities, evaluating QM findings, and maintaining current knowledge of **accreditation** standards. The second component consists of providing information and feedback regarding the QM process, serving as a continuous-improvement leader/facilitator, providing education to the organization regarding continuous-improvement methods, functioning as quality-improvement expert, and establishing self as mentor to unit-based QM coordinators or TQM teams — in short, serving as a consultant.

According to Parisi, Johnson, and Keill (1993), the quality professional must possess an exceptional degree of management ability and skills in areas such as resource management, information management, and problem solving. Additionally, because these position holders usually are accountable for facilitating continuous-improvement teams, they should possess effective interpersonal and group skills. Advanced formal education in health care and a strong experiential base is preferred for the individual in this role. Parisi and others consider the baccalaureate degree as a minimal requirement for those holding key QM positions. Graduate education is highly preferred because these roles require advanced knowledge of organizational behavior, systems theory, information management, and the change process, as well as superb communication and problem-solving skills. It is also important that the QM professional have past work experience that includes a strong clinical and leadership base.

Staff Nurses

Although professional staff nurses are accountable to the public for the quality of nursing care, previous to the advent of TQM, staff nurses usually held passive roles in the actual QA process. At most, these professionals would participate in data collection for QA studies and provide input for planning improvement actions.

In the TQM environment, staff nurses participate in the decision making affecting them and their work environment. They are involved in work-process teams, often with professionals from other departments. Nurses frequently serve as leaders or members of continuous-improvement teams. Nurses' involvement in these teams is crucial because they function as patient advocates while providing a strong clinical base for the other team members.

In addition to formal education in the management of quality, staff nurses need further education and in-house training on TQM philosophy and continuous-improvement concepts in order to fully participate in quality processes in the changing environment. The organization usually establishes educational programs for these individuals to prepare them for their roles in the new organization.

The Nurse Manager

The nurse manager holds a pivotal position in the QM environment. Much like the CEO and CNE, the nurse manager models the new philosophy to immediate staff as well as to the organization at large. Additionally, the nurse manager is accountable for the unit-based QM plan — its implementation and evaluation. The nurse manager maintains ultimate accountability for identification of problems and opportunities to improve care, while taking the appropriate actions to actually improve care. The nurse manager often is a member of the quality-improvement team and may act as the team leader. The nurse manager must have a strong knowledge of quality-improvement methods and the ability to act in a consultative role to nursing staff regarding the improvement process.

The nurse manager's current function in quality endeavors is quite different from that of past manager's involved in QA. Previously, nurse managers played active parts in the QA process on the unit level. They were accountable for the unit-based QA and its subsequent implementation and evaluation. It was often the nursing QA coordinator, however, who held the function of QA process expert and consultant.

In addition to in-house training on TQM philosophy and continuous-improvement concepts, it is strongly recommended that nurse managers have advanced formal education. This education ideally consists of a baccalaureate degree in nursing, and graduate education in nursing administration or business. Ideally this preparation will include at least the key concepts of the quality-management specialty. This background is necessary because the nurse manager in today's complex environment is required to possess an expert level of management competencies as well as superb interpersonal skills.

The Role of Professional Organizations in the Improvement of Quality of Care

Professional organizations assume a strong position in the development of quality-improvement environments in health-care settings. Most notably, the American Nurses Association *Standards of Clinical Nursing Practice* (1991) is just one of many documents delineating the professional responsibilities of nurses in various roles and settings. The standard addressing quality of care, as shown in Table 30-2, specifically defines the role component and guides the practice of the professional nurse in the quality improvement of nursing practice.

In sum, it becomes clear that an early definition of the quality component of the nurse's role is essential. The clarification of role behaviors in the form of professional standards, expectations, and subsequent evaluation is essential to the establishment of a quality environment .

Related Positions

It is desirable that risk managers have a major role in TQM. Their primary role is to evaluate situations and implement strategies to prevent or minimize the occurrence of injury or loss in the health-care organization. These individuals also serve as safety consultants and educators to the organization. Additionally, the risk manager maintains a current knowledge of regulations, such as safety codes and rules, and interprets these regulations for the organization. These individuals often serve as members on continuous-improvement teams. Their presence is valuable because they provide expert knowledge related to their specific role. (See Chapter 29 for a detailed discussion of risk management and its role relationships to QM.)

The role of the utilization manager (utilization review coordinator) is to monitor the medical necessity of care to ensure that the care will be appropriately reimbursed.

Table 30-2 • **STANDARDS OF PROFESSIONAL PERFORMANCE**

Standard I. Quality of Care

THE NURSE SYSTEMATICALLY EVALUATES THE QUALITY AND
EFFECTIVENESS OF NURSING PRACTICE.

Measurement Criteria

1. The nurse participates in quality of care activities as appropriate to the individual's position, education, and practice environment. Such activities may include:
   • Identification of aspects of care important for quality monitoring.
   • Identification of indicators used to monitor quality and effectiveness of nursing care.
   • Collection of data to monitor quality and effectiveness of nursing care.
   • Analysis of quality data to identify opportunities for improving care.
   • Formulation of recommendations to improve practice or client outcomes.
   • Implementation of activities to enhance the quality of nursing practice.
   • Participation on interdisciplinary teams that evaluate clinical practice or health services.
   • Development of policies and procedures to improve quality of care.

2. The nurse uses the results of quality-of-care activities to initiate changes in practice.

3. The nurse uses the results of quality-of-care activities to initiate changes throughout the health care delivery system, as appropriate.

Reprinted with permission from Standards of Clinical Nursing Practice, *p. 13. Copyright 1991, American Nurses Association, Washington, DC.*

These individuals have broad knowledge regarding reimbursement guidelines, and they act as reimbursement consultants to the organization. The role of the utilization manager frequently includes key TQM components such as continuous-improvement team leadership or membership. (See Chapter 27 for a detailed discussion of utilization management and its role relationships to QM.)

There are various other organizational roles that deal somewhat specifically with the management of quality. The infection control manager and the safety manager roles embody implicit and explicit references to the management of quality. Certainly, the prevention of infections and of accidents is by its very nature a standard related to the improvement of care quality.

QUALITY-MANAGEMENT ROLES: FUTURE TRENDS AND ISSUES

An objective of QM in health care is to continue to promote the active involvement of all members of the health-care team in quality-improvement activities. Leaders will continue to empower staff to take advantage of opportunities to improve processes, thereby improving organizational performance and customer satisfaction. The demand for cost containment will continue to be one of the greatest challenges to the health-care worker of the future.

The health-care team will assume a most important role in the future of QM as they work as a unit to improve quality while reducing costs of services. Ideally, this team will no longer work as a separate departmental entity in their efforts to address quality. Interdisciplinary work teams that include physicians and address cross-departmental patient-care issues as a whole rather than on a departmental, fragmented, or turf-bound basis, will become more predominant.

Most individuals currently involved in quality-improvement efforts obtain QM-related knowledge and skills from seminars or on-the-job training. With the likely increased emphasis on QM in the future, it will be necessary to ensure that QM concepts are somehow integrated into formal programs of study.

Larson (1992) states, "Nursing educators must lay the foundation for competence in assessing and assuring quality by instilling the idea that every nurse is accountable for professional practice. Socialization to the role of evaluation must begin as early as possible" (p. 226). Undergraduate educators currently are grappling with what students need to know about QM, and whether a complete course of study is indicated or whether QM should be integrated into the overall undergraduate program.

Similar issues, as discussed by Schmele (1992), are relevant to graduate education. There is a need for all advanced practitioners to have a knowledge base that will support their ability to evaluate and improve their own practice. Further, the increasingly interdisciplinary nature of patient care requires a systems view rather than a fragmented, and sometimes competitive, guarding of turf. It would seem that advanced education providing opportunites for interdisciplinary approaches to improvement of patient-care quality and organizational performance would serve as a basis for effective functioning in the work setting. The issue remains whether or not it is adequate to integrate a knowledge base about the management of quality throughout a curriculum or whether there needs to be a specialized approach to the science of QM. There may also be a need for specialized QM courses for those who will function in key roles as QM specialists. From all appearances, the science of QM in health care will continue to rapidly emerge during the decade ahead. This presents a challenge to colleges and universities — to ensure adequate preparation to meet the role demands of the future.

CONCLUSION

The promotion of quality and the prevention of "unquality" is inherent in every role in an organization committed to TQM. As previously discussed, this role is more specifically delineated in some positions than in others. Ironically, at the present time, a majority of the QM role components deal with preventing unquality rather than promoting quality. The ideal scenario of the future, however, is one wherein quality is so much a part of everyone's role that work processes are done correctly the first time. Thus, roles created to prevent and deal with unquality may tend to disappear.

In light of the move toward role transition in response to the QM philosophy, the need to understand the process of role transition and the subsequent need for role development becomes apparent. In the future, new QM roles will appear, some roles will be redefined, and each employee's role will embody a clearer accountability for quality. This context creates the need to deliberately plan role changes in order to lessen role stress and enhance productivity and quality of care.

REFERENCES

Agency for Health Care Policy and Research. (May, 1994). AHCPR invites proposals to evaluate guideline effects. *Research Activities, 174,* 15.

American Nurses Association. (1991). *Standards of Clinical Nursing Practice.* Kansas City, MO: Author.

Arnold, W. (1993). The leader's role in implementing quality improvement. Walking the talk. *Quality Review Bulletin, 19*(3), 79–82.

Benner, P. (1985). *From novice to expert: Excellence and power in clinical nursing.* Reading, MA: Addison-Wesley.

Hardy, M., & Hardy, W. (1988). Role stress and role strain. In M. Hardy & M. Conway (Eds.), *Role Theory: Perspectives for Health Professionals* (2nd ed., pp. 159–239). Norwalk, CT: Appleton & Lange.

Hurley-Wilson, B. (1988). Socialization for roles. In M. Hardy & M. Conway (Eds.), *Role Theory: Perspectives for Health Professionals* (2nd ed., pp. 73–110). Norwalk, CT: Appleton & Lange.

Jaeghers, S. (1991). TQM: A CEO's perspective. *The Quality Letter for Healthcare Leaders, 3*(8), 11–13.

Kibbee, P. (1988). An emerging professional: The Quality Assurance nurse. *The Journal of Nursing Administration, 18*(4), 30–33.

Kuhn, A. (1974). *The logic of social systems.* San Francisco: Jossey-Bass.

Larson, E. (1992). Teaching Quality Assurance: The undergraduate student/faculty experience. In C. Meisenheimer (Ed.), *Improving quality: A guide to effective programs* (pp. 226–259). Gaithersburg, MD: Aspen.

Masters, F., Acquaye, M., MacRobert, M., & Schmele, J. (1990). Role development: The nursing Quality Assurance coordinator. *Journal of Nursing Quality Assurance, 4*(2), 51–62.

McLaughlin, C., & Kaluzny, A. (1990). Total Quality Management in health: Making it work. *Health Care Management Review, 15*(3), 7–14.

Parisi, L., Johnson, T., & Keill, P. (1993). The nursing quality professional: A role in transition. *Journal of Nursing Care Quality, 7*(4), 1–5.

Schmele, J. A. (1992). Teaching Quality Management: The graduate experience. In C. Meisenheimer (Ed.), *Improving quality: A guide to effective programs* (pp. 260–281). Gaithersburg, MD: Aspen.

ADDITIONAL READING

Hardy, M., & Conway, M. (Eds.). (1988). *Role theory: Perspectives for health professionals* (2nd ed.). Norwalk, CT: Appleton & Lange.

Largen, C. W. (1994). Bringing quality to the customer: A new paradigm for quality managers. *Journal of Nursing Care Quality, 8*(2), 81–84.

Norman, D. K., Randall, R. S., & Hornsby, B. J. (1990). Critical features of a curriculum in health care quality and resource management. *Quality Review Bulletin, 6*(9), 317–336.

U.S. Department of Health and Human Services. (1993, April). *AHCPR fact sheet* (AHCPR Publication No. 93-0055). Washington, DC: Author.

Verhey, M. P., & Haw, M. B. (1994). Teaching Quality Management in a nursing graduate program: A collaborative university-agency quality team. *Journal of Nursing Care Quality, 8*(4), 48–54.

Laura L. Cross

CHAPTER *31*

Legal Implications of Quality Management

INTRODUCTION

The legal system's impact on the delivery of health care has greatly increased over the past two decades. The development of **Quality-Management (QM)** programs has mirrored that impact. Although originally unrelated, the two are now closely intertwined. The focus of this chapter is the legal system as it applies to health-care delivery and the implications for QM.

SOURCES OF THE LAW

The law generally can be defined as a set of rules or principles that command or restrain people or entities from doing certain things. These rules or principles have four primary sources. The law in any given case generally looks like a jigsaw puzzle, with various pieces from different sources. Generally, there are gaps or missing pieces of law for any given situation.

Constitutions

The most fundamental and overriding source of law is *constitutions* — both federal and individual state constitutions. In general, a constitution delineates an individual's rights, as well as differentiates the responsibilities of the various branches of government. While the federal constitution is the law of the land, each state also has its own constitution. The federal constitution sets out the basic, or minimum, rights. A state's constitution can provide for greater rights but cannot fall below the minimum provided in the federal constitution. The federal constitution can be amended, but such amendments are difficult to pass because ratification by two-thirds of the states is required. State constitutions are generally more readily amended by popular vote of the citizens of the state voting in a general election.

Statutes

The second source of law is *statutes*. Also termed *codes* in some jurisdictions, these are rules set down in print form by the legislative branch of a state or the federal government. Federal statutes are established by Congress; state statutes are established by the various state legislatures. After statutes are enacted, they can be amended or repealed.

Regulations

Regulations are the third source of law. Regulations are developed by government officials to implement state statutes. Hundreds of proposed and final regulations are issued by the federal and state governments every working day. These regulations are developed by various agencies. Most are adopted following a prescribed comment and objection period. There are regulations that address almost every aspect of our daily lives; many of these are unknown to most of us.

Common Law

The fourth source of law is the *common law*. The common law includes principles, usages, and rules that do not rely for their authority on any expressed declaration such as a statute, code, or constitution. The common law is based on court decisions. Past cases become precedents for future cases that rest on similar facts and are interpreted according to the same reasoning. The common law represents a gradual accumulation of decisions. Some of the decisions are based on long-term custom or are guided by principles of fairness.

All of the states except Louisiana adopted the English common law; Louisiana adopted the Napoleonic Code, which codifies the French common law. Each state has developed its own common law based on its adopted precedent. Thus, the common law may differ greatly among various states. There is also a body of federal common law.

LEGAL THEORIES IMPOSING LIABILITY

A number of legal theories have been used successfully in recent years to impose liability on providers based on the care provided by another. The theory of *respondeat superior* holds that an employer is responsible for the acts or omissions of its employees. The *ostensible agency rule* provides that an entity may be liable for the acts or omissions of one who is not an employee, but appears to be one. Entities may also be found liable under a theory of *corporate liability*. Under the corporate liability theory, the corporation is held to be liable for allowing incompetent physicians or other health-care providers to provide services within the facility.

TYPES OF ACTIONS

The cause or type of action brought against the defendant in a lawsuit depends on which theory of liability is asserted. Most, if not all, jurisdictions, whether state or federal, allow for the assertion of more than one theory of liability against a defendant.

Actions are generally divided into civil, administrative, and criminal. The same conduct may give rise to claims under various theories of civil liability, as well as allegations of violation of administrative and criminal law. Criminal and administrative prosecutions for alleged misconduct are tried separately from civil lawsuits.

Like criminal law, administrative law falls under the category of public law. Administrative law differs from criminal law mainly in that the activities defined are in the form of regulations established by an administrative or bureaucratic agency. Violation of a regulation generally carries with it imposition of a penalty in the form of restricting or restraining a provider's right to practice. This restriction may pass through to the individual if the agency **licenses** practitioners or to the facility if the agency regulates the licensing of agencies.

The burden of proof used by licensing agencies generally is a preponderance of the evidence. The burden of proof in criminal cases is "beyond a reasonable doubt." Therefore, it is not unusual for misconduct that violates a criminal law to result in loss of license but not be prosecuted as a criminal violation because there is not sufficient evidence to meet the higher burden of proof.

Various civil theories may be alleged in the same civil lawsuit. Such theories may include violation of constitutional rights, breach of contract, or tort. *Tort law* deals with a legal wrong committed by one person on the person or property of another. It is not based on any contractual obligation, but on the breach of some duty. It may be based on the breach of a private duty or the infraction of some public duty. As an example, a person who fails to stop his automobile at a stop sign would violate a public law. Civil liability for damage incurred in an automobile collision caused by the failure to stop would fall on the driver, who breached his duty by failing to stop at the stop sign.

Malpractice is professional negligence or unreasonable lack of skill. Malpractice differs from other torts in that providers are held to a higher duty or **standard** of care based on their superior knowledge and skill. The standard of care is often set by the profession rather than the public. Because of the superior knowledge and skill inherent in the service, the exact duty of care or standard to which the defendant should be held is not easily determined by a lay person serving as either a judge or the jury. Therefore, the court must rely on "expert witnesses" who are knowledgeable in the field to interpret the standard of practice for the particular case. The expert witness assists the court in determining whether or not the defendant's conduct fell below that standard and whether the negligent act was the cause of the alleged injury. Although this sounds simple, difficulty arises when the court hears conflicting testimony by expert witnesses who may represent differing, though legitimate, schools of thought or application of standards.

STANDARDS OF PRACTICE

Traditionally, the standard of practice within any area was the standard of practice in that community. Under this local community doctrine, it became increasingly difficult to obtain an objective expert witness from the community. Many jurisdictions have eliminated the "locality rule" and adopted a national standard that looks to what a prudent and competent peer of the defendant would do under the same or similar circumstances. The community where the defendant practices has become one of many factors used in determining whether the defendant's conduct measures up to the professional standard that society would expect. The actual standard of practice is generally a national standard; this allows experts from all over the country to testify in any given case.

According to the individual case, Joint Commission on Accreditation of Healthcare Organizations (Joint Commission) standards, standards developed by professional organizations, policies and procedures, equipment literature, drug information, textbooks, journals, and other learned treatises may be used to establish the standard of care. There are more than 20,000 health-care standards, guidelines, laws, and regulations published by some 500 organizations and agencies, which are listed in the *Health Care Standards Directory* (1993).

Severe problems occur when an entity has established its own policies and procedures that it failed to meet. In such a case the defendant has established the standard of practice that was not met. Similarly, professional organization standards that are truly aspirations rather than accomplishable standards establish a standard that may be used against a practitioner. Providers of health care should carefully monitor which standards are adopted and be sure that only attainable standards are adopted.

CLINICAL-PRACTICE GUIDELINES

The federal government is now involved in establishing standards through its Clinical Practice Guidelines Program sponsored by the **Agency for Health Care Policy and Research (AHCPR)**. This agency was established in 1989 by Congress to develop and disseminate guidelines to assist patients and practitioners in making decisions about dealing with various clinical conditions. Based on scientific evidence and the judgment of clinical experts, **interdisciplinary** panels develop guidelines for practice related to specific **outcomes**. The first three sets of guidelines released deal with acute pain, urinary incontinence, and prevention of pressure sores (Agency for Health Care Policy and Research [AHCPR], 1993). Nurses have substantial responsibility for each of these conditions. Other conditions for which guidelines are being developed include Alzheimer's disease and related dementias, unstable angina, low-back problems, management of cancer-related pain, cardiac rehabilitation, heart failure, HIV, quality determinants of mammography, otitis media in children, sickle cell disease, treatment of pressure ulcers, and post-stroke rehabilitation (Jacox, 1993). These guidelines will be very strong evidence of the standard of care for the conditions addressed. (See Chapter 9 for additional information on the AHCPR guidelines.)

COMPUTERIZED PROGNOSTICATORS

With the introduction of computers into everyday aspects of life, it naturally follows that computers will be used to determine measures of care. The best-known computer prognosticator is the APACHE system. APACHE is an acronym for acute, physiology, age, and chronic health evaluation. Its methodology was originally developed in 1978 by Dr. William Knaus and a team of researchers at George Washington University in Washington, DC (Knaus et al., 1991). Now in its third generation, the APACHE system can be used as a means of evaluating an intensive care unit's performance in terms of traditional mortality and length-of-stay data. The system is also used to evaluate resource consumption, appropriateness of bed use, and unit efficiency.

There are a number of other computerized programs that can establish standards of practice. The HELP program developed at the University of Utah and marketed by the 3M Company analyzes patient information such as lab results and drugs taken and issues alerts if anything seems wrong. The Gofer System developed by Regenstrief Institute in Indianapolis is a program that is supposed to cut back on unnecessary lab work simply by letting doctors know how likely it is that a given test will come back with an uneventful result. The Quick Medical Reference (QMR) is sold by Camdat. This program suggests possible diagnoses when symptoms are entered. Massachusetts General Hospital has developed DXplain, which similarly proposes diagnoses based on input of particular symptoms. Continued development and expanded use of such computerized standards of practice will certainly occur. And while they rely on probabilities rather than facts, computerized standards will certainly become more important in QM. (See Chapter 25 for a detailed discussion on the use of computers to support QM.)

LAWS AND STANDARDS APPLICABLE TO QUALITY MANAGEMENT

Traditionally, QM activities were directed primarily in the area of peer review. More recently, however, programs and policies have been designed to measure and improve general quality of care. As these activities have developed, it has become evident that laws and standards are needed to support QM activities.

Peer-Review Laws

Many states have had peer-review laws in effect for several years (Ala. Code §§ 34-24-58 et al.). Federal peer-review law was enacted with the Health Care Quality Improvement Act of 1986 (HCQIA). The purpose of the HCQIA is three-fold: first, improve the overall quality of health care; second, restrict the ability of incompetent physicians to move from state to state without disclosure or discovery of past performance; and third, encourage and protect good faith participation in peer-review activities by practitioners. The HCQIA requires physicians and facilities to report payments made on behalf of practitioners as a result of medical malpractice actions and claims. It also requires reporting of adverse actions taken regarding the license or clinical privileges of physicians and dentists. The HCQIA establishes a national data bank to serve as a national source of information regarding physicians, dentists, and other health-care practitioners. The reporting requirements apply to hospitals; health-care entities; boards of medical examiners; and professional societies of physicians, dentists, and other licensed health-care practitioners. The requirements also apply to insurance companies and other individuals and entities making payment with respect to medical malpractice actions or claims. Reports of information relating to nonphysician health-care providers is discretionary under the HCQIA. Disclosure of information reported to the data bank is limited by the HCQIA. In addition, the HCQIA provides protections and immunities, with certain limited exceptions, from damages and antitrust liability for good faith participation in reporting peer-review matters.

Medicare and Medicaid Patient and Program Protection Act

The Medicare and Medicaid Patient and Program Protection Act of 1987 is designed to protect Medicare and Medicaid beneficiaries from poor-quality or unnecessary services. Combined with the HCQIA, it provides for mandatory and discretionary exclusions from participation in the Medicare and Medicaid program of practitioners whose misconduct is reported to the national data bank.

Peer Review Improvement Act

The Peer Review Improvement Act of 1982 authorizes professional review organizations (PROs) to contract for the review of services provided to Medicare beneficiaries. The PRO's review is to determine (1) reasonableness and medical necessity of the services provided; (2) whether the quality of services provided meets professionally recognized standards; and (3) whether services could have been effectively provided more economically on an outpatient basis or at an inpatient facility of a different type. The PRO develops **criteria** that identify the **norms** of care, diagnosis, and treatment typical to the locality. The PRO, however, may consider national standards where deemed appropriate. Where there has been a substantial failure to comply with statutory requirements, sanctions may be imposed, including exclusion from participation in the Medicare program. The law provides for immunity from civil and criminal liability for persons providing pertinent information to a PRO. Professional review organizations are not subject to the Freedom of Information Act (5 U.S.C.S. § 552) and the information provided to them is protected from disclosure.

The PRO system is now under its Fourth Scope of Work. Under the new contracts, PROs will use Uniform Clinical Data Sets (UCDS), a computerized review process. This system will attempt to identify variant medical practice behavior and outcomes through computerized screening of selected medical records (PRO Fourth Scope of Work Draft, 1992). Copies of the UCDS software are commercially available for facilities and providers to use to review their own services.

Joint Commission Standards

The Joint Commission continually revises its standards to encourage health-care entities to implement policies and procedures that identify and resolve patient-care problems. In an effort to increase provider **accountability** to **consumers**, the Joint Commission now discloses the number and nature of substantive complaints filed against **accredited** facilities. Upon request of any consumer (including lawyers), the Joint Commission will specifically disclose any complaints of patients or employees, as well as whether it has issued any Type 1 recommendations. A Type 1 recommendation indicates a violation of Joint Commission's formal standards. The Joint Commission will not reveal the number or nature of Type 1 recommendations — simply whether any Type 1 recommendations have been made.

HEALTH-CARE REFORM

National standard setting and increased emphasis on quality analysis are mainstays of health-care reform. Without such measures, rationing without consideration of outcomes will occur. Information about the effectiveness of health plans based on established criteria will be available to consumers and utilized by providers to market services. Compliance with nationally set standards will protect providers who meet the standards but do not offer all available treatment from liability.

CONFIDENTIALITY OF QUALITY-MANAGEMENT INFORMATION

When it comes to disclosure of QM data, two diametrically opposed concepts come into play. First, the judicial system's search for truth is aided by making all information readily available to lawyers. On the other hand, some information must be kept confidential in order for society's systems to function. To maintain the confidentiality of information, lawyers look for privileges established by the law. There are four major privileges: (1) physician/patient; (2) attorney/client; (3) attorney work product; and (4) peer-review or morbidity/mortality studies. For any of these privileges to apply, the communication must originate in confidence; the confidentiality of the communication must be essential to retain the function of the communication; and the injury from the disclosure must outweigh the benefits that would be gained from the correct disposition of the litigation (Wigmore, 1961). These privileges are established by statutes in some states and recognized by common law in others. The extent and dimensions of the privilege and what is required to maintain the privilege are questions of state law.

INVESTIGATIONS

An important part of any QM program is having in place not only a compliance program but also an investigation-response program. Far too often providers fail to recognize the risk presented every time public auditors or investigators arrive at the business. When facing an inquiry, health-care providers should at a minimum: (1) identify the investigator; (2) ascertain the true purpose of the investigation; and (3) control the flow of information.

Identify the Investigator

Accurate identification of the investigator can tell the provider a great deal about the nature of the problem and how to respond to it. Records that investigators are unquestionably entitled to review can be identified, as can material that the investigator need not be given. The Federal Bureau of Investigation (FBI) is responsible for investigating violations of federal criminal statutes including Medicare fraud statutes. The FBI does not conduct civil investigations. Federal Bureau of Investigation agents will ask to conduct interviews or will serve a grand jury subpoena. Contact with the FBI should always be handled by counsel experienced in criminal matters. Federal Bureau of Investigation involvement is a sure sign that matters already have advanced to a serious point.

Agents of the Office of the Inspector General (OIG) are authorized to investigate fraud and abuse in Medicare and state Medicaid programs. They can demand access to relevant records. The OIG can issue subpoenas for records and obtain statements of witnesses under oath. An OIG inquiry may lead to administrative monetary penalties or exclusion from Medicare/Medicaid programs. Agents of the OIG may also assist a federal grand jury with a criminal investigation.

A majority of states have created state Medicaid fraud-control units. Initial contact from a fraud unit often is made by an auditor. The fraud unit agent may demand relevant records and documents, which are to be released within the requirements of state law and regulations. The fraud units may also conduct grand jury investigations.

Ascertain True Purpose

If asked, investigators may disclose the reason for their investigation, as well as their objective. No matter what they say, however, it must be assumed that the inquiry is not routine. If investigators are unwilling to disclose the purpose of the inquiry, assume the worst and proceed as if it is a criminal investigation.

An internal investigation may be indicated. If so, it should be conducted under the direction of legal counsel to ensure that the internal investigation is protected by the attorney/client privilege. No matter what the purpose of the investigation, informal communication between employees and investigators should be discouraged.

Control the Flow of Information

Investigators are, needless to say, looking for information. The relevant information may be documents, billing records, or testimony from witnesses. Care should be taken not to obstruct the flow of appropriate information while protecting privileged information. Interviews and testimony must be handled carefully. Employees must be allowed to speak with an investigator but are under no obligation to do so. It is common to require that all requests for interviews be made through counsel. Further, individuals have a constitutional right not to testify against themselves. Providers must realize that interview statements ultimately may become evidence in a criminal trial or administrative proceeding. If an employee is a target or likely target of a criminal investigation, she should seek separate legal counsel. In many cases, an employer will pay for an employee's separate counsel. When separate counsel is in place, a joint defense agreement can be reached so that all represented parties can continue to communicate and devise strategy without compromising privileged communications.

An established compliance program with policies to deal with investigations has become a necessity in this age of accountability.

CONCLUSION

As the emphasis on QM continues to grow, it is likely that the legal implications of QM will similarly continue to grow. Quality-management professionals will need to work closely with legal counsel to understand the evolving impact of the law on health-care delivery. While the principles of QM may lead to better patient care, they may also lead to more legal battles for health-care providers. The current tort system itself may need alteration to allow for real improvement of the quality of health care.

REFERENCES

Abelson, R. (1992, July 20). What have I got, doc? *Forbes*, 308–310.

Agency for Health Care Policy and Research. (1993). *Clinical Practice Guidelines.* Silver Spring, MD: AHCPR Clearinghouse. (Free copies can be obtained by calling 1-800-358-9295 or by writing to Center for Research Dissemination and Liaison, AHCPR Clearinghouse, P. O. Box 8547, Silver Spring, Maryland 20907.)

Ala. Code §§ 34-24-58; Alaska Stat. § 18.23.020; Ariz. Rev. Stat. Ann. §§ 36.445.02; Ark. Stat. Ann. §§ 82-3201 *et seq.*; Cal. Civ. Code §§ 43.7 and 43.8; Colo. Rev. Stat. §§ 12-36.5-101 *et seq.*; Conn. Gen. Stat. § 38-19a; Del. Code Ann. title 24, § 1768; D.C. Code Ann. § 32-503; Fla. Stat. Ann. §§ 768.40 and 395.0115; Ga. Code Ann. §§ 31-7-132; Haw. Rev. Stat. § 663-1.7; Idaho Code Ann. § 39-1392c; Ill. Stat. Ann. ch. 111 1/2, § 151.2; Ind. Code Ann. § 34.4-12.6-3; Kan. Stat. Ann. § 65-442; Ky. Rev. Stat. Ann. § 311.377; La. Rev. Stat. Ann. § 44:7D; Me. Rev. Stat. Ann. titles 32, § 3293 and 24, § 2511; Md. Health Occ. Code §§ 14-601 and 14-603; Mass. Gen. Laws Ann. ch. 231, § 85N; Mich. Stat. Ann. § 14.15 (16244); Minn. Stat. Ann. §§ 145.61 and 145.63; Miss. Code Ann. § 41-63-5; Mo. Ann. Stat. § 537.035; Mont. Code Ann. § 37-2-201; Neb. Rev. Stat. § 71.147.01; Nev. Rev. Stat. § 630-364; N.H. Rev. Stat. Ann. § 507:8-c; N.J. Stat. Ann. § 2A:84A-22.9; N.M. Stat. §§ 41-9-1 through 41-9-4; N.Y. Educ. Law § 6527(3); N.C. Gen. Stat. § 131E-95; N.D. Cent. Code § 23-01-02.1; Ohio Rev. Code Ann. §§ 2305.24, 2305.25 and 2305.28; Okla. Stat. Ann. title 63, § 1-1709; Or. Rev. Stat. § 41.675(4); Pa. Stat. Ann. titles 62, § 444.2 and 63, § 425.3; R.I. Gen. Laws Ann. § 5-37.3-7; S.D. Codified Laws Ann. § 36-4-25; Tenn. Code Ann. §§ 63-6-219 and 63-5-131; Tex. Rev. Civ. Stat. art. 4447d(3); Utah Code Ann. §§ 26-25-1; 26-25-2 and 58-12-2; Vt. Stat. Ann. title 26, § 1442; Va. Code Ann. §§ 8.01-581.13, 8.01-581.16 and 8.01-581.19; Wash. Rev. Code Ann. §§ 4.24.240, 4.24.250 and S.B. No. 5972; W. Va. Code Ann. § 30-3c-2; Wis. Stat. Ann. § 146.37; and Wyo. Stat. Ann. §§ 35-2-603 and 35-17-106.

Freedom of Information Act, 5 U.C.S. § 552.

Health Care Quality Improvement Act of 1986, 42 U.S.C. § 11101 *et seq.* (1986).

Health Care Standards Directory (1993). PA: ECRI. (For information contact Circulation Department, 5200 Butler Pike, Plymouth Meeting, PA 19462, 1-610-825-6000.)

Jacox, A. (1993, January). Improving quality through clinical practice guidelines. *The American Nurse, 25*(1), 12.

Knaus, W. A., Wagner, D. P., Draper, M. S., Zimmerman, J. E., Bergner, M., & Bastos, P. G. (1991). The APACHE III prognostic system. *Chest, 100*(6), 1619–1636.

Medicare and Medicaid Patient and Program Protection Act of 1987, Pub. L. 100-93 (August 18, 1987).

Peer Review Improvement Act of 1982, 42 U.S.C. §§ 1320c *et seq.* (1982).

PRO Fourth Scope of Work Draft (April 28, 1992). 8 Wigmore on Evidence, § 2-285 (1961).

ADDITIONAL READING

American Hospital Association (1993, August 30). Standard treatment protocols can be used to manage costs, quality. *American Hospital Association News,* 6.

Couch, J. B. (1988). Legal aspect of the medical staff peer review process. Legally permissible uses of mandated health data disclosure. *Quality Assurance & Utilization Review, 3*(4), 124–126.

Couch, J. B. (1988). Legal aspect of the medical staff peer review process. The third revolution in health care — a public policy and legal analysis. *Quality Assurance & Utilization Review, 4*(2), 56–58.

Darby, M. (1993, August). Special report: Lawyers turn to practice guidelines applications to defend doctors in malpractice lawsuits. *Managed Care Law*, S1–S3.

Fox, J. G. (1993, August 5). Interview: Health policy researcher John E. Wennberg. *Hospitals and Health Networks*, Vol. 67, No. 15.

Freed, G. L. (Ed.) (1993). Influence of standard of care on claims payment. *Medico-Legal Watch, 2*(4), 19.

Hamilton, C. L. (1993). The law, ethics, and total quality. In A. F. Al-Assaf & J. A. Schmele (Eds.), *The textbook of total quality in healthcare* (pp. 173–189). Delray Beach, FL: St. Lucie Press.

Kjervik, D. K. (1994). Advance directives. In J. McCloskey & H. K. Grace (Eds.). *Current issues in nursing* (pp. 752–757). St. Louis: Mosby.

Leone, A., Jr. (1993). Medical practice guidelines are useful tool in litigation. *Medical Malpractice Law & Strategy, 10*(6), 1, 4–6.

Stewart, D. O., & Fee, M. K. (1991 September). Coping with investigators & investigations. *CARING Magazine, 10*(9) 32–35.

Truhe, J. V., Jr. (1993). Quality assessment in the '90s: Legal implications for hospitals. *Journal of Health and Hospital Law, 26*(6), 171–180.

Wilging, P. R. (1992). OBRA as a measure of quality. (*National League for Nursing Publications*, 41-2440), 21–25.

Joe B. Hurst
Mary Keenan
John Minnick

CHAPTER *3 2*

Health-Care Polarities:
Quality and Cost

INTRODUCTION

Health-care institutions are obliged to provide patients with high-quality care, staffs with professional development, and their field of endeavor with adequate research. At the same time, health-care institutions are plagued with rising costs, payment regulations, competition for patients, and public pleas for economizing. Most often, repeated campaigns to accomplish one goal or the other struggle to achieve one final resolution of the conflicts that they pose.

Administrators and financial people usually campaign for cost reduction and often order the same cost-containment measures throughout the organization or system. Operational managers often respond to such crusades with open and covert resistance, because most practitioners regard certain allocations of time, materials, and technological procedures as essential to **quality** care.

Any efforts to produce notable and lasting breakthroughs on the cost and quality front will prove limited and probably unsuccessful because people view these two as separate problems to be solved in some sequence of priorities. They do not understand precisely how their daily activities influence both at the same time.

Everyone needs a new perspective on the quality-cost relationship, which will enable them to handle it not as a problem to be solved once and for all, but as a polarity to be managed collaboratively as time goes on. Viewing the poles as independent, static sets of solutions to separate problems overlooks their interdependence in the common field they influence, and hides the predictable "flow" of polarities over time. Furthermore, both "front-office" and operational health-care administrators need suggestions for a definite course of action to handle this flow.

Note: This chapter is reprinted with permission from *Nursing Management, 23*(9), 40–43, September 1992.

POLARITIES: STRUCTURE AND FLOW

Two opposing but interdependent concepts that occupy the same field of interest constitute a polarity (Johnson, 1989).

For example, suppose a hospital's field of concern is maintaining a leading position in the community. Keeping a staff who delivers excellence care may require expensive outlays in high technology to satisfy their rising practice **standards** and expectations. Providing for a steady flow of patients may require contracting with insurers at discounted rates for services to satisfy their actuarial assumptions and plans. Thus, maintaining the hospital's position produces a flow of consequences between the poles of continually improving patient care and reducing care costs.

Ranged within the field of such spheres of influence as cost and quality are the upside (positive **outcomes**) of actions toward each pole, and the downside (negative outcomes) of such actions away from the each pole.

A fully equipped and staffed Level III nursery would enhance regional access to high-tech care (upside for quality) but would expose the hospital to heavier financial risks (downside for cost). Closing a maternity services unit would reduce the hospital's exposure to many revenue and liability risks (upside for costs) but would diminish availability of that kind of care in the community (downside for quality).

Thus, a polarity's structure consists of polar opposites on a horizontal axis across a field that can be then vertically divided into four quadrants of consequences: two upside and two downside (see Figure 32-1). Poles A and B are interdependent to the

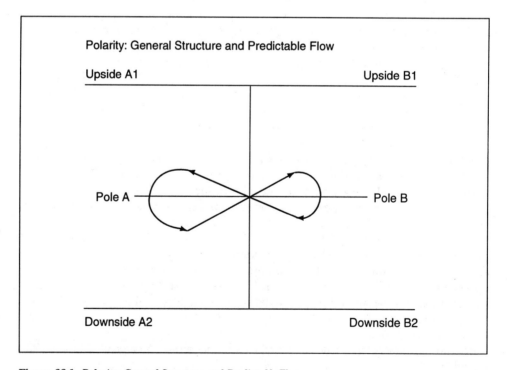

Figure 32-1 *Polarity: General Structure and Predictable Flow*

extent that overemphasizing one to the exclusion of the other will lead to downside outcomes. Under that circumstance, a shift toward the opposite pole would be appropriate. Notice that polarities naturally flow from the downside of one pole toward the upside of the other; then toward the downside of the second pole; then toward the upside of the first pole; and, finally, back to the downside where it all began.

Unmanaged polarities have an "infinite-type swing" to them. While these swings may be quite limited, they may also move deeply into downside outcomes and then back into upside outcomes. Such movements can occasionally cause disruptions of operating efficiencies. When such polar opposites as quality and cost are approached as separate problems to be solved — as they usually are — the results tend to reflect less time spent in the upside quadrants and more time spent in the downside ones. Because staffs "choose up sides" blindly and contend for prior consideration, many times they settle for the downside of either or both poles. Hospitals, or any institution for that matter, cannot afford these deep or prolonged swings because they waste not only money and time, but also energy, material, and morale.

LINING UP: ACTORS AND OUTCOMES

Concerted actions to move from the downside of one pole to the upside of the other is called *crusading*. *Crusaders* are energizers for change. Because of this, they concentrate their attentions on the downside outcomes of one pole and the upside outcomes of the other. This focus usually gives them an accurate enough, but very incomplete picture of the polarity. They are "blind" to other possible consequences.

Those who do focus on those other outcomes are *tradition-bearers* (Hurst, Johnson, Spencer, & VanderVeen, 1990; Johnson, 1992). They want to keep the upside benefits that crusaders are willing to trade off, and avoid the downside consequences of the goal toward which the crusaders are moving.

By contending with one another to win everyone over to accurate but incomplete views of what is so and what is possible, both crusaders and tradition-bearers deepen the swings of the polarity pendulum. Over time, their temporary successes and failures in controlling the field produce more downside effects. A more logical option would be for them to collaborate on sensing the beginning of downside outcomes early, then acting to shift attentions toward the opposite pole as soon as possible. By teaming up to maximize the upsides and minimize the downsides of both poles, they would develop a broader view of the polarity. They also would become accustomed to tolerating small swings of emphasis when needed. In this way, everyone could experience the upside of both poles more often and more intensively.

When the interested actors label the poles with as neutral terms as possible, the upsides and downsides can be charted in the quadrants of a polarity diagram. Because they are identifying interdependent, although opposing, goals or activities, the poles can clearly outline consequences that the actors detail in upside and downside quadrants (see Figure 32-2).

Emphasizing outcomes is essential because many people concentrate on the decisional and performance procedures that they can control, over any concerns about the consequences of particular actions that they advocate. A clear, comprehensive view of the situation requires that everyone involved considers both the short- and long-term results of emphasizing either or both poles.

Upside A1	Upside B1
• more satisfied patients • higher patient census • more qualified staff • high morale • rise in reputation • program expansion • fewer lawsuits • high accreditation	• expenditures within budget norms • higher return rates on capital • targeted outreach • resource conservation • satisfactory revenue streams and low debt service • efficient staffing • targeted high-tech investments and sharing arrangements
A Quality ———————————————	——————————————— **Cost B**
• expenditures exceed budget • lower return rates on capital • generalized outreach • resource waste • uncertain revenue streams and high debt service • inefficient staffing • heavy dependence on costly in-house technology	• more dissatisfied patients • lower patient census • more staff turnover • low morale • reputation loss • fewer programs • more lawsuits • accreditation losses
Downside A2	**Downside B2**

Figure 32-2 *The Quality of Care and Cost Containment Polarity*

THE QUALITY AND COST POLARITY

While managers could start with any quadrant from any pole, a "breakdown" in obtaining upside results presents a valuable opportunity to look at what is working and not working, as well as what is missing (Heidegger, 1972; Winograd & Flores, 1986). Any of the negative quality outcomes listed in the downside (overemphasis on costs) quadrant B2, Figure 32-2, raises questions about patient-care quality, which would serve as a point of departure for questioning its relationship to emphasizing cost influences.

Quadrant A1, Figure 32-2, lists the upside consequences of emphasizing quality. Organizations often express these as expectations, and many institutions indeed accomplish them — unfortunately sometimes at the cost of raising prices or increasing the fiscal burdens of debt.

Quadrant A2, Figure 32-2, lists the downside consequences of overemphasizing quality to the exclusion of fiscal considerations. The appearance of any of these consequences greatly concerns administrators and staff members who are **accountable** for the financial viability of the entire organization. These individuals generally tend to view quality as an end that clinicians achieve by spending large amounts of money.

Finally, the upside consequences of cost-reduction programs are listed in quadrant B1, Figure 32-2. Their presence signals security to finance officers and risk-averse administrators. Nevertheless, successes in cost containment stimulate pressures to expend more on practitioners' working environment and to improve patient-care access and options.

The interdependence of the poles in real-life situations leads to a predictable flow from pole to pole, downside to upside to downside and return. People who crusade or tradition-bear for some pole and wind up in the downside of that or the other pole often assess the experience as a failure — especially when it is a deep, prolonged swing. The more people treat polarities as independent problems to be solved or decisions to be made once and for all, the more they set themselves and their institutions up for a frustrating working environment.

BUILDING COLLABORATION

Polarities present those persons in charge of the organization's mission and vision statements with a new challenge. Rather than static states to attain, leaders have to envision the future in terms of well-managed dynamic polarities. With personnel at all levels, these leaders also need to communicate the full nature of any polarity, or related set of polarities, that affects the working environment. This includes clear and comprehensive delineation of the upside and downside outcomes of *both* poles.

People tend to focus on the downside of one pole and the upside of the other. A full view of any polarity requires listening carefully to the "opposite" perspective for additional accuracy and completeness. In practical terms, this means managers must acknowledge the downside of crusading efforts and the upside of tradition-bearing efforts.

After that, concerted action for the future needs requires team building that commits the entire staff to doing what it takes to maximize the upside effects of both poles, even though some actions taken more toward their historically least-preferred pole. Sometimes, people sense a change in focus toward one pole or the other as inconsistent with policies or goals to which they believe they are committed. In the polarity context, that shift in emphasis can be viewed as a trade-off and cooperative move in a needed direction for some productive or necessary period of time. In this context, they realize there will be a reciprocal shift back for the good of all over the long term.

In confronting the polarity of cost containment and quality of service, it is crucial to acknowledge that the organization's people can be both the greatest resource and the biggest block to desired breakthroughs. Listening to those most concerned about and sensitive to the downside issues of either pole is one way to determine the position of the entire organization, or some department within it, at any particular moment. Rather than regarding such persons as complainers and adversaries, the wise manager listens to them as expert consultants about outcomes of particular actions on their field of activity.

Hearing points of view to which one is most deaf, dumb, blind, and then expressing them as well as — or better than — their advocates might is a great art that requires determined practice. It means actively listening for grounds for collaborating, rather than for points of resistance. Taking such a lead in sharing all the concerns for down-side and upside consequences genuinely persuades crusaders and tradition-bearers to form productive partnerships. These gradually replace destructive battles for dominance over resources.

"Difficulty in isolating a problem is often due to the tendency to spend a minimum of effort on a problem definition in order to get to the important process of solving it" (Adams, 1985, p. 23). Following the latest fad or joining the current crusade tends to obscure people's vision of potential and desired results, to prevent reflection on cogent issues, and to impede collaborative group and individual action. Identifying polarities and diagramming their components can help avoid such pitfalls of inadequate problem definition and open up a whole new range of projects for further collaboration. With this form of analysis, both individuals and groups can collaborate on identifying (1) the key elements of troublesome dilemmas, (2) associated decisions to be made, and (3) action steps to be taken.

With respect to group dynamics, Zander (1982) has cautioned, "members are often more concerned with their own personal needs and rights than with those of the organization" (p. xi). Polarity identification and management promotes team building to overcome this inclination. As concerned parties grapple with the actual elements of "views and sides" of polarities affecting their work, they openly come to terms with one another's particular interpretations as well as the perspectives they share in common. After the polarity has been defined to general satisfaction, sharing within the group increases and allows the group to envision the future, deal with individual agendas, and make long-term plans for managing the polarity more effectively.

Every narrow problem solution begets two or more new problems (Weisbord, 1987). Polarity analysis either prevents such specific focusing or provides a larger context for handling new problems as they emerge. Finally, polarity management, by eliciting the positions of opposing advocates, tends to tie each person's needs and interests to those of others and the organization as a whole. This opens a context previously not fully available through which partners can fruitfully collaborate time and again.

REFERENCES

Adams, J. L. (1985). *Conceptual blockbusting: A guide to better ideas.* New York: W. W. Norton Co.

Heidegger, M. (1972). *On time and being.* New York: Harper and Row.

Hurst, J. B., Johnson, B., Spencer, J., & VanderVeen, C. (1990). *Managing polarities effectively: Workbook.* Toledo, OH: Human Resource Development Center, University of Toledo at Seagate.

Johnson, B. (1989). *How polarities work: Managing unsolvable problems.* Presentation to the XLV General Assembly of the Interamerican Press Association.

Johnson, B. (1992). *Polarity management: An alternative to the problem solving paradigm.* Amherst, MA: Human Resource Development Press.

Weisbord, M. R. (1987). *Productive workplaces.* San Francisco: Jossey-Bass, Inc.

Winograd, T., & Flores, F. (1986). *Understanding computers and cognition: A new foundation for design.* Norwood, NJ: Ablex Publishers.

Zander, A. (1982). *Making groups effective.* San Francisco: Jossey-Bass, Inc.

ADDITIONAL READING

Bueno, M. M., & Fralic, M. F. (1994). Balancing cost and quality. In J. McCloskey & H. K. Grace (Eds.), *Current issues in nursing* (4th ed., pp. 490–500). St. Louis, MO: Mosby.

Crosby, P. B. (1979). *Quality is free.* New York: New American Library.

Fleming, S. T., & Boles, K. E. (1994). Financial and clinical performance: Bridging the gap. *Health Care Management Review, 19*(1), 11–17.

Hopkins, G., & Doggett, S. (1993). Enhancing hospital cash flow through improved medical records processing. *Quality Management in Health Care, 1*(2), 23–33.

Hutton, J. (1994). Economic evaluation of healthcare: A half-way technology. *Health Economics, 3*(1), 1–4.

Manus, D. A., Werner, T. R., & Stout, R. J. (1994). Using measurement and feedback to reduce health care costs and modify physician practice patterns. *Quality Management in Health Care, 2*(2), 48–60.

Rosenstein, A. H. (1994). Cost-effective health care: Tools for improvement. *Health Care Management Review, 19*(2), 53–61.

Seever, J. D., Neuman, B. R., & Boles, K. E. (1992). Accounting for the cost of quality. *Healthcare Financial Management, 46*(9), 29–37.

Smeltzer, C. H. (1993). Lessons learned: Implementing cost reductions and enhancing quality. *Nursing Economics, 11*(6), 373–375.

Smith, K., & Wright, K. (1994). Informal care and economic appraisal: A discussion of possible methodological approaches. *Health Economics, 3*(3), 137–148.

June A. Schmele

CHAPTER *33*

The Future:
Trends, Issues, and Opportunities

INTRODUCTION

The last decade of this century has evoked a flurry of proactivity as society, organizations, and health-care entities have made concerted efforts to prepare for the next century. It is not just the end of the decade or the end of the century, but the end of the millennium. Naisbitt and Aburdene (1990) state, "For centuries that monumental, symbolic date has stood for the future and what we shall make of it. In a few short years that future will be here" (p. xvii). The value of envisioning the future, while looking at the past, is to proclaim the present in the fullest way possible in order to accomplish a predetermined vision. It is hoped that the present will manifest the vision of the future and, one day, will make a timely and respectable contribution to the past.

There is no question that the current times bear witness to some of the most rapid, unprecedented, and often turbulent changes that the universe, society, organizations, and individuals have ever experienced. It is recognized that a perturbation at any level of the system will directly or indirectly, and in varying degrees, affect the other systems levels as well. It is the author's observation that most of the trends of the future seem to relate at some level of the system to either **structure**, **process**, or **outcome**, or any combination thereof. Perhaps the message here is that **quality** is in some way a part of every aspect of society and its organizations. For these reasons, the purpose of this chapter is to raise the level of conscious awareness regarding trends and issues that will impact the future. The chapter presents an overview of the major trends that are impacting society, organizations (and, most specifically, health-care organizations), and, ultimately, the state of the art in **Quality Management (QM)**.

Recognizing that futurism and the study of its various aspects are in themselves very complex areas of exploration, this chapter presents an overview. Efforts have been made to cite some of the best-known experts. There are a number of challenging and exciting books in the popular press, written by "presentists" looking at the future and futurists looking at both the present and the future. In addition, this chapter cites several classic documents that represent not only the present, but that provide a map to the future — especially for the 1990s and on into the next century. There are common threads that weave throughout these thoughtful writings; thus, readers are encouraged to peruse them.

MAJOR SOCIETAL TRENDS

According to Curtin (1994), it is important to differentiate between trends and fads. She states that a fad is "a novelty: something new that catches our attention" (p. 7). A fad lacks deep roots and may or may not work. On the other hand, a trend "has deep demographic, scientific, sociologic, financial, and maybe even political roots" (p. 7).

Readers will be familiar with the megatrends of the 1980s, as predicted by Naisbitt (1982). As these trends have come to pass, they have impacted, and continue to impact, the present. According to Naisbitt and Aburdene (1990) the megatrends of the 1990s provide a new frame of reference that offers structure to vast amounts of seemingly unrelated data reflecting the context of the present day. These megatrends are identified as:

1. The Booming Global Economy of the 1990s;
2. A Renaissance in the Arts;
3. The Emergence of Free Market Socialism;
4. Global Lifestyles and Cultural Nationalism;
5. The Privatization of the Welfare State;
6. The Rise of the Pacific Rim;
7. The Decade of Women in Leadership;
8. The Age of Biology;
9. The Religious Revival of the New Millennium;
10. The Triumph of the Individual. (p. xix)

Several of these megatrends have direct, and sometimes indirect, international implications that lead to a global society. Naisbitt (1994) describes a global paradox, which suggests that as a system grows larger, the parts (or individuals) become more important, and, thus, the present opportunities for individuals are greater than during any other time in history. Considering Curtin's previously cited definition of a trend, it bears emphasis that the aforementioned overarching trends have had and will have far-reaching implications at every societal and individual level.

A second noted futurist, Alvin Toffler, recently completed the fourth volume in a series wherein he has projected societal changes, most of which have occurred over a twenty-five-year period (Toffler & Toffler, 1993). New projections are currently being offered that extend well beyond today's date. When the present and future are considered within a longitudinal perspective, the essence of the trends that influence society are more easily seen. He suggests that it is necessary to consider the resulting changes from the standpoint of what happens to individuals and organizations when there is abrupt transformation in the whole of society. In keeping with his longitudinal view of change, Toffler presents a model that shows interconnectedness and a conceptual whole. His first book, *Future Shock* (1971), deals with the process of change and its effect on people and organizations. The 1980s are reflected in *The Third Wave* (Toffler, 1980), which focuses on the direction of change and where it is taking individuals, organizations, and society. *Powershift* (Toffler, 1990) deals with the control of change and addresses the question of who will have the power to shape this change. Toffler identifies the major universal bases of power as violence, money, and information. In the current environment, he contends that the power of information, and ultimately knowledge, is the key power base of the future. His major thesis is that power is possessed by those who have the ability to gain and use information at all levels of the system — from individual to global. The recognition of this power shift is especially important because of the many and varied implications of a rapidly expanding information age. According to Toffler and Toffler (1993), "a revolutionary new economy is arising based on knowledge, rather than conventional raw materials and physical labor" (p. 5). It is noteworthy that Toffler, like Naisbitt, observes that the vast amount of unrelated information and knowledge is unmanageable without an overarching framework to identify patterns and the forces that shape them.

Anyone in the field of QM certainly recognizes that vast amounts of data do not automatically become information, much less knowledge. According to Susser (1993), the major functions of data are assessment, explanation, evaluation, and prediction. Therefore, a challenge of the future becomes one of collecting and managing vast amounts of data for one or more of these four functions. This data, with appropriate management and analyses, will then become information and, ultimately, knowledge that can be used as a basis for decision making.

A rapidly developing major value that is impacting decision making and organizational change is the recognition of the **consumer** as a vital source of information and knowledge. Although this recognition may have been, and may still be, market driven, the momentum of the consumer movement is just beginning. The wants and needs of the consumer, coupled with the availability of information and the competitiveness of the marketplace, promise to be one of the major shaping forces of renewed organizations. Consumers' voices and purchasing power will be increasingly strong forces in the determination of what constitutes quality. *The Popcorn Report* (1992) is one example of predicting future consumer behavior in order to prepare for the marketplace of the present. Popcorn, well recognized for her predictions, offers the following trends for the 1990s:

- Cocooning (stay at home syndrome);
- Fantasy Adventure (emotional escape);
- Small Indulgences (reward for self);
- Egonomics ("me-ness");
- Cashing Out (leaving the corporate world);

- Dam-Aging (refusal to be bound by traditional age limits);
- Staying Alive (hyper-quest for health);
- The Vigilante Consumer (consumers on their own product-investigation);
- 99 Lives (super-person);
- S.O.S. (Save our Society) (p. xiii).

Through their long-term explorations of change and trends, Toffler, Naisbitt, Popcorn, and others have offered frameworks that provide some order, direction, and degree of predictability. The work of Wheatley (1992), however, suggests that very rapid and sometimes tumultuous changes are antecedents to chaos, which she defines as total unpredictability. Wheatley and others suggest the valid presence and place of chaos in the regeneration of changing systems. According to Flower (1993), "chaos seems to be a critical part of the process by which living systems constantly recreate themselves in their environment" (p. 50). In an interview with Flower, Wheatley notes that there is some reassurance in knowing that we can expect chaos as "the final state in a system's moves away from order. Not all systems move into chaos. If a system is dislodged from its stable state, it moves first into a period of oscillation, swinging back and forth between different states. If it moves from this oscillation, the next state is full chaos, a period of total unpredictability. But in the realm of chaos, where everything should fall apart, the strange attractor comes into play" (Flower, 1993, p. 52). The next stage will then bring about a new order.

The technology perhaps most related to bringing order to the chaos of information overload is that of the computer, which transforms data, work, and learning in order to provide meaning to the whole. With its multitude of ever-expanding capabilities, the future of computer science is mind boggling. Denning (1993), a computer expert, proposes that the major computer growth areas of the future will be hardware, software, data (mega amounts), work (long-distance collaboration), publishing (electronic distribution), and research.

Technical advances such as world systems of communications, data, and networks, to name just a few, are leading to the recognition of unprecedented activity in global marketplaces. As a result, trade entities are being led to consider the examples of other countries in the search for quality. The International Standards (ISO 9000) and their implementation provide one example of the global recognition of the nature of quality and the subsequent promulgation of universal **standards**. Although the current major emphasis of ISO 9000 is industrial, it is recognized that the movement is equally as applicable in health care and other service arenas (Arnold, 1994). Another example is the increasingly popular technique of **benchmarking**, which leads us to determine what others are doing best in order that we may become better ourselves.

Styles (1994), who has long emphasized the importance of recognizing global influences, calls for a summit on "the world as a classroom at which we exchange information about our activities and interests and plans . . ." (p. 507). With an emphasis on international health care and nursing, she proposes that the next century be known as the International Century. It is evident that preparation for the future includes the encouragement of international mobility and interchange through the growth of technology and political alignments.

ORGANIZATIONAL TRENDS

A dramatic paradigm shift, or new way of looking at things, is taking place not only in society, but in organizations as well. The previously discussed societal changes, coupled with the dysfunctionality of many organizational bureaucracies of the past and new visions of the future, necessitate a rapid organizational response to environmental changes. These changes are being approached on a continuum from tinkering to starting over.

Hammer and Champy (1993) suggest that the most effective organizational renewal may sometimes necessitate a starting over, which they term *reengineering*. They propose a radical new conceptual approach to rid the world of old anachronistic organizations that do not have the capabilities to respond to the current environmental forces of **customers**, competition, and change. The increasingly popular term *reengineering* is used to define a "fundamental and radical redesign of business processes to achieve dramatic improvements in critical, contemporary measures of performance, such as cost, quality, service, and speed" (Hammer & Champy, 1993, p. 32). Hammer and Champy advocate that the key to successful reengineering is the willingness to start over from scratch, with a blank piece of paper. For most persons, this is a disruptive and revolutionary idea that will require risk taking, vision, and effective leadership.

In agreement with Toffler, Drucker, in his book *Managing for the Future* (1992), emphasizes that the 1990s and beyond will comprise a knowledge society. Organizations will become more information based and, thus, will need to restructure around information. He conveys the importance of recognizing that the workforce is increasingly made up of knowledgeable workers who require a different type of leadership than that of the past. Drucker states that "The foundation of effective leadership is thinking through the organization's mission, defining it, and establishing it, clearly and visibly" (p. 121). Drucker also emphasizes the importance of creating "human energies and human vision" (p. 122) within a framework of trust. Kouzes and Posner (1993) suggest that the discipline of credibility (consistency between words and deeds) is increasingly important to employees who are looking for leaders who will actually do what they speak.

In Deming's forward to *The Trust Factor* (Whitney, 1994) he emphasizes that "trust is mandatory for the optimization of a system" (p. viii). Whitney, considered a corporate-turnaround specialist, recognizes that institutionalized mistrust is a major impediment to effective organizations. He calls for an executive wake-up call and the infusion of win-win organizational transactions in order for organizations to survive and accomplish their purpose.

Peter Senge (1990) is just one of many who have heard the wake-up call. He has popularized the concept of the learning organization, which is an organization "where people continually expand their capacity to create the results they truly desire, where new and expansive patterns of thinking are nurtured, where collective aspiration is set free, and where people are continually learning how to learn together" (p. 3). Senge proposes that five component technologies provide the essential dimensions of a learning organization: systems thinking, personal mastery, mental models (how we see the world), shared visions, and team learning. Senge and his associates have further advanced this theory into a practice application of the new discipline of the learning organization (Senge, Roberts, Ross, Smith, & Kleiner, 1994).

Another who has responded to the wake-up call is Stephen Covey (1989), who exemplifies a strong commitment to the current trend toward individual empowerment. He is also a noted expert in the field of leadership development. *Principle-centered Leadership* (Covey, 1991) advances the idea that true empowerment results from a congruence of principles (why) and practices (what) at four levels (personal, interpersonal, managerial, and organizational). Covey's principle-centered leadership paradigm includes key principles of trustworthiness, trust, empowerment, and alignment. He proposes that the internalization of principle-centered leadership depends on appropriate value-based prioritization and a subsequent congruent management of time (Covey, Merrill, & Merrill, 1994). This leadership paradigm shift from "control" to "release" is in keeping with the movement to empower workers in **Total-Quality-Management (TQM)** environments.

Ideally, total-quality environments will be made up of empowered employees and team-motivated leaders. Katzenbach and Smith (1993) contend that teams are vital to the future of successful organizations. The critical elements in the definition of a team are worth emphasizing in order to exploit the essence rather than simply the structure of team. "A team is a small number of people with complimentary skills who are committed to a common purpose, performance goals, and approach for which they hold themselves mutually accountable" (p. 45). The presence of the word *common* in the operationalization of teams is essential if team functions are to be maximized. The scholar in QM is well aware of the major role of teams in the current and future pursuit of quality. According to Katzenbach and Smith, "Teams will be the primary building blocks of company performance in the organizations of the future" (p. 173).

Longitudinal views of society and organizations have great merit for those who are attempting to envision the future. Just as Toffler and Naisbitt have responded with views of the future and projected megatrends of the current decade and beyond, Tom Peters has studied the megatrends in organizations. His book titles themselves capture the essence of the megatrend evolution changing organizational systems. The first of Peters's trilogy, *In Search of Excellence* (1982), denounces the model of modern management and calls for recognition of the customer, humanistic concern for employees, and a bias for action. His next volume, *Thriving on Chaos* (1987), is a plea for leadership and organizational flexibility, which may lead to the disorganization of the old system and a subsequent ability to renew. In accord with Wheatley, this chaos, or unpredictability, is an antecedent to the formation of new systems that will respond to the needs of the current and future age. In response to the chaos, Peters proposes a new type of *Liberation Management* (1992) wherein the leader responds to what Peters calls the "Necessary Disorganization of the Nanosecond Nineties" (xxxiii). Like Popcorn, Peters proposes that "fashion" is the key word. Fashion manifests itself in the explosiveness of the changing service and product markets with their accompanying competitiveness and the need for ever more rapid responses. In keeping with Drucker, Peters proposes that it is time for organizations to prepare to abandon everything they do. He insists that organizations need to go *beyond* the recent and prevailing movements of management change, centralization, empowerment, loyalty, disintegration, reengineering, learning, TQM, and change. Peters (1994) recognizes the worth of these organizational thrusts, but insists that it is time to move beyond them and into a time of constant revolution.

As a summary of the previously discussed currents, the work of Burris (1993), a futurist and technology forecaster, capsulizes the shifting societal and organizational forces that will direct both the organizations of the future and their quests for quality (see Table 33-1).

Table 33-1 • THE SHIFTING FOCUS

Corporate Culture

From	To
Status quo	Rapid change
Industry performance	Individual action
Incremental innovation	Fundamental change
Expansion	Consolidation
Sameness	Redirection
Corporate groups	Partnerships
New technology as a cost	New technology as a necessity
Cost/growth/control	Quality/innovation/service
Bottom line of last quarter	Global market share

Management

From	To
Management	Leadership
Cheerleaders	Visionaries
Focus on process	Focus on strategy
Manage by control	Manage by commitment
Decision by command	Decision by consensus
Accepting the status quo	Taking risks
Reacting to change	Initiating change
Managing today's crisis today	Managing tomorrow's opportunities today
Solving today's problems today	Solving tomorrow's problems today
Individual work	Teamwork
Controlling others	Empowering others
Negative reinforcement of bad behaviors	Positive reinforcement of good behaviors
Fixing the blame	Fixing the problem
Taking credit	Giving acknowledgments
Periodic improvement	Continuous improvement
Organization man	Migrant professional
Centralized decision making	Decentralized decision making
Reward and promote by seniority	Reward and promote by performance

Table 33-1 • **THE SHIFTING FOCUS** *(continued)*

Human Resources

From	To
Focus on task	Focus on process
Job titles	Job skills
Individual values	Shared values
Isolated specialists	Multiskilled generalists
Work with your hands	Work with your brains
Workers' gloves protect hands	Workers' gloves protect product
Upgrading technology	Upgrading people
Periodic training	Just-in-time training
Job security	Job adaptability
Guarantee your employment	Guarantee your employability
Organization man	Migrant professional
Retirement at age 65	Reengagement several times in a life

Price versus Speed

From	To
Price	Speed
Pay for products	Pay for time
Value material wealth	Value free time

Information

From	To
Access to capital	Access to information
More information	Focused information
Static information	Dynamic information
Automation and support	Integration and coordination
Focus on new technology	Focus on new applications of technology

Computers

From	To
Information Age	Communication Age
Collecting information	Sharing information
Words and numbers	Data, voice, and video
Data processing	Decision processing
Fit user to interface	Fit interface to user
Nice-to-have features	Need-to-have features
Client server to mainframe	Client server using UNIX
Proprietary systems	Open systems
Gigabits	Terabits
Character interface	Graphic-user interface
Profits from hardware	Profits from software
Programming by programmers	Programming by users
Repair national *infra*structure	Repair national *info*structure
Paper used for information storage	Paper used for information display

Table 33-1 • **THE SHIFTING FOCUS** *(continued)*

Manufacturing

From	To
Sell what they make	Make what sells
Premanufacture to anticipate sales	Manufacture when ordered
Predemand manufacturing	On-demand manufacturing
Mass production	Lean production
Large inventory	Just-in-time inventory
Long cycle times	Short cycle times
Mastery of the art of replication	Mastery of the art of innovation
Focus on what to make	Focus on how to make it
Quality manufacturing	Flexible manufacturing
Focus on quality	Focus on design
Design for assembly	Design for disassembly
Upgrade internal *infra*structure	Upgrade internal *info*structure
Build a better product	Build a better path to the customer
Employees as assemblers	Employees as problem solvers
Mass production (common products)	Customized mass production (common products with unique features)

Globalization

From	To
Design for assembly	Design for disassembly
Foreign competition invades manufacturing	Foreign competition invades services
Thinking global	Being global
Focus on internal market	Focus on global market
Global competition	Global collaboration
Independence	Interdependence

Cultural Barriers to International Marketing

From	To
(Most culture bound)	*(Least culture bound)*
Consumer products	Industrial products
Established product categories	New products and categories
Simple technology	Complex technology
Items used in home	Items used away from home

National Focus: United States versus Japan and Germany

United States Focus	*Japan and Germany Focus*
Financially driven	Large industry groups
Short-term focus	Long-term focus
Antagonistic toward rivals	Collaboration with rivals

Industry

From	To
Litigation	Mediation and arbitration

Table 33-1 • **THE SHIFTING FOCUS** *(continued)*

Logistics

From	To
Goods	Services

Television News

From	To
Report on something that has happened	Report on something that is happening

Environment

From	To
Town dumps	Regional landfills
Dumping	Waste reduction and recycling

Electronic Data Interchange (EDI)

From	To
Big-unit shipments	Small-unit shipments
Managing inventory	Managing information

Appendix D "The Shifting Focus" from Technotrends *by Daniel Burrus with Roger Gittines. Copyright 1993 by Daniel Burrus. Reprinted by permission of HarperCollins Publishers, Inc.*

QUALITY

Juran (1993) proposes that the twentieth century is the Century of Productivity and that the twenty-first century will be the Century of Quality. Covey (1991) states that "quality is widely seen as the key to American economic survival and success . . . Total Quality represents the century's most profound, comprehensive alteration in management theory and practice" (p. 261). He points out that the paradigm of Total Quality means continuous improvement in four areas:

1. Personal and professional development;

2. Interpersonal relations;

3. Managerial effectiveness;

4. Organizational productivity. (pp. 250-251)

The comprehensiveness of the four areas of improvement imply a total or complete response to the call to quality.

Crosby (1992), well known as one of the fathers of the TQM movement, coins the term "completeness" to describe quality for the twenty-first century. "Quality (meaning getting everyone to do what they have agreed to do) is the skeletal structure of an organization; finance is the nourishment; and relationships are the soul. All of this comes together in what I call *Completeness*" (pp. xiii–xiv). Crosby insists that quality, which he defines as conformance to requirements, is a part of the organizational philosophy, which becomes the way of operating the organization, rather than an add-on system. Crosby believes that the goal ought to be for zero defects and states that "the purpose of completeness is to avoid problems and guarantee success" (p. 19).

Perhaps one of the greatest contrasts to a zero-defect system is that of the federal government. Still, in 1993 the *National Performance Review* began the national move toward quality in this greatest of all bureaucracies. In his report, Gore (1993) proposes major reforms to reinvent government so that it will work better and cost less. Gore's landmark report proposes four major tenets that are basic to TQM and quality improvement in any organization:

1. cutting red tape

2. putting customers first

3. empowering employees to get results

4. cutting back to basics (producing better government for less)

There is little doubt in anyone's mind regarding the monumental and long-term nature of these proposals, as well as the national ramifications of the changes implied. The changes are regarded by some to represent a national move toward TQM. It is clear that this report has the capacity and potential to provide guidance to the federal government and other levels of government at least for the next decade and beyond.

It is likely that the move toward health-care reform will direct many organizations well into the next century. It is recognized that in addition to the increasing cost of health care, there exist other major trends, which often are referred to as social problems. These problems will need to be dealt with over time in order to bring about effective health-care reform. The social problems that Goltschalk and Teymour (1992) identify appear to be increasing in importance, and, in some instances, severity:

- economic questions
- decreased social services for the disadvantaged
- environmental destruction
- substance abuse
- family violence
- chaos in schools
- deterioration of the core socioeconomic framework of society

It is very clear that most, if not all, social conditions impact health care to a greater or lesser degree. It is this environment of widespread social need and the presence of an inadequate and outmoded health-care delivery system that has prompted the United States to embark on the monumental task of health-care reform. (See Chapter 11 for a discussion of this topic.) The author is hopeful that a response to these major societal problems will be found implicitly, if not explicitly, within the critical principles of the health-reform movement:

- creating security
- controlling costs
- expanding choices
- enhancing quality
- reducing bureaucracy (*The President's Health Security Plan*, 1993)

These critical principles of the health-care reform plan can be considered attributes or direct reflections of quality.

The well-known American Nurses Association document *Nursing's Agenda for Health Care Reform* (1991) advances several premises that contain both implicit and explicit directions for the quality of care within the framework of reform. Careful examination of these premises demonstrates that they are either structure, process, or outcome characteristics of quality:

- Equitable access to essential services for all citizens.
- Prominent role of primary health care.
- Consumers must be the central focus.
- Consumers must have access to qualified providers and a variety of delivery arrangements.
- Consumers must assume greater responsibility for care.
- Health-care services must be restructured and balance established between illness and wellness care.
- Health-care system must ensure appropriate and effective care through efficient use of resources.
- A standardized package of services must be provided and financed through integration of public and private resources.

These premises are likely to remain in the forefront as major components of the quality that will be inherent in health-care reform at a national level.

At the international level, a major study done by the American Quality Foundation and Ernst & Young (1992), the *International Quality Study* (IQS) of health care, focused on QM as it is practiced in hospitals in Japan, Germany, Canada, and the United States. Data was gathered to reflect and compare the past, present, and future in the four countries; thus worldwide trends showing large scale changes in the hospital environment were uncovered. Select findings in major areas included:

1. The customer is not the driving force behind quality performance; quality is defined from the provider's perspective.
2. There is a lack of leadership for quality initiatives.
3. Process improvement in health care is surpassed by industry, although major emphases in health care are anticipated.
4. Human-resource practices directed toward greater employee participation in quality improvement are planned.
5. A strategic emphasis on quality is evidenced in hospital operations and structures.

In order to determine the response of hospitals to the TQM movement, the Baxter Foundation funded a national survey of quality-improvement activities ("The Quality March," 1993). This survey showed that the major barriers inhibiting quality-improvement activities were lack of strong commitment and support from senior managers and the inability and inadequacy of the infrastructure to respond to the quality-improvement movement.

A third major study of national scope was funded by the Eastman Kodak Company and carried out by the Healthcare Forum Leadership Center (1992). The prominent issue is conveyed in the title of the study: "Bridging the Leadership Gap in Healthcare." Major findings were:

- Leaders identified a major gap between present leadership practices and those that will be required in the twenty-first century.

- By the year 2001, transformational values and competencies (mastering change, systems thinking, shared vision, continual quality improvement, redefining health care, and serving the public) will be critical.

- Leaders desire community-based care that is universal, cost efficient, and preventative in nature.

- Leaders are concerned that less desirable scenarios (continued growth/high tech or hard times/government control) will occur.

ISSUES

It is evident from the foregoing discussion that several major issues will require attention in order to bring about a transformed health-care system. One of these issues deals with the need to redefine health care and differentiate it from ill care, which is currently generally considered medical care. According to Schoor (1993),

> Health care is the generic term. Medical care is part of health care.
> Nursing care is part of health care. Social work, psychotherapy,
> dietetics, occupational therapy; the list of disciplines that make up
> health care could go on and on . . . As long as the term "medical
> care" is used to subsume the work of all other health care
> providers, their work will be considered ancillary to that of the
> physician. (pp. 294–295)

The importance of differentiating between health care and medical care has greater implications than the implied power struggle and turf-guarding. According to noted health-care futurist Leland Kaiser (1994), health is an outcome that occurs when everything works. He further proposes that major determinants of health are sanitation, nutrition, lifestyle, education, and income. Kaiser advocates that although the medical care in the American system is the best in the world, we do not have a health-care system. He further states that there is almost no relationship between medical care and health; thus hospitals and medical care do not necessarily improve health care. The essential challenge remains that of lowering the amount of disease in the population and improving the health state of the population. This, of course, implies a major impetus on preventive care.

In addition to changing the emphasis from illness care to prevention, there are a number of other public-health issues that have emerged with the debates regarding health-care reform. These include the question of how the mandate for public health, including financing, is to be carried out in a reformed system. A related issue is that of differentiation or integration of roles and responsibilities within the private and public sectors. Kaiser (1994) suggests that to be effective, reform will need to begin at the local level where health is considered something that a community does. The first step is organizing networks from all sectors of the community and its organizations, such as businesses, hospitals, and schools, to mention just a few. The community organization will then decide what the health-care needs are and how the available resources may be brought to bear. The key, says Kaiser, is the goal-directed interaction of the community members, with an openness to creating new forms of care delivery at the local level. Only after this is accomplished can state and national reform take place.

Ziegenfuss (1993) puts forth the following key questions, which will spawn other important issues regarding health-care reform and quality:

1. Will quality improvement be a part of the reform?

2. What technical quality-improvement processes will be built into the reform proposals?

3. On which level of the system will policies for health quality be formulated?

4. Will adequate legal protection be provided for organizations that identify targets for improvement?

5. Who will lead the policy-level quality movement during health care reform?

Many have an additional serious concern regarding the lack of ethical imperatives within the driving forces of the new health-care vision. Consequently, it has been suggested that there needs to be a three-dimensional view of quality, which includes the components of ethics, amenities, and clinical perspectives (Brobst, 1992).

In order to deal with the aforementioned and other issues, Berwick (1992) proposes the need for "systemness" as boundaries in the health-care system are redrawn. Berwick, like Kaiser, suggests that ways to achieve this are to:

1. solicit the community to identify healthcare needs

2. refine information systems

3. develop forms for community planning

4. improve human-resource development

5. strive for consistency in methods of quality improvement

6. correlate financing with the purpose of the system

7. place increased emphasis on learning

Goldsmith (1992), health-care consultant and futurist, envisions that health care of the future will be to predict and manage care. This implies that treatment will take place before acuity occurs. "The paradigm of diagnosis and treatment will be replaced by one of prediction and early-stage management of illness, rendering much of our current armada of diagnostic and curative technologies obsolete" (p. 19). One wonders why we are not responding to this need at the present time given that we now have the capabilities to predict many illnesses that are known to be based on lifestyle patterns of behavior. Perhaps the reason is two-fold: first, funding is not readily available for prevention and second, the impetus has been on medical care rather than health care.

PREDICTIONS

Curtin (1994) offers predictions about the hospital-based integrated health-care networks of the future. She suggests that there will be:

- offsite ER
- offsite and onsite ambulatory surgery
- integrated subacute services
- access to nontraditional therapies
- case management
- benchmarking based on outcome
- health promotion, fitness, and education
- telecommunication linkage with doctors' offices, homes, payers, and regulatory bodies

Changes in health-care delivery will necessitate major role changes. Goldsmith (1992) envisions mobile skill clusters, multiskilled workers, health-information specialists, acceptance of advanced nurse practitioners, and an increased number of specialists in gerontology. It is likely that the configuration of the delivery system at the local and community level will drive the development of a cadre of new, innovative, and entrepreneurial health-care roles.

In response to the prediction of changing roles, the goal of the Pew Health Foundations Commission report *Healthy America: Practitioners for 2005* (1991) is to assist professional schools in developing health-care professionals who will have the expanded knowledge and skills needed to meet the rapidly changing health-care needs. The Pew report categorizes these needs into five broad forces that will shape the future and direct the preparation of practitioners:

- efficiency and effectiveness through coordinated care
- diversity and aging in the population
- the expansion of science and technology
- consumer empowerment
- values shaping health care

The Pew Commission has enumerated the competencies that will be needed in order to respond to these forces and meet the rapidly changing health-care needs of society. O'Neil's report (1993) summarizes the competencies as follows:

1. care for the community's health
2. provide contemporary clinical care
3. participate in the emerging system and accommodate expanded **accountability**
4. ensure cost-effective care and use technology appropriately
5. practice prevention and promote healthy lifestyles

6. involve patients and families in the decision-making process

7. manage information and continue to learn

In addressing the challenges proposed in the Pew report, it is essential to also emphasize the changing roles in leadership. The previously mentioned Leadership Gap Studies (Healthcare Forum Leadership Center, 1992) proposed that the most critical transformational leadership competencies needed for the year 2001 will be:

- the ability to master change

- systems thinking

- shared vision

- continuous improvement of quality

- redefinition of health care

- the serving of public/communities

Narrowing the gap between current leadership practice and future requirements presents a major challenge to those in the health-care field. The essence of the challenge is to develop futuristic leadership competencies that will mesh with the health-care opportunities that are being articulated.

OPPORTUNITIES

Healthy People 2000 (U.S. Department of Health and Human Services, 1990) is the national initiative directed toward the improvement of the nation's health during the current decade. This comprehensive set of objectives for improved health care is based on the following societal beliefs that have emerged in the past fifteen years:

- Increased individual health consciousness and subsequent recognition of health is a personal responsibility.

- The most vulnerable are entitled to good health.

- Every citizen is entitled to the benefits of good health.

- The promotion of a culture of healthy living is a necessity.

- Prevention of disease and promotion of healthy lifestyles is a necessity.

As the culmination of many years of collaboration between national organizations and the United States Government, twenty-two major areas of clinical focus for health-care objectives have been enumerated. The articulation of these topical areas will continue to direct public and private efforts to improve health care in the 1990s and beyond.

In keeping with the aforementioned objectives, Kaiser (1994) believes that the key to the reform of the health-care system is the local community. It is here that members will come together to plan for an integrated delivery network model that includes such entities as the doctor, nurse, insurance company, community, hospital, and others. One of the areas of greatest need, therefore, is the establishment of accountability for the health of the community. Kaiser proposes that each of us, as part of the community, is "the problem, the solution, and the resource" and, therefore, is challenged to be an inventor of the future. Thus, the questions we should ask are:

"What is our vision of health care?"

"What is a healthy community?"

"With the resources we have, how can we get there?"

"What role do I play in this?"

Newly formed community organizations will assess areas of unmet needs as well as available resources, and will make community-based resource-allocation decisions. In this scenario, the hospital will no longer function as a place, but rather will be an entity where the people are. This hospital without walls will then become the geographic area of accountability, which will extend to schools, churches, homes, and the workplace to improve health. Kaiser touts the capitated managed-care system as one of the greatest breakthroughs in health care. He believes that the next two to three years will constitute an open window of time during which local prototypes and demonstration projects will be developed and tested.

In the future, the model of care delivery will be one wherein decentralized primary care is available to the neighborhood so that everyone can reach a primary caregiver. There is no one system that is best; it is, therefore, desirable that each community sculpt an individualized delivery network. During a three-to-four year period of redefining and reshaping, Kaiser predicts turbulence and turmoil followed by a Golden Age of Medicine and Health in the next century. He also predicts that during this time there will most definitely be an improvement of the quality of care. Kaiser summarizes the dimensions of the paradigm shift from the more stable times of the past to the quantum leaps of today, which will direct the reshaping of the health-care system of the future (see Table 33-2).

Table 33-2 • **CHANGING PARADIGMS FOR CHANGING TIMES**

Old Paradigm	New Paradigm
Exclusive	Inclusive
Isolation	Networking
Bottom line	Community good
Competition	Collaboration
Outer	Inner
Curing	Healing
Disease	Health
Local	Regional (planetary)
Coming to us	Going to them
Hospital with walls	Hospital without walls
Profitable	Ethical
Institutional resources	Community resources

Table 33-2 • **CHANGING PARADIGMS FOR CHANGING TIMES** *(continued)*

Old Paradigm	New Paradigm
Historical	Futuristic
Status quo	Innovative
Physician centered	Patient centered
Disease as pathology	Disease as transformation
Federal responsibility	Local responsibility
Greed	Sacrifice
Self interest	Community interest
Boxes	Circles
Left brain	Right brain
Treatment	Prevention
Middle years	Early and late years
Licensure	Competence
Material	Spiritual
Logic	Imagination
Functional architecture	Healing architecture
Scientific method	Intuitive method
High tech	High touch
Separative	Integrative
Science	Spirituality
Scarcity	Abundance
Procedure	Outcome
Centralized	Decentralized
Old metaphors	New metaphors
Exploitation	Ecology
Family as onlookers	Family as participants
Litigation	Conciliation
Hospital as business	Hospital as community resource

Reprinted from L. Kaiser, Keynote address at AWHONN Meeting, Reno, Nevada, June 1993, with permission of Leland Kaiser. Copyright 1993.

CONCLUSION

The current state of the health-care delivery system, with its many "unquality" attributes, as well as the social forces shaping the future of health care, offer an unprecedented challenge. The health-care delivery system of the future is yet to be invented.

The challenge of health-care reform has unfrozen the former ways of doing things and has opened the door for innovative approaches to improve health. Almost all of the recommendations for a reformed health-care system include either explicit or implicit attributes or characteristics of quality.

The quality movement in health care has gained considerable momentum. If this momentum can be coupled with the objectives of health-care reform, and if major **stakeholders** can be involved in a win-win situation, the power source directing the reshaping of the health-care system will know no bounds. The science of Quality Management (QM) has tended to take on the characteristics of a specialty, which the author believes will be manifested in a multitude of facilitative QM roles for experts during at least the next decade. The greatest credit to quality managers in the next century, however, would be to work themselves out of their jobs and bring about the demise of QM departments. In their place would be leaders and caregivers who perceive that managing quality of care is an integral component of their roles.

REFERENCES

American Nurses Association (1991). *Nursing's agenda for health care reform.* Kansas City, MO: Author.

American Quality Foundation and Ernst & Young (1992). *International quality study.* Cleveland, OH: Authors.

Arnold, K. L. (1994). *The manager's guide to ISO 9000.* New York: The Free Press.

Berwick, D. W. (1992). Seeking systemness. *Healthcare Forum Journal, 35*(2), 22–24.

Brobst, K. (1992, August). Reforming health care from experience. *Quality Review Bulletin, 18*(8), 275–277.

Burris, D. (1993). *Technotrends.* New York: Harper Collins.

Covey, S. R. (1989). *The 7 habits of highly effective people.* New York: Simon & Schuster.

Covey, S. R. (1991). *Principle-centered leadership.* New York: Simon and Schuster.

Covey, S. R., Merrill, A. R., & Merrill, R. R. (1994). *First things first.* New York: Simon and Schuster.

Crosby, P. B. (1992). *Completeness: Quality for the 21st century.* New York: Dutton.

Curtin, L. L. (1994). Editorial opinion: Learning from the future. *Nursing Management, 25*(1), 7–9.

Denning, P. J. (1993). An end and a beginning. *American Scientist, 81*(5), 416–418.

Drucker, P. F. (1992). *Managing for the future.* New York: Truman Talley Books.

Flower, J. (1993). The power of chaos. *Healthcare Forum Journal, 36*(5), 48–55.

Goldsmith, J. C. (1992). The reshaping of healthcare. *Healthcare Forum Journal, 35*(3), 19–41.

Goltschalk, J., & Teymour, L. (1992). Envisioning the future: Challenges in community health nursing. *Journal of Nursing Administration, 20*(6), 11–12.

Gore, A. (1993). *The Gore report on reinventing government.* New York: Times Books.

Hammer, M., & Champy, J. (1993). *Reengineering the corporation.* New York: Harper Collins.

Healthcare Forum Leadership Center. (1992). *Bridging the leadership gap in healthcare.* San Francisco: The Healthcare Forum.

Juran, J. M. (1993, July–August). Made in U.S.A.: A renaissance in quality. *Harvard Business Review*, 42–50.

Kaiser, L. R. (1994, January 5). *Healthcare: Future trends and its impact on business.* Presented at Oklahoma Business Health Institute, Oklahoma City, OK.

Katzenbach, J., & Smith, D. (1993). *The wisdom of teams.* Boston: Harvard Business School Press.

Kouzes, J. M., & Posner, B. Z. (1993). The credibility factor. *Healthcare Forum Journal, 36*(4), 16–24.

Kouzes, J. M., & Posner, B. Z. (1993). *Credibility: How leaders gain and lose it, why people demand it.* San Francisco: Jossey-Bass.

Naisbitt, J. (1982). *Megatrends.* New York: Warner Books.

Naisbitt, J. (1994). *Global paradox.* New York: Wilham Marrow.

Naisbitt, J., & Aburdene, P. (1990). *Megatrends 2000.* New York: Avon.

O'Neil, E. H. (1993). *Health professions education for the future: Schools in service to the nations.* San Francisco: Pew Health Profession Commission.

Peters, T. J. (1982). *In search of excellence.* New York: Harper & Row.

Peters, T. J. (1987). *Thriving on chaos: Handbook for a management revolution.* New York: Harper and Row.

Peters, T. J. (1992). *Liberation Management.* New York: Alfred A. Knopf, Inc.

Peters, T. J. (1994). *Tom Peters seminar.* New York: Vintage Books.

Pew Health Professions Commission (1991). *Healthy America: Practitioners for 2005.* Dunham, NC: Author.

Popcorn, F. (1992). *The Popcorn report.* New York: Harper Collins. *The President's health security plan: Preliminary summary.* (1993). Springfield, VA: U.S. Department of Commerce. (NTIS No. PB 93-234979)

The Quality March: National Survey Profiles Quality Improvement Activities. (1993, December 5). *Hospitals and Health Networks*, 52–55.

The Quality March: National Survey Profiles Quality Improvement Activities. (1993, December 20). *Hospitals and Health Networks*, 40–42.

Schoor, T. (1993). The term is "health care." *Nursing and Health Care, 14*(6), 294–295.

Senge, P. M. (1990). *The fifth discipline: The art and practice of learning organization.* New York: Doubleday.

Senge, P. M., Roberts, C., Ross, R. B., Smith, B. J., & Kleiner, A. (1994). *The fifth discipline fieldbook.* New York: Doubleday.

Styles, M. (1994). The world as a classroom. *Nursing and Health Care, 14*(10), 507.

Susser, M. (1993). From information to knowledge: Assimilating Public Health data. *American Journal of Public Health, 83*(9), 1205.

Toffler, A. (1971). *Future shock.* New York: Bantam Books.

Toffler, A. (1980). *The third wave.* New York: Bantam Books.

Toffler, A. (1990). *Powershift.* New York: Bantam Books.

Toffler, A., & Toffler, H. (1993). *War and anti-war.* Boston: Little, Brown and Co.

U.S. Department of Health and Human Services, Public Health Service (1990). *Healthy People 2000.* Washington, DC: U.S. Government Printing Office.

Wheatley, M. (1992). *Leadership and the new science: Learning about organizations from an orderly universe.* San Francisco: Berrett-Koehler.

Whitney, J. O. (1994). *The trust factor.* New York: McGraw-Hill.

Ziegenfuss, J. T. (1993). Editorial: Policy questions regarding quality and health care reform. *American Journal of Medical Quality, 8*(4), 171.

ADDITIONAL READING

Baker, R. (1993). Avedis Donabedian: An interview. *Quality in Health Care, 2*(1), 40–46.

Barker, J. A. (1992). *Paradigms.* New York: Harper Collins.

Covey, S. (1994). *Reflections for highly effective people.* New York: Simon and Schuster Trade.

Curtin, L. L. (1992). Editorial opinion: Signs of things to come. *Nursing Management, 23*(7), 7–8.

Curtin, L. L. (1994). Learning from the future. *Nursing Management, 25*(1), 7–9.

Hagland, M. M., & Cerne, F. (1993, March 20). Fast forward into the future. *Hospitals,* 26–28.

Kaiser, L. R. (1992). The hospital as a healing place. *Healthcare Forum Journal, 35*(5), 39–40.

Kaiser, L. R. (1993, June). Goodbye Newton . . . hello quantum: Changing paradigms for changing times. Keynote address presented at the Association of Women's Health, Obstetric, and Neonatal Nurses, Reno, Nevada.

Scherer, J. L. Healthcare reform: Nursing's vision of change. (1993, April 20). *Hospitals,* 20–26.

GLOSSARY

accountable — To be answerable to someone for something.

accreditation — A voluntary process that verifies that acceptable standards of a bonified accrediting agency have been met.

Agency for Health Care Policy and Research (AHCPR) — A recently established component of the United States Public Health Service the programs of which are directed toward the improvement of quality, appropriateness, effectiveness, and access to health-care services.

Baldrige Award — *See* **Malcolm Baldrige National Quality Award.**

benchmark — A reference point signifying the highest mark of quality of certain goods, services, or processes used as a comparison point for quality in like organizations or situations.

cause and effect diagram — *See* **fishbone diagram**.

certification — A process that designates an entity as worthy of recognition, either in a particular field as an individual or in a specific program in an organization.

common cause variation — The expected aberration in process data that occurs by chance and may not call for remediation unless there is a desire to improve the process.

consumer — *See* **customer**.

consumerism — The preservation, safeguarding, and enhancement of the rights and interests of those who purchase goods and services.

Continuous Quality Improvement (CQI) — A collaborative team process, usually interdisciplinary and statistically supported, used to systematically respond to discrete opportunities for improvement. (Continuous quality improvement is sometimes referred to in a general way to imply a state of constant betterment of some component of quality.)

control chart — A line graph or run chart with three additional statistically determined horizontal lines depicting an average, an upper, and a lower limit in order that a judgment can be made about whether or not a process is within control; one of the commonly used CQI tools.

criteria — A measurable statement that addresses the intent of the standard and reflects the level of accomplishment of that standard.

customer — Also known as *consumer,* a role taken on when one is the recipient of goods, services, or information; frequently referred to as internal or external consumer. (*See* **internal consumer** and **external consumer**.)

evaluate — To determine the worth of.

external consumer — Also known as *external customer,* those individuals or entities outside of an organization who are recipients of goods, services, or information provided by the organization.

fishbone diagram — Also known as a **cause and effect diagram** or an *Ishikawa diagram;* a commonly used graphic quality-improvement tool where the problem is pictured as the head of a fish, and the various causes of the problem are depicted by branches originating from the backbone, and are generally categorized as equipment, procedures, quality, or people.

flow chart — A graphic depiction of the step-by-step sequence of activities making up an organizational or work process; one of the commonly used CQI tools.

gatekeeper — A primary-care professional, generally a physician, who has the function of regulating the use of health-care services during an episode of care.

guidelines — Authoritative statements describing recommended courses of action for specific clinical situations, technical conditions, or patient populations.

histogram — A bar graph displaying the frequencies of events or measurements; one of the commonly used CQI tools.

indicator — Objective, measurable criteria showing the degree to which a standard has been met. (Use of this term sometimes implies the tool or instrument that contains all of the individual criterion measures.)

interdisciplinary — The collaboration of two or more disciplines in the accomplishment of a common goal, generally referred to in the context of patient care.

internal consumer — Also known as *internal customer,* those individuals or entities within an organization who are recipients of goods, services, or information provided by other individuals or entities who are part of that same organization.

intradisciplinary — The collaboration of two or more members of the same discipline in the accomplishment of a common goal, generally referred to in the context of patient care.

ISO 9000 — A system of international recognition of quality to be accomplished through the meeting of global standards. The major current focus is industrial, however the standards are also applicable to health-care organizations.

Kaizen — Japanese expression for continuous effort to improve all work and organizational processes.

licensure — The lawful authorization to provide a particular service, either at an individual or institutional level.

Malcolm Baldrige National Quality Award — A prestigious, highly competitive national quality award recognizing organizations that excel in the categories of leadership, information and analysis, strategic quality planning, human resource utilization, quality assurance of products and services, quality results, and customer satisfaction.

monitor — To critically observe.

multidisciplinary — The working together of two or more disciplines, such that each discipline carries out its own specific function; generally referred to in the context of patient care.

norm — The customary acceptable level of quality as measured by criteria for a given region, locale, or institution.

outcome — End result.

Pareto chart — Also known as *pareto diagram,* a bar graph or histogram that displays data with decreasing frequencies from left to right and also exhibits a superimposed line graph to represent the cumulative frequencies; one of the commonly used CQI tools.

process — An activity or series of activities directed toward a specific outcome.

Program Evaluation (PE) — A systematic assessment of the value, worth, or merit of an organized, goal-directed set of activities; generally used as a basis for decision making.

quality — Level of excellence, value, or worth; conformance to standards that are either implicit or explicit.

Quality Assessment and Improvement (QA&I) — A systematic process wherein there is a data-based, judgmental appraisal of a selected element of care and subsequent betterment; a term that is gaining common usage as a replacement term for the traditional term, *Quality Assurance (QA).*

Quality Assurance (QA) —The classic or traditional programs that organizations have used to assess, monitor, and improve quality. These programs are usually directed toward the meeting of external requirements called for by accreditation or certification processes.

Quality Management (QM) — An umbrella term encompassing all systematic approaches to the assessment and improvement of quality.

registration — The formulation of a list of individuals who have met the prescribed requirements of the licensing process, for example registered nurses (RNs).

run chart — A line graph that depicts a data trend over a period of time; one of the commonly used CQI tools.

scatter diagram — A graphic display of data obtained from two variables that may relate to each other; data from one variable is placed on the x axis and data from a second variable is placed on the y axis, thus demonstrating whether or not there is a correlation between the variables; one of the commonly used CQI tools.

sentinel event — Signifies an untoward or undesirable happening or an effect that acts as a trigger point calling for an in-depth investigation of the cause.

special cause variation — An unexpected aberration in process data; calls for problem-solving activity to remedy the specific cause, but may not improve overall process.

stakeholders — Persons having a vested interest in a specific program or venture.

standard — A broad statement of agreed-upon quality for a given element of care.

structure — Resources such as staff, physical facilities, and technology that are used in the delivery of a service.

supplier — Role taken on when an individual or entity is the provider of goods, services, or information.

threshold — A pre-established trigger point used to evaluate data and determine whether or not a specific measure of quality is within control.

Total Quality Management (TQM) — A leadership paradigm that subscribes to quality as a driving value for the organization; this value is operationalized by top-down total employee commitment and participation in consumer-focused continuous quality improvement of all work processes throughout the organization.

variance — Lack of compliance with a norm that implies quality.

INDEX

evolution of, 106–7
Florence Nightingale, sanitation program, 105–6
formative issues, defined, 104
fourth generation focus, 110
history of, 105–7
indicators, 109
introduction, 104–5
measureability/feasibility, 115
measurement, emphasis on, 106
measure *vs.* evaluate, 106
policy space, 108
role of the evaluator, 121–22
  active-reactive-adaptive stance, 122
stakeholder, 108, 110
summative evaluation, defined, 104
third generation focus, 109–10
types of
  implementation/accountability and monitoring
      study, 116–18
    acceptability/accountability issues, 117
    coverage, 116
    overcoverage, 117
    parameters, establishing, 116
    participation bias *vs.* coverage efficiency, 118
    program bias, 116, 117
    undercoverage, 116–17
  intervention/impact model, 110, 113–15
    action hypothesis, 115
    causal hypothesis, 113–14
    intervention hypotheses, 114–15
    inventory of existing information, 113
    model for a Kangaroo Care Program, 115f
  outcome impact/utility study, 118–21
    cost-benefit analysis, 120–21
    cost effectiveness analysis, 120
    cost-efficiency study, 121
    defining success, 119
    goals and objectives, 118
    program delivery to target population, 118–19
    program efficiency, 119
    randomization of clients, 119
  planning study or needs assessment, 110, 111–12
Prophylactic antibiotics, for SSI prevention, 513
Prospective data, 423
Prospective Payment System (PPS), 375, 498
  for Medicare/Medicaid, 21, 176
Provider
  acceptance of consumer role, 12
  accountability, 11
  -client mutuality, 12–13, 15
  perspective, 11
Provincial Health Advisory committee, 253
Psychiatric facilities, accreditation of, 291, 292
Public-assistance system, 201–2
Public Health and Marine Hospital Services, 192
Puerperal fever, triumph over, 159–60
Purchasing cooperatives, 179, 181
Pure Food and Drug Law, passage of, 4
Purpose, in QM and TQM, compared, 359t

Q

Qualcare Scale, 382
Qualitative data, data sources, 416–17
Quality
  deficiencies in, causes of, 93
  defined, 330
  definitions of, 10, 38
  in health-care, defining, 129
  and nursing care, concept analysis of
    antecedents and consequences of quality, 48
    caring, 36

conclusion, 48–49
data analysis framework, 37
health, 36
identification and selection of the data sample,
    37–38
identification of the concept to be analyzed, 37
introduction, 35–36
outcome attributes/criteria, 45–47
process attributes/criteria, 43–45, 46t
purpose of concept analysis, 36–37
reassurance, 36
related concepts, 41–42
related terminology, 42
structural attributes/criteria, 42–43, 44t
surrogate terms, 41
themes
  applications, 38
  interpretations, 38–40
    customer value, 40
    excellence, 38–39
    fitness for purpose and conformance to
        standards, 39
    ideal, 39
    meeting the customer's requirements,
        39–40
    satisfying need, 40
  summary of, 40–41
types of, balancing, 330
Quality Assessment and Improvement (QA&I), 91,
    345
  and risk-management programs, comparison of,
      523–24
Quality Assurance (QA), 104, 132
  application to nursing research, 483t
  and CQI, comparison, 512t
  growth of, 1970s, 147–50
  in hospitals, 71
  and infection control, 510–11, 511
  model by Lang, 148–49
  models: industrial model *vs.* health-care model,
      88–103
    analytic tools for problem solving, 96
    conclusion, 102–3
    contextual quality, 92
    epidemiological perspective, 96, 97
    introduction, 88
    lessons we could learn, 97–98
    long-range developments, 101–2
    methods of QA and improvement, 95–97
    nature of quality, 88–90
      responsibilities for managing cost/quality
          relationship, 90
      responsibilities toward individuals, 89
      responsibilities toward society, 90
    nature of the quality problem: goals and causes,
        92–93
    overemphasis on vocabulary, 97
    peripheral quality, 92
    Quality Assessment and Improvement (QA&I),
        91, 345
    scope of quality, 91–92
    statistical control, 97
    strategies of QA and improvement, 93–95
    tabular summary
      methods of quality monitoring, 100t
      nature of quality, 98–99t
      nature of the quality problem, 99t
      scope of quality, 99t
      some conclusions, 101t
      strategies of QA and improvement, 99–100t
total quality, 91, 92